CURRENT REVIEW OF

Minimally INVASIVE SURGERY

CURRENT REVIEW OF

Minimally INVASIVE SURGERY

Edited by
DAVID C. BROOKS, MD

Associate Professor of Clinical Surgery
Harvard Medical School
Brigham and Women's Hospital
Boston, Massachusetts

With 44 Contributors

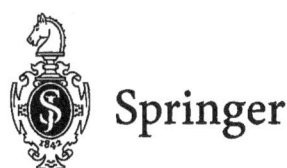 Springer

Current Medicine, Inc.
400 Market Street, Suite 700
Philadelphia, PA 19106

Director, Product Development: Lori J. Bainbridge
Developmental Editor: Elizabeth Rexon
Art Director: Paul Fennessy
Design: Patrick Ward
Layout: Christine Keller-Quirk, Erika Mangan, and Patrick Ward
Illustration Director: Ann Saydlowski
Illustrators: Beth Starkey, Lisa Weischedel, and Debra Wertz
Production Manager: Lori Holland
Typesetter: Ryan Walsh

ISBN 978-1-4612-7247-2   ISBN 978-1-4612-1692-6 (eBook)   SPIN 10645056
DOI 10.1007/978-1-4612-1692-6

5 4 3 2 1

Although every effort has been made to ensure that drug doses and other information are presented accurately in this publication, the ultimate responsibility rests
with the prescribing physician. Neither the publishers nor the author can be held
responsible for errors or for any consequences arising from the use of the information contained therein. Any product mentioned in this publication should be used
in accordance with the prescribing information prepared by the manufacturers.
No claims or endorsements are made for any drug or compound at present under
clinical investigation.

Contributors

JOSEPH F. AMARAL, MD
Associate Professor of Surgery
Department of Surgery
Brown University
Rhode Island Hospital
Providence, Rhode Island

JORGE BALLI, MD
Assistant Professor of Surgery
Department of Surgery
Hospital San José - ITESM
Monterrey, Mexico;
Texas Endosurgery Institute
San Antonio, Texas

K. BHAVANI-SHANKAR, MD
Fellow
Department of Anesthesia
Harvard Medical School
Brigham and Women's Hospital
Boston, Massachusetts

DAVID C. BROOKS, MD
Associate Professor of Clinical Surgery
Department of Surgery
Harvard Medical School
Brigham and Women's Hospital
Boston, Massachusetts

L. MICHAEL BRUNT, MD
Associate Professor
Department of Surgery
Washington University School of Medicine
St. Louis, Missouri

MARK P. CALLERY, MD
Associate Professor
Department of Surgery and Cell Biology
University of Massachusetts Medical School
University of Massachusetts Medical Center
Worcester, Massachusetts

FRANK H. CHAE, MD
Assistant Professor
Department of Surgery
University of Colorado School of Medicine
Denver, Colorado

ALBERT K. CHIN, MD
Vice President of Research and Founder
Guidant Corporation, Origin Medsystems Inc.
Menlo Park, California

JOHN MORGAN COSGROVE, MD
Assistant Professor of Surgery
Department of General Surgery
Albert Einstein College of Medicine
Bronx, New York;
Director of Laparoscopy/Minimally Invasive
  Surgery
Long Island Jewish Medical Center
New Hyde Park, New York

MALCOLM M. DeCAMP, JR., MD
Assistant Professor of Surgery
Department of Thoracic Surgery
Harvard Medical School
Brigham and Women's Hospital
Boston, Massachusetts

TIMOTHY M. FARRELL, MD
Endoscopic Surgery Fellow
Department of Surgery
Emory University School of Medicine
Atlanta, Georgia

STEVEN J. FISHMAN, MD
Instructor in Surgery
Department of Surgery
Harvard Medical School
Children's Hospital
Boston, Massachusetts

RAJA M. FLORES, MD
Fellow
Department of Thoracic Surgery
Harvard Medical School
Brigham and Women's Hospital
Boston, Massachusetts

MORRIS E. FRANKLIN, JR., MD
Professor of Surgery
Department of Surgery
University of Texas Health Sciences Center,
  San Antonio
Director, Texas Endosurgery Institute
San Antonio, Texas

GEORGE GALLOS, BS
Medical Student
Albert Einstein College of Medicine
Bronx, New York

SHAWN M. GARBER, MD
Adjunct Instructor/Fellow
Department of Surgery
The George Washington University Medical
  Center
Washington Institute of Surgical Endoscopy
Washington, DC

JOHN G. HUNTER, MD
Professor
Department of Surgery
Emory University School of Medicine
Atlanta, Georgia

PATRICK G. JACKSON, MD
Clinical Fellow in Surgery
Harvard Medical School
Massachusetts General Hospital
Boston, Massachusetts

MICHAEL T. JAKLITSCH, MD
Instructor of Surgery
Department of Thoracic Surgery
Harvard Medical School
Brigham and Women's Hospital
Boston, Massachusetts

FERENC A. JOLESZ, MD
Professor in Radiology
Department of Radiology/MRI
Harvard Medical School
Brigham and Women's Hospital
Boston, Massachusetts

JOHN J. KELLY, MD
Assistant Professor
Department of Surgery
University of Massachusetts Medical School
University of Massachusetts Medical Center
Worcester, Massachusetts

KENNETH A. KERN, MD
Associate Professor of Clinical Surgery
Department of Surgery
University of Connecticut School of
  Medicine
Farmington, Connecticut;
Attending Surgeon
Hartford Hospital
Hartford, Connecticut

JOACHIM KETTENBACH, MD
Research Fellow
Image-Guided Therapy Program
Department of Radiology
Harvard Medical School
Brigham and Women's Hospital
Boston, Massachusetts;
Instructor
University Hospital of Vienna
Vienna, Austria

RON KIKINIS, MD
Assistant Professor
Department of Radiology
Harvard Medical School
Brigham and Women's Hospital
Boston, Massachusetts

MARY E. KLINGENSMITH, MD
Senior Resident
Department of Surgery
Harvard Medical School
Brigham and Women's Hospital
Boston, Massachusetts

MICHAEL F. KUTKA, MD
Fellow
Department of Surgery
Johns Hopkins University Medical School
Baltimore, Maryland

D.E.M. LITWIN, MD, FRCSC
Associate Professor
Department of Surgery
University of Massachusetts Medical School
Director, Minimally Invasive Surgical Services
University of Massachusetts Medical Center
Worcester, Massachusetts

WILLIAM E. LORENSEN, MS
GE Corporate Research and Development
Niskayuna, New York

KEVIN R. LOUGHLIN, MD
Associate Professor
Department of Urology
Harvard Medical School
Brigham and Women's Hospital
Boston, Massachusetts

ROBERT C. McINTYRE, JR., MD
Assistant Professor
Department of Surgery
University of Colorado School of Medicine
University Hospital
Denver, Colorado

TAKAO OHKI, MD
Assistant Professor
Chief, Endovascular Program
Department of Surgery
Division of Vascular Surgery
Albert Einstein College of Medicine
Montefiore Medical Center
Bronx, New York

MICHAEL P. O'LEARY, MD, MPH
Assistant Professor
Department of Surgery
Harvard Medical School
Department of Urology
Brigham and Women's Hospital
Boston, Massachusetts

CLAUDE H. ORGAN, JR., MD
Professor of Surgery
Department of Surgery
University of California Davis
Alameda County Medical Center
Oakland, California

JOSEPH B. PETELIN, MD
Clinical Associate Professor
Department of Surgery
University of Kansas School of Medicine
Shawnee Mission, Kansas

DAVID W. RATTNER, MD
Associate Professor of Surgery
Harvard Medical School
Massachusetts General Hospital
Boston, Massachusetts

JONATHAN M. SACKIER, MB, CHB, FRCS
Professor of Surgery
Department of Surgery
The George Washington University Medical
  Center
Washington Institute of Surgical Endoscopy
Washington, DC

ROBERT L. SOARES, JR., MD
Clinical Instructor
Department of Surgery
Brown University
Rhode Island Hospital
Providence, Rhode Island

NATHANIEL J. SOPER, MD
Professor
Department of Surgery
Washington University School of Medicine
Barnes-Jewish Hospital
St. Louis, Missouri

RICHARD A. STEINBROOK, MD
Assistant Professor
Department of Anesthesia
Harvard Medical School
Anesthesiologist
Brigham and Women's Hospital
Boston, Massachusetts

GREGORY V. STIEGMANN, MD
Professor
Department of Surgery
University of Colorado School of Medicine
Head, Division of GI, Tumor, and Endocrine
  Surgery
University Hospital
Denver, Colorado

MARK A. TALAMINI, MD
Associate Professor
Department of General Surgery
Johns Hopkins University Medical School
Johns Hopkins Hospital
Baltimore, Maryland

EDMUND K.M. TSOI, MD
Assistant Clinical Professor of Surgery
Department of Surgery
University of California Davis
Alameda County Medical Center
Oakland, California

FRANK J. VEITH, MD
Professor
Department of Surgery
Albert Einstein College of Medicine
Montefiore Medical Center
Bronx, New York

WILLIAM M. WELLS III, PHD
Assistant Professor
Department of Radiology
Harvard Medical School
Brigham and Women's Hospital
Boston, Massachusetts

Preface

In the 4 years since the first edition of this book was published, there have been major advances in minimally invasive surgery. The excitement that general surgeons first experienced with laparoscopic cholecystectomy has been transplanted into a variety of other specialties, all of which have found innovative applications for minimally invasive surgery. Many of the lessons learned in general surgery continue to be applicable, including the importance of sound technical training, the necessity for strict credentialing, and the significance of outcome measurement. All of these areas are mandatory in order that we rationally develop and implement new procedures.

This new edition evaluates a variety of the "traditional" general surgical laparoscopic procedures, such as cholecystectomy and common duct exploration, esophageal fundoplication and myotomy, bowel resection, appendectomy, and so forth. Likewise, the chapters on urologic and pediatric surgical procedures have been updated. Additionally, in the past decade, anesthesia for minimally invasive procedures has become far more sophisticated and the lessons learned in this area are detailed in a new chapter. These lessons, combined with what we have learned about the physiologic changes that accompany laparoscopy, both in the acute operating room setting as well as the short- and immediate-term effects on the immune system, are discussed in detail. The field of gasless laparoscopy is explored thoroughly, and new advances in suturing and tissue approximation are discussed in detail. Finally, medical malpractice suits associated with laparoscopic or minimally invasive procedures have increased dramatically over the past 6 to 8 years, recently surpassing obstetrical suits. A new chapter discusses the implications of medicolegal aspects of minimally invasive surgery.

In the technical arena there have been advances in a number of areas, which only a few years ago were unheard of. To this end there are new chapters on surgery of the thyroid and parathyroid glands, the adrenal and pancreas, and bariatric surgery. Additionally, entirely new disciplines such as minimally invasive vascular surgery and virtual imaging are included.

The revolution in surgical care that began with the introduction of laparoscopic cholecystectomy 10 years ago has thoroughly changed the way we perform surgery. These changes have not always been as we forecasted, or in the areas in which we forecasted change. Nevertheless, as the revolution proceeds, we continue to challenge surgical dogma in an effort to improve outcomes while diminishing the trauma of surgery. This edition hopes to provide a guide to these changes.

David C. Brooks, MD
Boston, Massachusetts

Contents

Laparoscopic Cholecystectomy

Nathaniel J. Soper

CHAPTER

1

E. Mühe [1] of Böblingen, Germany, performed the first laparoscopic cholecystectomy in 1985. However, most authors have given credit to Phillipe Mouret of Lyon, France, who in 1987 facilitated the procedure by rotating the entire right lobe of the liver in a cephalad direction with traction applied to the gallbladder itself. This maneuver allowed the gallbladder and porta hepatis to be viewed from a telescope placed at the umbilicus and directed cranially toward the undersurface of the liver. Surgeons in Paris and Bordeaux subsequently learned the procedure and initiated the first clinical series of laparoscopic cholecystectomies [2,3]. This procedure was first performed in the United States in mid-1988 by surgeons in private practice [4]. Academic medical centers were slower to accept laparoscopic cholecystectomy, but many large clinical series were reported over the following years [5–13]. Laparoscopic cholecystectomy was adopted at a rate unprecedented in American surgery because of our free-market medical system, the preference of patients for "less invasive" procedures, and the marketing effort by individuals and hospitals. Laparoscopic cholecystectomy rapidly became the new "gold standard" therapy for symptomatic cholelithiasis [6,14•].

Laparoscopic cholecystectomy has many potential advantages over traditional, "open" cholecystectomy [15,16•,17]. Postoperative pain and intestinal ileus are diminished, and the multiple small incisions are more appealing cosmetically than the large incision used during traditional cholecystectomy. The patient usually can be discharged from the hospital within 24 hours of operation and return to full activity within a few days [18,19]. The small size of the fascial incisions also allows rapid return to heavy physical labor. These factors lead to an overall decrease in the cost of the procedure [20–22]. Laparoscopic cholecystectomy does have several disadvantages. Patients must be acceptable candidates for general anesthesia. Three-dimensional depth perception is limited by the monocular image of the video telescope, and the operative field being viewed is not determined by the surgeon. Some patients may be excluded from undergoing this therapy because of their anatomy or intra-abdominal adhesions. The common bile duct is more difficult to visualize and instrument during laparoscopy than during traditional open surgery. In addition, it is technically difficult to remove the gallbladder from the fundus to the infundibulum, and control of brisk hemorrhage is diminished using laparoscopy compared with laparotomy.

Many of these limitations are under active investigation. Three-dimensional video systems are being developed and marketed. Robotic camera holders have been developed that allow the surgeon to control the camera position remotely and easily program the mechanical arm to return to set positions [23]. Pneumoperitoneum can be avoided altogether with various designs of abdominal retractors [24]. Unfortunately, acquiring these new technologies is often costly. This chapter reviews the current status of laparoscopic cholecystectomy, focusing on preoperative, intraoperative, and postoperative considerations.

PREOPERATIVE CONSIDERATIONS
Indications
Several studies have documented an increased frequency of cholecystectomy since the introduction of the laparoscopic technique [25,26•]. It is unclear whether patients

simply are more willing to undergo a minimally invasive procedure rather than suffer biliary pain or if the indications for cholecystectomy have become more liberal with the advent of laparoscopy.

In general, patients should have documented cholelithiasis and symptoms attributable to a diseased gallbladder. Gallbladder discomfort is typically severe, recurrent upper abdominal pain, which often radiates to the back. Attacks frequently occur after fatty meals and may awaken the patient at night. Patients with gallstones and porcelain gallbladder, immunosuppression, or limited access to modern medical care may be considered for laparoscopic cholecystectomy despite their lack of biliary symptoms. Patients with no stones but typical biliary symptoms also may benefit from cholecystectomy. Recent studies suggest that symptoms develop in less than 20% of individuals with asymptomatic gallstones over a prolonged period and that the risk of "prophylactic" operation outweighs the potential benefit of surgery [27,28].

In an individual with typical biliary colic, the only diagnostic test necessary is a high-quality ultrasound. This study demonstrates the size and number of the stones, thickness of the gallbladder wall, pericholecystic fluid collections, sludge, polyps, and diameter of the common bile duct. It also may give clues to nonbiliary disorders such as hepatic lesions or fatty infiltration, masses in the pancreas, or renal tumors. When ultrasound is negative and typical biliary symptoms persist, cholecystokinin-stimulated biliary scintigraphy demonstrating a low gallbladder ejection fraction with or without reproducing pain after cholecystokinin administration suggests acalculous cholecystitis, which generally responds to cholecystectomy [29]. If atypical symptoms are present, a more extensive work-up, including upper gastrointestinal contrast radiographs or endoscopy, computerized tomography, or cardiac evaluation, may be appropriate.

Contraindications

Preoperative evaluation should determine the presence of biliary and nonbiliary conditions that may adversely affect the outcome of laparoscopic cholecystectomy [30]. Absolute contraindications (Table 1-1) include inability to tolerate general anesthesia, uncorrectable coagulopathy, diffuse peritonitis, "frozen" abdomen, or gallbladder cancer. Numerous relative contraindications, which primarily are dictated by the surgeon's philosophy and experience, also exist. Many of the relative contraindications shown in Table 1-1 previously had been considered to be absolute.

Patients with morbid obesity are rarely denied the benefits of laparoscopic surgery [31]. Longer trocars may be useful to traverse the anterior abdominal wall, and higher insufflation pressures may be required to obtain an adequate working space.

Despite scattered reports of laparoscopic cholecystectomies having been performed during pregnancy [32], the effects of the prolonged carbon dioxide pneumoperitoneum on the fetus are unknown, and the position of the gravid uterus itself may present a problem. We have performed eight laparoscopic cholecystectomies during the second trimester. Open insertion of the initial port is recommended to avoid accidental injury to the uterus. Hyperventilation and monitoring of the end-tidal CO_2

concentration help minimize both maternal and fetal acidosis. Insufflation pressures kept below 12 mm Hg obviate respiratory problems and compromised venous return. Monitoring fetal heart sounds is done in consultation with an obstetrician.[33]. To date, all of these pregnancies have resulted in normal deliveries of healthy infants. For the novice laparoscopic surgeon, however, it would certainly be wise to avoid potentially difficult cases.

Operating room preparation

Set-up of the operating room equipment and personnel requires consideration. Laparoscopic biliary surgery requires more personnel than open operations. The surgeon stands to the left of the patient for cross-table access to the right upper quadrant. The French prefer to operate in the lithotomy position, with the surgeon standing or sitting between the patient's legs [2,3]. The first assistant stands to the patient's right to manipulate the gallbladder and provide exposure. A laparoscopic videocamera operator stands below the surgeon and assumes the important responsibility of "being the surgeon's eyes." The camera operator must maintain the proper orientation of the camera and scope (particularly if an angled laparoscope is used), keep the surgeons' instruments in the center of the video monitor, follow (or guide) all instruments as they enter or exit the operative field, and assist with instruments or trocar valves as needed. No sharp or pointed instruments should be moved unless they are under direct vision. The camera operator also must take care of any obstruction to vision, such as wiping off condensation or blood that may cloud the lens. Condensation on the lens itself can be minimized by heating the laparoscope's tip in warm water or applying an antifog solution to the lens before inserting the laparoscope into the abdominal cavity. A hot plate on the operating room table heats sterile water to 38°C

Table 1-1

Contraindications to laparoscopic cholecystectomy

Absolute	Relative
Unable to tolerate general anesthesia	Acute cholecystitis with suspected empyema
Uncorrected coagulopathy	Biliary fistula
Suspected carcinoma	Morbid obesity
Generalized peritonitis	Previous upper abdominal surgery
Other conditions requiring laparotomy	Cirrhosis/portal hypertension
	Severe obstructive lung disease
	Pregnancy
	Possible malignancy
	Immunosuppression/hypercortisolism
	Uncertain diagnosis
	Unreducible abdominal/inguinal hernia
	Umbilical abnormalities
	Abdominal aortic/iliac aneurysm

and is readily available to rewarm the lens whenever the scope is outside the abdomen.

PREOPERATIVE CARE AND ANESTHESIA

As for any abdominal operation, patients are fasted from midnight before the operation. Patients without other major medical problem are admitted to the hospital the morning of the operation and given a preoperative sedative and H_2-receptor antagonist. All patients are administered a single dose of intravenous antibiotics, usually a first-generation cephalosporin. On the patient's arrival in the operating room, sequential compression stockings are placed on both legs to avoid blood pooling in the lower extremities because of the reverse Trendelenburg position. We have not routinely used minidose heparin, but this can be used safely in patients at risk for venous thromboembolism. After the induction of anesthesia, an orogastric tube is placed to decompress the stomach. The abdomen is prepared in standard fashion, except that particular care is taken to clean the umbilicus of all detritus.

Although diagnostic laparoscopy can be performed with either local or regional anesthesia, laparoscopic cholecystectomy generally is performed using inhalation anesthesia and controlled ventilation. Important considerations for optimal anesthetic management are adequate depth of anesthesia, complete muscle relaxation, administration of amnesics, and administration of antiemetics such as metoclopramide or a scopolamine patch before the operation concludes. Patient monitoring during therapeutic laparoscopy using general anesthesia includes electrocardiography, blood pressure, precordial stethoscope, airway pressure, and capnography (specifically to assess end-tidal CO_2 concentration). Invasive monitoring (*eg*, arterial line, Swan-Ganz catheter) may be indicated in selected high-risk individuals [34,35].

There are scattered reports of laparoscopic cholecystectomy using thoracic epidural (*ie*, bupivicaine) anesthesia supplemented with intravenous sedation and local anesthetics. Referred shoulder pain may be troublesome with this technique, but it can be diminished by slowly insufflating the peritoneal cavity and maintaining a lower abdominal pressure (*ie*, <10 mm Hg). Regional anesthesia may be appropriate for high-risk patients or those who are highly motivated to avoid a general anesthetic. We use general anesthesia in all cases, however, because of the potential need for rapid conversion of the procedure to an open laparotomy. Postoperative pain is best avoided by preincisional, subcutaneous injection at the cannulation sites with a long-acting local anesthetic; a 0.5% bupivacaine solution usually is used, to a maximum dose of 0.5 mL/kg [36].

CREATION OF PNEUMOPERITONEUM AND TROCAR INSERTION

A pneumoperitoneum, which is established by instilling gas, usually is used to allow visualization of the abdominal cavity. Recently, devices that elevate the abdominal wall by external retraction to create the working space have been described [24,37,38]. This technology would potentially eliminate the adverse local and systemic effects of pneumoperitoneum, and it would allow the use of instruments free of the design limitations imposed by maintenance of an air-tight system. This novel instrumentation ultimately may replace peritoneal insufflation for abdominal wall lift during laparoscopy. However, many surgeons find exposure of the right upper quadrant to be suboptimal using these devices. Prospective, randomized trials are necessary to assess whether perioperative pain or morbidity is altered by these traction devices.

For diagnostic laparoscopy, both CO_2 and nitrous oxide are applicable. Nitrous oxide usually is not used to create the pneumoperitoneum for laparoscopic cholecystectomy; despite being nonflammable, it supports combustion. Carbon dioxide has the advantage of being noncombustible and is eliminated rapidly from the body; most CO_2 disappears within 4 hours after the operation. Absorption of CO_2 from the blood ordinarily is rapid and safe, without formation of gas emboli even when infused directly into a systemic vein at a rate of less than 1 L/min [39]. However, absorption may lead to hypercapnia in patients with chronic obstructive pulmonary disease [40]. Also, CO_2 is converted to carbonic acid on the moist peritoneal surfaces and therefore may cause mild postoperative discomfort. Because of these adverse effects, ongoing studies are now establishing whether other gases (*eg*, helium, argon) may be preferable for use during laparoscopic surgery [41].

The pneumoperitoneum can be established by either a closed or an open technique. In the closed technique, CO_2 is insufflated into the peritoneal cavity through a needle, and the initial laparoscopic trocar and sheath are placed blindly into the abdominal cavity. In the open technique, a small incision is made, and a laparoscopic sheath without the sharp trocar (Hasson cannula) is inserted under direct vision into the peritoneal cavity (Fig. 1-1*A–D*). The pneumoperitoneum is then established only after ensuring safe peritoneal entry. There are advantages and disadvantages to both techniques, and surgeons performing laparoscopy should learn both and use them selectively.

We now perform open insertion on a routine basis. This technique is particularly helpful in patients with previous periumbilical incisions, those in whom insertion of the Veress needle is not performed satisfactorily, and those with large (*ie*, >2.5 cm) gallstones or acute cholecystitis.

TECHNIQUE

During laparoscopic cholcystectomy, a 10.5-mm laparoscope is inserted into the abdomen. The retroperitoneum immediately posterior to the umbilicus and the pelvis is first viewed to assure that no injury has resulted from insertion of the trocar or sheath. The pelvic viscera are examined for other pathologic abnormalities before evaluating the upper abdomen. The anterior surface of the intestines, omentum, and stomach also are examined for abnormalities. The patient is then placed in a reverse Trendelenburg position of 30° to 40° while the table is rotated to the patient's left by 15° to 20°. Repositioning the patient intraoperatively is facilitated with a motorized surgical table. This maneuver generally allows the colon and duodenum to fall away from the liver edge. The falciform ligament and

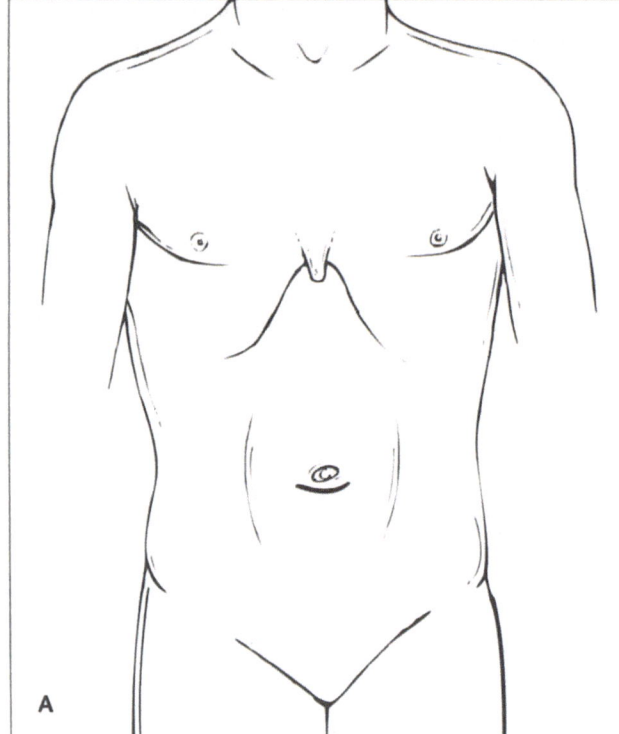

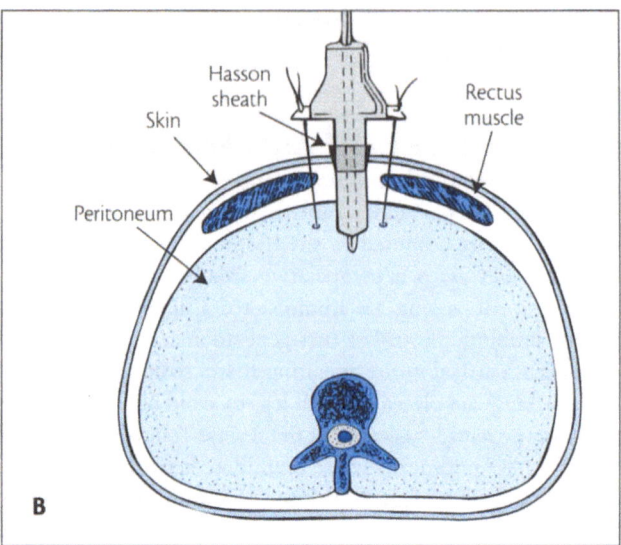

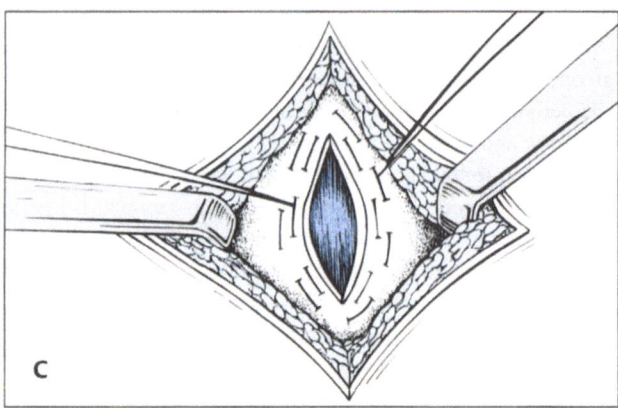

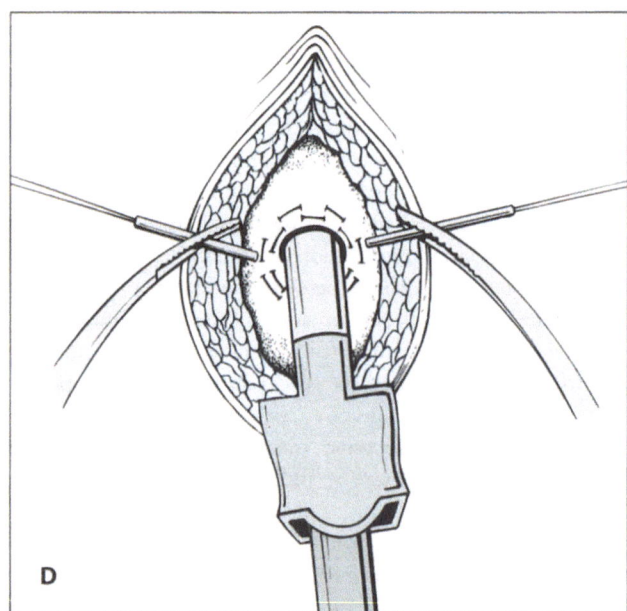

Figure 1-1 Techniques for open insertion of the initial laparoscopic sheath. **A**, Site of skin incision. **B**, Placement of Hasson sheath through the abdominal wall and secured in place with sutures between the fascia and the wings of the sheath. **C** and **D**, An alternative technique using a standard laparoscopic sheath and two concentric, purse-string sutures placed in the abdominal fascia. (*From* Soper [15]; with permission.)

both lobes of the liver are closely examined for pathology. The inferior margin of the liver is then visualized to determine the location of the gallbladder. The gallbladder usually can be seen protruding beyond the edge of the liver, but it sometimes is not visible without carefully elevating the liver, taking down adhesions, or both.

At this point, the two small, accessory, subcostal ports in the right upper quadrant are placed under direct vision. The first trocar is placed in the anterior to middle axillary line between the twelfth rib and the iliac crest. This sheath should be placed inferior (*ie,* caudad) to the gallbladder fundus and liver edge. A second 5-mm port is then inserted under direct vision approximately midway between the axillary sheath and the xiphoid process. It should be possible to avoid major abdominal wall blood vessels during trocar insertion by combining transillumination of the

abdominal wall and direct examination of the parietal peritoneum. Grasping forceps are placed through these two sheaths, and the gallbladder is secured. Standing at the right side of the table, the assistant manipulates the lateral grasping forceps, which are used to elevate the liver edge to expose the fundus of the gallbladder. Standing at the left of the patient, the surgeon uses dissecting forceps to raise a serosal "fold" of the most dependent portion of the fundus. The assistant's heavy grasping forceps are then locked onto this fold using either a spring or ratchet device. Using this axillary grasping forceps, the fundus of the gallbladder is pushed in a lateral and cephalad direction, causing the entire right lobe of the liver to roll cephalad. Successful performance of this maneuver is important to expose the porta hepatis and gallbladder. In patients with high- or low-lying livers, the positioning of these trocars is quite different from that in the "standard" patient.

In patients with a fixed cirrhotic liver or a heavy friable liver caused by fatty infiltration, this maneuver may be difficult.

In patients with few adhesions to the gallbladder, pushing the fundus cephalad exposes the entire gallbladder, cystic duct, and porta hepatis. Most patients, however, have adhesions between the gallbladder and the omentum, hepatic flexure, or duodenum. These adhesions generally are avascular and may be lysed bluntly by grasping with a dissecting forceps at their site of attachment to the gallbladder wall and gently "stripping" them down toward the infundibulum. Vascular adhesions may be divided with a hook cautery. After exposing the infundibulum, blunt grasping forceps are placed through the midclavicular trocar for traction on the neck of the gallbladder. The operative field is thereby established, and the final working port is then inserted.

The last 10- to 11-mm trocar is placed through a transverse skin incision in the midline of the epigastrium. In general, this is placed 5 cm below the xiphoid process, but the position depends on the location of the gallbladder as well as the size of the medial segment of the left liver lobe. When uncertain about the appropriate position for this trocar, a Veress needle may be placed at the proposed site to ascertain whether its location and angle of insertion are optimal. The trocar is then inserted with a "drilling" motion, the surgeon angling its tip just to the right of the falciform ligament while aiming toward the gallbladder.

The basic positions for placement of the various ports are shown in Figure 1-2. Accessory sheaths should be separated as far as possible so that the external portions of the instruments do not cross or interfere with one another. The orientation of the laparoscope generally is parallel to that of the cystic duct when the fundus is elevated, whereas the instruments placed through the axillary and epigastric sheaths enter the abdomen at right angles to this plane. Finally, the midclavicular sheath is anterior to the gallbladder, making the instruments passing through it perpendicular to the cystic duct. Thus, all of the accessory sheaths are placed at right angles to the axis of the cystic duct, while the surgeon's vision is directed parallel to its axis. The French prefer to elevate the liver lobe with a rod placed in a medial right subcostal position and operate through a left paramedian port while the surgeon stands between the patient's abducted legs [2,3].

Having established the positions of the sheaths, the first assistant places the fundus and infundibulum of the gallbladder under tension away from the common bile duct in a superior and lateral direction. Then either a "one-handed" or "two-handed" dissection technique may be used depending on whether the surgeon or the assistant manipulates the gallbladder infundibulum. With the fundus and neck of the gallbladder under tension, fine-tipped dissecting forceps are used to tease away the overlying fibroareolar structures from the gallbladder infundibulum and Hartmann's pouch. This is done with a blunt stripping action, always beginning on the gallbladder and pulling the tissue toward the porta hepatis.

During this initial dissection around the gallbladder neck, the peritoneum is lysed with the blunt dissector similar to the technique by which the peritoneum is incised and pushed bluntly with a Kittner dissector during a traditional open cholecystectomy. With the laparoscopic dissection visualized under two-dimensional optics, it is vital to identify clearly the structures contained within two triangles: the hepatocystic triangle, and its reverse side. The hepatocystic triangle is the ventral aspect of the area bounded by the cystic duct, hepatic duct, and liver edge. The reverse side of the triangle is the dorsal aspect of this space.

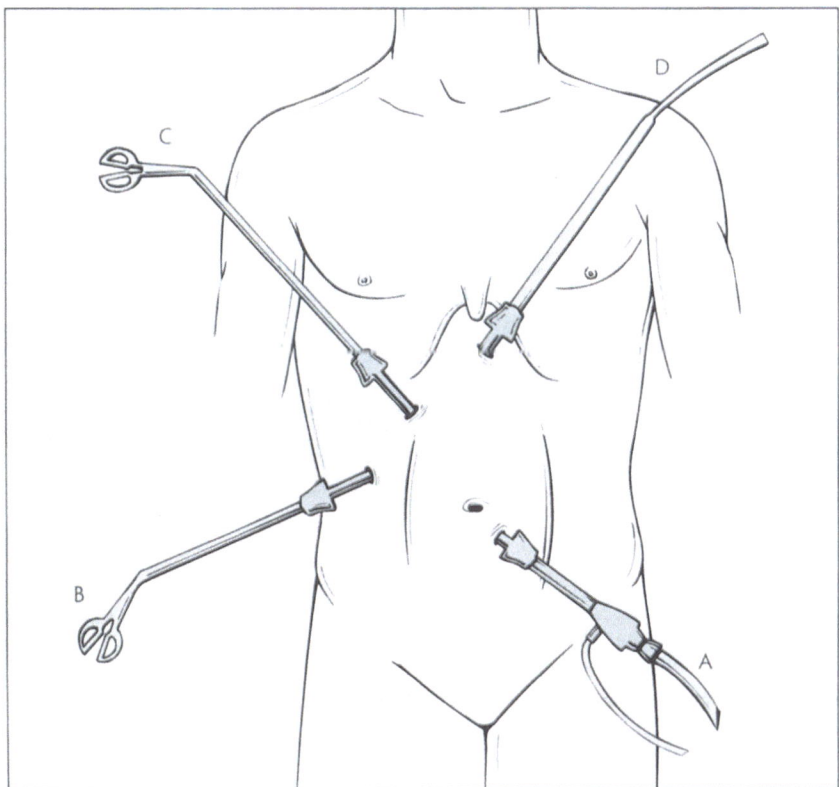

Figure 1-2 Positions for insertion of the initial (*A*) and accessory sheaths (*B, C,* and *D*) for biliary surgery. (*From* Soper [15]; with permission.)

This triangle is placed on tension and maximally exposed by retracting the gallbladder infundibulum inferiorly and laterally while pushing the fundus superiorly and medially (Fig. 1-3*A*). A lymph node usually overlies the cystic artery, and a brief application of electrical current occasionally is required to obtain hemostasis as the lymph node is swept away. The assistant then stretches the infundibulum of the gallbladder superiorly and medially while pushing the fundus superiorly and laterally, thereby exposing the reverse side of the hepatocystic triangle, an area defined by the cystic duct, the inferior lateral border of the gallbladder, and the right lobe of the liver (Fig. 1-3*B*). Further blunt dissection is used to identify precisely the junction between the infundibulum and the origin of the cystic duct.

Identification of this junction is the critical maneuver in the operation; certainly, no structure should be sharply divided until the cystic duct is clearly identified. The strands of peritoneal, lymphatic, neural, and vascular tissue are stripped away from the cystic duct to gain as much length as possible. Curved dissecting forceps are helpful in creating a "window" around the posterior aspect of the cystic duct to isolate the duct (Fig. 1-3). Alternatively, the tip of a hook-shaped cautery probe can be used to encircle and expose the duct. The cystic artery may be separated from the surrounding tissue by similar blunt dissection either at this time or later depending on its anatomic location. In the usual position, the cystic duct is dissected and divided first, because it is the structure presenting most anteriorly in the field. If the cystic artery crosses anterior to the duct, the artery may require dissection and division before the cystic duct can be approached. An additional maneuver that often helps during dissection of the duct is to use the blunt, concave blade of the spatula-tipped cautery. Gentle irrigation through its central lumen while pushing away the periductal structures aids in

precise visualization. Dissection of the neck of the gallbladder away from its bed with identification of two structures (cystic duct and artery), and *only* two structures traversing the hepatocystic triangle exposes the "critical view" of safety to prevent duct misidentification [42•].

After initial dissection of the cystic duct, cholangiography with or without intracorporeal ultrasonography may be performed. We routinely perform laparoscopic ultrasonography to teach surgical residents ultrasound interpretation and as part of an ongoing investigational study. Besides accurately locating stones in the gallbladder and common bile duct, ultrasonography delineates anatomy and pathology of the porta hepatis [43]. Cholangiography also may be performed selectively or routinely. In our operating suite, cholangiographic images are transmitted in real time to the radiology reading room for confirmatory interpretation. An intercom system permits the surgeon and radiologist to discuss any problems encountered during cholangiography. We perform cholangiography through the cystic duct, although other techniques may be applicable. In brief, the dissecting forceps is used to squeeze the cystic duct gently in the direction of the gallbladder, thereby "milking" cystic duct stones back into the gallbladder. A clip applier placed through the epigastric sheath is used to apply a single clip at the junction of the cystic duct and the gallbladder. A scissors inserted through the axillary or midclavicular trocar is used to incise the anterolateral wall of the cystic duct, and a 4- or 5-F catheter is inserted into the duct and fixed in place. The cholangiogram should be scrutinized to ascertain the following:

1. The size of the common bile duct,
2. The location of the junction between the cystic duct and the common bile duct,

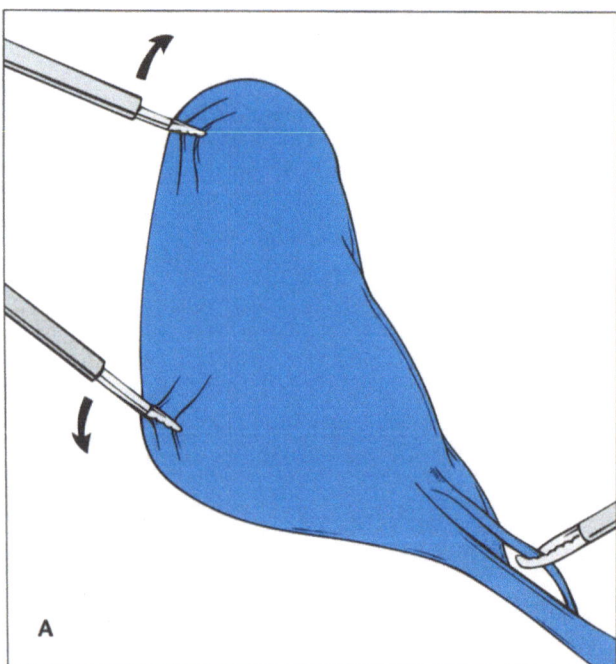

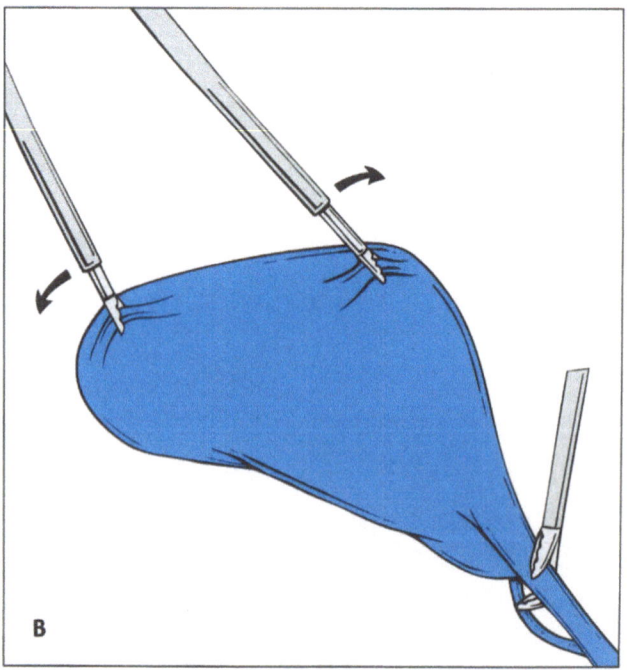

Figure 1-3 The hepatocystic triangle. **A,** The triangle is exposed by manipulating the gallbladder with traction applied by the assistant's grasping forceps. The surgeon's curved instrument is encircling the cystic artery; the cystic duct is anterior. *Arrows* indicate vector of forceps movement. **B,** The reverse (dorsal aspect) of the hepatocystic triangle is displayed. *Arrows* indicate vector of forceps movement (*From* Soper [15]; with permission.)

3. The presence of intraluminal filling defects,
4. Free flow of contrast media into the duodenum,
5. The anatomy of the proximal biliary tree, and
6. Aberrant biliary radicles entering the gallbladder directly.

After removing the cholangiocatheter the cystic duct is incised and "milked" to remove stones contained within it that could subsequently migrate into the common duct if not addressed. The cystic duct is then clipped twice near its junction with the common bile duct and divided. The posterior jaw of the clip applier must be visualized before applying each clip to avoid injuring surrounding structures. Great care should be taken so that the common bile duct is not "tented up" into the clip. If the cystic duct is particularly large or friable, it may be preferable to replace the clips with a preformed loop ligature or suture.

Attention is then directed to the cystic artery. The infundibulum of the gallbladder is placed on tension, and the cystic artery is dissected bluntly from the surrounding tissue. The surgeon must ascertain that the structure is the cystic artery and not the right hepatic artery looping up onto the neck of the gallbladder, as sometimes may be seen. After an appropriate length of cystic artery has been separated from the surrounding tissue, it is clipped and divided sharply. Clips should be fastened at right angles to the artery and clearly include the whole structure to avoid later slippage. Electrocautery should not be used for this division, because the current may be transmitted to the proximal clips, leading to subsequent necrosis and hemorrhage. A common error is to dissect and divide the anterior branch of the cystic artery after mistaking it for the main cystic artery. This may result in hemorrhage from the posterior branch during dissection of the gallbladder fossa.

Now, the ligated stumps of the duct and cystic artery are examined to assure that neither bile nor blood has leaked, that the clips are securely placed, and that the clips compress the entire lumen of the structures without impinging on adjacent tissue. To avoid injury to structures in the porta hepatis, no dissection is undertaken medial to the stumps. A suction-irrigation catheter is used to remove any accumulated debris or blood from dissection of the duct and artery. The heavy grasping forceps traversing the midclavicular trocar are repositioned on the proximal end of the gallbladder at Hartmann's pouch. The infundibulum is retracted superiorly and laterally, and it is distracted anteriorly away from its hepatic bed. The surgeon uses the dissecting forceps to thin out the tissue tethering the neck of the gallbladder and to assure that no other sizable tubular structures traverse the space. Dissection of the hepatic fossa is then initiated using a thermal source to divide and coagulate small vessels and lymphatics. Occasionally, a larger blood vessel or aberrant small bile duct will require placement of a clip for control.

Once the appropriate plane has been identified, separation of the gallbladder from its bed is performed usually with electrocautery (Fig. 1-4). Extensive cauterization often creates smoke, which periodically must be released through a port valve. With the tissue connecting the gallbladder to its fossa placed under tension, the surgeon uses an electrocautery spatula or hook in a gentle, sweeping motion with low wattage (*ie*, 25 to 30 W) to coagulate and divide this tissue. Using the cautery probe, the surgeon also can perform blunt dissection, pushing the tissue to facilitate exposure of the proper plane. Hemorrhage from the liver bed or gallbladder occasionally obscures precise identification of the anatomy. Tears in the gallbladder wall may be clipped or loop ligated to prevent further bile leakage. Small liver lacerations frequently stop with direct pressure, further electrocauterization, or application of a topical hemostatic agent. Frequent irrigation during this dissection clarifies visualization of the plane.

Dissection of the gallbladder fossa continues from the infundibulum to the fundus, intermittently moving the midclavicular grasping forceps to a position closer to the plane of dissection, allowing for maximal countertraction. The dissection proceeds until the gallbladder is attached by only a thin bridge of tissue. At this point, before losing visualization of the operative field afforded by cephalad traction applied to the gallbladder, the hepatic fossa and porta hepatis are again inspected for hemostasis and bile leakage. The clips are reinspected to ensure that they did not inadvertently dislodge during dissection of the gallbladder fossa. Small bleeding points are coagulated with the electrocautery, and the right upper quadrant is liberally irrigated and aspirated dry. The final attachments of the gallbladder are lysed and the liver edge examined again for hemostasis.

After performing cholecystectomy, the gallbladder is removed from the abdominal cavity. Although costly and usually unnecessary, the gallbladder may be placed in a plastic pouch to assist with its extraction. We recommend bagging the gallbladder if it is purulent, fragmented, perforated with multiple small stones, or suspicious for carcinoma. The gallbladder usually is removed through the umbilicus, because there are no muscle layers and

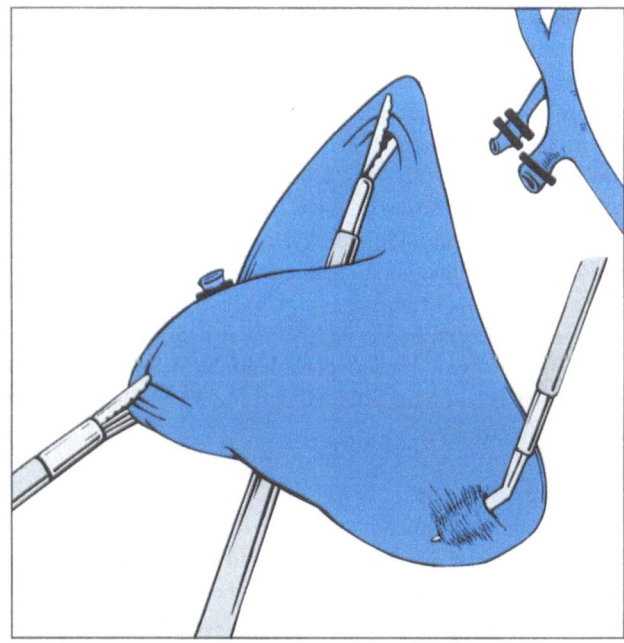

Figure 1-4 Separation of the gallbladder from its bed by dissection with a blunt-tipped, thermal energy probe. The neck of the gallbladder is placed on traction in a superior direction, then twisted to the left and right to place tension on the junction between the gallbladder and hepatic fossa. (*From* Soper [15]; with permission.)

only one fascial plane to traverse. Also, if the fascial opening needs to be enlarged because of large or numerous stones, extending the umbilical incision causes less postoperative pain than enlarging the subxiphoid entry site. The laparoscope is removed from the umbilical port and placed into the epigastric sheath. The pelvis and lower abdomen are inspected for evidence of unappreciated injury to the bowel, bladder, or retroperitoneal blood vessels, and the umbilical trocar insertion site is examined for hemorrhage. Large "claw" grasping forceps are then introduced through the umbilical sheath and guided to the right upper quadrant. The assistant presents the gallbladder neck into the jaws of the grasper so that it is aligned parallel to the axis of the forceps. The assistant then releases the gallbladder, and its infundibulum is pulled up into the umbilical sheath. The forceps, sheath, and gallbladder neck are then retracted as a unit through the umbilical incision. The neck of the gallbladder is thus exposed on the anterior abdominal wall, with the distended fundus remaining within the abdominal cavity.

If the gallbladder is not distended with bile or stones, it can be simply withdrawn with gentle traction. In most cases, a suction catheter is introduced into the gallbladder to aspirate bile and small stones. Also, a stone forceps can be placed into the gallbladder to extract or crush calculi if necessary. Occasionally, the fascial incision must be dilated or extended to deliver larger stones. The laparoscopic sheaths are opened to deflate the abdomen. If this is not done, a partial vacuum is formed that may carry omentum or small intestine into the cannulation site during removal of the sheath, thereby increasing the risk of herniation and intestinal injury. Placing the patient in a slight Trendelenburg position as well as high-volume manual ventilation may facilitate the escape of CO_2 trapped under the diaphragm. The sheaths are then removed.

Each incision is infiltrated with a 0.5% bupivicaine solution and irrigated with saline solution. The fascia of the umbilical incision is closed with one or two large, absorbable sutures. Failure to approximate adequately the fascial edges has resulted in incisional herniae. The skin of the subxiphoid and umbilical incisions is closed with subcuticular absorbable sutures, and Steri-strips (3M Health Care, St. Paul, MN) are applied to each incision. Ideally, an intramuscular or intravenous nonsteroidal anti-inflammatory agent such as ketorolac tromethamine (Torodol; Syntex, Palo Alto, CA) is given 30 minutes before extubation and before skin closure to alleviate diaphragmatic irritation and postoperative discomfort. A loading dose of 30 to 60 mg followed by 15 to 30 mg every 6 hours is very effective [44].

Anatomic hazards

The surgeon performing laparoscopic cholecystectomy must be aware of anatomic hazards that may lead to complications. The common bile duct may be "tented-up" because of the vigorous superolateral traction placed on the gallbladder, making it susceptible to injury during placement of the clips. Likewise, dissection in the region of the lateral wall of the common bile duct may cause bleeding from its nutrient vessels. Also, application of electrocautery in this area must be avoided, because subsequent devascularization and stricture may occur.

Absent or extremely short cystic ducts may lead to two potential problems. First, the surgeon must recognize this anomaly and not mistake the common bile duct for the cystic duct. Second, it may be extremely difficult to occlude the cystic duct with a clip of insufficient length. The surgeon may need to convert to an open cholecystectomy in these circumstances or possibly to close a small portion of gallbladder infundibulum with a laparoscopic suture.

Aberrant bile ducts may be present as well. If they are not recognized and ligated, direct communications between the biliary system and the gallbladder may lead to postoperative bile collections [11]. Aberrant origin of the right hepatic duct is not uncommon and must be ruled out in every case. Anomalous hepatic and cystic arteries also may be present. The most frequent anomaly in our experience is a right hepatic artery that loops up onto the infundibulum of the gallbladder. In this situation, the cystic artery must be dissected up onto the gallbladder wall, clipped, and divided to allow the hepatic artery to retract away from the operative field.

Finally, patients with a large left hepatic lobe may pose special problems. The epigastric trocar must be placed in an appropriate location so that instruments enter the operative field from an angle that does not lacerate the left liver lobe. If needed, an extra 5-mm port can be placed for insertion of a blunt probe to retract the left hepatic lobe during the operation.

Conversion to an open operation

Surgeons performing laparoscopic cholecystectomy should not hesitate to convert to a traditional, open cholecystectomy if the anatomy is unclear or complications arise (Table 1-2). It is better to open one too many than to open one too few. Some complications requiring laparotomy are obvious, such as massive hemorrhage, bowel perforation, or major injury to the bile duct. An additional indication for open laparotomy is anatomy that because of inflammation, adhesions, or anomalies cannot be delineated. Fistulas between the biliary system and bowel are rare but generally require laparotomy for optimal management. Finally, the demonstration of potentially resectable carcinoma dictates open exploration.

Acute cholecystitis

Acute cholecystitis may be treated within the first 72 hours of presentation, or it may be allowed to "cool down" and an elective laparoscopic cholecystectomy performed 6 to 8 weeks following the acute attack. Intervention during the early phase reveals an inflamed, thick-walled, tensely distended organ. To gain purchase for the grasping forceps, it may be necessary to decompress the gallbladder by aspirating it with a large-gauge needle. As long as the inflammation is limited to the gallbladder, laparoscopic cholecystectomy usually is technically feasible. If inflammation extends to the porta hepatis, however, great care must be taken with the operation. The normally thin, minimally adherent tissue investing the cystic duct and artery is markedly thickened and edematous, and it may not readily separate from these structures with the usual blunt dissection techniques. The duct wall also may be edematous, making its external diameter similar to that of the gallbladder neck and common bile duct. If the anatomy is unclear, cholangiography must be performed before clipping or dividing the tissue. When acute inflammation has been present for several days or weeks before the operation, the pericholecystic tissue planes may be obliterated by thick, "woody" tissue that is impossible to dissect bluntly. The surgeon therefore may need to convert to an open cholecystectomy if laparoscopic surgery is initiated during this subacute phase.

The ability to perform laparoscopic cholecystectomy should not influence the management of patients with acute cholecystitis [45]. Antibiotics and bowel rest are initiated on the patient's admission to the hospital, and the operation is undertaken within 24 to 48 hours. There is no harm in inserting the laparoscope and assessing the right upper quadrant. The subcostal working ports are placed and the initial dissection performed. If the anatomy is obliterated, a laparotomy is performed; if laparoscopic dissection is possible, the operation is completed. The decision to convert to an open operation is a matter of judgment based on the existing anatomy and the surgeon's experience. Several authors have reported performing laparoscopic cholecystectomy in the face of acute inflammation [46–48]. Sometimes the edema of the tissue planes actually may aid in the dissection of the gallbladder from its fossa. Despite a greater incidence of conversion to open surgery, the procedure may be completed safely in most patients.

Intraoperative gallbladder perforation

Perforation of the gallbladder with bile or stone leakage can be a distressing problem, but it should not require conversion to an open cholecystectomy. Perforation may occur secondary to traction applied by the grasping forceps or because of thermal injury during removal of the gallbladder from its bed. Almost one third of our patients have had some intraoperative spillage of bile or stones.

Patients with an intraoperative bile leak have not experienced an increased incidence of infection or prolongation of hospitalization or postoperative disability [49]. The only difference between patients with and without bile leakage has been that the operating time of those with a perforation is approximately 10 minutes longer, presumably because of the time spent cleaning

up the operative field. When perforation does occur, the bile should be aspirated completely and irrigation used liberally. The stones should be retrieved and removed if at all possible. When treated in this manner, gallbladder spillage results in no adverse short- or long-term complications. Escaped stones composed primarily of cholesterol pose little threat of infection. Pigment stones frequently harbor viable bacteria, however, and may potentially lead to subsequent infectious complications if allowed to remain in the peritoneal cavity [50].

POSTOPERATIVE CARE

Following laparoscopic cholecystectomy, patients may be observed in the hospital or discharged later that day. We routinely keep patients overnight to monitor for immediate complications. It seems reasonable to perform this operation on an outpatient basis for responsible individuals who live with another person near the hospital and those without evidence of acute cholecystitis, urinary retention, or persistent nausea. Orders are written for antiemetics and analgesics as needed. The patient is allowed clear liquids in the immediate postoperative period and advanced to a regular diet as tolerated. Nausea and shoulder pain because of diaphragmatic irritation may occur early in the first postoperative day. No activity restrictions are placed on the patient, because functional status depends entirely on the degree of abdominal tenderness, which usually subsides by the second or third postoperative day. The patient may return to work as soon as the abdominal discomfort is tolerable but is encouraged to do so within 1 week. We routinely evaluate patients 1 month after the operation, or sooner should they have cause for concern.

RESULTS
Author's personal series

Between November 1989 and September 1997, more than 3500 laparoscopic cholecystectomies were performed at Washington University's affiliated hospitals. Among the author's personal series of 1150 laparoscopic cholecystectomies, there has been a conversion rate of 2.3% and one mortality; our early results have been reported previously [6]. Cumulatively, major morbidity has occurred in 0.39% of patients. The postoperative course in most patients has been uneventful, with 95% being discharged from the hospital within 24 hours of surgery and only 10% requiring parenteral narcotics after leaving the recovery room. Similarly, the duration of disability is minimal; the average postoperative interval for return to full activity is 8 days. These results compare favorably with those of traditional open cholecystectomy, after which hospitalization for 3 to 5 days and return to work at 1 month after surgery are standard [18].

Other reported series

Our data reflect those from most series of laparoscopic cholecystectomies reported to date (Table 1-3). Mortality is rare after this procedure and usually attributed to unrelated events. Death resulting from bile duct or intestinal injury, however, has been reported [12]. The conversion rate from laparoscopic to open operation ranges from 1.8% to 8.5% and generally is greater early

Table 1-2

Reasons for conversion to open cholecystectomy

Known or suspected injury to major blood vessel, viscus, or bile duct

Unclear anatomy

Unexpected pathology not amenable to laparoscopic management

Common bile duct stone unable to be removed laparoscopically, with little chance of subsequent endoscopic extraction (Billroth II anastomosis, duodenal diverticulum, previously failed endoscopic retrograde cholangiopancreatography)

Failure to progress in the dissection

Table 1-3

Compiled results of laparoscopic cholecystectomy

Study	Patients, n	Conversions, %*	Mortality, %	Major complications, %	Bile duct injuries, %
Southern Surgeons Club [7]	1518	4.7	0.07	1.5	0.5
Cuschieri et al. [10]	1236	3.6	0.00	1.6	0.3
Soper et al. [6]	618	2.9	0.00	1.6	0.2
Spaw et al. [5]	500	1.8	0.00	1.0	0.0
Wolfe et al. [12]	381	3.0	0.90	3.4	0.0
Bailey et al. [8]	375	5.0	0.30	0.6	0.3
Graves et al. [13]	304	6.9	0.00	0.7	0.3
Peters et al. [11]	283	2.8	0.00	2.1	0.4
Schirmer et al. [9]	152	8.5	0.00	4.0	0.7

*Conversions to an open laparotomy.

in the surgeon's experience with the procedure. Major complications such as bile duct injury are relatively rare in series of cases performed by surgeons who have been performing laparoscopic cholecystectomy since its description. If bile duct injury occurs, however, a coordinated effort by radiologists, endoscopists, and surgeons is necessary to optimize patient management [42•,51].

National Institutes of Health consensus development conference

Because of the prevalence of gallstones in the US population, the resulting cost borne by the health-care system, and the rapid employment of laparoscopic cholecystectomy, the National Institute of Diabetes and Digestive and Kidney Diseases held a consensus development conference entitled Gallstones and Laparoscopic Cholecystectomy on September 14–16, 1992 [52]. This conference evaluated and compared the data available on laparoscopic cholecystectomy versus traditional surgical and nonsurgical treatments of gallstones. The consensus panel was comprised of surgeons, endoscopists, hepatologists, gastroenterologists, radiologists, epidemiologists, and representatives of the general public, and it considered the scientific evidence presented by a number of experts in relevant fields. The panel's conclusions included the following:

1. Most asymptomatic patients with cholelithiasis should not be treated, but once symptoms develop, treatment should be initiated promptly.
2. Laparoscopic cholecystectomy has become the treatment of choice for many patients, because it offers decreased pain and disability and the potential for substantial cost savings. However, the outcome of laparoscopic cholecystectomy is greatly influenced by the surgeon's training, experience, skill, and judgment.
3. Open cholecystectomy is a safe and effective operation for symptomatic gallstone disease and remains the standard against which new treatments should be judged; conversion from laparoscopic to open cholecystectomy should not be considered a complication of laparoscopic cholecystectomy.
4. Nonresective therapies for gallstones have limited clinical applicability and require further development.
5. Management of common bile duct stones depends on the local availability of technical expertise; valid treatment options include preoperative, intraoperative, or postoperative identification and removal of stones.
6. Future research should focus on refining the techniques of laparoscopic cholecystectomy and laparoscopic common bile duct exploration to maximize their safety and cost-effectiveness.
7. Strict guidelines for training in laparoscopic surgery and determination of competence as well as monitoring for quality should be developed and implemented promptly.
8. Safe, noninvasive, cost-effective strategies to prevent gallstones should actively be sought.

CONCLUSIONS

Laparoscopic management of gallstones has rapidly become the new gold standard for therapy in the United States and throughout the world. Most cases of symptomatic gallstones can be treated laparoscopically. Occasionally, anatomic or physiologic considerations will preclude the laparoscopic approach, and conversion to an open operation in such cases reflects sound judgment and should not be considered a complication.

ACKNOWLEDGMENT

The author gratefully acknowledges the Washington University Institute for Minimally Invasive Surgery, as funded by a grant from Ethicon-Endosurgery, Inc.

REFERENCES AND RECOMMENDED READING

Recently published papers of particular interest have been highlighted as:

- •   Of interest
- ••   Of outstanding interest

1. Mühe E: Die erste Cholecystektomie durch das Laparoskop. *Langenbecks Arch Klin Chir* 1986, 369:804.

2. DuBois F, Icard P, Berthelot G, et al.: Coelioscopic cholecystectomy: preliminary report of 36 cases. *Ann Surg* 1990, 211:60–62.

3. Perissat J, Collet D, Belliard R: Gallstones: laparoscopic treatment—cholecystectomy, cholecystostomy, and lithotripsy. *Surg Endosc* 1990, 4:1–5.

4. Reddick EJ, Olsen DO: Laparoscopic laser cholecystectomy: a comparison with mini-lap cholecystectomy. *Surg Endosc* 1989, 3:131–133.

5. Spaw AT, Reddick EJ, Olsen DO: Laparoscopic laser cholecystectomy: analysis of 500 procedures. *Surg Laparosc Endosc* 1991, 1:2–7.

6. Soper NJ, Stockmann PT, Dunnegan DL, et al.: Laparoscopic cholecystectomy: the new "gold standard?" *Arch Surg* 1992, 127:917–921.

7. The Southern Surgeons Club: A prospective analysis of 1518 laparoscopic cholecystectomies. *N Engl J Med* 1991, 324:1073–1078.

8. Bailey RW, Zucker KA, Flowers JL, et al.: Laparoscopic cholecystectomy: experience with 375 consecutive patients. *Ann Surg* 1991, 214:531–540.

9. Schirmer BD, Edge SB, Dix J, et al.: Laparoscopic cholecystectomy: treatment of choice for symptomatic cholelithiasis. *Ann Surg* 1991, 213:665–676.

10. Cuschieri A, DuBois F, Mouiel J, et al.: The European experience with laparoscopic cholecystectomy. *Am J Surg* 1991, 161:385–387.

11. Peters JH, Gibbons GD, Innes JT, et al.: Complications of laparoscopic cholecystectomy. *Surgery* 1991, 110:769–778.

12. Wolfe BM, Gardiner BN, Leary BF, et al.: Endoscopic cholecystectomy: an analysis of complications. *Arch Surg* 1991, 126:1192–1196.

13. Graves HA, Ballinger JF, Anderson WJ: Appraisal of laparoscopic cholecystectomy. *Ann Surg* 1991, 213:655–662.

14.• Soper NJ, Brunt ML, Kerbl K: Laparoscopic general surgery. *N Engl J Med* 1994, 330:409–419.

Overview of the rapid progress of laparoscopy and its impact on general surgery.

15. Soper NJ: Laparoscopic cholecystectomy. *Curr Probl Surg* 1991, 28:585–655.

16.• McMahon AJ, Russell IT, Baxter JN, et al.: Laparoscopic versus minilaparotomy cholecystectomy: a randomized trial. *Lancet* 1994, 343:135–138.

Rigorous comparison demonstrating shorter hospital stay and quicker return to normal activity after laparoscopy in the United Kingdom.

17. Schmieg RE Jr, Schirmer BD, Combs MJ, et al.: Recovery of gastrointestinal motility after laparoscopic cholecystectomy. *Surg Forum* 1993, 44:135–136.

18. Soper NJ, Barteau JA, Clayman RV, et al.: Laparoscopic vs. standard open cholecystectomy: comparison of early results. *Surg Gynecol Obstet* 1992, 174:114–118.

19. Barkun JS, Barkun AN, Sampalis JS, et al.: Randomized controlled trial of laparoscopic vs. mini-cholecystectomy. *Lancet* 1992, 340:1116–1119.

20. Anderson ER, Hunter JG: Laparoscopic cholecystectomy is less expensive than open cholecystectomy. *Surg Laparosc Endosc* 1991, 1:82–84.

21. Fisher KS, Reddick EJ, Olsen DO: Laparoscopic cholecystectomy: cost analysis. *Surg Laparosc Endosc* 1991, 1:77–81.

22. Bass EB, Pitt HA, Lillemoe KD: Cost-effectiveness of laparoscopic cholecystectomy versus open cholecystectomy. *Am J Surg* 1993, 165:466–471.

23. Sackier JM, Wang Y: Robotically assisted laparoscopic surgery. *Surg Endosc* 1994, 8:63–66.

24. Banting S, Shimi S, Velpen GV, Cuschieri A: Abdominal wall lift: low pressure pneumoperitoneum laparoscopic surgery. *Surg Endosc* 1993, 7:57–59.

25. Legorreta AP, Silber JH, Costantino GN, et al.: Increased cholecystectomy rate after the introduction of laparoscopic cholecystectomy. *JAMA* 1993, 270:1429–1432.

26.• Steiner CA, Bass EB, Talamini MA, et al.: Surgical rates and operative mortality for open and laparoscopic cholecystectomy in Maryland. *N Engl J Med* 1994, 330:403–408.

Interprets the increasing rate of laparoscopic cholecystectomy in Maryland to reflect a lower threshold among both patients and physicians for surgical intervention.

27. Gracie WA, Ransohoff DF: The natural history of silent gallstones: the innocent gallstone is not a myth. *N Engl J Med* 1982, 307:798–800.

28. Ransohoff DF, Gracie WA, Wolfenson LB, et al.: Prophylactic cholecystectomy or expectant management for silent gallstones: a decision analysis to assess survival. *Ann Intern Med* 1983, 99:199–204.

29. Jones DB, Soper NJ, Brewer JD, et al.: Chronic acalculous cholecystitis: Laparoscopic treatment. *Surg Laparosc and Endosc* 1996, 6:114–122.

30. Soper NJ: Effect of nonbiliary problems on laparoscopic cholecystectomy. *Am J Surg* 1993, 165:522–526.

31. Unger SW, Scott JS, Edelman DS: Laparoscopic approach to gallstones in the morbidly obese patient. *Surg Endosc* 1991, 5:116–117.

32. Soper NJ, Hunter J, Petrie RH: Laparoscopic cholecystectomy in pregnancy. *Surg Endosc* 1992, 6:115–117.

33. See WA, Soper NJ: Selection and preparation of the patient for laparoscopic surgery. In *Essentials of Laparoscopy*. Edited by Soper NJ, Odem RR, Clayman RV, and McDougall EM. St. Louis: Quality Medical Publishing; 1994:6–7.

34. Monk TG, Weldon BC: Anesthetic considerations for laparoscopic surgery. In Essentials of Laparoscopy. Edited by Soper NJ, Odem RR, Clayman RV, and McDougall EM. St. Louis: Quality Medical Publishing; 1994:24–33.

35. Gravenstein JS, Paulus PA, Hayes TJ: Carbon dioxide and monitoring. In *Capnography in Clinical Practice*. Edited by Gravenstein JS, Paulus PA, and Hayes TJ. Boston: Butterworth Publishers; 1989:3–10.

36. Tverskoy M, Cozacor C, Ayache M, et al.: Postoperative pain after inguinal herniorrhaphy with different types of anesthesia. *Anesth Analg* 1992, 74:495–498.

37. Kitano S, Tomikawa M, Iso Y, et al.: A safe and simple method to maintain a clear field of vision during laparoscopic cholecystectomy. *Surg Endosc* 1991, 6:197–198.

38. Hashimoto D, Nayeem SA, Kajiwara S, et al.: Laparoscopic cholecystectomy: an approach without pneumoperitoneum. *Surg Endosc* 1993, 7:54–56.

39. Graff TD, Arbgast NR, Phillips OC, et al.: Gas embolism: a comparative study of air and carbon dioxide as embolic agents in the systemic venous system. *Am J Obstet Gynecol* 1959, 78:259–265.

40. Fitzgerald SD, Andrus CH, Baudendistel LJ, *et al.*: Hypercarbia during carbon dioxide pneumoperitoneum. *Am J Surg* 1992, 163:186–190.

41. Leighton TA, Bongard FS, Liu SY, *et al.*: Comparative cardiopulmonary effects of helium and carbon dioxide pneumoperitoneum. *Surg Forum* 1991, 42:485–487.

42.• Strasberg SM, Hertl M, Soper NJ: An analysis of the problem of biliary injury during laparoscopic cholecystectomy. *J Am Coll Surg* 1995, 180:101-125.
Biliary injury is more common with laparoscopic, than with open cholecystectomy. The causes, means of prevention, and management of these bile duct injuries are discussed in detail.

43. Yamamoto M, Stiegmann GV, Durham J, *et al.*: Laparoscopy-guided intracorporeal ultrasound accurately delineates hepatobiliary anatomy. *Surg Endosc* 1993, 7:325–330.

44. Albala DM, Clayman RV: Postoperative care. In *Essentials of Laparoscopy.* Edited by Soper NJ, Odem RR, Clayman RV, and McDougall EM. St. Louis: Quality Medical Publishing; 1994:210–212.

45. Hermann RE: Surgery for acute and chronic cholecystitis. *Surg Clin North Am* 1990, 70:1263–1275.

46. Cooperman AM: Laparoscopic cholecystectomy for severe acute, embedded, and gangrenous cholecystitis. *J Laparosc Endosc Surg* 1990, 1:37–40.

47. Reddick EJ, Olsen D, Spaw A, *et al.*: Safe performance of difficult laparoscopic cholecystectomies. *Am J Surg* 1991, 161:377–381.

48. Unger SW, Edelman DS, Scott JS, *et al.*: Laparoscopic treatment of acute cholecystitis. *Surg Laparosc Endosc* 1991, 1:14–16.

49. Soper NJ, Dunnegan DL: Does intraoperative gallbladder perforation influence the early outcome of laparoscopic cholecystectomy? *Surg Laparosc Endosc* 1991, 1:156–161.

50. Stuart L, Smith AL, Pellegrini CA, *et al.*: Pigment gallstones form as a component of bacterial microcolonies and pigment solids. *Ann Surg* 1987, 206:242–249.

51. Soper NJ, Flye MW, Brunt LM, *et al.*: Diagnosis and management of biliary complications of laparoscopic cholecystectomy. *Am J Surg* 1993, 165:663–669.

52. National Institutes of Health Consensus Development Conference Statement on Gallstones and Laparoscopic Cholecystectomy. *Am J Surg* 1993, 165:390–398.

Laparoscopic Choledocholithotomy

Joseph B. Petelin

Choledocholithiasis is present in approximately 10% of patients who present for cholecystectomy [1,2]. Definitive treatment of these patients includes not only cholecystectomy, but also clearance of the entire ductal system. This has presented a technical challenge to the biliary tract surgeon since the earliest days of biliary tract surgery. Indeed, while Langenbuch performed the first cholecystectomy in July 1882, the first successful common duct exploration was not performed until 8 years later, in January 1890 by Courvoisier [3]. One hundred years later, in the late 1980s, laparoscopic cholecystectomy was introduced and soon became the standard of care. While many early observers believed that a laparoscopic approach to common bile duct exploration would present insurmountable technical difficulties, the pioneers in this field quickly developed numerous laparoscopic techniques for treating common duct pathology. Laparoscopic common bile duct exploration has been effectively employed in thousands of cases, albeit by a relatively small percentage of the practicing biliary tract surgeons today. The reasons for this lack of application of laparoscopic ductal exploration are many, and too complicated to permit a full discussion here. Nevertheless, a brief review of the recent history of biliary tract surgery is enlightening.

In the 100 years preceding the introduction of laparoscopic cholecystectomy, surgeons were expected to clear the common ductal system in approximately 90% of cases where they attempted common duct exploration. That is to say, the literature prior to 1990 suggested that a 5% to 10% failure rate of common bile duct exploration was expected [4,5••,6]. However, since the advent of laparoscopic cholecystectomy, most surgeons have more or less abrogated their intraoperative responsibility for doing a complete job, *ie*, returning the biliary tract to its normal healthy status without ductal calculi. Instead, they have relied more and more on alternative and additional interventional methods (endoscopic retrograde cholangiopancreatography [ERCP], dissolution agents, and lithotripsy) to handle these problems [7]. While these other techniques are certainly useful in managing complicated biliary tract problems, they are not without cost, morbidity, mortality, and significant lifestyle disruption.

Appropriate management of biliary tract pathology must, now and in the future, not only consider the ultimate outcome, but also the efficiency, efficacy, and cost of the methods employed to achieve that endpoint, *ie*, clearance of the ductal system. The laparoscopic solution to this problem has proved to be the safest, most cost-effective, and efficient means of returning the patient to his or her former lifestyle with the least financial or social disruption (Petelin, Paper presented at the Society of American Gastrointestinal Endoscopic Surgeons Annual Meeting, 1994).

Choledocholithotomy may involve the application of a number of technical maneuvers. These maneuvers include administration of glucagon, dilatation of the distal common bile duct, balloon catheter manipulation, basket manipulation, with or without fluoroscopic guidance, and choledochoscopic manipulations [8–17]. All of these techniques presuppose that intraoperative cholangiography (IOC) has been performed, whether or not preoperative ductal evaluation (chemical, radiographic, or endoscopic retrograde cholangiography [ERC]) has been used to evaluate or treat the common duct pathology prior to that time.

This chapter explores the techniques and technology currently available for laparoscopic treatment of common duct pathology. During the past few years, the general approach to the patient with choledocholithiasis has solidified, and a number of techniques have been repeatedly demonstrated to be effective. However, even as this material is being published, new developments will occur that may render some of these seemingly leading-edge concepts and technologies obsolete. The reader is encouraged to entertain these ideas with this in mind: That which is state of the art today, will most likely not be state of the art tomorrow.

PATIENT MANAGEMENT

Clinical situations that can arise may be divided into two main groups: those situations in which choledocholithiasis is suspected preoperatively, and those in which it is discovered intraoperatively.

When common bile duct stones are suspected preoperatively, the clinician must decide whether to attempt ductal treatment, *ie*, ERCP and extraction with or without sphincterotomy (ERC +/- S) before operation, or to proceed directly with laparoscopic cholecystectomy and laparoscopic common duct exploration (LCDE) [8]. ERC +/- S has been shown to be successful in clearing the common duct in over 90% of cases [18••,19–21]. Similarly, LCDE is successful in clearing the duct in over 90% of cases as well [9,10,22–24]. The choice of clearance method will be based on the local availability of expert endoscopists capable of a high degree of success with ERC +/- S, the availability of laparoscopic and choledochoscopic equipment, the surgeon's own expertise in laparoscopic surgery, and the general condition of the patient [5••,7,18••,25]. The surgeon must realize, however, that ERC +/- S is not without its own set of complications. Morbidity and mortality have been reported at 5% to 19% and 1.3%, respectively [26,27].

When common bile duct stones are discovered intraoperatively, the decision is much easier to make. The surgeon either proceeds with LCDE, converts the case to "open" common duct exploration and choledocholithotomy, or leaves the stones in place for subsequent ERC +/- S [5••,8,14]. Although any of these alternatives are acceptable, the latter two are more costly and associated with increased morbidity. It would seem wise in most situations, therefore, to attempt LCDE unless the patient's condition warrants termination of the anesthetic as soon as possible. If LCDE is unsuccessful or not attempted, then the decision regarding conversion to "open" common duct exploration versus postoperative ERC +/- S will depend on the local availability of expert endoscopists. These considerations are graphically demonstrated in Figure 2-1.

Indications

An abnormal intraoperative cholangiogram or sonogram is the most common indication for laparoscopic common bile duct exploration. Preoperative studies, including unexplained elevated liver function tests, a dilated ductal system, sonographic evidence of bile duct stones, scintigraphic, endoscopic, or radiographic evidence of common bile duct obstruction, or history of biliary pancreatitis may also warrant laparoscopic common bile duct exploration.

Contraindications

The strongest contraindication to laparoscopic manipulation of the common bile duct is lack of training of the surgeon. Inability of the surgeon to perform the maneuvers required for common bile duct exploration, absence of any of the noted

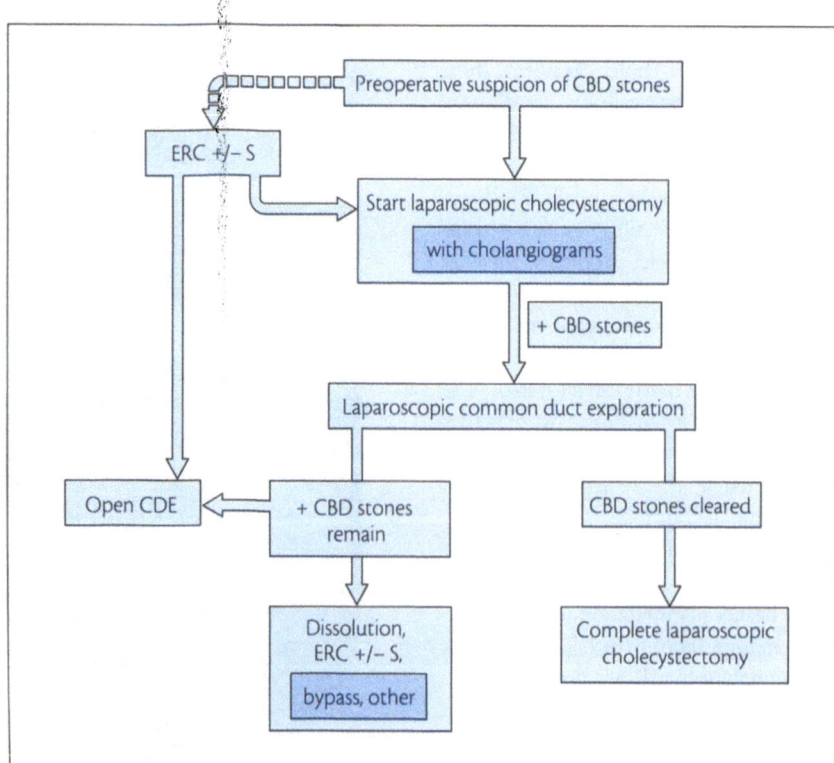

Figure 2-1 Protocol for management of common bile duct stones. CBD—common bile duct; CDE—common duct exploration; ERC +/- S—endoscopic retrograde cholangiopancreatography and extraction with or without sphincterectomy.

indications listed above, instability of the patient, and local conditions in the porta hepatis that would make exploration hazardous are the primary contraindications to laparoscopic common bile duct exploration. Additionally, as will be explained below, there are relative contraindications to specific approaches to ductal exploration. In these situations, either a transcystic approach or a direct choledochotomy approach may be preferred over the other.

EQUIPMENT

In addition to the basic set of equipment used to perform laparoscopic cholecystectomy, a number of other instruments are required to facilitate LCDE. Some or all of the following items may be required for ductal exploration:

1. 14-Gauge intravenous (IV) catheter, 2 inches in length
2. Glucagon, 1 to 2 mg (given IV by the anesthetist)
3. Balloon-tipped catheters (4 F preferred over 3 F and 5 F)
4. Segura-type baskets (4-wire, flat, straight in-line configuration)
5. 0.035-Inch diameter long guidewire
6. Mechanical "over-the-wire" dilators (7 to 12 F)
7. High pressure "over-the-wire" pneumatic dilator
8. IV tubing (for saline instillation through the choledochoscope)
9. Atraumatic grasping forceps (for choledochoscope manipulation)
10. Flexible choledochoscope with light source (smaller < 3 mm diameter, with > 1.1 mm working channel preferred)
11. Second camera
12. Second monitor (or second viewing area on the primary laparoscopic monitor)
13. Video switcher (for simultaneous same-monitor display of choledochoscopic, fluoroscopic, and laparoscopic images)
14. High pressure irrigator (eg, Waterpik; Teledyne, Fort Collins, CO)
15. Electrohydraulic lithotripter
16. Absorbable suture (polyglycolic acid suture, 4-0 or 5-0 size)
17. T-tube (transductal) or C-tube (transcystic)
18. Stent (straight, 7 F or 10 F)
19. Sphincterotome (for antegrade sphincterotomy)

A standard 2-inch long 14-gauge IV catheter is used to gain access to the peritoneal cavity for intraoperative cholangiography. This device presents a "5th" port for introduction of the cholangiography catheter, and subsequently, balloon catheters and baskets [28].

Fogarty embolectomy catheters are often useful for LCDE. A standard vascular-type of catheter is preferred because the "biliary" Fogarty is not long enough. Most commonly, a 4-F size proves adequate, but occasionally 3-F and 5-F models may be required.

Stone retrieval baskets are usually essential. These are available in straight and helical configurations with either flat or round wires. The straight flat wire basket, with its natural ability to expand the duct, presents large interstices for stones to

enter the basket. The round wire helical basket is used by those who prefer a twisting maneuver to capture stones while trolling through the duct. It should be noted, however, that while the basket is in the channel of the scope twisting maneuvers are quite difficult to achieve. Although I prefer a 4-wire straight basket, each surgeon will develop his own preferences. Models with variations of the distal tip offer a wide variety of baskets from which to choose.

A flexible choledochoscope is necessary to perform LCDE in approximately 60% of cases. The most versatile scopes feature a maximum outside diameter of 3 mm, tip deflection in at least one direction, a working channel of > 1 mm, excellent optics, and camera-ready capability. The scope requires a light source with automatic intensity control (Fig. 2-2).

Although not absolutely essential, a second camera directly connected to the scope significantly improves the performance of LCDE. This allows the surgeon to use both hands during the manipulation, since he or she doesn't have to hold the scope to his or her eye during the exploration. Projection of the choledochoscopic image onto the video monitor allows other members of the operative team to assist more effectively. Obviously, this either requires an additional monitor or video mixing equipment.

A video mixer is a useful adjunct in this setting. Using a picture-in-picture effect, both the laparoscopic and choledochoscopic images may be viewed on the same monitor simultaneously. This device reduces clutter in the operating room since it eliminates the need for an additional trolley and monitor. It also improves the efficiency of the operating surgeon since he can direct his gaze at one monitor, instead of alternating it between two [22,29].

Lithotripters may be used to disintegrate large or impacted stones in the ductal system. Electrohydraulic and laser models are available, but the latter are prohibitively expensive. The energy from either of these sources is delivered to the stone via wires or optical fibers introduced through the working channel of the choledochoscope. I find both types to be of limited value in most cases because they multiply the debris present within the duct when fragmentation occurs. Nevertheless, in the infrequent case of impaction of a stone, they can be very useful [15,18••].

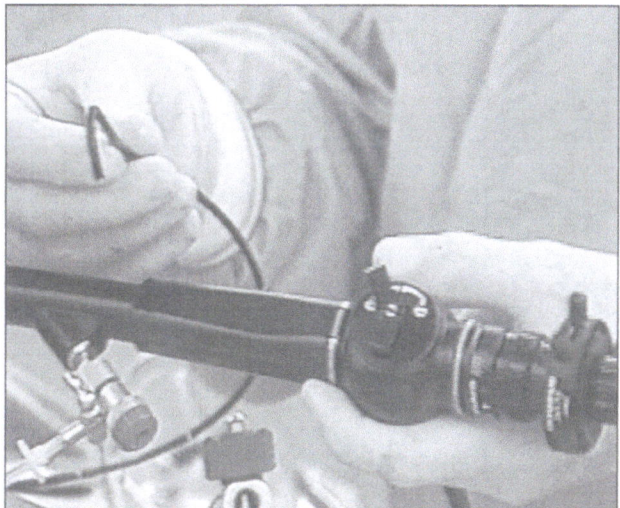

Figure 2-2 Flexible choledochoscope: the Olympus URF P2 (Melville, NY).

Dilators are often used to enlarge the cystic duct to a 12-F diameter to allow easy introduction and manipulation of the choledochoscope. Graduated over-the-wire mechanical dilators have the advantage of being inexpensive and readily available in most urology departments. Pneumatic dilators, while slightly more expensive, allow excellent control of the dilatation process.

In cases where choledochotomy is necessary, a laparoscopic scalpel or scissors is necessary to open the duct [8,29]. Standard T-tubes suffice for subsequent drainage of the duct, and are most easily introduced through a 10-mm portal using an 8-mm introduction sleeve [30,31]. Laparoscopic needle holders facilitate closure of the choledochotomy.

Storage

It is wise to have all of these materials, including balloon-tipped catheters and baskets, located on a cart or trolley in the department, so that in the case of an abnormal cholangiogram, they may be accessed without delay. This cart should be placed near the operating room where the common duct exploration is being performed (Fig. 2-3).

Intraoperative location

A separate Mayo stand, placed either at the foot of the table or preferentially near the patient's left shoulder, to the right of the surgeon, is useful for storing the choledochoscope and related equipment in the sterile field (Fig. 2-4). The various cables, catheters, and tubes used in the duct exploration should be routed so as to minimize clutter in the operative field. Additionally, nursing staff or biomedical engineering personnel should be available to connect the choledochoscope to its light source, the choledochoscopic camera to its processing unit, and the video cable to the appropriate location on the video mixer or monitor.

These considerations are often overlooked in most operating theaters, resulting in a chaotic environment when LCDE becomes necessary. Prior time spent in planning for equipment preparation and placement during LCDE scenarios is well worth the effort, and should be given the same importance as

preparation of the surgeon's skills to carry out the maneuvers once the equipment is available.

SURGICAL APPROACH

Laparoscopic common bile duct exploration may be accomplished through the cystic duct or through a choledochotomy. The surgeon must select the route of access: transcystic or choledochotomy. In addition to stone size, the anatomic definition of the triangle of Calot, including the cystic duct–common duct junction, the course of the cystic duct, and the diameter of each of the ducts affect this decision. If a transcystic approach appears feasible, it is usually tried before choledochotomy, because it is less invasive and is associated with better patient satisfaction.

In most cases, transcystic ductal exploration is possible and highly successful. In others, choledochotomy is necessary or even the preferred route. Table 2-1 summarizes characteristics that are helpful in making the determination.

Negative influences listed in this table have a more profound impact on selection of the access route than positive or neutral ones [32]. The techniques discussed below may be used with either access route, although there is usually less morbidity with the transcystic approach.

OPERATIVE TECHNIQUES
Ductal imaging

Intraoperative imaging of the ductal system is an integral part of managing choledocholithiasis. The surgeon should be facile with his or her favorite method: percutaneous cholangiography, portal cholangiography, or intraoperative ultrasonography. Fluoroscopic imaging has become the gold standard for intraoperative radiologic evaluation, because it is faster than other methods, more detailed, and allows surgeon interaction with the images in real time, *ie*, the surgeon can scan the ductal system by moving the C-arm while injecting contrast material (Fig. 2-5).

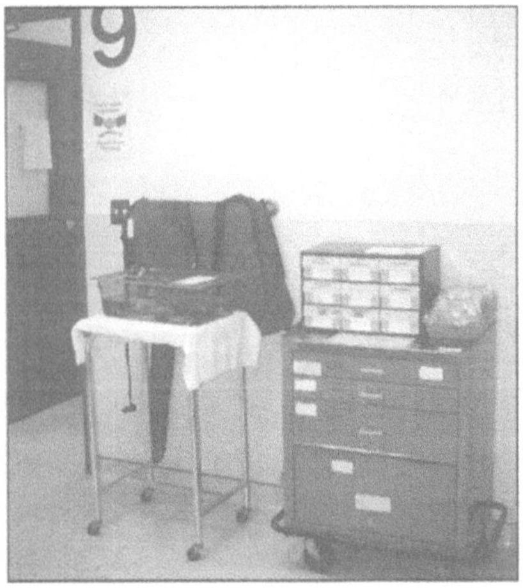

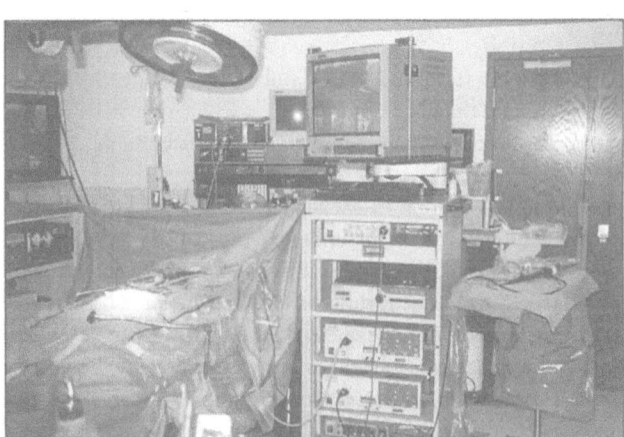

Figure 2-3 The common bile duct exploration storage cart should be located near the operating room where the duct exploration is being performed.

Figure 2-4 The sterile Mayo stand containing the choledochoscope, basket, balloon catheter, and dilators is located adjacent to the left-sided monitor trolley. It is simply moved adjacent to the patient's left shoulder, in front of the trolley, when needed for duct exploration.

Percutaneous cholangiography

A 14-gauge IV needle/catheter is inserted through the abdominal wall approximately 3 cm medial to the midclavicular port. It is directed toward the cystic duct orifice. The needle is removed and the catheter is used as a sleeve for introduction of the cholangiogram catheter. The catheter is grasped with forceps introduced through the medial epigastric port and placed into the cystic duct. It is fixed into position with a clip applied transversely across the axis of the catheter at its insertion point into the cystic duct.

I prefer this technique because it does not require removal of forceps controlling the gallbladder from another port (as is needed in the portal technique). This sleeve also acts as a "miniport" that may be used for introduction of balloons and baskets during common bile duct exploration.

Portal cholangiography

This method of cholangiogram catheter introduction requires removal of an existing instrument from one of the ports, usually the midclavicular port. The catheter is introduced through this port freely or with an applicator that directs it into the cystic duct. Some applicator models also fix the catheter into the cystic duct [33]. The major disadvantage of this technique is that it uses an existing port that would otherwise be used by an instrument to provide exposure in the porta hepatis.

Intraoperative sonography

Some authors have advocated the use of intraoperative laparoscopic sonography to evaluate the ductal system, liver, and surrounding structures for abnormalities. Here the sonographic probe is inserted through a 10-mm port and is placed in direct contact with the tissues. Proponents of this technology indicate that it is faster and more accurate than cholangiography. Critics have argued that fluoroscopic imaging is not only faster than sonographic imaging but doesn't require additional equipment expense, and that cholangiographic films may be used as "maps" of the ductal anatomy in cases where intense inflammation obscures visual cues. Widespread use of this technology for ductal evaluation has not occurred.

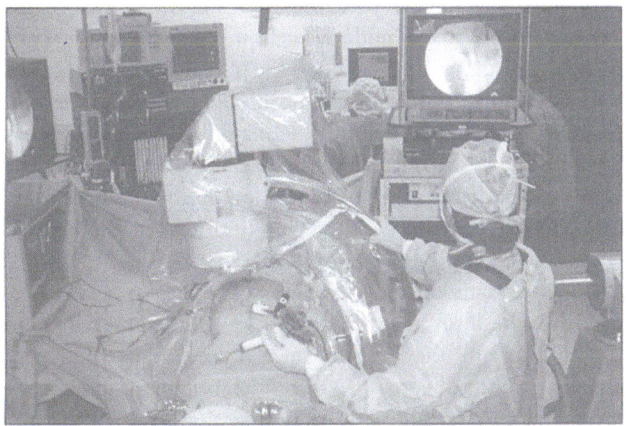

Figure 2-5 Fluoroscopic cholangiography.

Table 2-1

Factors influencing duct exploration approach

Factor	Transcystic approach	Choledochotomy approach
Single stone	+	+
Multiple stones	+	+
Stones < 6 mm diameter each	+	+
Stones > 6 mm diameter each	-	+
Intrahepatic stones	-	+
Diameter of cystic duct < 4 mm	-	+
Diameter of cystic duct > 4 mm	+	+
Diameter of common duct < 6 mm	+	-
Diameter of common duct > 6 mm	+	+
Cystic duct entrance: lateral	+	+
Cystic duct entrance: posterior	-	+
Cystic duct entrance: distal	-	+
Inflammation: mild	+	+
Inflammation: marked	+	-
Suturing ability: poor	+	-
Suturing ability: good	+	+

+, Positive or neutral effect; -, negative effect.

Preparation of the porta hepatis

Dissection

When abnormal cholangiograms are obtained, dissection of the porta hepatis is usually carried out more thoroughly in preparation for laparoscopic duct exploration than it is for routine laparoscopic cholecystectomy. In general, the dissection of the triangle of Calot should be approached from lateral to the neck of the gallbladder and carried toward the cystic duct–common duct junction as the anatomy is further defined. This is required because access to the cystic duct–common duct junction or the anterior surface of the common duct itself is usually necessary for ductal exploration. Intraoperative cholangiography provides a "map" that proves useful in this sometimes tedious dissection.

Although some dissection in the triangle of Calot will have occurred prior to the initiation of cholangiograms, further delineation of the anatomy in this area is usually required in order to pursue common duct exploration. The lateral aspect of the infundibulum of the gallbladder and the cystic duct is approached first (Fig. 2-6) [34]. The peritoneum in this area is incised and reflected. This displays the cystic duct–common duct junction, and in some instances allows the surgeon to "unwrap" a posteriorly located junction. Occasionally, the lateral peritoneal attachments of the duodenum must also be severed, ie, the Kocher maneuver, in order to achieve this effect. This facilitates introduction of instruments into the common duct via the cystic duct. The importance of these maneuvers cannot be overestimated.

The triangle of Calot is then approached again. During dissection of the triangle of Calot, the location of the common duct may be temporarily demonstrated by depressing the duodenal sweep inferiorly with atraumatic forceps introduced through the midclavicular port. This stretches the common duct into a taught band, which is easily identified. If the cystic artery has not yet been divided, and if it obscures visualization of the common hepatic duct, then it may be divided at this time. Extension of the incision in the peritoneum lying medial to the neck of the gallbladder is also helpful in some cases. This often allows the extrahepatic ductal system to be delivered into a more anterior location as the gallbladder is displaced toward the right hemi-diaphragm. Dissection must be done carefully here in order to avoid hemorrhage from small vessels on or around the common duct.

Dilatation of the cystic duct

Although some authors prefer common duct access via a choledochotomy [23,35,36], laparoscopic common duct exploration may be carried out through cystic duct access in over 90% of the cases [8–10,15]. When choledochoscopic maneuvers are needed, the cystic duct will need to accept a 9- or 10-F diameter scope. If the duct is not already large enough for scope insertion, it may be dilated either with mechanical over-the-wire graduated dilators or with pneumatic dilators.

In either case, a guidewire (0.028 inch or 0.035 inch) is first inserted through the midclavicular port, through the cystic duct, and into the common duct. If graduated dilators are used, a 9-F size is usually the first to be advanced over the wire into the duct. I have found that if a 9-F dilator will not relatively easily enter the cystic duct, then the likelihood of dilatation to a large enough diameter, 11 or 12 F, is low. Each successively larger dilator is advanced over the wire until the duct is patulous enough to accept the scope [8,22,25].

If a pneumatic dilator is employed, it may also be advanced over the wire into the cystic duct. Then, while observing both the monitor and the pressure gauge on the screw-type syringe attached to the dilator, the dilatation balloon is filled. It is important to closely observe the physical changes in the duct while the dilatation proceeds, so that injury to the cystic duct–common duct junction may be avoided (Fig. 2-7).

After either of these maneuvers, the guidewire may be removed or left in place for subsequent guidance of the choledochoscope. The dilatation equipment should remain sterile, however, so that it is available in the uncommon case where it might be needed again for dilatation.

Choledochotomy

If the cystic duct cannot be dilated enough to accept passage of the scope or the largest common duct stone, or if intrahepatic pathology is suspected, then choledochotomy may be necessary.

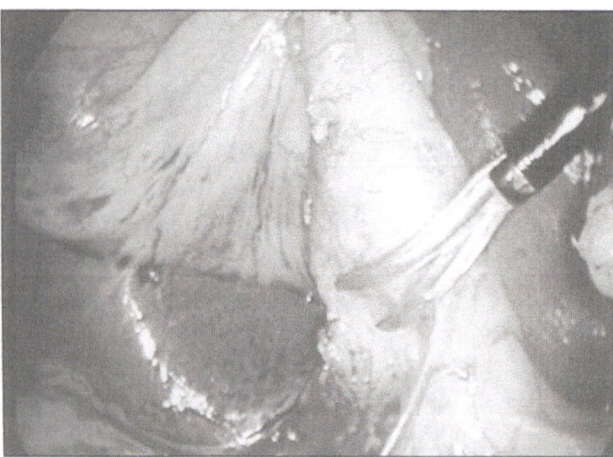

Figure 2-6 Dissection is first performed lateral to the infundibulum of the gallbladder. (*See* Color Plate.)

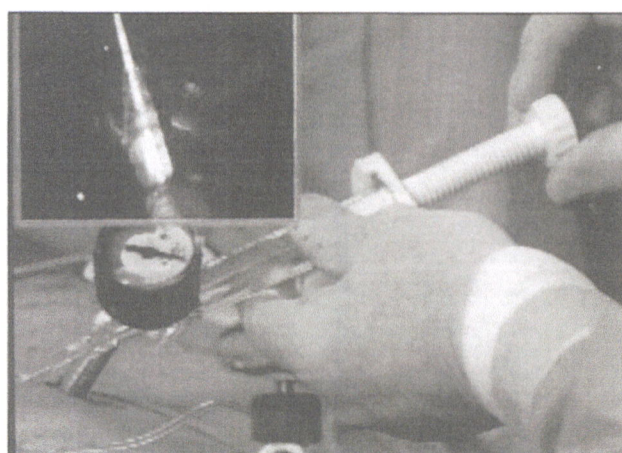

Figure 2-7 Pneumatic dilation of the cystic duct using a microvasive dilator.

This may be accomplished with a laparoscopic scalpel, scissors, or contact tip laser inserted through the medial epigastric port. A longitudinal incision approximately 1 cm in length, or as long as the largest stone, is sufficient. This limits the amount of time spent later in closing the choledochotomy. Stay sutures, which are commonly used in open common duct exploration, are not necessary for laparoscopic common duct exploration.

Irrigation techniques

When very small stones (< 2 mm in diameter), sludge, or sphincter spasm is suspected to be responsible for lack of flow of contrast into the duodenum, glucagon, 1 to 2 mg, may be administered intravenously by the anesthetist in order to relieve sphincter pressure. This is combined with transcystic flushing of the duct with saline or contrast material in an attempt to force the debris into the duodenum. The progress, or lack thereof, is monitored fluoroscopically. Surgeons should not expect this method to be successful in clearing stones 4 mm and larger from the duct. This often yields a normal cholangiogram [14].

Balloon techniques

The next step involves the use of a standard 4-F Fogarty balloon catheter. It is inserted into the abdomen through the 14-gauge sleeve used to perform the percutaneous cholangiograms. This 14-gauge sleeve is located 3 cm medial to the midclavicular port [8,28]. Forceps introduced through the medial epigastric port guide the catheter into the common duct through the cystic duct. The catheter is advanced into the duodenum if possible. The balloon is inflated and the catheter is withdrawn until resistance is met at the sphincter; the duodenum is observed to move with the catheter at this point. The balloon is deflated, the catheter is withdrawn 1 cm, and the balloon is reinflated. This should position it in the most distal portion of the duct, just proximal to the sphincter. The catheter is then withdrawn through the cystic duct, using the forceps from the medial epigastric port. Although it would seem unlikely for the stones or debris to be preferentially directed out of the cystic duct rather than into the common hepatic duct, the surgeon is frequently rewarded with delivery of this material from the cystic duct ori-

fice. It can then be removed with forceps introduced through the medial epigastric port. The surgeon must use great care and gentle manipulations with the catheter in order to avoid perforation of the ductal system during these maneuvers, especially when a stone is impacted in the distal duct.

Whereas in most cases the balloon catheter technique is employed without choledochoscopic or fluoroscopic monitoring, either of these devices may aid in exact localization of the stone and the balloon. If a choledochoscope is used, the balloon-tipped catheter must be inserted alongside the scope because the working channel of the scope is not large enough to accept the catheter. This obviously requires either a cystic duct of large diameter or insertion through a choledochotomy.

In some cases, stones defy capture with a basket, even under direct vision through the choledochoscope. Here, a balloon-tipped catheter may be used in conjunction with the choledochoscope. It is inserted alongside the scope (not in the scope channel) (Fig. 2-8). It is advanced past the stone, inflated, and withdrawn toward the scope. The entire scope-stone-balloon ensemble is then withdrawn through the ductal orifice. This technique is especially useful when dealing with intrahepatic stones. Baskets are less useful in the intrahepatic ductal system because they cannot be fully deployed in the narrow diameter hepatic radicles.

Basket techniques

Stone retrieval baskets may also be inserted through the 14-gauge sleeve used for cholangiography. The basket is advanced into the common duct through the cystic duct, using forceps introduced through the medial epigastric port. If no fluoroscope is used during this maneuver, the surgeon must estimate the location of the basket tip in the common duct. Estimation can be relatively accurate when the length of the duct has already been measured with the balloon-tipped catheter. When the basket is located in the distal common duct, it is opened and the entire basket unit is moved back and forth in small increments while slowly withdrawing it as the wires of the basket are being closed. Capture of a stone is identified when the basket fails to close completely. The device is removed through the cystic duct, and the stones are delivered from the abdomen as described above. Great care must be exercised with this method so that accidental "capture" of the papilla of Vater does not occur.

A more accurate method of determining the exact location of the stones and the basket employs a fluoroscope [9]. In the contrast-filled common duct, the manipulations required for stone capture with the basket may be monitored in real time. This technique, however, requires positioning of the fluoroscope in such a way as to avoid interference with movements of the forceps in the medial epigastric port. In some individuals, especially the obese, adequate fluoroscope position cannot be achieved. The surgeon must then decide whether to pursue basket extraction without it, or use a choledochoscope to monitor the procedure.

Choledochoscopic techniques

The conservative measures described above are usually employed while the choledochoscope and its related equipment are being prepared. In many hospitals this usually requires 20 to 30 minutes if the scope has not already been sterilized. (The choledochoscope

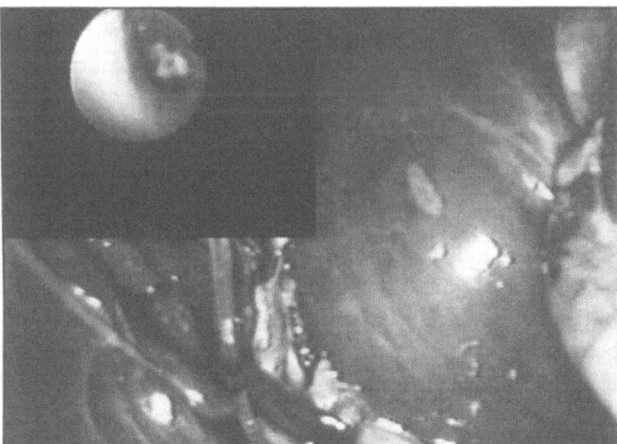

Figure 2-8 Fogarty balloon catheter manipulation alongside the choledochoscope in the hepatic ductal system. (*See* Color Plate.)

may be either gas sterilized on the day before surgery or soaked in gluteraldehyde for 20 minutes at the time of the procedure.)

The choledochoscope is inserted through the midclavicular port, with or without wire guidance, into the cystic duct or the choledochotomy (Fig. 2-9). The choledochoscopic and laparoscopic images must be kept in view, either on separate monitors or preferably on the same screen with a video mixer. At the level of the skin, the surgeon initially uses an atraumatic forceps inserted through the medial epigastric port to help guide the scope into the common duct. Saline instillation through the working channel of the scope should be employed at this time in order to expand the common duct and provide for better visualization. Once a sufficient length of the choledochoscope is present within the common duct, the forceps is withdrawn. Further manipulations require the surgeon to use both hands on the scope in most cases. One hand controls twisting maneuvers on the body of the scope at the cannula site, while the other holds the scope head and directs the tip of the scope with the deflection lever located there.

As the common duct is negotiated, stones, debris, or other pathology become visible. The distal portion of the common bile duct is usually the easiest to inspect and treat. If a cystic duct approach is employed, access to the proximal ductal system is usually not possible unless the cystic duct is very short or patulous and oriented at 90° to the common duct. If a choledochotomy has been prepared, the scope may be directed either into the proximal system or the distal bile duct.

If the surgeon experiences difficulty in traversing the cystic duct–common duct junction, further dissection along the lateral border of the cystic and common bile duct, or a Kocher maneuver, may be necessary. Occasionally this will allow the junction to "unwrap," thereby providing a less convoluted path into the common duct.

In most cases, stones identified with the choledochoscope will require entrapment in a basket for removal through the cystic duct or the choledochotomy. I believe that these are the most difficult maneuvers associated with laparoscopic common duct exploration. They often require the help of the scrub nurse or an assistant.

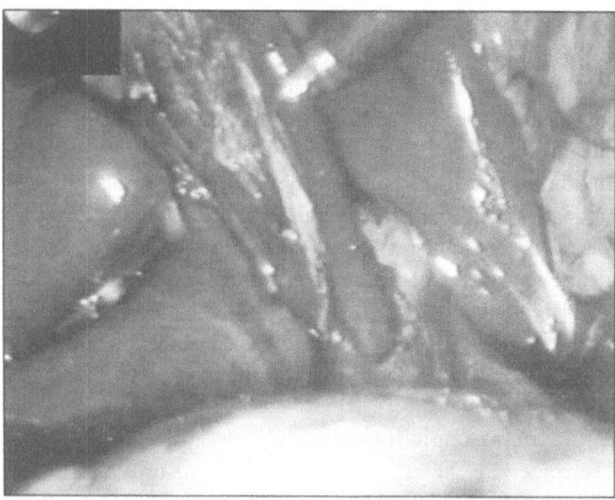

Figure 2-9 Insertion of the choledochoscope into the cystic duct. (*See* Color Plate.)

The scope is manipulated by the surgeon so that the stone is in direct view. Control of the body of the scope is then transferred to the assistant. It is essential that he or she provide the same amount of torque on the scope at the level of the midclavicular cannula as the surgeon had applied prior to the transfer. Although simple in concept, this step can become one of the most frustrating of the entire LCDE. The assistant must understand the importance of keeping the stone in view, and must direct undivided attention to the monitor providing the choledochoscopic view. Otherwise the location of the stone will be lost. If this happens after the basket is inserted into the working channel of the scope, it is very difficult to manipulate the scope to find it again without removing the basket from the channel. This difficulty occurs because most scopes use the working channel to provide the saline instillation that dilates the duct. With the basket in the channel, very little, if any, saline is delivered into the duct, and its lumen collapses. This problem becomes compounded when multiple stones are present in the duct, since their manipulation and capture usually produces minute debris that "clouds" the fluid in the duct. This cloudiness, combined with loss of the exact location of the stone, make it nearly impossible to capture the stone. In this case, the basket will need to be removed so that saline instillation through the basket channel may be used to clear the fluid in the duct. Obviously, inefficient manipulations performed at this time create more debris and decrease the likelihood of a successful LCDE.

After transfering the body of the scope to the assistant, with the stone in direct view, the surgeon temporarily interrupts the saline instillation and inserts the basket into the working channel of the scope. Once the basket is located in the channel, the saline may once again be allowed to flow, although the amount that will actually enter the channel will be limited because of the presence of the basket. The basket is then advanced until its tip is seen protruding from the tip of the choledochoscope. The basket is advanced past the stone and then it is opened. It is withdrawn back to the stone in order to attempt capture. If this is unsuccessful, as it usually is on the first few passes, the basket must be moved back and forth past the stone until it drops into the interstices. In some cases, this maneuver must be combined with twisting of the scope body or tip deflection in order to capture the stone. The basket is then slowly closed around the stone to secure it. This step usually requires the entire basket ensemble to be advanced as the wires are being closed, because closure usually withdraws the wires toward the scope and may dislodge the stone from its position in the basket.

Lithotripsy

The primary indication for intraoperative lithotripsy continues to be an impacted stone that defies less aggressive removal techniques. Intraoperative electrohydraulic or laser lithotripsy techniques have been used sporadically since the introduction of laparoscopic common bile duct exploration. Laser lithotripters are far too expensive to encourage widespread implementation; electrohydraulic lithotripters (EHL) are much less expensive, and consequently have been used somewhat more frequently. EHL devices must be used with great caution because they may cause unwanted ductal damage if the tip of the EHL probe is not accurately applied to the stone. However, with careful, direct visualization and application of EHL energy to the stone surface, stones may be safely fragmented without undue risk [15,18••].

I have also found that application of a pulsatile saline jet, *eg,* Waterpik, through the working channel of the scope may be useful in freeing debris from the duct wall. Because there are no ready-made adapters for such devices to connect to the scope, the surgeon will have to configure his own if he elects to use this modality.

Sphincterotomy and drainage procedures

Laparoscopic antegrade sphincterotomy was first described by DePaula in Brazil in 1993 [37•]. In this technique, a sphinc-terotome is passed through the working channel of the chole-dochoscope and through the sphincter. The cutting action of the device is monitored by simultaneous side-viewing endoscopy of the duodenum. While this technique achieves excellent results as a drainage procedure, it is logistically quite difficult to accomplish. It requires more equipment and an additional endoscopic team to be present in an already crowded operating theater. Endoscopists report that it more difficult to perform this procedure with the patient supine rather than in the typical prone position. Surgeons indicate that excessive air insufflation by the endoscopist hampers laparoscopic visualiza-tion and manipulation. For all these reasons, laparoscopic ante-grade sphincterotomy has not gained widespread acceptance. Gagner and coworkers [38•] have employed endoscopic retro-grade sphincterotomy at the same time as the LCDE, but again this has not gained widespread acceptance.

In patients with an impacted distal stone, a stone or stones located distal to a stricture, or dramatically dilated ducts with multiple stones, a choledochoenterostomy may be indicated. This may be accomplished laparoscopically, but it requires sig-nificant advanced laparoscopic suturing skills.

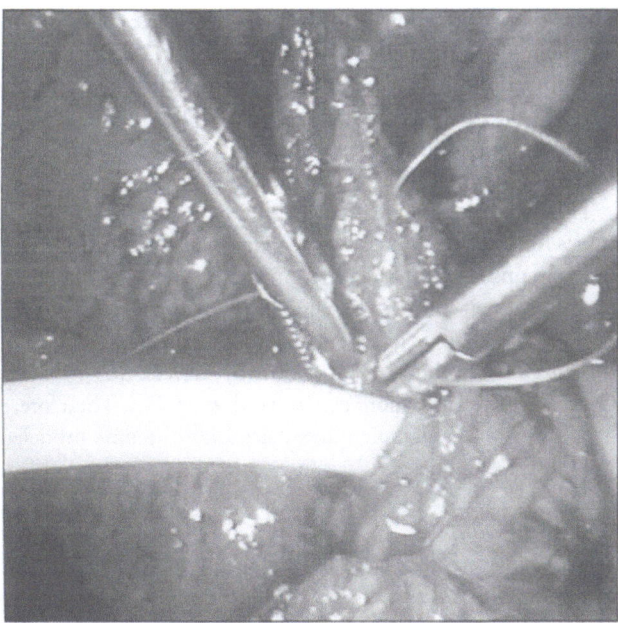

Figure 2-10 The choledochotomy is closed around the T-tube with absorbable 4-0 or 5-0 suture. (*See* Color Plate.)

Completion cholangiography and cholecystectomy

After the common duct exploration has been completed, cholangiograms should be repeated in order to ensure that the duct is cleared. If a transcystic duct LCDE approach has been used, then the cholangiogram catheter is reinserted into the cystic duct and the films are repeated. If choledochotomy has been made, then the cholangiograms may be obtained through the T-tube. If for some reason the duct is still not cleared, the surgeon must decide whether to proceed with LCDE, convert to open CDE, consider choledochoenterosto-my, or leave the stones in place for subsequent treatment with ERC +/- S.

Leaving the porta hepatis

Ligation of the cystic duct

The cystic duct stump must be occluded with either clips or ligatures or sutures. In cases where the cystic duct is rather dilated, > 6 mm, or where subsequent ERC +/- S is contem-plated, it is wise to use a ligature, in addition to clips, to secure the stump. In these instances, the ligature should be applied first, then the clips. This should decrease the likelihood of a stump leak.

T-tube or C-tube placement

If a choledochotomy has been used to gain access to the com-mon duct, it is usually closed over a T-tube after the ductal exploration is complete. A 14-F T-tube is prepared by remov-ing the back wall of the T portion. It is then loaded into an 8-mm cylinder and delivered through the 10-mm medial epigas-tric portal into the peritoneal cavity [8,27]. The entire T-tube is placed into the abdomen, and then the T is inserted into the common duct. This usually requires some effort, but it is not much more difficult than in open surgery. After the tube is in the duct, the outlying portion is temporarily occluded at its tip with a hemoclip or ligature; this prevents bile drainage into the peritoneal cavity while the remainder of the cholecystectomy is completed. This clip is later removed just prior to delivery of the tube through the abdominal wall.

The choledochotomy is closed with 4-0 or 5-0 Vicryl suture (Fig. 2-10) [8]. Either interrupted or continuous suture may be used, although the former is usually easier for the novice to complete. The magnification afforded by the laparoscope and camera allows more precise placement of the sutures than in open surgery. The suture is secured with intracorporeal ligation techniques rather than extracorporeal techniques because of the fragility of the duct. The closure may be tested for water tight-ness by temporarily advancing the end of the tube out of one of the 5-mm portals and injecting saline in the same fashion as would be done in open surgery. It is usually necessary to replace the tube into the peritoneal cavity until the cholecystectomy is completed so that the portal is available for retracting forceps and the tube itself does not limit access to the porta hepatis. While the tube is completely inside the peritoneal cavity, its tip should remain occluded with a clip or ligature. Alternatively, the choledochotomy may be closed and a transcystic tube, a C-tube, may be inserted to decompress the common bile duct and provide access for subsequent cholangiography [39].

Primary closure of the choledochotomy

The rationale for T-tube use developed for three primary reasons: 1) decompression of the duct, in the case of residual distal obstruction; 2) ductal imaging in the postoperative period; and 3) provision of an access route for removal of residual common duct stones, should they be left after common bile duct exploration [40].

T-tube placement during open surgery can be difficult at times. This difficulty may become even more pronounced in laparoscopic surgery [41,42]. Numerous gadgets and techniques have been suggested to facilitate this maneuver, but surgeon patience and practice are the most important requirements [43–49]. Most authors prefer a longitudinal choledochotomy, a 14-F latex T-tube (or larger), and ductal closure with an absorbable fine suture such as 4-0 or 5-0 polyglycolic acid. Although silicone T-tubes have been used by some authors, they are often not preferred because they do not excite the degree of tissue reaction necessary to produce a tract to the surface in the case of persistent bile leakage after removal. Silicone T-tubes, however, have been associated with less bacterial contamination than Latex T-tubes [50–56].

Management of T-tubes in the postoperative period may be associated with bacteremia, dislodgment of the tube, obstruction by the tube, or fracture of the tube [41,42,57]. Some authors recommend broad-spectrum antibiotic coverage while the T-tube is in situ [58]. T-tube cholangiography should be performed before removal of the tube. Removal of T-tubes has been suggested as early as 4 days postoperatively, and as long as 6 weeks postoperatively [59]. Between these two extremes lies the most appropriate management plan. Removal of T-tubes has been associated with bile leaks, peritonitis, and reoperation [54–56,58,60–62].

Despite the advantages of T-tube drainage, and because of the potential complications of T-tube placement, primary closure of the common bile duct without drainage has been advocated by some authors in open biliary tract surgery [40,50–56,63,64]. Shorter operative times and length of hospital stay have been observed with primary closure. No increase in bile leak or peritonitis has been noted with primary closure in the open literature. Higher patient satisfaction has been associated with primary closure.

In my series, primary closure of the choledochotomy laparoscopically did not result in any complications. There was no incidence of bile leak, peritonitis, or clinical evidence of retained bile duct stones. Patients reported a higher degree of comfort and satisfaction than those in whom T-tubes had been placed.

Drain placement

While drains are not routinely placed after uncomplicated laparoscopic cholecystectomy, they are more commonly used after laparoscopic common bile duct exploration. A drain may be indicated in cases where intense inflammation, infection, or contamination is present, where a choledochotomy has been performed, or where tissue integrity may be questionable. When indicated, a closed system suction drain is inserted through a 10-mm port into the porta hepatis and is usually brought out through the abdominal wall through one of the 5-mm port sites.

Biliary bypass

Surgical biliary bypass may be indicated for patients with a dramatically dilated common bile duct, multiple common duct stones, nonremovable impacted distal common duct stones, retained common duct stones not amenable to ERC +/- sphincterotomy, and obstruction secondary to tumor. Three laparoscopic operations have proven feasible: cholecystoenterostomy, choledochoduodenostomy, and choledochoenterostomy. Cholecystoenterostomy requires patency of the cystic duct [65]. All of these procedures have been performed in the laboratory and in patients [66–68].

These procedures require advanced technical skills including laparoscopic suturing and knotting. Therefore, they should only be attempted by surgeons with proficiency in these techniques. In skilled hands, patency rates, morbidity, and mortality compare favorably with open techniques.

AVOIDANCE AND MANAGEMENT OF COMPLICATIONS
Failure to clear the common duct

There are numerous reasons for inability to clear the common duct of its obstruction. These include intense inflammation in the porta hepatis, obesity, intrahepatic stones, impacted stones, stones distal to a stricture, inadequate equipment, and surgeon inexperience.

The most important of these is surgeon inexperience. While it may be difficult to gain actual laparoscopic common bile duct exploration experience, surgeons who practice routine intraoperative cholangiography are using many of the same maneuvers that are used for transcystic ductal exploration, such as catheter and basket insertion into the ductal system. This should make them somewhat more adept at transcystic LCDE techniques than those who don't practice routine cholangiography. Participation in a laparoscopic common bile duct exploration course or a laparoscopic fellowship are indispensable in providing the training needed to perform successful LCDE.

Completion cholangiography is essential to document the status of the ductal system after LCDE. Intraluminal opacities or failure of contrast to pass into the duodenum is usually indicative of retained intraductal material.

The surgeon should make his or her best effort to remove the stones from the duct by using the maneuvers described above. If these are unsuccessful, then the surgeon must decide whether to convert to open common bile duct exploration or resort to postoperative endoscopic retrograde techniques for stone removal. It should be noted, however, as shown by Traverso [69], that the latter is significantly more expensive than LCDE. Therefore, it behooves the laparoscopic biliary surgeon to become proficient in LCDE techniques.

Bile leak

Bile leak may emanate from the gallbladder bed, the cystic duct orifice used for LCDE, the cystic duct–common duct junction, or the common duct itself. This may be the result of dissection and manipulation of these structures during LCDE.

Good visualization and gentle tissue handling techniques may help reduce the incidence of this problem. Additionally, the cystic duct must be secured adequately. This may require suture ligation in cases where the cystic duct is large, thickened, or short, significant distal common duct manipulation was used, or where recent pancreatitis may cause temporary distal ductal hypertension. Suture ligation of the cystic duct stump should be considered in cases where the surgeon suspects that postoperative ERCP may be required.

Postoperative fever, excessive bilious drain output, ileus, and elevated liver function studies may indicate a bile leak. A radionuclide scan may confirm the presence of a leak, and the possibility of a distal obstruction in the common bile duct. Sonography or CT scanning of the abdomen may help localize a bile collection if there is one.

If a drain is already in place, and if there is no evidence of distal obstruction of the common bile duct, observation, intravenous fluids, and antibiotic coverage may be all that is necessary. If no drain is in place, and if a bile collection is localized, then radiographically directed placement of a drain may be adequate to allow a period of observation. The surgeon should not wait an excessively long time to intervene if there is no indication that the leak will seal itself or if generalized peritonitis is present.

Abscess

Patients requiring LCDE are often older, with more intense gallbladder inflammation than those requiring laparoscopic cholecystectomy. Hence, they may be more prone to the development of postoperative infectious problems at the surgical site. Prophylactic antibiotics are essential here, and when acute or gangrenous cholecystitis or cholangitis is documented, therapeutic antibiotic coverage should be continued into the postoperative period.

The perihepatic space should also be thoroughly freed of debris and stones prior to completion of the case. In patients in whom there is severe inflammation or there has been spillage of bile or stones, placement of a closed system suction drain may be prudent.

Postoperative fever, tachycardia, ileus, and abdominal pain usually signal the presence of a problem at the surgical site. Sonography or CT scanning may confirm the presence of an abscess. Intravenous antibiotics are usually necessary here. Radiographically directed percutaneous drain placement may be the first interventional step in management. If this is not successful in reducing or eliminating the above symptoms, surgical intervention is warranted.

Common duct injury

Improper identification of the anatomy during dissection may lead to injury to the duct. This may be more likely in cases where there is intense inflammation in the porta hepatis. During the ductal exploration, aggressive manipulation of instruments or the duct may lead to ductal injury. A thorough knowledge of the anatomy, as seen laparoscopically, is essential. Intraoperative cholangiography via the cystic duct or the gallbladder if necessary may provide clues as to the location of the duct.

Introduction of instruments into the common bile duct must be done gently. This is especially true when using baskets in the ductal system because they may puncture the duct more easily than larger more blunt instruments. Similarly, application of electrohydraulic lithotripsy to stones in the duct must done accurately and under direct vision in order to avoid injury to the duct wall.

The best time to recognize this injury is at the time of surgery, when it can be either repaired primarily or bypassed if necessary. Unfortunately, most injuries are not recognized at this time but present themselves later with fever, tachycardia, abdominal pain, ileus, and jaundice. At that point, after stabilization of the patient, referral to a center specializing in reconstructive biliary tract surgery is the best option.

Pancreatitis

Pancreatitis may be caused preoperatively by the stones themselves. Intraoperatively it may be caused by manipulation of the distal duct. Baskets, balloons, or the scope may cause such injury. Gentle techniques are the rule here in order to minimize the occurrence of this problem.

Some authors have advocated high-pressure balloon dilatation of the sphincter of Oddi. While this technique may occasionally be successful, it commonly causes hyperamylasemia or frank pancreatitis. It is therefore not widely recommended.

Passage of the choledochoscope into the duodenum is also a potentially hazardous practice and should only be used when necessary to gently push debris into the duodenum, or when the orifice into the duodenum is widely patent, such as after preoperative sphincterotomy or intraoperative intravenous glucagon administration.

Pancreatitis may present postoperatively with excessive abdominal or back pain, fever, ileus, anorexia, or failure to thrive. The diagnosis may be confirmed with amylase measurement. CT scanning of the abdomen may be necessary if the patient does not improve with intravenous fluids, NPO (nothing by mouth) status, and nasogastric suction. Antibiotics may be required if pancreatic abscess is suspected or confirmed with CT scanning.

RESULTS

Thousands of successful laparoscopic common bile duct explorations have been reported since the introduction of laparoscopic cholecystectomy in the late 1980s. During this time techniques have evolved that enhance the likelihood of success of the procedure. In experienced hands successful ductal clearance rates exceed 90% [8–10,15,22,30,32,35–37,70–77]. Morbidity rates have been low in these series. Mortality has occurred in less than 1% of patients. An overview of the result of some larger series in shown in Table 2-2.

Access route

Most laparoscopists have generally preferred the transcystic route for ductal exploration when it is feasible. In most series it is successful in 80% to 90% of cases [22,73,74]. In some authors' experience, eg, Franklin and coworkers [77], the type and size of the ductal stones dictates the need for a transductal approach in approximately 90% of cases. As discussed above, there are well-defined criteria that should lead a surgeon to one or the other approach.

Operative times

Laparoscopic choledocholithotomy takes longer than straight-forward laparoscopic cholecystectomy. The mean operative times for some of the larger series are: DePaula, 110 minutes; Petelin, 120 minutes; and Phillips, 136 minutes (Personal communication). Not all reported series in the literature listed operative times. Assuming that mean operative time for laparoscopic cholecystectomy in less than 1 hour, it appears that LCDE adds approximately 1 hour or more to the procedure time. Interestingly, this added time is not solely due to technical manipulations, but includes equipment set-up time and often the need to perform additional surgery. It is also noted that these patients are often older, with more chronic changes in the tissues in the porta hepatis, making dissection more difficult [22,73,74].

Length of stay

Whereas the length of stay for laparoscopic cholecystectomy is generally less than 24 hours, the length of stay for patients undergoing LCDE ranges from 1.3 to 7 days, depending on the access route, whether or not a T-tube was placed, and whether or not a biliary enteric anastomosis was created. For transcystic LCDE, the mean length of stay is 1.5 days in reports of larger series.

Complications

Morbidity associated with LCDE occurs in approximately 8% to 10% of patients, and includes those problems typically asso-ciated with general surgery and laparoscopy: nausea, diarrhea, ileus, ecchymosis, atelectasis, fever, phlebitis, urinary retention, urinary tract infection, wound infection or inflammation, biliary leak, dislodged T-tube, subhepatic fluid collection, pulmonary embolus, and myocardial infarction. It is generally believed that the incidence of complications is less with a laparoscopic approach than an open approach to common bile duct stones.

Mortality associated with LCDE is 0% to 1% in the hands of experienced laparoscopic biliary tract surgeons. This incidence is similar to that found in open surgery and relates more to the general health status of these patients than to laparoscopic common bile duct exploration.

The author's experience

From September 21, 1989 through February 20, 1997, 2255 patients presented to me with symptomatic biliary tract disease. Laparoscopic cholecystectomy was attempted in 2229 of them (99%), and completed in 2215 (99%). Open cholecystectomy was performed in 26 patients for the following reasons: hospital or insurance company mandate (five patients), presence of common bile duct stones (four patients), concomitant surgery (eight patients), obesity (two patients), and severity of illness/general condition (seven patients).

Intraoperative cholangiograms were performed in 2108 patients (95%). Abnormalities were found in 236 (13%) of these cholangiograms. This represents 11% of the entire group of 2229 patients. Abnormal cholangiograms were managed primarily with LCDE in 211 (89%) of patients, postoperative ERC in 19 (8%) of patients, and conversion to open CDE in six (3%) of patients.

Thirty-six patients (1.6%) underwent preoperative ERCP, and 28 patients (1.3%) underwent postoperative ERCP.

Table 2-2

Results of laparoscopic common bile duct exploration

Study and year*	Total LCDE cases, n	Transcystic route, n(%)	Choledochotomy route, n(%)	Total successful clearance, n(%)	Mortality, n(%)
Petelin [8], 1991	22	20(91)	1(5)	19(86.36)	0(0)
Shapiro et al. [70], 1991	16	15(94)	1(6)	16(100)	0(0)
Hunter [9], 1992	20	20(100)	0(0)	17(85)	0(0)
Petelin [22], 1993	77	75(97)	2(3)	74(96.1)	1(1.3)
Fielding and O'Rourke [71], 1993	21	20(95)	1(5)	17(80.95)	0(0)
Fletcher [72], 1993	12	12(100)	0(0)	8(66.67)	0(0)
DePaula et al. [73], 1994	119	107(90)	12(10)	108(90.76)	1(0.84)
Phillips et al. [74], 1994	120	111(93)	9(8)	112(93.33)	1(0.83)
Dion et al. [75], 1994	59	18(31)	41(69)	52(88.14)	0(0)
Ferzli et al. [76], 1994	24	13(54)	11(46)	24(100)	0(0)
Franklin et al. [77], 1994	113	2(1.8)	111(98)	112(99.12)	1(0.88)
Petelin [32], 1996	197	173(88)	24(12)	189(95.94)	1(0.51)

*Some authors listed more than once to show series evolution over time.

Laparoscopic common bile duct exploration (LCDE) was attempted in 218 patients, and completed successfully in 210 patients (96%).

Mean operating time for all patients undergoing laparoscopic cholecystectomy with or without cholangiograms or LCDE was 68 minutes (range, 17 to 421), and mean length of stay was 23.6 hours (range, 1 to 622). Mean operating time for patients not undergoing LCDE was 61 minutes (range, 17 to 410), and mean length of stay was 21 hours (range, 1 to 622).

Ductal exploration was performed via the cystic duct in 186 patients (85%), and through a choledochotomy in 32 patients (15%). T-tubes were used in patients in whom there was concern for possible retained debris or stones, distal spasm, pancreatitis, or general poor tissue quality secondary to malnutrition or infection.

In patients where choledochotomy was used, placement of a T-tube occurred in 21 (66%), and primary closure without a T-tube occurred in 11 (34%). Mean operative times for patients undergoing transcystic duct exploration was 118 minutes (range, 32 to 345). Mean length of stay for patients undergoing transcystic ductal exploration was 41 hours (range, 1.5 to 540). Mean operative time for patients undergoing choledochotomy without T-tube drainage was 187 minutes (range, 104 to 355), and mean length of stay was 57 hours (range, 19 to 216). Mean operative time for patients undergoing choledochotomy with T-tube placement was 177 minutes (range, 74 to 395), and mean length of stay was 88 hours (range, 16 to 288).

In the group of patients in whom T-tubes were placed, two patients had a known retained stone and one had an undetected retained stone. In one of the patients with a known retained stone the ductal exploration was terminated because of septic complications and instability in the operating room. In both of these patients, and in the third patient, the retained stones were later removed by ERC +/- S. There were no complications in the group of patients who underwent choledochotomy and primary ductal closure without T-tube placement. There were no bile leaks, no retained stones, no sepsis, and no subsequent operations.

CONCLUSIONS

During the past 8 years a comprehensive laparoscopic solution to the problem of common bile duct stones has been developed. The success rate among accomplished laparoscopists should approach 90% or better. This compares favorably with treatment expectations in the prelaparoscopic era. Nevertheless, it is unlikely that a surgeon who has had little or no formal training in advanced laparoscopic biliary tract surgery will successfully and safely complete laparoscopic common bile exploration routinely. If a surgeon has not had enough training, or if his performance does not meet the standards listed above, he should consider other options for the patient, and should set a plan for becoming more proficient.

Biliary tract surgeons practicing in this era should have the ability to treat all benign biliary tract pathology laparoscopically in one setting, not requiring a series of patient manipulations.

REFERENCES AND RECOMMENDED READING

Recently published papers of particular interest have been highlighted as:

* • Of interest
* •• Of outstanding interest

1. Nahrwold D: The biliary system. In *Textbook of Surgery*, edn 14. Edited by Sabiston X. Philadelphia: WB Saunders; 1991:1042–1075.

2. Way LW, Admirand WJ, Dunphy JE: Management of choledocholithiasis. *Ann Surg* 1972, 176:347–359.

3. Beal J: Historical perspective of gallstone disease. *Surg Gynecol Obstet* 1984, 158:181–189.

4 Escat J, Fourtanier G, Maigne C, *et al.*: Choledochoscopy in common bile duct surgery for choledocholithiasis: a must. *Am Surg* 1985: 51(3):166–167.

5.•• Fink AS: Current dilemmas in management of common duct stones. *Surg Endosc* 1993, 7:285–291.
An excellent review of the past and current status of the treatment of common duct calculi, including references to open CDE, LCDE, and ERC +/- S.

6. Pappas TN, Slimane TB, Brooks DC: 100 Consecutive common duct explorations without mortality. *Ann Surg* 1990, 211:260–262.

7. Fink AS: To ERCP or not to ERCP? That is the question. *Surg Endosc* 1993, 7:375–376.

8 Petelin J: Laparoscopic approach to common duct pathology. *Surg Laparosc Endosc* 1991, 1:33–41.

9. Hunter J: Laparoscopic transcystic common bile duct exploration. *Am J Surg* 1992, 163:53–58.

10. Carroll BJ, Phillips EH, Daykhovsky L, *et al.*: Laparoscopic choledochoscopy: an effective approach to the common duct. *J Laparoendosc Surg* 1992, 2:15–21.

11. Sackier JM, Berci G, Pas-Partlow M: Laparoscopic transcystic choledochotomy as an adjunct to laparoscopic cholecystectomy. *Am Surg* 1991, 57:323–326.

12. Jacobs M, VCerdeja JC, Goldstein HS. Laparoscopic choledocholithotomy. *J Laparoendosc Surg* 1991, 1:79–82.

13. Quattlebaum JK, Flanders HD: Laparoscopic treatment of common bile duct stones. *Surg Laparosc Endosc* 1991, 1:26–32.

14. Appel S, Krebs H, Fern D: Techniques for laparoscopic cholangiography and removal of common duct stones. *Surg Endosc* 1992, 6:134–137.

15. Birkett D: Technique of cholangiography and cystic-duct choledochoscopy at the time of laparoscopic cholecystectomy for laser lithotripsy. *Surg Endosc* 1992, 6:252–254.

16. Fletcher D, Jones RM, O'Riordan B, Hardy KJ: Laparoscopic cholecystectomy for complicated gallstone disease. *Surg Endosc* 1992, 6:179–182.

17. Dion YM, Morin J, Dionne G, Dejoie C: Laparoscopic cholecystectomy and choledocholithiasis. *Can J Surg* 1992, 35:67–74.

18.•• Arregui M, Davis CJ, Arkush AM, Nagan RF: Laparoscopic cholecystectomy combined with endoscopic sphincterotomy and stone extraction or laparoscopic choledochoscopy and electrohydraulic lithotripsy for management of cholelithiasis with choledocholithiasis. *Surg Endosc* 1992, 6:10–15.
An excellent overview of the evolving relationship of ERCP, laparoscopic cholecystectomy, and common duct exploration. The authors review the literature regarding ERCP and laparoscopic common duct exploration, present their results, and anticipate their movement away from ERCP as laparoscopic common duct exploration techniques improve.

19. Cotton PB: Endoscopic management of bile duct stones (apples and oranges). *Gut* 1984, 25:587–597.

20. Carr-Locke DL: Acute gallstone pancreatitis and endoscopic therapy. *Endoscopy* 1990, 22:180–183.

21. Vitale GC, Larson GM, Wieman TJ, *et al.*: The use of ERCP in the management of common bile duct stones in patients undergoing laparoscopic cholecystectomy. *Surg Endosc* 1993, 7:9–11.

22. Petelin J: Laparoscopic approach to common duct pathology. *Am J Surg* 1993, 165:487–491.

23. Franklin ME, Pharand D: Laparoscopic common bile duct exploration. *Surg Laparosc Endosc* 1994, 4(2):119–124.

24. Phillips E, Carroll BJ, Pearlstein R, *et al.*: Laparoscopic choledochoscopy and extraction of common bile duct stones. *World J Surg* 1993, 17:22–28.

25. Petelin J: Clinical results of common bile duct exploration. *Endosc Surg Allied Technol* 1993, 1:125–129.

26. O'Doherty D, Neoptolemos J, Carr-Locke D: Endoscopic sphincterotomy for retained common bile duct stones in patients with T-tube in situ in the early postoperative period. *Br J Surg* 1986, 73:454–456.

27. Broughman T, Sivak M, Herman R: The management of retained and recurrent bile duct stones. *Surgery* 1985, 98(4):746–751.

28. Petelin J: The argument for contact laser laparoscopic cholecystectomy. *Clin Laser Monthly* 1990, 71–74.

29. Petelin J: Laparoscopic common duct exploration. 16 minute comprehensive video presented at ACS Meeting, October, 1992. *American College of Surgeons Motion Picture Library*, 1992.

30. Kitano S, Iso Y, Moriyama M, Sugimachi K: A rapid and simple technique for insertion of a T-tube into the minimally incised common bile duct at laparoscopic surgery. *Surg Endosc* 1993, 7:104–105.

31. Mooney MJ, Deyo G, O'Reilly MJ: T-tube placement during laparoscopic cholecystectomy. *Surg Endosc* 1992, 6:32.

32. Petelin JB. Laparoscopic ductal stone clearance: transcystic approach. In *Bile Ducts and Bile Duct Stones*. Edited by Berci G, Cuschieri A. Philadelphia: WB Saunders; 1996:97–108.

33. Reddick EJ, Olsen DO, DAniell JF, *et al.*: Laparoscopic laser cholecystectomy. *Laser Med Surg News Adv* 1989, 38–40.

34. Klaiber C, Metzger A, Petelin J: Laparoscopic cholecystectomy. In *Manual of Laparoscopic Surgery*. Verlag Hans Huber Publishers; 1993:97–148.

35. Ferzli GS, Massaad A, Ozuner G, Worth MH: Laparoscopic exploration of the common bile duct. *Surg Gynecol Obstet* 1992, 174:419–421.

36. Stoker ME, Leveillee RJ, McCann JC, Maini BS: Laparoscopic common bile duct exploration. *J Laparoendosc Surg* 1991, 1:287–293.

37.• DePaula AL, Hashiba K, Bafutto M,*et al.*: Laparoscopic treatment of choledocholithiasis. *Surg Laparosc Endosc* 1993, 3:157–160.
In cases where a biliary drainage procedure is indicated, the authors perform antegrade sphincterotomy via the choledochoscope at the time of LCDE while the procedure is monitored with a side-viewing duodenoscope. This technique should avoid the potential problems of pancreatitis that could be induced from cannulation of the pancreatic duct during ERCP.

38.• Gagner M, Deslandres E, Pomp A, *et al.*: Double endoscopy: the role of intraoperative ERCP during laparoscopic cholecystectomy for choledocholithiasis. In *Proceedings of the III International Congress of Laparoscopic Surgery*. Brazil, 1993:126–127.
Simultaneous choledochoscopy and side-viewing duodenoscopy are used to perform ERCP at the time of laparoscopic cholecystectomy in cases where a drainage procedure is indicated. Avoids the need for a second procedure.

39. Shimi S, Banting Fracs S, Cuschieri A: Transcystic drainage after laparoscopic exploration of common bile duct. *Min Invas Ther* 1992, 1:273–276.

40. Williams JAR, Treacy PJ, Sidey CS, *et al.*: Primary duct closure versus T-tube drainage following exploration of the common bile duct. *Aust NZ J Surg* 1994, 64:823–826.

41. Bernstein DE, Goldberg RI, Unger SW: Common bile duct obstruction following T-tube placement at laparoscopic cholecystectomy. *Gastrointest Endosc* 1994, 40(3):362–365.

42. Elewaut A, de Vos M, Huble F, de Cock J: Unusual migration of a straight Amsterdam-type endoprosthesis for bile duct stones. *Am J Gastroenterol* 1989, 84(6):674–676.

43. Kram HB, Garces MA, Klein SR, Shoemaker WC: Common bile duct anastomosis using fibrin glue. *Arch Surg* 1985, 120:1250–1256.

44. Lange V, Rau HG, Schardey HM, Meyer G: Laparoscopic stenting for protection of common bile duct sutures. *Surg Laparosc Endosc* 1993, 3(6):466–469.

45. Kelly TR, Fink JA: A new inflatable T-tube for completion cholangiography. *Surg Gynecol Obstet* 1983, 157(4):374–376.

46. Jacob ET, Bronsther B: A double ballooned inflatable and collapsible T-tube for selective proximal or distal cholangiography. *Surg Gynecol Obstet* 1988, 166:85–86.

47. Fine AP: Laparoscopic, wire-guided insertion of biliary T-tubes. *Surg Laparosc Endosc* 1993, 3(2):147–148.

48. Kitano S, Iso Y, Moriyama M, Sugimachi K: A rapid and simple technique for insertion of a T-tube into the minimally incised common bile duct at laparoscopic surgery. *Surg Endosc* 1993, 7:104–105.

49. Lezoche E, Paganini AM, Guerrieri M: A new T-tube applier in laparoscopic surgery. *Surg Endosc* 1996, 10:445–448.

50. Lygidakis NJ: Choledochotomy for biliary lithiasis: T-tube drainage or primary closure-effects on postoperative bacteremia and T-tube bile infection. *Am J Surg* 1983, 146:254–256.

51. Lygidakis NJ: Operative risk factors of cholecystectomy-choledochotomy in the elderly. *Surg Gynecol Obstet* 1983, 157:15–19.

52. Lygidakis NJ: Incidence of bile infection in biliary lithiasis. Effects on postoperative bacteremia of choledochoduodenostomy, T-tube drainage, and primary closure of the common bile duct after choledochotomy–a prospective trial. *Am Surg* 1984, 50:236–240.

53. Koivusalo A, Makisalo H, Talja A, *et al.*: Bacterial adherence and biofilm formation on latex and silicone T-tubes in relation to bacterial contamination of bile. *Scand J Gastroenterol*, 1996, 398–403.

54. Horgan PG, Campbell AC, Gray GR, Gillespie G: Biliary leakage and peritonitis following removal of T tubes after bile duct exploration. *Br J Surg* 1989, 76:1296–1297.

55. Galan CP, Alonso AC: Bile leakage after removal of T tubes from the common bile duct. *Br J Surg* 1990, 77:1075.

56. Ryttov N, Rasmussen L, Pedersen SA, Oster-Jorgensen E: 99m Tc-labelled HIDA scintigraphy in assessment of bile leakage after removal of T tube from the common bile duct. *Br J Surg* 1989, 76:1319.

57. Thors H, Gudjonsson H, Oddsson E, Cariglia N: Endoscopic retrieval of a biliary T-tube remnant. *Gastrointest Endosc* 1994, 40:241242.

58. Gillatt DA, May RE, Kenedy R, Longstaff AJ: Complications of T-tube drainage of the common bile duct. *Ann R Coll Surg Engl* 1985, 67:369–371.

59. Norrby S, Heuman R, Anderberg B, Sjodahl R: Duration of T-tube drainage after exploration of the common bile duct. *Acta Chir Scand* 1988, 154:113–115.

60. Cohen Z, Rosenman H, *et al.*: Transient elevation of serum alkaline phosphatase after choledochotomy and T-tube placement. *J Clin Gastroenterol* 1986, 8(4):495–496.

61. Lygidakis NJ: Hazards following T-tube removal after choledochotomy. *Surg Gynecol Obstet* 1993, 163:153–155.

62. Thors H, Gudjonsson H, Oddsson E, Cariglia N: Endoscopic retrieval of a biliary T-tube remnant. *Gastrointest Endosc* 1994, 40:241–242.

63. Payne RA, Woods WGA: Primary suture or T-tube drainage after choledochotomy. *Ann R Coll Surg Engl* 1986, 68:196–198.

64. Shyr-Ming sheen C, Fong-Fu C: Choledochotomy for biliary lithiasis: Is routine T-tube drainage necessary? A prospective controlled trial. *Acta Chir Scand* 1990, 156:387–390.

65. Petelin JB, Lechleitner RA: Laparoscopic choledochotomy without T-tube drainage is effective and safe [abstract and poster]. *SAGES Annual Scientific Session*, 1997.

66. Tarnasky PR, England RE, Lail LM, *et al.*: Cystic duct patency in malignant obstructive jaundice. An ERCP-based study relevant to the role of laparoscopic cholecystojejunostomy. *Ann Surg* 1995, 221:265–271.

67. Schob OM, Schmid RA, Morimoto AK, *et al.* Laparoscopic Roux-en-Y choledochojejunostomy. *Am J Surg* 1997, 173:312–329.

68. Farello GA, Cerofolini A, Bergamaschi G, *et al.*: Choledochoduodenal anastomosis by laparoscopy. *J Chir Paris* 1993, 130:226–230.

69. Traverso LW: A cost-effective approach to the treatment of common bile duct stones with surgical versus endoscopic techniques. In *Bile Ducts and Bile Duct Stones*. Edited by Berci G, Cuschieri A. Philadelphia: WB Saunders; 1996:154–160.

70. Shapiro SJ, Gordon LA, Daykhovsky L, *et al.*: Laparoscopic exploration of the common bile duct: experience in 16 selected patients. *J Laparoendosc Surg* 1991, 6:333–341.

71. Fielding GA, O'Rourke NA: Laparoscopic common bile duct exploration. *Aust NZ J Surg* 1993, 63:113–115.

72. Fletcher DR: Common bile duct calculi at laparoscopic cholecystectomy: a technique for management. *Aust NZ J Surg* 1993, 63:710–714.

73. DePaula AL, Hashiba K, Bafutto M: Laparoscopic management of choledocholithiasis. *Surg Endosc* 1994, 8:1399–1403.

74. Phillips EH, Rosenthal RJ, Carroll BJ, *et al.* Laparoscopic transcystic duct common bile duct exploration. *Surg Endosc* 1994, 8:1389–1394.

75. Dion YM, Ratelle R, Morin J, *et al.* Common bile duct exploration: the place of laparosocpic choledochotomy. *Surg Laparosc Endosc* 1994, 6:419–424.

76. Ferzli GS, Massaad A, Kiel T, *et al.* The utility of laparoscopic common bile duct exploration in the treatment of choledocholithiasis. *Surg Endosc* 1994, 8:296–298.

77. Franklin ME, Pharand D, Rosenthal D: Laparoscopic common bile duct exploration. *Surg Laparosc Endosc* 1994, 2:119–124.

Anesthetic Considerations for Minimally Invasive Surgery

K. Bhavani-Shankar
Richard A. Steinbrook

CHAPTER 3

During the past decade, the scope of minimally invasive surgery has expanded from gynecologic surgery to include a variety of general as well as thoracic surgical procedures. This expansion has occurred principally because endoscopic surgery is less invasive than conventional open surgery (allowing for earlier recovery), there is less postoperative pain, and hospital stays and costs are minimized [1,2,3••,4,5•,6]. Minimally invasive surgery includes laparoscopic as well as mediastinal and thoracoscopic surgical procedures. Laparoscopic surgery involves intraoperative intraperitoneal gaseous insufflation of CO_2, often in reverse Trendelenburg position. Laparoscopic surgery is being performed with increasing frequency in elderly patients, patients with respiratory and cardiac diseases (American Society of Anesthesiologists [ASA] classes III and IV), in pregnant women, and in infants and children. Hemodynamic and respiratory alterations as a result of intraperitoneal CO_2 insufflation may be potentially deleterious in these patients. Therefore, to provide anesthesia safely it has become increasingly important to understand the physiologic consequences of intraperitoneal CO_2 insufflation in pregnant women, elderly patients with coexisting diseases, and infants and children [3••,7•,8••,9–11,12••,13–15,16••,17,18]. Further, a majority of patients undergoing endoscopic surgery are discharged on the same day, which mandates adequate control of postoperative pain and minimal postoperative nausea and vomiting (PONV). Hence, an understanding of the factors responsible for PONV and pain following laparoscopic surgery is also necessary.

In this chapter, we first consider the physiologic consequences of CO_2 insufflation in healthy adults and summarize anesthetic management for laparoscopic surgery. We then focus on the differences in physiologic responses to pneumoperitoneum in patients with cardiac or pulmonary disease, in pregnant women, and in infants and children—differences that influence anesthetic management. Finally, we include a brief review of anesthetic considerations for mediastinoscopy and thoracoscopy.

PHYSIOLOGIC CONSEQUENCES OF CO_2 PNEUMOPERITONEUM IN HEALTHY SUBJECTS
Cardiovascular system
Cardiovascular changes during laparoscopic surgery result from anesthetic agents, positive pressure ventilation, positional changes of the patient, and mechanical and neuroendocrine effects of the pneumoperitoneum and those of absorbed CO_2 (Table 3-1) (Fig. 3-1). Induction of anesthesia and positioning in reverse Trendelenburg (rT) prior to insufflation result in a 35% to 40% reduction in cardiac index (CI) and filling pressures of the heart (pulmonary artery occlusion pressure [PAOP]) and

Table 3-1

Physiologic consequences of carbon dioxide pneumoperitoneum

Cardiovascular	
Cardiac output	↓ 50%
Mean blood pressure	↑
Systemic vascular resistance	↑
Central venous pressure	↑
Pulmonary artery occlusive pressure	↑
Left ventricular wall stress	↑
Left ventricular systolic area	No change
Left ventricular diastolic area	No change
Respiratory	
Compliance	↓ 40%
Functional residual capacity	↓
Plateau pressure	↑ 40%–70%
PaO_2	Stable
CO_2 Delivery to lungs	↑ 30%
$PaCO_2$ (with hyperventilation)	Normal or ↑
$PaCO_2$–end-tidal PCO_2 gradient	Unchanged (3–5 mm Hg)
Gastrointestinal	
Postoperative emesis	↑ 42%–61%

central venous pressure [CVP]) [8••,19]. A further reduction in CI to 50% occurs during the initial phase of CO_2 insufflation in rT as a result of increased intra-abdominal pressure [19]. Increased abdominal pressure produces an initial transient increase in venous return due to compression of the abdominal capacitance vessels. This is followed by a decrease in the venous return from the lower limbs as a result of an impedance to the venous flow in the abdomen (biphasic effect on venous return) resulting in a reduction in the CI [20,21]. The increased abdominal pressure also compresses the arterial tree, increasing systemic vascular resistance (SVR) and mean arterial blood pressure (MAP) [8••,19–21]. Increases in MAP are associated with an increase in left ventricular wall stress [22]. Further, the increased abdominal pressure is also partially transmitted to the cardiac chambers, causing an increase in cardiac filling pressures (PAOP, CVP), which were markedly reduced by the induction of anesthesia and by positioning in rT [8••,10,19]. The increase in filling pressures, however, is not associated with increases in left ventricular systolic and diastolic areas (LVESA or LVEDA) as measured by transesophageal echocardiography (TEE) [22]. The reduction in CI following CO_2 insufflation may be avoided by performing CO_2 insufflation in the supine position, when no changes in ejection fraction, heart rate, LVEDA, and LVESA occur [22]. However, subsequent positioning in rT following insufflation resulted in reduced LVEDA and probably CI as well [22]. Further investigations are required to confirm these findings [8••,22].

A gradual restoration of CI and a partial restoration of SVR begins 10 to 15 minutes after the induction of pneumoperitoneum [8••,10,19]. Neurohumeral responses to laparoscopic cholecystectomy (increases in vasopressin, dopamine, cortisol, adrenaline, noradrenaline, and renin) and the effects of absorbed CO_2 (catecholamine response initiated by hypercarbia) play an important role in the restoration of CI and in minimizing the adverse hemodynamic effects of increased intra-abdominal pressure [8••,23,24]. Direct vasodilatory effects of CO_2 also decrease SVR. Thus, the net effects of pneumoperitoneum and hypercarbia during laparoscopy usually include increases in SVR, MAP, left ventricular wall stress, CVP and PAOP, and decreases in CI.

Lung function and gas exchange

Laparoscopic surgery affects functional residual capacity (FRC), compliance, oxygenation, and CO_2 homeostasis. Induction of anesthesia reduces FRC and compliance by about 20% [25]. CO_2 Insufflation further reduces FRC and compliance. Plateau pressure increases 40% to 70% [19,26] during insufflation, corresponding to a 30% to 50% reduction in compliance [26,27]. Sudden changes in plateau pressure are indicative of serious complications, such as pneumothorax, during surgery [28].

In healthy patients, PaO_2 is stable despite changes in compliance and cardiac output, as discussed previously [19]. Oxygen delivery, however, declines due to the decrease in CI, resulting in lactic acidosis [29]. CO_2 Homeostasis is a major concern during laparoscopy [8••]. Hypercarbia occurs as result of CO_2 absorption and inadequate gas exchange consequent to low compliance. The delivery of CO_2 to the lungs can increase by 30% during the first 30 minutes [30]. Appropriate increases in minute volume in healthy patients (12% to 16%) maintains $PaCO_2$ within acceptable limits [17,19]. The normal gradient of 3 to 5 mm Hg between $PaCO_2$ and end-tidal PCO_2 ($PETCO_2$) remains unchanged even during CO_2 insufflation [17]. Further, prolonged insufflation does not significantly affect the reliability of $PETCO_2$ monitoring in predicting $PaCO_2$ in healthy ASA I and II subjects [17,31,32].

ANESTHETIC MANAGEMENT
Healthy adults

Although epidural anesthesia has been used for laparoscopic tubal ligations [33], endotracheal general anesthesia is the technique most commonly used in laparoscopic procedures. Laparoscopic surgeries are usually short procedures performed on day-surgery patients. Therefore, a technique that allows rapid emergence is preferred (Table 3-2). Propofol induction, short-acting narcotics, benzodiazepines, muscle relaxants, and inhalation agents with low blood–gas solubility serves this purpose well. Stomach decompression by an oral-gastric tube is recommended to protect the stomach from instrument injury and also to improve the surgical field.

As patients may be discharged home on the day of surgery, prevention of nausea and vomiting and adequate pain control play a major role in the postoperative period. PONV prolongs recovery time, delays patient discharge, and increases hospital

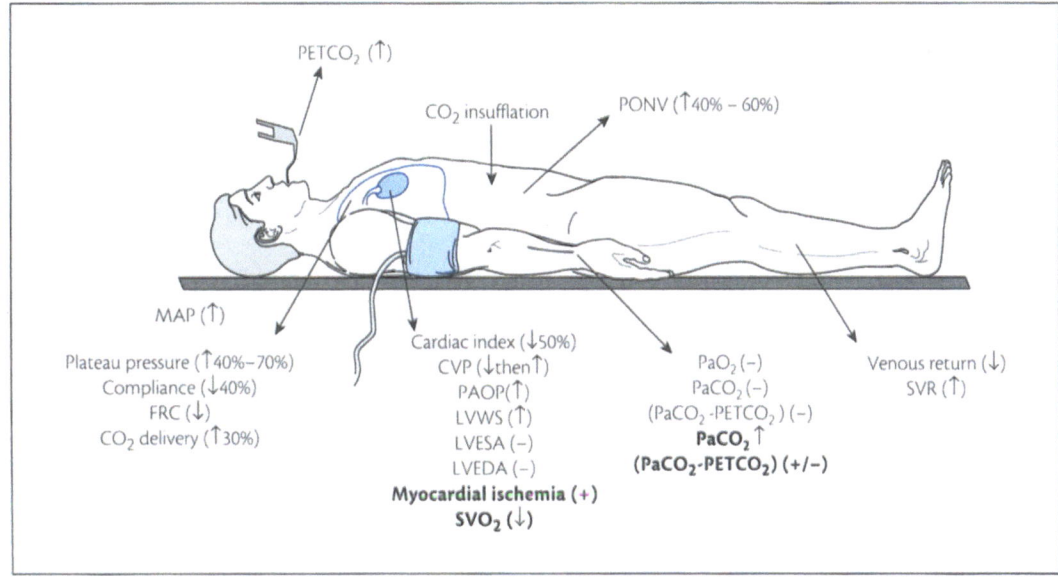

Figure 3-1 Physiologic changes during pneumoperitoneum in healthy subjects. Additional changes that may occur in American Society of Anesthesiologists class III/IV subjects are shown in **bold**. CVP—central venous pressure; FRC—functional residual capacity; LVEDA—left ventricular end-diastolic area; LVESA—left ventricular end-systolic area; LVWS—left ventricular wall stress; MAP—mean arterial pressure; PAOP—pulmonary artery occlusion pressure; PETCO$_2$—end-tidal PCO$_2$; PONV—postoperative nausea and vomiting; SVO$_2$—mixed venous oxygen saturation; SVR—systemic vascular resistance.

costs. Inadequate relief of postoperative pain from tissue trauma at the operating site, as well as shoulder pain induced by irritation of the diaphragm by residual subdiaphragmatic CO$_2$, may result in considerable postoperative discomfort and thus delay patient discharge.

The highest incidence of postoperative emesis (up to 61%) was reported in women undergoing laparoscopic surgery [34–36]. In addition, there are several predisposing factors to PONV, such as age (occurs more often in younger than older patients, with peak incidence between the ages of 11 and 14 years); gender (three times as common in female patients); obesity (positive correlation between body weight and postoperative emesis); history of motion sickness; previous PONV; high level of preoperative anxiety; gastroparesis; preanesthetic narcotic premedication; gastric distention from vigorous positive pressure ventilation; use of nitrous oxide, ketamine, etomidate, neostigmine; as well as duration of surgery [34,37,38••]. Every effort should be made to manipulate factors under the control of the anesthesiologist that influence postoperative emesis.

Because laparoscopic surgery is associated with a 42% increase of PONV, we often use antiemetic prophylaxis [37]. Four major neurotransmitter systems (dopaminergic, histaminic [H$_1$], cholinergic muscarinic, and 5-hydroxytryptamine$_3$ [5-HT$_3$]) appear to play important roles in mediating the emetic response [34,39]. Several antiemetic medications active at these receptors, used either alone or in combination, have been used to reduce PONV following laparoscopy. We have found that droperidol, 0.625 mg intravenously (IV), in combination with metoclopramide, 10 mg IV, is more effective in preventing postoperative nausea than ondansetron, 4 mg IV, in patients undergoing laparoscopic cholecystectomy, with no differences in time to discharge [40].

Table 3-2

Anesthetic management for laparoscopic surgery in healthy adults

Premedication: midazolam, 1–2 mg IV; fentanyl, 50–100 µg IV

Induction: propofol, 150–200 mg IV

Monitoring: continuous ECG, capnography, pulse oximetry, inspired oxygen, intermittent noninvasive blood pressure

Ventilatory adjustments: to keep end-tidal PCO$_2$ between 32 and 40 mm Hg

Maintenance: isoflurane or desflurane in oxygen/air, additional fentanyl as needed

Neuromuscular blockade: pancuronium, cisatracurium, or vecuronium

Orogastric tube: following induction

Local infiltration: bupivacaine, 0.25% infiltration at the operative sites

Insufflation pressures: no more than 12–15 mm Hg

Antiemetics: metoclopramide, 10 mg and/or droperidol, 0.625 mg, IV, during anesthesia

Supplementary analgesics: ketorolac 30 mg IV before the completion of surgery

End of anesthesia: antagonize neuromuscular block with glycopyrrolate, 0.5–1 mg IV, neostigmine, 2.5–5 mg IV

Postoperative analgesia: fentanyl and ketorolac supplements, if needed

Postoperative antiemetics: ephedrine, 50 mg intramuscular or ondansetron, 4 mg IV, if needed

ECG—electrocardiogram; IV—intravenous.

The effect of nitrous oxide on PONV following laparoscopic surgery is controversial. Havorka and coworkers [36] did not find increased incidence of PONV following nitrous oxide use during laparoscopic surgery. Conversely, studies showed the incidence of nausea and vomiting to be lower in patients who received no nitrous oxide than in patients who received nitrous oxide for general anesthesia for laparoscopic surgery [35,41]. The proposed mechanisms of nausea and vomiting following nitrous oxide includes central effects on opioid receptors, sympathetic nervous system stimulation, and subsequent catecholamine release, bowel distention (200% increase in intestinal gas volume following 4 hours of 70% inspired nitrous oxide in oxygen), and increased middle ear pressure [42–44]. Further, the gaseous distention of the bowel by the diffusion of nitrous oxide may be a hindrance for good surgical visibility, particularly during prolonged surgery [44]. Therefore, we avoid nitrous oxide use during general anesthesia.

All opioids, regardless of their route of administration, can produce nausea and vomiting. This effect is partly caused by stimulation of µ-opioid receptors in the area postrema (chemoreceptor trigger zone in the medulla). Opioids also contribute to nausea and vomiting via delayed gastric emptying, sensitization of vestibular-induced emesis, and release of vasopressin. Opioid administration also stimulates serotonin release, although this is not a major pathway [45]. It is essential, however, that pain be adequately controlled because postoperative pain correlates highly with nausea. Anderson and Krohg [46] found that pain occurred alone as a postoperative symptom relatively rarely, affecting only 10% of their patients after abdominal surgery, whereas pain with nausea coexisted in 59% of their subjects. The mechanisms by which pain can induce nausea and vomiting include stimulation of the visceral nociceptors and peripheral and central sensitization of the reflex by a variety of chemical mediators. Because pain also increases central nervous system arousal, patients may be aware of nausea caused by other factors. Substituting injectable nonsteroidal anti-inflammatory drugs for opioids as analgesic agents may avert some of the undesirable features of narcotics, particularly respiratory depression and postoperative emesis, while also providing adequate pain relief [34,47–49]. Intraperitoneal installation of local anesthetic has been proposed as an alternative method for analgesia following laparoscopy. Twenty milliliters of 0.5% lidocaine instilled intraperitoneally provided 5 hours of significant pain reduction compared with a control group without lidocaine; however, potentially toxic levels of local anesthetics were produced in the plasma of those patients receiving the lidocaine [50,51].

Sedation suppresses PONV, whereas rapid awakening may enhance the risk of this complication. Awake patients are more likely to experience nausea, which occurs before the emetogenic anesthetic effects have waned. Movement also plays a role in producing PONV through a variety of mechanisms, such as prolonged recumbence increasing vestibular discharge, or postural hypotension resulting in decreased blood flow to chemoreceptor trigger zones when sitting or standing upright [52].

Etomidate and ketamine are associated with increased incidence of PONV, whereas propofol is associated with a lower incidence of PONV compared with other intravenous agents [53–56]. The rapid recovery characteristics in addition to antiemetic properties of propofol make it a preferred agent for general anesthesia for laparoscopic surgery. Further, propofol can be given postoperatively for its direct antiemetic effect. Using propofol as a sedative at a dose of 10 to 20 mg, Borgeat and coworkers [57] reported reduction of vomiting in 81% of patients versus 35% of placebo-treated control subjects.

Elderly and ASA III and IV patients

Elderly patients frequently have hypertension, stable coronary artery disease, congestive heart failure, or preexisting lung diseases, such as chronic obstructive pulmonary disease (COPD). In patients with mild heart disease or those with clinically severe systemic diseases (ASA III or IV), the pattern of changes in CI, MAP, and SVR is qualitatively very similar to that of healthy patients [8••,10,58,59]. The most striking features are the considerable initial reduction in CI occurring simultaneously with large increases in PAOP, MAP, and SVR followed by a recovery of the CI similar to healthy subjects. Left ventricular stroke work index is also increased, causing an increase in myocardial oxygen demand [9]. During CO_2 insufflation, mixed venous oxygen saturation may increase or decrease. The latter is accompanied by a greater reduction in CI than the former, with a higher MAP and reduced oxygen delivery [59].

Depending on the severity of associated cardiovascular disorders, anesthesia can be induced with etomidate (0.3 mg/kg, with fentanyl 2 to 3 µg/kg). The reduction in CI may be corrected by volume loading.

The deleterious effects of positioning in rT and the creation of pneumoperitoneum are well tolerated in healthy patients, but can lead to serious morbidity and mortality in patients with limited cardiopulmonary reserve [7,8••]. We recommend gradual abdominal insufflation to 10 to 12 mm Hg followed by a limited 10° head-up tilt to ensure cardiovascular stability.

Patients with cardiovascular disease are at risk for myocardial ischemia during laparoscopy due to the increase in myocardial wall tension caused by increased MAP and SVR, especially in the presence of tachycardia. The decrease in CI observed in ASA III and IV patients can result in insufficient tissue oxygen delivery and a reduction in mixed venous oxygen saturation [59]. The clinical management of ASA III and IV cardiac patients should include continuous monitoring of ST segment changes and, possibly, invasive hemodynamic monitoring. TEE , if available, is useful to monitor regional wall motion [22]. Arterial cannulation will give beat-to-beat information on MAP and facilitate arterial blood–gas sampling when required. The PAOP does not accurately reflect ventricular filling volume in these patients during CO_2 insufflation. An increase in PAOP or CVP during constant CO_2 insufflation, however, may be indicative of myocardial ischemia or dysfunction. One has to recognize limitations of PAOP in that several factors, such as changes in depth of anesthesia or pulmonary compliance, may affect PAOP. Under these circumstances, cardiac output may be more informative [8••]. Mixed venous oxygen saturation may be another useful parameter to monitor, as mixed venous desaturation in ASA III and IV patients has been reported [59]. Patients with coronary artery disease maintain satisfactory hemodynamic function with isoflurane and narcotic supplementation, but may require vasoactive or inotropic drugs [60].

Hypercarbia can result in pulmonary vasoconstriction and may worsen preexisting pulmonary hypertension. Intracranial pressure can increase due to an increase (by 50%) in blood flow velocity through middle cerebral artery as a result of increases in $PaCO_2$ [61]. Hyperventilation may not normalize $PaCO_2$ in ASA III and IV patients [62]. Factors that indicate increased risk of hypercarbia with acidosis (pH < 7.35) during laparoscopy are low preoperative values of forced expiratory volume in 1 second (FEV_1) and vital capacity (VC), and high ASA (III or IV) scores [63]. Age alone does not predispose to respiratory acidosis [63].

Concerns regarding hypercarbia during CO_2 insufflation have led to the evaluation of alternative techniques, such as helium insufflation, nitrous oxide insufflation, and gasless endoscopic surgery. Helium gas emboli and combustibility of nitrous oxide, however, limit their safe use. The normal gradient of 3 to 5 mm Hg between $PaCO_2$ and $PETCO_2$ is markedly increased during laparoscopy in ASA III and IV patients [8••,62]. Prolonged intra-abdominal insufflation with CO_2 in anesthetized and mechanically ventilated patients during upper abdominal laparoscopic surgery does not significantly affect the reliability of $PETCO_2$ monitoring in predicting $PaCO_2$ in healthy ASA I and II subjects and elderly patients [17,31,32]; however, in ASA III and IV patients, $PETCO_2$ may not reflect changes in $PaCO_2$ during insufflation due to changes in alveolar dead space consequent to reduced cardiac output, increased ventilation–perfusion mismatching, or both [62,64]. Therefore, direct arterial $PaCO_2$ monitoring is recommended in patients with significant cardiorespiratory diseases. Thus, an arterial line is reasonable to monitor $PaCO_2$ in ASA III and IV patients for three reasons: 1) end-tidal PCO_2 is not a reliable index of $PaCO_2$, 2) the normal gradient of 3 to 5 mm Hg between $PaCO_2$ and $PETCO_2$ is increased, and 3) even with normal $PETCO_2$, achieved by increasing minute volume, $PaCO_2$ may be high as 50 mm Hg.

Impedance of venous return and stasis as a result of increased abdominal pressure may increase the risk of deep venous thrombosis and pulmonary embolism. We recommend the use of compression boots during surgery and early postoperative ambulation to help prevent venous thrombosis.

Pregnant women

Pregnancy is associated with a variety of physiologic changes (Table 3-3) that significantly alter responses to intraperitoneal gaseous insufflation as well as to anesthesia [3••]. Pneumoperitoneum during laparoscopy is associated with an increase in peak airway pressure, a decrease in total lung compliance, and an increase in airway resistance. Head-down tilt, which is occasionally used during this procedure, will increase the intrathoracic pressure even further and can reduce the effective ventilation. This obviously depends on the degree of abdominal insufflation. Decreased FRC and increased oxygen demand will make the parturient more prone to hypoxic episodes. Furthermore, the supine position will decrease the PaO_2 significantly, particularly in the presence of increased abdominal pressure. Hyperventilation, which might be used to keep the $PaCO_2$ normal during insufflation, may reduce uteroplacental perfusion [65]. Any increase in maternal $PaCO_2$ or decrease in PaO_2 will directly affect fetal well-being [66].

The enlarged gravid uterus can cause aortocaval compression while parturients lie in the supine position. This effect will be exaggerated in patients with increased intra-abdominal pressure for any reason. The drop in blood pressure may also be exaggerated with rT tilt, which will reduce the uteroplacental blood flow and thus cause fetal acidosis. Parturients will need higher doses of α- and β-mimetic agents to maintain normal blood pressure. Increased blood volume and decreased colloid oncotic pressure, as well as the presence of an enlarged uterus, can increase the risk of pulmonary complications.

Surgery can be performed with minimal threat to fetal viability during the second trimester or after the 10th week of gestation (Table 3-4) [3••]. To minimize the risk of pulmonary acid aspiration, all pregnant patients should receive an oral nonparticulate antacid (eg, sodium citrate, 30 mL) as well as metoclopramide, 10 mg IV. An H_2-receptor antagonist may be administered orally the night before surgery as well. Routine sedatives are minimized to avoid unnecessary fetal exposure to these drugs. Opioids are considered safe and may be used as needed [67]. Fetal heart rate and uterine activity should be evaluated preoperatively in all patients at 16 weeks or older gestational age. Tocolytic drugs are not administered prophylactically, as they are rarely necessary and are frequently associated with significant side effects. However, they are administered if

Table 3-3

Physiologic changes of pregnancy

Respiratory	
Minute ventilation	↑ 50%
Tidal volume	↑ 40%
Respiratory rate	↑ 15%
$PaCO_2$	↓ 32 mm Hg
$PaCO_2$–end-tidal PCO_2	↓ -1–0.75 mm Hg
Functional residual capacity	↓
Oxygen consumption	↑ 15%–20%
Mixed venous oxygen content	↓
Arteriovenous oxygen difference	↑
Cardiovascular	
Cardiac output	↑ 40%
Heart rate	↑ 10–15 beats
Stroke volume	↑
Systolic blood pressure	No change
Diastolic blood pressure	↓ 1–15 mm Hg
Supine hypotensive syndrome	Present
Gastrointestinal	
Motility	↓
Food absorption	↓
Lower esophageal sphincter tone	↓
Gastric acid secretion	↑

Table 3-4

Anesthetic management of pregnant patients for laparoscopy

Position: left or right uterine displacement

Premedication: oral sodium citrate, 30 mL; metoclopramide, 10 mg intravenous

Induction: rapid sequence; sodium pentathol and succinylcholine

Ventilatory adjustments: to keep end-tidal P_{CO_2} between 32–34 mm Hg

Positioning: gradual changes to reverse Trendelenburg

Fetal heart rate monitoring: ±16 weeks, pre- and immediate postoperative period

Insufflation technique: open trocar technique

Tocolysis: terbutaline, 0.25 mg subcutaneous, if needed

Hypotension: increments of ephedrine, 5–10 mg

Postoperative period: left/right uterine displacement, oxygen supplements, fetal heart rate monitoring

indicated. Terbutaline, 0.25 mg subcutaneously, remains the drug of choice [3••].

Parturients should be maintained in left or right lateral tilt for uterine displacement to minimize the effect of aortocaval compression during surgery, as well as in the postoperative period. Induction of general anesthesia should be rapid sequence (sodium pentathol, 4 mg/kg, and succinylcholine, 1 mg/kg) with cricoid pressure to minimize the risk of pulmonary aspiration. A relatively small endotracheal tube (7 mm) is desirable to minimize the risk of traumatizing edematous upper airway mucosa. An open trocar insertion technique is used for CO_2 insufflation [68]. Peritoneal insufflation pressure should be kept as low as possible, not only to minimize compression of the inferior vena cava, but also to minimize cephalad displacement of the diaphragm. Further, all positional changes should be gradual to minimize the adverse effects of positional changes on the cardiac output. Minute ventilation should be increased during peritoneal CO_2 insufflation to maintain PET_{CO_2} around 32 mm Hg [3••]. There are no published studies of the relationship between PET_{CO_2} and $PaCO_2$ in pregnant subjects. Studies in pregnant ewes have suggested that PET_{CO_2} is not an adequate guide to predict $PaCO_2$ during laparoscopic surgery in parturients [66,69]. However, caution is necessary regarding the use of capnographic data from gravid ewes to draw inferences about parturients [70•]. During general anesthesia, for example, the preinsufflation arterial to end-tidal P_{CO_2} ($PaCO_2$–PET_{CO_2}) in pregnant ewes ranges from 6 to 15 mm Hg [66,69], whereas the gradient in pregnant humans varies from -1 to 0.75 mm Hg [71,72]. In fact, PET_{CO_2} often exceeded $PaCO_2$ in anesthetized pregnant women, which may relate in part to a steeper slope of phase III (alveolar plateau) in capnograms of pregnant versus nonpregnant subjects [71–73]. Thus, it seems conceivable that the physiologic consequences of pneumoperitoneum could be different in parturients as compared with pregnant ewes [70•].

We have used PET_{CO_2} (32 to 36 mm Hg) to guide ventilation during laparoscopic operations in pregnant women, with no untoward effects on the mother or baby [3••]. Further, we used transcutaneous P_{CO_2} (tcP_{CO_2}) monitoring to trend changes in $PaCO_2$ during laparoscopic cholecystectomy in a parturient while maintaining PET_{CO_2} at 32 mm Hg (Fig. 3-2) [74]. The maximum observed increase in tcP_{CO_2} was about 6 to 7 mm Hg during laparoscopy. This observation corresponds to a $PaCO_2$ of 40 mm Hg. A change in maternal $PaCO_2$ of 6 to 7 mm Hg produces a change of less than 0.1 in fetal pH, which is probably within safe limits, as it is generally believed that fetal pH greater than 7.25 is considered not worrisome, and isolated fetal hypercarbia and concomitant low pH is not as detrimental to the fetus as the presence of metabolic acidosis consequent to hypoxia [66,75]. Further, a mild fetal acidosis may benefit the fetus by improving tissue oxygen unloading by right-shifting the fetal hemoglobin dissociation curve [66,75]. Although long-term effects of a transient episode of fetal acidosis during pregnancy are unknown, it may be considered benign, as evidenced by successful outcome following laparoscopic surgery in several parturients (no spontaneous abortions, preterm labors, or premature deliveries reported in 67 parturients) [2,3••,4,5•,6]. Conversely, excessive hypercarbia ($PaCO_2$ > 60 mm Hg) in parturients has been associated with decreased uterine and umbilical circulation and fetal heart rate changes [76–78]. Hence, the tcP_{CO_2} monitor, if available, can provide important information about maternal $PaCO_2$.

Although fetal heart rate can be monitored from the 16th gestational week onward, continuous fetal heart rate monitoring during laparoscopic surgery is usually not performed because of the proximity of the periumbilical trocar site to the optimal site for fetal heart monitoring. Alternatively, continuous transvaginal Doppler monitoring may be performed. If fetal heart rate monitoring is not performed during surgery, it should be monitored immediately before and after the surgical procedure. Postoperative supplemental oxygen therapy during transport and the postoperative period until full recovery should be provided to avoid hypoxemia. Further, transport in lateral position is recommended to minimize the risks of aspiration and aortocaval compression.

Infants and children

Pediatric patients tolerate pneumoperitoneum as well as do adults (Table 3-5) [11,12••,13,79–82]. Pneumoperitoneum causes an immediate reduction (29% to 33%) in dynamic thoracic compliance with an increase of airway pressures by 18% to 20 % [12••]. Physiologic dead space remains unchanged [12••]. Hypercapnia occurs in 14% to 21% and is caused by peritoneal absorption of CO_2 [12••]. However, arterial P_{CO_2} can remain in the physiologic range by compensatory hyperventilation (plus 25% of physiologic tidal volume) [12••]. There is no significant decrease in PaO_2 during CO_2 insufflation. The systolic pressure increases by 10% and diastolic pressure by 32% at 5 minutes following CO_2 insufflation. The PET_{CO_2} returns to baseline values 4 to 9 minutes following termination of CO_2 insufflation [11].

General endotracheal anesthesia can be safely administered for endoscopic surgery in pediatric patients. As in adults, ventilation

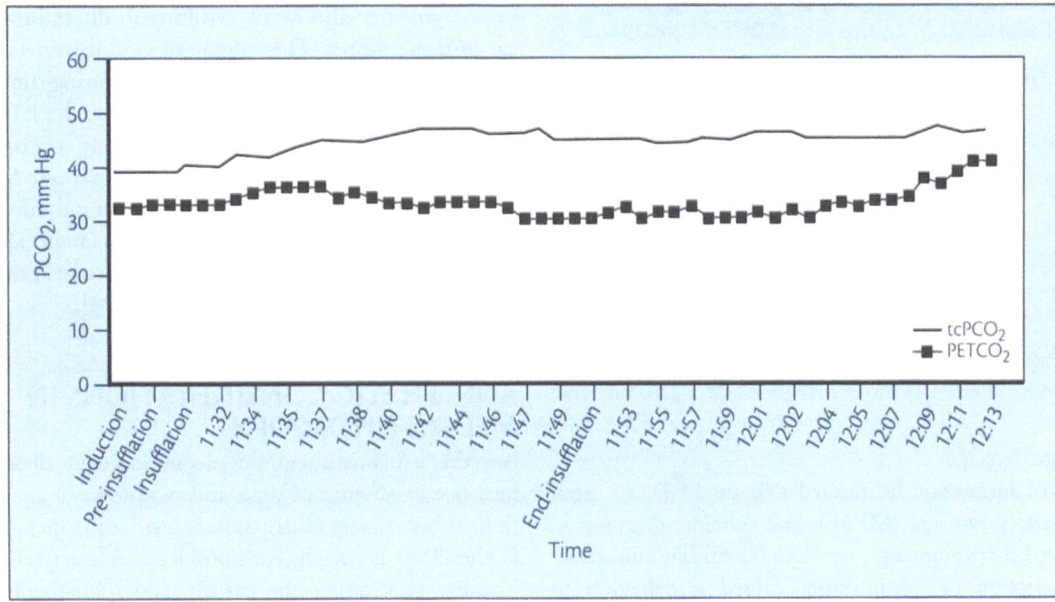

Figure 3-2 Transcutaneous carbon dioxide measurements (tcPco$_2$) during laparoscopic cholecystectomy in a pregnant patient. Minute ventilation was adjusted to maintain end-tidal Pco$_2$ (PETco$_2$) at 32 mm Hg. tcPco$_2$ Increased by 6 to 7 mm Hg (corresponding to an estimated Paco$_2$ of 39–40 mm Hg) during co$_2$ insufflation. tcPco$_2$ Returned to baseline after 1 hour following anesthesia.

is increased to prevent hypercarbia on CO_2 insufflation. If Jackson-Reese modification of Ayre T piece is used, it is also necessary to increase fresh gas flows to minimize rebreathing. Capnography has been shown to be an excellent guide to monitor Paco$_2$ [11,12••].

COMPLICATIONS OF LAPAROSCOPIC SURGERY

Table 3-6 lists complications associated with laparoscopy. Patients undergoing laparoscopic surgery are at risk for several potentially life-threatening complications. These complications include venous air embolism, pneumothorax, subcutaneous emphysema (SCE), hemodynamic compromise secondary to increased intra-abdominal pressure, cardiac dysrhythmia, and unrecognized hemorrhage [16••]. Cardiac arrest is a rare complication. The risk of death associated with laparoscopic tubal ligations is approximately four in 100,000 procedures [83].

Pneumothorax

A study of pneumothorax revealed that it is more likely to occur on the right side during laparoscopic cholecystectomy (20 reported cases, with two reported cases of bilateral pneumothoraces) [16••], whereas it occurred on the left side when surgery was performed around the esophagus [16••]. The three most important consistent signs were 1) increase in PETco$_2$, 2) increase in airway pressure and decrease in dynamic compliance, accompanied by 3) decreased arterial oxygen saturation [16••]. A decrease in MAP suggests development of tension pneumothorax. The diagnosis is usually confirmed by auscultation of the chest and, if possible, by an immediate radiologic examination. Thoracocentesis will provide immediate relief and further confirmation. The suspected mechanism

of pneumothorax during laparoscopic abdominal surgery include diaphragmatic defects resulting from improper closure of the communications between pleural and peritoneal cavities, migration of the gas through venacaval openings, or through ruptured falciform ligaments [16••]. Appropriate management includes discontinuation of peritoneal insufflation and release of pneumoperitoneum. Positive end-expiratory pressure (PEEP) may hasten resorption of gas [28]. Thoracocentesis is rarely necessary.

Carbon dioxide embolism

Small CO_2 emboli occur during laparoscopy and can be detected by TEE [16••]. Such microemboli may increase PETco$_2$ with no hemodynamic consequences. Macroemboli sufficient to cause a gas "lock" result in classic signs of embolism, *ie*, precipitous reduction in PETco$_2$, "mill-wheel murmur," hypotension, and desaturation. Three important factors play a role in determining the severity of gas embolism [16••]. These factors are discussed in the following three sections.

Solubility of gas

Carbon dioxide is very soluble in blood, which has a huge buffering capacity; therefore, the median lethal dose for gas embolism is higher with CO_2 than with air (25 mL/kg vs 5 mL/kg, respectively).

Driving pressure

Driving pressure for embolization is the difference between intra-abdominal pressure and intravascular pressure. The pressure difference will determine the volume of gas introduced into the circulation. The CO_2 must come either from massive transperitoneal uptake or by intravenous injection under pressure to form a CO_2 "lock."

Table 3-5

Physiologic effects of pneumoperitoneum in children

Compliance	$\downarrow$ 29%–33%
Airway pressures	$\uparrow$ 18%–20%
Hyperventilation for normocapnia	$\uparrow$ 25%
Capnography	Reliable guide to $PaCO_2$
Systolic blood pressure	$\uparrow$ 10%
Diastolic blood pressure	$\uparrow$ 32%

Volume of gas injected

The effects of intravenously injected CO_2 on $PETCO_2$, mean pulmonary artery pressure (MPAP), and systemic pressures in the pig showed that volumes greater than 0.1 mL/kg/min, either by bolus injection or by infusion, caused a reduction in $PETCO_2$, an increase in MPAP, and hypotension. Smaller volumes resulted in insignificant changes in $PETCO_2$. The volume of CO_2 required for detection by TEE was 0.26 mL $\pm$ 0.24 mL/kg, whereas that required to change $PETCO_2$ was 0.66 $\pm$ 0.51 mL/kg [16••,84].

Management

The patient must be placed immediately in the left lateral head-down position, which will relieve the mechanical obstruction of the gas "lock" to blood flow through the right ventricular outflow tract. The change in the position places the outflow tract below the right atrium. Insufflation must be discontinued, pneumoperitoneum released, inspiratory oxygen concentration increased to 100%, and vasopressors administered to support the circulation, if needed. Aspiration of gas by large-bore catheters in the right heart and pulmonary artery may be of some value. Complete cardiopulmonary bypass may be required to evacuate the gas "lock" [16••].

Subcutaneous emphysema

Subcutaneous emphysema is not a serious complication, but it may be the harbinger of pneumothorax. In a review of 12 cases [16••], SCE was evident 45 minutes after the start of surgery, although it may appear later or only at the end of surgery. Frequently, it occurs during surgical manipulation around the esophagus [16••]. A consistent finding was sudden and brisk increase in $PETCO_2$ and very marked increase in $PaCO_2$ (as high as 100 mm Hg), coincident with the appearance of SCE in upper body (face, neck, and thorax) [16••]. An increased airway pressure and decreased compliance indicate the presence of pneumothorax.

The source of the SCE during laparoscopy may be either supradiaphragmatic (from direct injury) or infradiaphragmatic. CO_2 Can pass through the diaphragmatic foramina into the mediastinum and then into the subcutaneous tissue planes of the head and neck. Alternatively, the insufflated gas can track along a low-resistance conduit from the trocar into the subcutaneous tissue planes, driven by the insufflating pressure with improperly placed Veress needles. Inadvertent perforation of the diaphragm may also occur, resulting in direct introduction of gas into the thorax. The volume of CO_2 delivered to the lungs with SCE is twice as large as that during uncomplicated laparoscopy, resulting in markedly increased $PETCO_2$ [16••]. Subcutaneous emphysema is more likely to occur during lengthy procedures, particularly fundoplication. Management requires ruling out the presence of pneumothorax, increasing the ventilation by as much as 33% to maintain an acceptable $PETCO_2$ or $PaCO_2$, evaluating the upper airway at the end of the procedure, and reassuring the patient [16••].

ANESTHETIC CONSIDERATIONS IN MEDIASTINOSCOPY

Anesthetic management for mediastinoscopy depends on the presence or absence of signs and symptoms of airway obstruction. When airway obstruction is present preoperatively, general anesthesia is fraught with problems. Acute tracheal collapse, inability to ventilate the patient, and subsequent death have been reported [85].

In the absence of airway obstruction, general anesthesia is our technique of choice, with inhalational or intravenous agents or often a combination of the two. Innominate artery compression by the mediastinoscope is an important consideration. The danger of innominate artery compression is that falsely low blood pressure readings will be obtained. Several methods have been advocated to detect this complication: constant palpation of the right radial or carotid pulse, placement of a right indwelling radial artery catheter, or monitoring of the continuous plethysmographic tracing of a pulse oximeter [85,86]. Our practice is to record blood pressures with a cuff on the left arm while monitoring the plethysmographic tracing of a pulse oximeter on the right hand. If direct pressure monitoring is considered, we then insert the radial artery catheter into the left radial artery and apply the noninvasive cuff on the right arm.

Use of muscle relaxants provides the endoscopist with an operative field free from sudden movements that might lead to injury of the adjacent organs by the mediastinoscope. However, nondepolarizing muscle relaxants must be used judiciously in patients with potential myasthenic syndromes.

Anesthetic management is more controversial in the presence of airway obstruction secondary to compression by mass, and depends on whether tissue diagnosis exists. In the presence of a tissue diagnosis, it may be advisable to proceed with preoperative chemotherapy, radiotherapy, or both to shrink the tumor and decrease the degree of obstruction, and thereby reduce the likelihood of airway complications [87]. Without tissue diagnosis, the most prudent management in the presence of airway compression would be to obtain percutaneous needle biopsy under local analgesia, followed by radiation and then general anesthesia for mediastinoscopy [88].

In case of extrathoracic variable obstruction, the airway is secured via fiberoptic intubation under topical anesthesia, or through a tracheostomy or cricothyroidotomy, performed under local anesthesia. Intrathoracic obstructing masses create the most challenging management dilemmas for three reasons. First, the extent of airway compromise may be difficult to assess.

Second, the tumor may compress distal trachea and both mainstream bronchi, so that introduction of endotracheal tube distal to the compromised area is not feasible. Last, positive pressure ventilation and muscle relaxation will worsen the intrathoracic obstruction because the distending, negative intrathoracic pressure generated by spontaneous inspiration is lost. Endotracheal intubation should be performed in the spontaneously breathing patient and anesthetic technique should preserve spontaneous ventilation during maintenance. If muscle relaxation or positive pressure ventilation become unavoidable, collapse of the airway may ensue. Under these circumstances, if an endotracheal tube or a rigid bronchoscope does not provide adequate patency of airway, the only recourse would be rapid institution of partial cardiopulmonary bypass [85,89]. In the case of an intrathoracic obstructing mass involving the trachea and only one of the main stem bronchi, a double-lumen endotracheal tube may provide a patent airway.

Pneumothorax and hemorrhage are the most common complications during mediastinoscopy. The occurrence of pneumothorax during mediastinoscopy must be anticipated. It may be prudent to avoid the routine use of nitrous oxide, which may increase the size of the pneumothorax and lead to tension pneumothorax. Typed and cross-matched blood should be available, as there is a possibility of sudden and massive hemorrhage. Placement of an intravenous catheter in a lower extremity will ensure venous access below the level of obstruction in the presence of superior vena caval obstruction. Other complications associated with mediastinoscopy are recurrent laryngeal nerve injury, esophageal injury, chylothorax, air embolism, and hemiparesis [85].

ANESTHETIC CONSIDERATIONS IN THORACOSCOPY

Thoracoscopy may be diagnostic as well as therapeutic. Diagnostic indications are biopsy of lesions of lung and pleura, diagnosis of cardiac herniation after pneumonectomy, and identification of the origin of a bronchopleural fistula. Therapeutic indications include chemical pleurodesis for recurrent pneumothorax, drainage of pleural effusions and empyema, and, more recently, lung volume reduction surgery. Thoracoscopy can be performed under either general or regional anesthesia.

Regional anesthesia consists of performing intercostal nerve blocks at least two segments above and below the level of the anticipated operative site. Visceral pleura requires topical application of local anesthetics. Cough reflex is obtunded by intravenous narcotics or alternatively by stellate ganglionic block [85]. The major disadvantage of regional anesthesia is that the patient has to breathe spontaneously while the operative lung is collapsed. Although this may be tolerated for short periods of time, it is not advisable for longer procedures.

A double-lumen endotracheal tube is recommended if general anesthesia is chosen. This allows deflation of the lung on the operative side. General anesthesia for thoracoscopy can be accomplished with short-acting intravenous agents and inhalational

Table 3-6
Complications of laparoscopy

Cardiovascular
  Decreased venous return/hypotension
  Hemorrhage
  Venous air embolism
  Cardiac arrhythmia
  Myocardial infarction
  Aortofemoral occlusion
  Deep vein thrombosis
  Cardiac arrest

Respiratory
  Hypercarbia
  Pneumothorax
  Subcutaneous emphysema
  Atelectasis
  Pneumonia

agents to allow for rapid emergence, as in day-surgical patients. This also ensures prompt recovery of airway reflexes. Supplementary epidural anesthesia is performed preoperatively to provide postoperative analgesia for patients having lung volume reduction surgery to improve breathing and facilitate coughing. Patients are observed in the recovery room for pneumothorax, postoperative bleeding, and sudden pulmonary decompensation.

CONCLUSIONS

In the future, anesthesiologists will encounter with increasing frequency infants and children, pregnant patients, and patients with cardiovascular and respiratory disorders requiring anesthesia for endoscopic surgery. Laparoscopic surgery can be performed safely in these patients provided anesthesiologists take appropriate precautions. Peritoneal insufflation of CO_2 in parturients and patients with cardiovascular and respiratory disorders may result in an exaggerated fall in cardiac output, hypercarbia, and respiratory acidosis. Therefore, anesthesiologists should minimize the adverse effects of CO_2 insufflation by additional monitoring as appropriate, using lower peritoneal insufflation pressures, making gradual changes in positioning, and observing for complications. Laparoscopic surgery is associated with certain life-threatening complications, such as pneumothorax, subcutaneous emphysema, and embolism. Vigilance, therefore, is necessary to diagnose these complications before they have produced profound deleterious effects on an already compromised cardiovascular and respiratory system. With such precautions, anesthesia for endoscopic surgery can be performed safely in parturients and children as well as patients with cardiorespiratory disorders, thus allowing these groups to benefit from minimally invasive surgery.

REFERENCES AND RECOMMENDED READING

Recently published papers of particular interest have been highlighted as:

•   Of interest

••   Of outstanding interest

1. Soper NJ, Brunt LM, Kerb K: Laparoscopic general surgery. *N Engl J Med* 1994, 330:409–419.

2. Curete MJ, Allen D, Josloff RK, *et al*.: Laparoscopy during pregnancy. *Arch Surg* 1996, 131:546–550.

3.•• Steinbrook RA, Brooks DC, Datta S: Laparoscopic cholecystectomy during pregnancy. *Surg Endosc* 1996, 10:511–515.

With appropriate attention to the altered physiology of pregnancy, laparoscopic cholecystectomy can be performed safely and effectively during pregnancy.

4. Eichenberg RJ Vanderlinden J, Bianchi MC, *et al*.: Laparoscopic cholecystectomy in the third trimester of pregnancy. *Am Surg* 1996, 62:874–877.

5.• Lanzafame RJ: Laparoscopic cholecystectomy during pregnancy. *Surgery* 1995, 118:627–631.

Based on the review of 46 cases of laparoscopic cholecystectomy during pregnancy, the author concludes that laparoscopic cholecystectomy is safe during pregnancy when undertaken by the skilled laparoscopic surgeon.

6. Soper NJ, Hunter JG, Petrie RH: Laparoscopic cholecystectomy during pregnancy. *Surg Endosc* 1992, 6:115–117.

7.• Dhoste K, Lacoste L, Karayan J, *et al*.: Hemodynamic and ventilatory changes during laparoscopic cholecystectomy in elderly ASA III patients. *Can J Anaesth* 1996, 43:783–788.

Gradual abdominal insufflation to 12 mm Hg followed by a limited 10° head-up tilt is associated with cardiovascular stability in elderly ASA III patients.

8.•• Wahba RWM, Berque F, Kleiman SJ: Cardiopulmonary function and laparoscopic cholecystectomy [review article]. *Can J Anaesth* 1995, 42:51–63.

This excellent article reviews extensively the cardiopulmonary changes during pneumoperitoneum in healthy patients as well as in patients with cardiac and respiratory disorders.

9. Feig BW, Berger DH, Dupuis JF, *et al*.: Hemodynamic effects of CO_2 abdominal insufflation (CAI) during laparoscopy in high-risk patients. *Anesth Analg* 1994, 78:S109.

10. Fox LG, Hein HAT, Gawey BJ, *et al*.: Physiologic alterations during laparoscopic cholecystectomy in ASA III & IV patients [abstract]. *Anesthesiology* 1993, 79:A55.

11. Hsing CH, Hseu SS, Tsai SK, *et al*.: The physiological effect of CO_2 pneumoperitoneum in pediatric laparoscopy. *Acta Anaesthesiol Scand* 1995, 33:1–6.

12.•• Resinoso-Barbero F, Diez A, Paz JA, *et al*.: Physiopathologic implications of the anesthesiologic management of pediatric laparoscopic surgery. *Rev Esp Anestesiol Reanim* 1995, 42:277–282.

Discusses the physiologic consequences of pneumoperitoneum in children and concludes that laparoscopic surgery in children diminishes thoracic distensibility and causes hypercapnia, making it necessary to measure $PETCO_2$ to regulate ventilation.

13. Ikeya K, Kashimoto S, Takahashi M, *et al*.: Anesthetic management of laparoscopic ovarian cystectomy in a 2-year-old child. *Masui* 1994, 43:778–780.

14. Fahy BG, Barnas GM, Flowers JL, *et al*.: The effects of increased abdominal pressure on lung and chest wall mechanics during laparoscopic surgery. *Anesth Analg* 1995, 81:744–750.

15. Cunningham AJ, Brull SJ: Laparoscopic cholecystectomy: anesthetic implications. *Anesth Analg* 1993, 76:1120–1133.

16.•• Wahba WM, Tessler MJ, Kleiman SJ: Acute ventilatory complications during laparoscopic upper abdominal surgery. *Can J Anaesth* 1996, 43:77–83.

Immediate recognition of the three complications (pneumothorax, subcutaneous emphysema, CO_2 embolism) requires continuous monitoring of $PETCO_2$, arterial saturation, airway pressure, and an index of pulmonary compliance.

17. Wahba RWM, Mamazza J: Ventilatory requirements during laparoscopic cholecystectomy. *Can J Anaesth* 1993, 40:206–210.

18. Wittgen CM, Andrus CH, Fitzgerald SD, *et al*.: Analysis of the hemodynamic and ventilatory effects of laparoscopic cholecystectomy. *Arch Surg* 1992, 126:997–1001.

19. Joris JL, Noirot DP, Legrand MJ, *et al*.: Hemodynamic changes during laparoscopic cholecystectomy. *Anesth Analg* 1993, 76:1067–1071.

20. Breton G, Poulin E, Fortin C, *et al*.: Evaluation clinique et hemodynamique des cholecystectomies par voie laparoscopique. *Ann Chir* 1991, 45:783–790.

21. Reid CW, Martineau RJ, Hull KA, Miller DR: Haemodynamic consequences of abdominal insufflation with CO_2 laparoscopic cholecystectomy [abstract]. *Can J Anaesth* 1992, 39:A132.

22. Cunningham AJ, Turner J, Rosenbaum S, Rafferty T: Transoesophageal echocardiographic assessment of haemodynamic function during laparoscopic cholecystectomy. *Br J Anaesth* 1993, 70:621–625.

23. Aoki T, Tanil M, Takahashi K, *et al*.: Cardiovascular changes and plasma catecholamine levels during laparoscopic surgery. *Anesth Analg* 1994, 78:S8.

24. Felber AR, Blobner M, Goegier S, *et al*.: Plasma vasopressin in laparoscopic cholecystectomy [abstract]. *Anesthesiology* 1993, 79:A32.

25. Wahba RWM: Perioperative functional residual capacity. *Can J Anaesth* 1991, 38:384–400.

26. Makinen MT: Dynamic lung compliance during laparoscopic cholecystectomy. *Anesth Analg* 1994, 78:S261.

27. Feinstein R, Ghouri A: Change in pulmonary mechanics during laparoscopic cholecystectomy. *Anesth Analg* 1993, 76:S102.

28. Chiche JD, Joris J, Lamy M: PEEP for treatment of intraoperative pneumothorax during laparoscopic fundoplication [abstract]. *Br J Anaesth* 1994, 72:A38.

29. Joris J, Honore P, Lamy M: Changes in oxygen transport and ventilation during laparoscopic cholecystectomy [abstract]. *Anesthesiology* 1992, 77:A149.

30. Wurst H, Schulte-Steinberg H, Finsterer U: Pulmonary CO_2-elimination in laparoscopic cholecystectomy: a clinical study. *Anaesthetist* 1993, 42:427–434.

31. Nyarwaya JB, Mazoit JX, Samii K: Are pulse oximetry and end-tidal carbon dioxide tension monitoring reliable during laparoscopic surgery? *Anaesthesia* 1994, 49:775–778.

32. Baraka A, Jabbour S, Hammoud R, *et al*.: Can pulse oximetry and end-tidal capnography reflect arterial oxygenation and carbon dioxide elimination during laparoscopic cholecystectomy? *Surg Laparosc Endosc* 1994, 4:353–356.

33. Ciofolo MJ, Clergue F, Seebacher J, *et al*.: Ventilatory effects of laparoscopy under epidural anesthesia. *Anesth Analg* 1990, 70:357–361.

34. Watcha MF, While PF: Postoperative nausea and vomiting. *Anesthesiology* 1992, 77:162–184.

35. Alexander GD, Skupski JN, Brown EM: The role of nitrous oxide in postoperative nausea and vomiting [abstract]. *Anesth Analg* 1984, 63:175.

36. Havorka J, Korttila K, Erkola O: Nitrous oxide does not increase the incidence of nausea and vomiting after gynecological laparoscopy. *Can J Anaesth* 1989, 36:145–148.

37. Andrews PLR: Physiology of nausea and vomiting. *Br J Anaesth* 1992, 69:2S–19S.

38.•• Philip BK: Etiologies of postoperative nausea and vomiting. *Pharm Ther* 1997, 22:18S–25S.
Postoperative nausea and vomiting is a common problem that is growing in significance with the growth of ambulatory surgery. It is precipitated by a multitude of factors related to patient, procedure, and anesthetic agents.

39. Kapur PA: The big 'little problem'. *Anesth Analg* 1991, 73:243–245.

40. Steinbrook RA, Freiberger D, Gosnell JL, Brooks DC: Prophylactic antiemetics for laparoscopic cholecystectomy: ondansetron versus droperidol plus metoclopramide. *Anesth Analg* 1996, 83:1081–1083.

41. Lonie DS, Harper JN: Nitrous oxide anaesthesia and vomiting. *Anaesthesia* 1986, 41:703–707.

42. Jenkins JC, Lahay D: Central mechanisms of vomiting related to catecholamine response: anaesthetic implications. *Can Anaesth Soc J* 1971, 18:434–441.

43. Perreault L, Normandin N, Plamondon L, *et al.*: Middle ear pressure variations during nitrous oxide-oxygen anesthesia. *Can Anaesth Soc J* 1982, 29:428–434.

44. Egar EI II, Saidman LJ: Hazards of nitrous oxide anesthesia in bowel obstruction and pneumothorax. *Anesthesiology* 1965, 26:61–66.

45. Bhandari P, Bingham S Andrews PLR: The neuropharmacology of loperamide-induced emesis in the ferret: the role of the area postrema, vagus, opiate, and 5-HT$_3$ receptors. *Neuropharmacology* 1992, 31:735–742.

46. Anderson R, Krohg K: Pain as a major cause of postoperative nausea. *Can Anaesth Soc J* 1976, 23:366–369.

47. Ding Y, Terkonda R, White PF: Use of ketorolac and dezocine as alternatives to fentanyl during outpatient anesthesia [abstract]. *Anesth Analg* 1992, 74(suppl):S67.

48. Watcha MF, Jones MB, Lagueruela R, *et al.*: A comparison of ketorolac and morphine when used during pediatric anesthesia [abstract]. *Anesthesiology* 1991,75:A942.

49. Buckley MMT, Brogden RN: Ketorolac: a review of pharmacodynamic and pharmacokinetic properties and therapeutic potential. *Drugs* 1990, 39:86–109.

50. Helvacioglu A, Weis R: Operative laparoscopy and postoperative pain relief. *Obstet Gynecol* 1986, 67:447–479.

51. Spielman FJ, Hulka JF, Ostheimer GW, Mueller RA: Pharmacokinetics and pharmacodynamics of local analgesia for laparoscopic tubal ligations. *Am J Obstet Gynecol* 1983, 146:821–824.

52. Rothenberg DM, Parnass SM, Litwak K, *et al.*: Efficacy of ephedrine in the prevention of postoperative nausea and vomiting. *Anesth Analg* 1991,72:58–61.

53. Korttila K, Ostman P, Faure E, *et al.*: Randomized comparison of recovery after propofol-nitrous oxide versus thiopentone-isoflurane-nitrous oxide anaesthesia in patients undergoing ambulatory surgery. *Acta Anaesthesiol Scand* 1990, 34:400–403.

54. Doze VA, Westphal LM, White PF: Comparison of propofol with methohexital for outpatient anesthesia. *Anesth Analg* 1986, 65:1189–1195.

55. Watcha MF, Simeon RM, White PF, Stevens JL: Effect of propofol on the incidence of postoperative vomiting after strabismus surgery in pediatric outpatients. *Anesthesiology* 1991, 75:204–209.

56. Chettleborough MC, Osborne GA, Rudkin GE, *et al.*: Double-blind comparison of patient recovery after induction with propofol or thiopentone for day-case relaxant general anaesthesia. *Anaesth Intens Care* 1992, 20:160–173.

57. Borgeat A, Wilder-Smith OHG, Saiah M, Rifat K: Subhypnotic doses of propofol possess direct antiemetic properties. *Anesth Analg* 1992, 74:539–541.

58. Iwase K, Takenaka H, Yagura A, *et al.*: Hemodynamic changes during laparoscopic cholecystectomy in patients with heart disease. *Endoscopy* 1992, 24:771–773.

59. Safran D, Sgambati S, Orlando R III: Laparoscopy in high-risk cardiac patients. *Surg Gynecol Obstet* 1993, 176:548–554.

60. Duale C, Bazin JE, Ferrier C, *et al.*: Hemodynamic effects of laparoscopic cholecystectomy in patients with coronary disease [abstract]. *Br J Anaesth* 1993, 72:A31.

61. Litwin DEM, Girotti MJ, Poulin EC, *et al.*: Laparoscopic cholecystectomy: trans-Canada experience with 2201 cases. *Can J Surg* 1992, 35:291–296.

62. Feig BW, Berger DH, Dougherty TB, *et al.*: Pulmonary effects of CO_2 abdominal insufflation (CAI) during laparoscopy in high-risk patients. *Anesth Analg* 1994, 78(suppl):S108.

63. Wittgen CM, Naunheim KS, Andrus CH, Kaminski DL: Preoperative pulmonary function evaluation for laparoscopic cholecystectomy. *Arch Surg* 1993, 128:880–885.

64. Monk TG, Weldon BC, Lemon D: Alterations in pulmonary function during laparoscopic surgery. *Anesth Analg* 1993, 76(suppl):S274.

65. Levinson G, Shnider SM, deLorimer AA, Steffenson JL: Effects of maternal hyperventilation on uterine blood flow and fetal oxygenation and acid-base status. *Anesthesiology* 1974, 40:340–347.

66. Hunter JG, Swanstrom L, Thornburg K: Carbon dioxide pneumoperitoneum induces fetal acidosis in a pregnant ewe model. *Surg Endosc* 1995, 9:272–279.

67. Martin LVH, Jurand A: The absence of teratogenic effects of some analgesics used in anaesthesia. *Anaesthesia* 1992, 47:473–476.

68. Brooks DC, Becker JM: A simplified technique for open laparoscopy using disposable trocar. *J Laparoendosc Surg* 1992, 2:357–359.

69. Cruz AM, Sutherland LC, Duke T, *et al.*: Intraabdominal carbon dioxide insufflation in the pregnant ewe. *Anesthesiology* 1996, 85:1395–1402.

70.• Bhavani Shankar K, Mushlin PS: Arterial to end-tidal carbon dioxide gradients in pregnant subjects. *Anesthesiology* 1997, 87:1596–1597.
Discusses the current status of capnography as a noninvasive monitor of $PaCO_2$ during laparoscopic surgery in parturients.

71. Bhavani-Shankar K, Moseley H, Kumar Y, *et al.*: Arterial to end-tidal carbon dioxide tension difference during anaesthesia for tubal ligation. *Anaesthesia* 1987, 42:482–486.

72. Bhavani-Shankar KB, Moseley H, Kumar Y, Vemula V: Arterial to end-tidal carbon dioxide tension difference during Caesarean section anaesthesia. *Anaesthesia* 1986, 41:698–702.

73. Bhavani-Shankar K, Moseley H, Kumar AY, Delph Y: Capnometry and anaesthesia. *Can J Anaesth* 1992, 39:617–632.

74. Bhavani-Shankar K, Steinbrook RA, Mushlin PS, Freiberger D: Transcutaneous PCO_2 monitoring during laparoscopic cholecystectomy in pregnancy. *Can J Anaesth* 1998, 45:164–169.

75. Harned HS, Rowshan G, MacKinney LC, Sugioka K: Relationship of PO_2, PCO_2, and pH to onset of breathing of the term lamb as studied by a flow-through cuvette electrode assembly. *Pediatrics* 1964, 33:672–681.

76. Ivankovic AD, Elam JO, Huffman J: Effect of maternal hypercarbia on the newborn infant. *Am J Obstet Gynecol* 1970, 107:939–945.

77. Newman W, Braid D, Wood C: Fetal acid-base status: 1. Relationship between maternal and fetal P_{CO_2}. *Am J Obstet Gynecol* 1967, 97:43–51.

78. Walker AM, Oakes GK, Ehrenkranz R, *et al.*: Effects of hypercarbia on uterine and umbilical circulations in conscious pregnant sheep. *J Appl Physiol* 1976, 41:727–733.

79. Pintus C, Coppola R, Talamo M, Perrelli L: Laparoscopic cholecystectomy in a 23-month-old infant. *Surg Laparosc Endosc* 1995, 5:148–150.

80. Radke M, Helms B, Czarnetzki HD, *et al.*: Laparoscopic cholecystectomy in a young girl. *J Pediatr Surg* 1994, 4:108–109.

81. Rosser JC Jr, Boeckman CR, Andrews D: Laparoscopic cholecystectomy in an infant. *Surg Laparosc Endosc* 1992, 2:143–147.

82. Holcomb GW, Naffis D: Laparoscopic cholecystectomy in infants. *Pediatr Surg* 1994, 29:86–87.

83. Peterson HB, DeStefano F, Rubin GL, *et al.*: Deaths attributable to tubal sterilization in United States, 1977 to 1981. *Am J Obstet Gynecol* 1983, 146:131–136.

84. Couture P, Boudreault D, Derouin M, *et al.*: Venous carbon dioxide embolism in pigs: an evaluation of end-tidal carbon dioxide, transesophageal echocardiography, pulmonary artery pressure, and precordial auscultation as monitoring modalities. *Anesth Analg* 1994, 79:867–873.

85. Ehrenwerth J, Brull SJ: Anesthesia for thoracic diagnostic procedures. In *Thoracic Anesthesia*, edn 2. Edited by Kaplan JA. New York: Churchill Livingstone; 1991:321–346.

86. Petty C: Right radial artery pressure during mediastinoscopy. *Anesth Analg* 1979, 58:428–430.

87. Piro AJ, Weiss DR, Hellman S: Mediastinal Hodgkin's disease: a possible danger for intubation anesthesia. *Int J Radiat Oncol Biol Phys* 1976, 1:415–419.

88. Neuman GG, Weingarten AE, Abramowitz RM, *et al.*: The anesthetic management of the patient with an anterior mediastinal mass. *Anesthesiology* 1984, 60:144–147.

89. Wilson RF, Steiger Z, Jacobs J, *et al.*: Temporary partial cardiopulmonary bypass during emergency operative management of near total tracheal occlusion. *Anesthesiology* 1984, 61:103–105.

Minimally Invasive Management of Esophageal Disease

Timothy M. Farrell
John G. Hunter

The esophagus is an innocuous component of normal gastrointestinal function that serves as a conduit between the oropharynx and stomach. However, when afflicted by disease, this simple muscular tube becomes a conspicuous source of morbidity and mortality. Until recently, operating on the esophagus required thoracotomy or laparotomy. Today, minimally invasive techniques are routinely applied for diseases of the foregut [1••] and in many cases have supplanted traditional methods by minimizing pain and recovery time.

GASTROESOPHAGEAL REFLUX DISEASE
Incidence and pathophysiology

Gastroesophageal reflux disease (GERD) accounts for 75% of esophageal pathology [2]. Forty percent of adult Americans suffer heartburn each month [3]; 7% endure daily symptoms [4]. Clinical manifestations of GERD typically include heartburn, regurgitation, and dysphagia, but also may encompass abdominal or chest pain, cough, hoarseness, asthma, belching, nausea, vomiting, odynophagia, dental erosions, and gastrointestinal bleeding.

Gastroesophageal reflux disease results from excessive retrograde passage of gastric contents into the esophagus. The predominant cause of pathologic reflux is lower esophageal sphincter (LES) dysfunction [5], usually manifesting as transient LES relaxations that are too long or too frequent [6,7]. Additional causes of GERD include poor salivary function, gastric herniation above the crural diaphragm [8], and esophageal or gastric dysmotility [9,10]. Pathologic findings range from subclinical esophagitis to ulceration, stricture, intestinal metaplasia (Barrett's esophagus), or adenocarcinoma.

Diagnostic evaluation

No constellation of symptoms is specific for GERD. Cholelithiasis, peptic ulcer disease, and even cardiac disease may mimic reflux. Symptomatic response to empiric antisecretory therapy (histamine antagonists, proton pump inhibitors) supports the diagnosis of GERD. Precise history and physical examination must be complemented by anatomic and physiologic foregut evaluation. Tests used to corroborate the diagnosis include barium swallow, esophagogastroduodenoscopy (EGD), esophageal manometry, 24-hour pH monitoring, and gastric emptying assessment.

Although barium swallow will demonstrate structural abnormalities associated with GERD, such as stricture, hiatal hernia, and esophageal shortening, we rely more heavily on EGD. EGD provides comparable anatomic information, but also allows mucosal survey for esophagitis, unrecognized malignancy, or gastric pathology. Biopsy is essential to identify Barrett's metaplasia, which indicates 30% to 40% increased risk

CHAPTER

4

for malignant transformation [11,12] and mandates long-term endoscopic surveillance [13].

Twenty-four-hour pH monitoring is the definitive test for acid reflux [14,15], and will document increased exposure of esophageal mucosa to gastric juice. Healthy individuals without heartburn have pH less than 4.0 for less than 4.2% of a 24-hour period [16]. Patients must suspend proton pump inhibitors at least 10 days prior to testing. This study may be omitted if EGD detects unambiguous evidence of severe reflux, such as erosive esophagitis [17].

Any patient considered for surgery requires an esophageal motility study [18] to characterize LES function and detect unsuspected functional disorders (achalasia, scleroderma) that may hinder propulsion of food through a surgical fundoplication. If esophageal body pressure is below 20 to 30 mm Hg, or if fewer than 60% to 80% of wet swallows induce peristalsis, we favor partial fundoplication.

A gastric emptying study is used selectively for patients with diabetes, peptic ulcer, prominent emesis, previous antireflux surgery, normal LES function, or bezoar. Although mildly abnormal gastric emptying is improved by fundoplication, severe impairment requires coincident pyloroplasty or pyloromyotomy.

Treatment options and surgical indications

The goals of treatment are to alleviate symptoms, promote healing of esophagitis, avoid disease progression, and prevent recurrence. Behavioral and dietary modifications, such as weight loss, smoking cessation, alcohol avoidance, decreased meal volume, and head of bed elevation are valuable [19]. Antacids, histamine antagonists, prokinetic agents, and proton pump inhibitors control symptoms in most patients. However, no medical option is curative, and patients with severe disease who cease medical therapy will likely develop recurrent symptoms [20].

The most frequent indication for operation is medically responsive GERD in patients who have residual symptoms such as regurgitation, or who are not willing to accept the expense of lifelong medical therapy. Surgery is also indicated for GERD patients with medically refractory symptoms, paraesophageal hernia, or complications such as recurrent aspiration, nonhealing esophageal ulcers, or peptic stricture.

The goal of surgery is to reproduce normal LES function, anchor the gastroesophageal junction within the abdomen, and obliterate any hiatal defect. Surgical management of GERD is safe and durable according to several large series, with 85% to 95% symptom control and acceptable morbidity and mortality [21–23]. Nissen fundoplication, the most popular antireflux operation, has been shown to be effective in comparative series [24].

Several years ago, open Nissen fundoplication was shown to be more effective than medical therapy for improving esophagitis, reducing esophageal exposure to acid, and controlling symptoms in veterans with severe or complicated GERD [25]. Proton pump inhibitors are more efficacious than other medical agents and appear safe for extended use thus far [26–28]. Laparoscopic antireflux surgery has presented an attractive alternative to lifelong medical therapy, especially for young patients. Economic comparison of contemporary treatment options for GERD found medical therapy to be less cost-effective than antireflux surgery after 1.4 years [29•].

The role of antireflux surgery for patients with Barrett's esophagus is still controversial. Because fundoplication does not cause regression of Barrett's metaplasia, and may not lessen the risk for malignant degeneration [30–33], clinicians hesitate to recommend surgery when symptoms are otherwise controlled. Recent evidence that nonacidic (duodenal) refluxate enhances Barrett's metaplasia suggests that LES reconstruction may be more protective than acid suppression alone against malignant transformation [34•,35–37].

Operative technique

The most popular antireflux operations are laparoscopic Nissen (360° wrap) and Toupet (270° wrap) fundoplications. Attention will be directed to our experience with these procedures.

Laparoscopic Nissen fundoplication

Under general endotracheal anesthesia, the patient is positioned with legs abducted by stirrups or a specially designed table. Pneumatic compression stockings, bladder catheter, and orogastric tube are placed. Pneumoperitoneum (15 mm Hg) is established by Veress or Hasson technique. A laparoscopic trocar (10 mm) is placed through the left rectus muscle 15 cm below the xiphoid process. A 45° oblique-viewing laparoscope is inserted that allows adequate visualization of the esophagus and retrogastric anatomy. A second trocar (10 mm) is inserted 10 cm from the xiphoid at the left costal margin to provide access for the surgeon's right hand. A third trocar (5 or 10 mm) is placed 15 cm from the xiphoid at the right costal margin, through which an expandable liver retractor is directed beneath the left lobe and immobilized by a table-mounted mechanical arm. The fourth trocar (5 mm) is angled right-to-left through the falciform ligament and beneath the liver edge to provide access for the surgeon's left hand. A fifth (5 mm) trocar is placed 20 cm from the xiphoid at the left costal margin for retraction.

The assistant retracts the gastroesophageal junction inferiorly by grasping epiphrenic fat with an atraumatic instrument. The surgeon uses electrocautery to open the gastrohepatic ligament cephalad to the hepatic branch of the vagus nerve, exposing the caudate lobe of liver and the right crus of the diaphragm. The peritoneal incision is extended across the phrenoesophageal ligament.

At this point, short gastric vessels are divided to mobilize the fundus off the left crus, and thereby facilitate retroesophageal dissection. The surgeon retracts the stomach to the patient's right and the assistant lifts the gastrosplenic omentum to expose the short gastric vessels (Fig. 4-1). The Harmonic scalpel (Ethicon Endosurgery, Cincinnati, OH) is used to control and divide these vessels, beginning 10 cm along the greater curvature and working back to the angle of His. Visualization of more proximal vessels often requires the first assistant to push the posterior gastric wall medially. Posterior attachments of the stomach must be divided back to the left crus to avoid tethering of the stomach and postoperative dysphagia [38].

The retroesophageal region is more accessible after greater curvature mobilization. The right crus is skeletonized along its medial border, sweeping inferiorly the hepatic branch of the vagus nerve. The plane between the right crus and the esophagus is developed (Fig. 4-2). The posterior vagus nerve, seen coursing through the mediastinum, is left with the esophagus. The surgeon passes a blunt grasper through the retroesophageal window created by crural dissection to emerge anterior to the left crus. Angling the 45° telescope usually allows direct visualization of this window. A 4-cm one-quarter-inch Penrose drain is drawn behind the esophagus, and its ends are clipped together. The assistant applies inferior traction using the Penrose. Circumferential dissection is continued up the mediastinal esophagus until its distal 3 cm will remain intraperitoneal and not withdraw into the hiatus when Penrose traction is released. During this dissection the esophagus is never grasped and electrocautery is used sparingly to avoid esophageal perforation or vagus nerve injury.

The orogastric tube is carefully replaced with a 60-F bougie. Bougie size is adjusted for children and adults with esophageal stricture. The crura are approximated with interrupted 0 nonabsorbable sutures (Fig. 4-3). Pledgets (1 cm²) are used routinely on the diaphragmatic closure. The fundus of the stomach is drawn behind the esophagus. If greater curvature mobilization is adequate, it will pass easily and not retract. A 2-cm fundoplication is created with three 2-0 nonabsorbable sutures on the left side of the esophagus. To prevent wrap slippage, each bite incorporates full-thickness fundus, partial-thickness esophagus, and full-thickness fundus. The fundoplication is secured to the posterior esophagus with a single 2-0 nonabsorbable "collar stitch" by rolling the gastroesophageal junction to the right (Fig. 4-4). The bougie is removed, the upper abdomen is irrigated, and the liver retractor is withdrawn. The pneumoperitoneum is released and instruments are removed. Incisions are closed with absorbable suture.

Laparoscopic Toupet fundoplication

Initial dissection and esophageal mobilization are identical to Nissen fundoplication. A Toupet fundoplication encompasses 270° posteriorly, and each arm of the fundus is secured to the esophagus with three 2-0 nonabsorbable sutures. Gastric bites are full-thickness and the esophageal bites are partial-thickness. The wrap is secured to the posterior esophagus by a "collar stitch" to prevent slippage (Fig. 4-5).

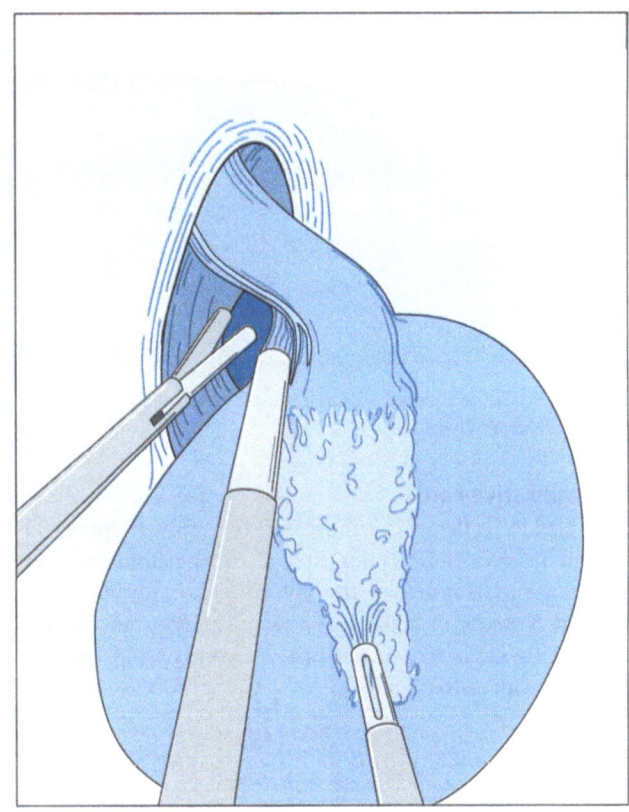

Figure 4-2 Dissection between the right crus and the esophagus. The posterior vagus nerve is usually left with the esophagus. (*Adapted from* Trus and Hunter [1••].)

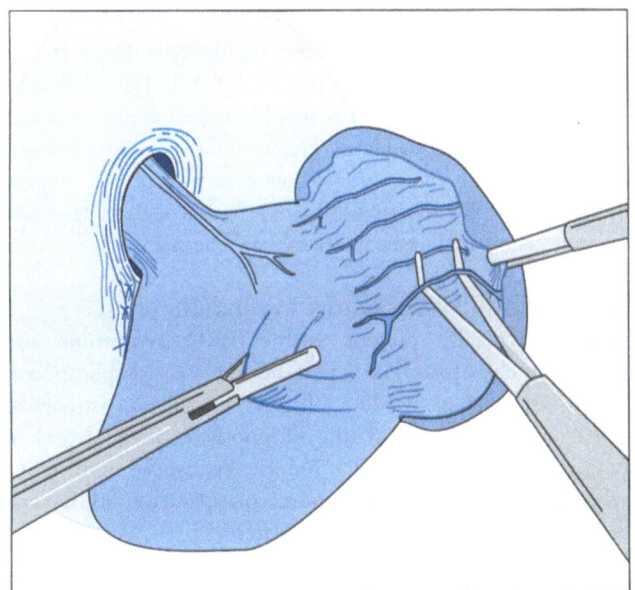

Figure 4-1 Division of the short gastric vessels. (*Adapted from* Trus and Hunter [1••].)

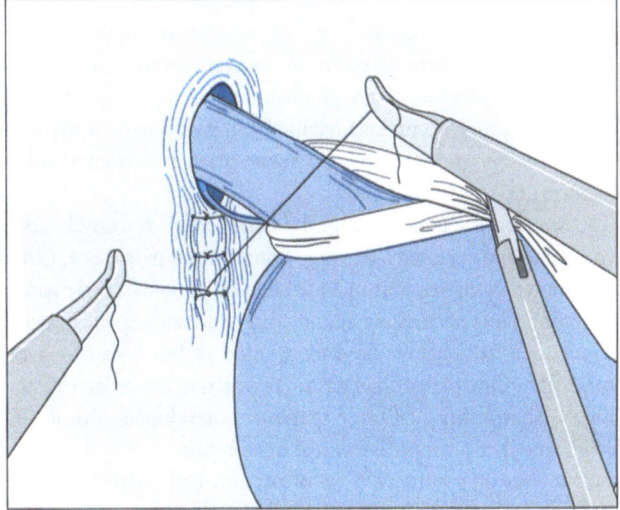

Figure 4-3 Crural closure is accomplished with heavy nonabsorbable suture. Pledgets are not shown. (*Adapted from* Trus and Hunter [1••].)

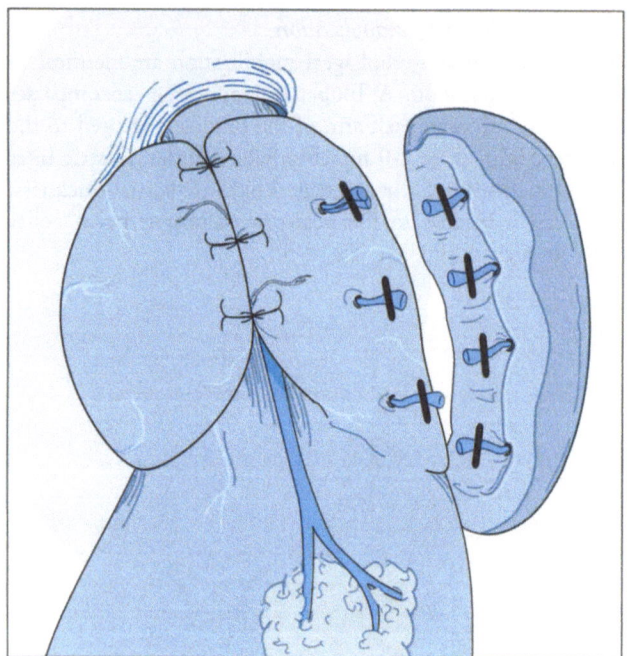

Figure 4-4 The completed Nissen fundoplication. (*Adapted from* Trus and Hunter [1··].)

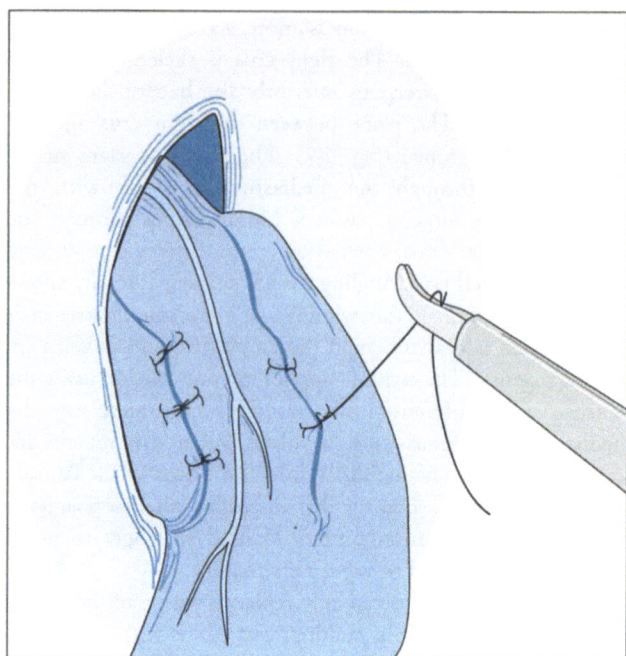

Figure 4-5 The completed Toupet fundoplication. (*Adapted from* Trus and Hunter [1··].)

Postoperative care

The bladder catheter is removed in the recovery room. The patient receives clear liquids after recovering from anesthesia and soft mechanical diet the following day. Regular diet is delayed 3 weeks to allow resolution of postoperative edema. Patients are discharged on the first or second postoperative day with no work restriction.

Outcomes

We recently reported 300 consecutive attempted laparoscopic fundoplications. Of these, four cases were converted to laparotomy because of adhesions from previous operation (*n*=3) or hepatomegaly (*n*=1). Mean operative time was 185 ± 51 minutes [39]. Median hospital stay was 2 days (range, 1–32). There was no mortality. One esophageal and four gastric perforations were recognized and repaired laparoscopically. Three pneumothoraces were noted in the recovery room, but only one became symptomatic. Although pneumothorax and subcutaneous emphysema may occur, and retained CO_2 may lengthen the need for ventilatory support, specific intervention is seldom required because CO_2 reabsorbs rapidly.

One acute paraesophageal herniation occurred after wretching and required laparotomy on postoperative day 4. Other self-limited complications included two pneumonias, three gastric dilatations, one necrotizing epididymitis, and one hepatic necrosis. Three more patients required reoperation within 1 year for wrap migration. One patient had gastric perforation a year later requiring laparotomy. One patient developed dumping syndrome that prompted eventual open repair.

One year after surgery, 93% of patients had good-to-excellent symptom relief and 4% reported only infrequent symptoms [40]. Of 55 patients who allowed repeat 24-hour pH study, 94% were normal and 6% mildly abnormal. Seventeen percent experienced

early dysphagia, but only 4% had persistent complaints at 1 year [41•]. Postoperative swelling is probably responsible for most postoperative dysphagia, so we remain diligent about creating "floppy wraps," with generous greater curvature mobilization and no more than 2-cm long fundoplication over 60-F bougie. If dysphagia persists after 4 weeks, dilatation is performed. Reoperation is seldom required. Results from other laparoscopic fundoplication series are comparable (Table 4-1) [42–45].

PARAESOPHAGEAL HERNIA
Incidence and pathophysiology

Hiatal hernias are usually of the sliding type (type I), the remainder are paraesophageal hernias [46,47]. Type II hernias contain gastric fundus or body that has migrated into the chest through the esophageal hiatus. Presence of the gastroesophageal junction within the sac is known as a type III hernia. Nontraumatic herniation outside the crural arch is rare, but when it occurs it is termed a "parahiatal" hernia.

Diagnostic and preoperative evaluation

Patients typically present with GERD symptoms and prominent chest pain. Thirty percent develop a complication of the disease, such as bleeding, obstruction, volvulus, strangulation, or perforation [48,49]. Diagnosis is made by chest radiograph or barium swallow. Given the association of reflux with paraesophageal herniation, preoperative EGD and esophageal manometry are appropriate.

Treatment options and surgical indications

No medical therapy diminishes the risk for the life-threatening complications of type II and III hiatal hernias, so prompt

Table 4-1

Results of laparoscopic fundoplication

Study	Patients, n	Conversion rate, %	Length of stay, d	Slippage, %	Disruption, %	Dysphagia, %	Heartburn, %
Weerts et al. [43]	132	3.3	2.8	—	0	5.4	0.8
Hinder et al. [44]	198	2.0	3	0	1	6.0	1.0
Jamieson et al. [45]	155	12.3	2.6	—	—	17.6	1.2
Anvari et al. [42]	168	2.3	2.5	1.2	—	2.4	0.6
Hunter et al. [40]	300	1.3	2.2	2	0.75	4.0	3.0

Table 4-2

Results of laparoscopic paraesophageal hernia repair with fundoplication

Study	Patients, n	Conversions, n	Deaths, n	Perforations, n	Wrap migration, n	Symptom free, %	Dilatation required, n	Second operation required, n
Perdikis et al. [54•]	65	2	0	3	1	92.5	4	3
Farrell and Hunter, unpublished results	62	1	2	4	2	100	1	5

elective repair is the standard of care. Laparoscopic repair of paraesophageal hernias has been reported [50–52]. We recommend coincident antireflux procedure because persistent symptomatic reflux will occur in 20% of cases if fundoplication is not performed [53].

Operative techniques

Patient preparation, positioning, and trocar locations are identical to fundoplication. Commonly, multiple adhesions must be divided to reduce the hernia sac from the mediastinum. During this dissection, it is possible to injure the mediastinal pleura and the vagus nerves, which often are displaced from the esophagus. Once the sac is separated from the crural ring, it is excised and removed. The hiatal defect is closed posterior to the esophagus by reapproximating the diaphragmatic crura with interrupted, pledgeted, 0-nonabsorbable sutures. Use of mesh is discouraged because of risk for excessive adhesion formation and esophageal erosion. After hernia reduction and repair, fundoplication is performed. Postoperative care is similar to that after fundoplication alone.

Outcomes

Sixty-two laparoscopic paraesophageal hernia repairs were attempted at our institution between February 1993 and July 1997. Mean operative time was 225 ± 78 minutes. Median hospital stay was 2 days (range, 1–127). Two intraoperative complications occurred. One steroid-dependent patient, who required conversion to laparotomy, had a protracted hospital course after esophageal laceration and pulmonary failure. One gastric lacer-

ation, which was recognized and repaired laparscopically, caused a 1-day discharge delay. Three gastroesophageal perforations presented on postoperative day 3 or 4. Of these, one patient with gastric necrosis died from sepsis after laparotomy, and two with esophageal perforations required thoracotomy for repair. Three patients suffered myocardial ischemia within 30 days of surgery, one of whom died. One patient developed esophageal stricture requiring dilatation. All patients were symptom free after surgery; however, two repairs prolapsed requiring reoperation after 6 and 16 months, respectively. Our results are similar to another large series (Table 4-2) [54•].

ACHALASIA AND OTHER MOTILITY DISORDERS

Incidence and pathophysiology

Achalasia is the most common esophageal motility disorder, with 0.5 new cases per 100,000 population per year [55]. Patients suffer slowly progressive dysphagia, frequent nocturnal regurgitation, and respiratory symptoms (cough, wheezing, aspiration, recurrent pulmonary infections) [56,57]. Symptoms are often present for years and are initially misdiagnosed in 50% of patients [58].

The pathophysiology of achalasia is unclear, but involves degeneration of Auerbach's plexus in the esophageal body and elevated LES resting pressure. Poor LES relaxation on swallowing results in gradual esophageal dilatation with progressive loss of peristalsis [59].

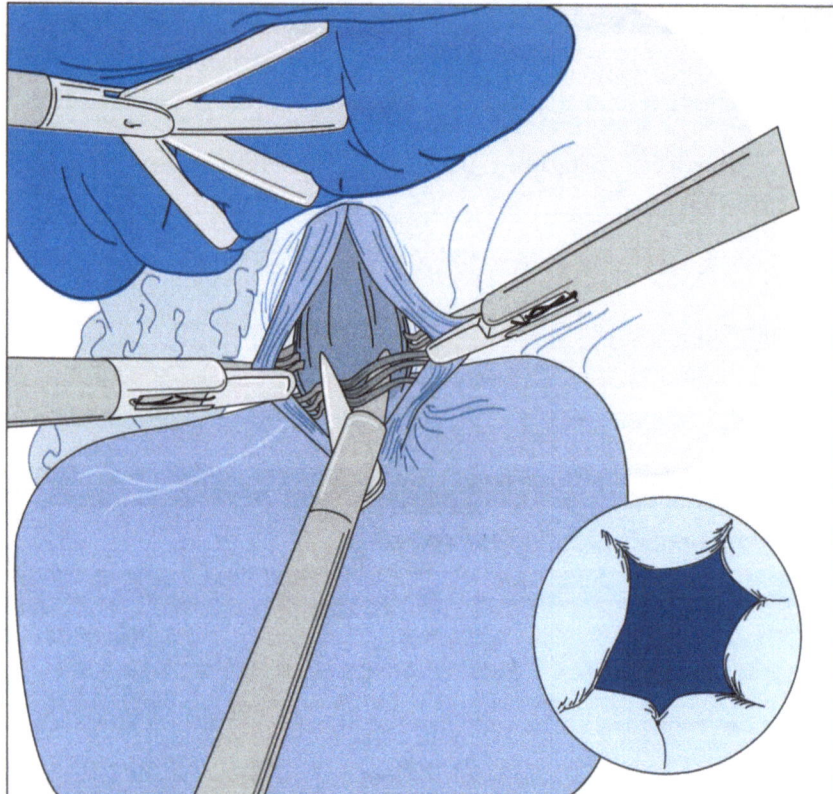

Figure 4-6 After blunt dissection of longitudinal muscle fibers, careful division of the circular muscle fibers with electrosurgical scissors reveals underlying esophageal mucosa. The *inset* demonstrates the endoscopic view after completion of the myotomy. (*Adapted from* Holzman *et al.* [72•].)

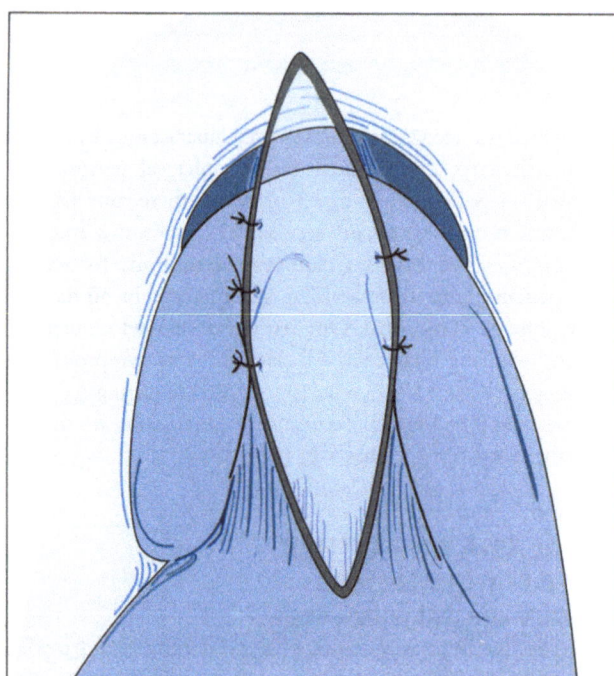

Figure 4-7 Completed Heller myotomy with Toupet fundoplication. (*Adapted from* Trus and Hunter [1••].)

Diagnostic evaluation

Barium swallow is a valuable diagnostic tool, typically displaying esophageal dilatation with "bird's beak" narrowing at the gastroesophageal junction. EGD is necessary to rule out tumor or peptic stricture, and most often discloses a patulous esophagus with retained food and secretions, and mucosal thickening. The most specific test is esophageal manometry. The LES resting pressure is elevated with incomplete or absent relaxation on swallowing, and the esophageal body is without primary peristalsis [60].

Treatment options and surgical indications

Because no cure is available, the goal of therapy for achalasia is to eliminate the functional gastroesophageal obstruction by reducing LES pressure. Medical options include nitrates and calcium channel blockers, but response is short-lived and associated with side effects [61]. Endoscopic injection of botlinum toxin [62,63] provides two thirds of patients short-term symptom relief (mean, 1.3 years) [64]. Mechanical treatments to overcome LES dysfunction include pneumatic balloon dilatation and surgical (Heller) cardiomyotomy. Both methods have high initial success in overcoming dysphagia, although dilatation carries four times greater risk for esophageal perforation [57,59]. Surgery provides more durable symptom relief according to retrospective (94% vs 81%) and prospective (95% vs 65%) studies of late outcomes [65,66]. Most gastroenterologists attempt dilatation initially, reserving surgical referral for treatment failures. Dissemination of minimally invasive methods may broaden the appeal of operative strategies for achalasia.

Operative techniques

Minimally invasive Heller myotomy may be performed by an abdominal [67] or thoracic [68,69] approach. Proponents of laparoscopy emphasize distal extension of the myotomy across the gastroesophageal junction and addition of fundoplication, which reduces postoperative reflux from 13.2% to 7.4% [70]. Thoracoscopic surgeons claim longer myotomy is achievable through the chest with less likelihood for subsequent reflux.

Laparoscopic Heller myotomy

Patient preparation, positioning, and trocar positions are similar to laparoscopic fundoplication. The procedure begins by opening the phrenoesophageal ligament and dissecting the diaphragmatic crura circumferentially away from the esophagus. Mobilization of short gastric vessels is accomplished to allow fundoplication after myotomy.

A longitudinal seromuscular incision is made above the gastroesophageal junction, to the left of the anterior vagus nerve. Longitudinal muscle fibers of the esophagus are separated by blunt dissection. The circumferential muscle fibers are carefully elevated and divided until mucosa is visualized. Electrosurgical scissors are used to extend the myotomy 6 cm proximally and 1 cm distally across the gastroesophageal junction (Fig. 4-6). The muscle edges are separated until exposed mucosa encompasses 40% of the esophageal circumference. Most perforations occur at the gastroesophageal junction, where mucosa and overlying muscle are intimately adhered. Instillation of methylene blue through the orogastric tube detects occult mucosal injury. A Toupet fundoplication is fashioned with the fundus anchored to the cut edges of the esophageal muscle to help maintain their separation (Fig. 4-7). Postoperative guidelines are similar to fundoplication.

Thoracoscopic Heller myotomy

After double-lumen endotracheal anesthesia, the patient is placed in a right lateral decubitus position, and the left lung is collapsed. A 10-mm port is placed at the midaxillary line in intercostal space six (ICS-6). The thoracoscope is inserted, and 5-mm ports are placed along the midaxillary line in ICS-3 and at the anterior and posterior axillary lines in ICS-4 or -5, creating a diamond configuration. The left lung is retracted cephalad and the inferior pulmonary ligament is divided to the inferior pulmonary vein. The mediastinal pleura overlying the esophagus is opened, with manipulation of an endoscope facilitating its exposure. The esophagus is longitudinally "scored" with electrocautery from the inferior pulmonary vein to the diaphragm. Hypertrophic esophageal muscle is divided down through the circular layer. A 7-cm myotomy is extended down the distal esophagus onto the gastroesophageal junction, which is visualized by pushing the diaphragm away while retracting the esophagus cephalad. Forty percent of the mucosal circumference is exposed to allow the distal esophagus to heal without stricture. LES patency by endoscopic view confirms adequate distal myotomy (Fig. 4-6 [inset]). A chest tube is left through the inferior trocar site and incisions are closed with absorbable suture.

Outcomes

We reported intermediate follow-up of our first 40 laparoscopic Heller myotomies (performed between July 1992 and November 1996) [71]. Thirty patients had been previously treated for achalasia, 21 with pneumatic dilation, one with botulinum toxin, six with dilatation and botulinum toxin, and two with transthoracic cardiomyotomy. Three patients had previous laparoscopic fundoplication for GERD. None required conversion to laparotomy. Mean operative time was 199 ± 36 minutes. Median hospital stay was 2 days (range, 1–13). Six intraoperative mucosal injuries were repaired primarily without event. Complications included two postoperative pneumonias and one delayed hemorrhage from an esophageal ulcer. Dysphagia was alleviated in all but four patients, and regurgitation in all but two. Our results are similar to other authors (Table 4-3) [72•,73,74•].

Other motility disorders

Diffuse esophageal spasm (DES) and nutcracker esophagus (NE) are less common causes of dysphagia and noncardiac chest pain. Esophageal manometry is the diagnostic test of choice. DES is characterized by simultaneous distal esophageal contractions in greater than 10% of wet swallows with intervening normal peristalsis. NE is diagnosed when mean peristaltic amplitude in the distal esophagus is greater than 180 mm Hg [75]. Initial therapy in both diseases is medical, with dilatation and cardiomyotomy reserved for failures. Although thoracoscopic esophageal myotomy (gastroesophageal junction to aortic arch) has been described for DES and NE [76], these conditions are best managed nonoperatively.

Epiphrenic esophageal diverticula are associated with the spasmodic esophageal motility disorders. If large, these may be removed during myotomy using a thoracoscopic stapling device.

Table 4-3

Results of minimally invasive Heller myotomy

Study	Patients, n	Operative approach, laparoscopy/ thoracoscopy	Conversions, n	Deaths, n	Perforations, n	Good-to-excellent symptom relief, %	Second operation required, n
Patti et al. [74•]	30	0/30	2	0	3	87	3
Raiser et al. [73]	39	35/4	0	0	7	62	3
Holzman et al. [72•]	10	7/3	1	0	1	90	1
Hunter et al. [71]	40	40/0	0	0	6	90	0

ESOPHAGEAL TUMORS
Benign tumors
Ten percent of esophageal neoplasms are benign. Leiomyomas are most common, and may be amenable to laparoscopic or thoracoscopic resection [77]. Tumor location dictates the appropriate approach. An endoscope is often required to locate the lesion intraoperatively. Trocar positions are similar to laparoscopic fundoplication or thoracoscopic Heller myotomy. Most leiomyomas will enucleate after longitudinal myotomy. If recent biopsy has engendered inflammation, resection and closure may be necessary. Methylene blue instillation via an oroesophageal tube will verify mucosal integrity after resection. The muscular layer is sutured closed and a chest tube is left if a thoracoscopic approach was used.

Malignant tumors
Lack of esophageal serosa and abundant periesophageal lymphatics permit early extraesophageal spread of malignancies. Prognosis for most esophageal cancers is poor, and operative approach (transthoracic or transhiatal) makes little difference in outcome [78–80]. The blind nature of transhiatal resection increases iatrogenic morbidity, but may decrease postoperative pulmonary dysfunction [81–83].

Thoracoscopy-assisted transhiatal esophagectomy
This two-stage technique [84–86] involves initial thoracoscopic esophageal dissection via the right chest, with subsequent patient repositioning for transhiatal esophagectomy and cervical anastomosis. Trocar locations are similar to thoracoscopic esophageal myotomy, except in the right chest. A flexible endoscope assists visualization and manipulation of the esophagus. The lung is retracted anteriorly and cephalad, and mediastinal pleura is divided from the azygous vein to the diaphragm. If necessary, the azygous vein is divided between ties or with a vascular stapler. The esophagus is encircled away from the tumor and retracted with a vascular tape. Blood vessels between the esophagus and the aorta are cauterized. Lymphatic tissues are kept in continuity with the esophagus. Once the entire thoracic esophagus is mobilized, a chest tube is placed and incisions are closed. The patient is repositioned supine, and transhiatal esophagectomy is performed, without need for blunt dissection, followed by cervical esophagogastric anastomosis.

Endoscopic microsurgical dissection of the esophagus
German surgeons have used minimally invasive techniques for dissection within the posterior mediastinum without thoracoscopy or blind dissection [87–89]. Endoscopic microsurgical dissection of the esophagus (EMDE) involves the use of a modified operating mediastinoscope, which consists of a light, an operating channel, and an olive-shaped tip that is grooved on one side. A cervical incision provides access to the esophagus at the thoracic inlet. The mediastinoscope is introduced and periesophageal tissues are circumferentially dissected to the diaphragm using electrocautery and suction. The cervical esophagus is divided, and the specimen is removed transabdominally, where a second operating team has mobilized the stomach for replacement of the esophagus. The gastric tube is drawn into the neck and anastomosis is accomplished.

Laparoscopy-assisted transhiatal esophagectomy
Small series of laparoscopic-assisted transhiatal esophagectomies have been reported. The laparoscope and instruments are passed through the hiatus, either after laparotomy [90,91] or via standard trocar locations [92,93]. Enthusiasts report less bleeding and improved lymphatic dissection when compared with conventional transhiatal esophagectomy.

Outcomes
Twenty-six cancer patients underwent attempted thoracoscopy-assisted transhiatal esophagectomy in one series [94]. There was one conversion to open thoracotomy for bleeding. There were no deaths. Postoperative complications included three pneumonias, two recurrent laryngeal nerve palsies, and one anastomotic leak. Median postoperative stay was 12 days (range, 9–30).

Early follow-up of 33 patients treated with EMDE has been presented [95]. Two cases were converted to thoracotomy, one for bleeding and one for bronchial infiltration of tumor. Of 31 remaining patients, two died of perioperative infections, nine suffered pulmonary complications, and one had myocardial infarction. Six patients developed radiographic fistulas at the esophagogastric anastomosis. Mean hospital stay was 24 days. In another series of 57 patients undergoing EMDE for esophageal carcinoma [96], one was converted to thoracotomy for a right main bronchus injury. Three patients died of gastric necrosis, cardiorespiratory failure, and pulmonary embolus, respectively. Three intraoperative esophageal lacerations occurred early in the series (5.3%), without subsequent mediastinitis.

Experience with laparoscopic-assisted transhiatal esophagectomy for cancer is limited. Japanese surgeons reported six patients with advanced esophageal cancer in whom periesophageal dissection was done after laparotomy using laparoscopic instruments through the esophageal hiatus [91]. There was no major bleeding, but two self-limited anastomotic leaks were detected postoperatively. All patients recovered normal swallowing function. A Brazilian surgeon reported 12 patients with 10 benign and two malignant esophageal tumors in whom completely laparoscopic transhiatal esophagectomy was attempted [92]. One case was converted to open technique for hepatic bleeding. Three minor pleural injuries occurred. One patient developed postoperative anastomotic leak with subsequent stenosis requiring endoscopic dilatation. No mortality occurred in this small series.

CONCLUSIONS
Although long-term follow-up is not yet available, present data suggest distinct advantages of minimally invasive versus traditional open approaches for certain diseases of the esophagus. Early patient mobilization after laparoscopic surgery for GERD and achalasia has improved patient satisfaction and shortened hospital stays compared with traditional surgery. Symptomatic response remains above 90% in most reports. The role of minimally invasive surgery for cancer is less well defined, because only small series are available to date. Controlled trials will resolve this issue.

REFERENCES AND RECOMMENDED READING

Recently published papers of particular interest have been highlighted as:
* • Of interest
* •• Of outstanding interest

1.•• Trus TL, Hunter JG: Minimally invasive surgery of the esophagus and stomach. *Am J Surg* 1997, 173:242–255.
Provides a contemporary review of minimally invasive foregut surgery.

2. DeMeester TR, Stein HJ: Surgical treatment of gastroesophageal reflux disease. In *The Esophagus*. Edited by Castell DO. Boston: Little-Brown; 1992:579–625.

3. Gallup survey on heartburn across America. Princeton: The Gallup Organization; 1988.

4. Spechler SJ: Epidemiology and natural history of gastro-oesophageal reflux disease. *Digestion* 1992, 51:24–29.

5. Stein HJ, Barlow AP, DeMeester TR, *et al.*: Complications of gastroesophageal reflux disease. *Ann Surg* 1992, 216:35–43.

6. Dodds WJ, Dent J, Hogan WJ, *et al.*: Mechanisms of gastroesophageal reflux in patients with reflux esophagitis. *N Engl J Med* 1982, 307:1547–1552.

7. Mittal RK, Holloway RH, Penagini R, *et al.*: Transient lower esophageal sphincter relaxation. *Gastroenterology* 1995, 109:601–610.

8. Mittal RK: The crural diaphragm, an external lower esophageal sphincter: a definitive study [editorial]. *Gastroenterology* 1993, 105:1565–1567.

9. Kahrilas PJ, Dodds WJ, Hogan WJ, *et al.*: Esophageal peristaltic dysfunction in peptic esophagitis. *Gastroenterology* 1986, 91:897–904.

10. Kahrilas PJ, Dodds WJ, Hogan WJ: Effect of peristaltic dysfunction of esophageal volume clearance. *Gastroenterology* 1988, 94:73–80.

11. Spechler SJ, Goyal RK: Barrett's esophagus. *N Engl J Med* 1986, 315:362–371.

12. Clark GW, Smyrk TC, Burdiles P, *et al.*: Is Barrett's metaplasia the source of adenocarcinomas of the cardia? *Arch Surg* 1994, 129:609–614.

13. Peters JH, Clark GW, Ireland AP, *et al.*: Outcome of adenocarcinoma arising in Barrett's esophagus in endoscopically surveyed and nonsurveyed patients. *J Thorac Cardiovasc Surg* 1994, 108:813–821.

14. Fuchs KH, DeMeester TR, Albertucci M: Specificity and sensitivity of objective diagnosis of gastroesophageal reflux disease. *Surgery* 1987, 102:575–580.

15. Johansson KE, Boeryd B, Fransson SG, *et al.*: Esophageal reflux test, manometry, endoscopy, biopsy, and radiology in healthy subjects. *Scand J Gastroenterol* 1986, 21:399–406.

16. Johnson LF, DeMeester TR: Twenty-four-hour pH monitoring of the distal esophagus. *Am J Gastroenterol* 1974, 62:325–332.

17. Waring JP, Hunter JG, Oddsdottir M, *et al.*: The preoperative evaluation of patients considered for laparoscopic antireflux surgery. *Am J Gastroenterol* 1995, 90:35–38.

18. Zaninotto G, DeMeester TR, Schwizer W, *et al.*: The lower esophageal sphincter in health and disease. *Am J Surg* 1988, 155:104–110.

19. Kitchin LI, Castell DO: Rationale and efficacy of conservative therapy for gastroesophageal reflux disease. *Arch Intern Med* 1991, 151:448–454.

20. Bell NJ, Hunt RH: Role of gastric acid suppression in the treatment of gastro-oesophageal reflux disease. *Gut* 1992, 33:118–124.

21. Low DE, Hill LD: Fifteen to 20-year results following the Hill anti-reflux operation. *J Thorac Cardiovasc Surg* 1989, 98:444–450.

22. Orringer MB, Skinner DB, Belsey RHR: Long term results of the Mark IV operation for hiatal hernia and analyses of recurrences and their treatment. *J Thorac Cardiovasc Surg* 1972, 63:25–33.

23. Peters JH, DeMeester TR: Gastroesophageal reflux. *Surg Clin North Am* 1993, 73:1119–1144.

24. DeMeester TR, Johnson LS, Kent AH: Evaluation of current operations for the prevention of gastroesophageal reflux. *Ann Surg* 1974, 180:511–525.

25. Spechler SJ: Comparison of medical and surgical treatment for complicated gastroesophageal reflux in veterans. *N Engl J Med* 1992, 326:786–792.

26. Dent J, Yeomans ND, Mackinnon M, *et al.*: Omeprazole v ranitidine for prevention of relapse in reflux esophagitis: a controlled double blind trial of their efficacy and safety. *Gut* 1994, 35:590–598.

27. Hallerback B, Unge P, Carling L, *et al.*: Omeprazole or ranitidine in the long-term treatment of reflux esophagitis. *Gastroenterology* 1994, 107:1305–1311.

28. Klinkenberg-Knol EC, Festen HP, Jansen JB, *et al.*: Long-term treatment with omeprazole for refractory reflux esophagitis: efficacy and safety. *Ann Intern Med* 1994, 121:161–167.

29.• Van Den Boom G, Go PM, Hameeteman W, *et al.*: Cost effectiveness of medical versus surgical treatment in patients with severe or refractory gastroesophageal reflux disease in the Netherlands. *Scand J Gastroenterol* 1996, 31:1–9.
Cost-analysis of medical versus surgical management of GERD.

30. Spechler SJ, Goyal RK: Barrett's esophagus. *N Engl J Med* 1986, 315:362–371.

31. Clark GW, Smyrk TC, Burdiles P, *et al.*: Is Barrett's metaplasia the source of adenocarcinomas of the cardia? *Arch Surg* 1994, 129:609–614.

32. Sagar PM, Ackroyd R, Hosie KB, *et al.*: Regression and progression of Barrett's oesophagus after anti-reflux surgery. *Br J Surg* 1995, 82:806–810.

33. Gore S, Healey CJ, Sutton R, *et al.*: Regression of columnar lined (Barrett's) oesophagus with continuous omeprazole therapy. *Aliment Pharmacol Ther* 1993, 7:623–638.

34.• Kauer WKH, Peters JH, DeMeester TR, *et al.*: Mixed reflux of gastric and duodenal juices is more harmful to the esophagus than gastric juice alone: the need for surgical therapy is re-emphasised. *Ann Surg* 1995, 222:525–533.
Analyzes the role of nonacidic duodenal refluxate in Barrett's metaplasia and suggests a possible advantage of antireflux surgery over medical therapy.

35. Caldwell MTP, Lawlor P, Byrne PJ, *et al.*: Ambulatory oesophageal bile reflux monitoring in Barrett's oesophagus. *Br J Surg* 1995, 82:657–660.

36. Vaezi MF, Richter JE: Synergism of acid and duodeno-gastro-oesophageal reflux in complicated Barrett's oesophagus. *Surgery* 1995, 117:699–704.

37. Gillison EW, DeCastro VAM, Nyhus LM, *et al.*: The significance of bile in esophagitis. *Surg Gynecol Obstet* 1972, 134:419–424.

38. Hunter JG, Swanstrom L, Waring JP: Patterns of dysphagia following laparoscopic antireflux surgery. *Ann Surg* 1996, 224:51–57.

39. Richardson WR, Hunter JG, Waring JP: Laparoscopic antireflux surgery. *Semin Gastrointest Dis* 1997, 8:100–110.

40. Hunter JG, Trus TL, Branum GD, *et al.*: A physiologic approach to laparoscopic fundoplication for gastroesophageal reflux disease. *Ann Surg* 1996, 223:673–687.

41.• Trus TL, Laycock WS, Branum G, *et al.*: Intermediate follow-up of laparoscopic antireflux surgery. *Am J Surg* 1996, 171:32–35.
Documents our series of laparoscopic antireflux operations and intermediate-term outcomes.

42. Anvari M, Allen C, Borm A: Laparoscopic Nissen fundoplication is a satisfactory alternative to long-term omeprazole therapy. *Br J Surg* 1995, 82:938–942.

43. Weerts JM, Dallemagne B, Hamoir E, *et al.*: Laparoscopic Nissen fundoplication: detailed analysis of 132 patients. *Surg Laparosc Endosc* 1993, 3:359–364.

44. Hinder RA, Filipi CJ, Wetscher G, *et al.*: Laparoscopic Nissen fundoplication is an effective treatment for gastroesophageal reflux disease. *Ann Surg* 1994, 220:472–483.

45. Jamieson GG, Watson DI, Britten-Jones R, *et al.*: Laparoscopic Nissen fundoplication. *Ann Surg* 1994, 220:137–145.

46. Harris DR, Graham TR, Galea M, *et al.*: Paraesophageal hernias: when to operate. *J R Coll Surg Edinb* 1992, 37:97–98.

47. Menguy R: Surgical management of large paraesophageal hernia with complete intrathoracic stomach. *World J Surg* 1988, 12:415–422.

48. Almond DJ, Bancewicz J: Paraesophageal hernia: the potential for disaster [case report]. *Br J Hosp Med* 1988, 40:221–222.

49. Skinner DB, Belsey RH: Surgical management of esophageal reflux and hiatus hernia: long term results of 1030 patients. *J Thorac Cardiovasc Surg* 1967, 53:33–54.

50. Kroger KE, Stone JM: Laparoscopic reduction of acute gastric volvulus. *Am Surg* 1993, 59:325–328.

51. Kuster GG, Gilroy S: Laparoscopic repair of paraesophageal hiatal hernias. *Surg Endosc* 1993, 7:362–363.

52. Cloyd DW: Laparoscopic repair of incarcerated paraesophageal hernias. *Surg Endosc* 1994, 8:893–897.

53. Williamson WA, Ellis FH, Streitz JM: Paraesophageal hiatal hernia: is an antireflux procedure necessary? *Ann Thorac Surg* 1993, 56:447–452.

54.• Perdikis G, Hinder, RA, Filipi CJ, *et al.*: Laparoscopic paraesophageal hernia repair. *Arch Surg* 1997, 132:586–590.
A large series of laparoscopic paraesophageal hernia repairs with intermediate-term outcomes.

55. Earlham RJ, Ellis FH, Nobrega FT: Achalasia of the esophagus in a small urban community. *Mayo Clin Proc* 1969, 44:478–483.

56. Reynolds JC, Parkman HP: Achalasia. *Gastroenterol Clin North Am* 1989, 18:223–255.

57. Ferguson MK: Achalasia: current evaluation and therapy. *Ann Thorac Surg* 1991, 52:336–342.

58. Rosenzweig S, Traube M: The diagnosis and misdiagnosis of achalasia. *J Clin Gastroenterol* 1989, 11:147–153.

59. Clouse RE: Motor disorders. In *Gastrointestinal Disease*, edn 4. Edited by Sleisinger MH, Fordtran JS. Philadelphia: WB Saunders Company; 1989:559–593.

60. Couturier D, Samama J: Clinical aspects and manometry criteria in achalasia. *Hepatogastroenterology* 1991, 38:481–487.

61. Short TP, Thomas E: An overview of the role of calcium antagonists in the treatment of achalasia and diffuse esophageal spasm. *Drugs* 1992, 43:177–184.

62. Pasricha PJ, Ravich WJ, Hendrix TR, *et al.*: Intrasphincteric injection of botulinum toxin for the treatment of achalasia. *N Engl J Med* 1995, 332:774–778.

63. Rollan A, Gonzalez R, Carvajal S, Chianale J: Endoscopic intrasphincteric injection of botulinum toxin for the treatment of achalasia. *J Clin Gastroenterol* 1995, 20:189–191.

64. Pasricha PJ, Rai R, Ravich WJ, *et al.*: Botulinum toxin for achalasia: long-term outcome and predictors of response. *Gastroenterology* 1996, 110:1410–1415.

65. Okike N, Spencer Payne W, Neufeld DM, *et al.*: Esophagomyotomy versus forceful dilatation for achalasia of the esophagus: results in 899 patients. *Ann Thorac Surg* 1979, 28:119–125.

66. Csendes A, Braghetto I, Henriques A, *et al.*: Late results of a prospective randomized study comparing forceful dilatation and esophagomyotomy in patients with achalasia. *Gut* 1989, 30:299–305.

67. Swanstrom LL, Pennings J: Laparoscopic esophagomyotomy for achalasia. *Surg Endosc* 1996, 9:537–540.

68. Pellegrini C, Wetter LA, Patti M, *et al.*: Thoracoscopic esophagomyotomy: initial experience with a new approach. *Ann Surg* 1992, 216:291–299.

69. Pellegrini C, Leichter R, Patti M, *et al.*: Thoracoscopic esophageal myotomy in the treatment of achalasia. *Ann Thorac Surg* 1993, 53:680–682.

70. Andreollo NA, Earlam RJ: Heller's myotomy for achalasia: is an added antireflux procedure necessary? *Br J Surg* 1987, 74:765–769.

71. Hunter JG, Trus TL, Branum GD, Waring JP: Laparoscopic Heller myotomy and fundoplication for achalasia. *Ann Surg* 1997, 225:655–664.

72.• Holzman MD, Sharp KW, Ladipo JK, *et al.*: Laparoscopic surgical treatment of achalasia. *Am J Surg* 1997, 173:308–311.
Well-presented technical details of laparoscopic cardiomyotomy.

73. Raiser F, Perdikis G, Hinder R, *et al.*: Heller myotomy via minimal-access surgery: an evaluation of antireflux procedures. *Arch Surg* 1996, 131:593–598.

74.• Patti MG, Pellegrini CA, Arcerito M, *et al.*: Comparison of medical and minimally invasive surgical therapy for primary esophageal motility disorders. *Arch Surg* 1995, 130:609–616.
Large series of thoracoscopic cardiomyotomies for achalasia with outcomes.

75. Stein HJ, DeMeester TR: Outpatient physiologic testing and surgical management of foregut motility disorders. *Curr Probl Surg* 1992, 29:413–555.

76. Shimi SM, Nathanson LK, Cuschieri A: Thoracoscopic long esophageal myotomy for nutcracker esophagus: initial experience of a new surgical approach. *Br J Surg* 1992, 29:533–536.

77. Everitt NJ, Glinatsis M, McMahon MJ: Thoracoscopic enucleation of leiomyoma of the esophagus. *Br J Surg* 1992, 79:643.

78. Fok M, Sin KF, Wong J: A comparison of the transhiatal and transthoracic resection for carcinoma of the thoracic esophagus. *Am J Surg* 1989, 158:414–419.

79. Gotley DC, Beard J, Cooper MJ, *et al.*: Abdominocervical (transhiatal) esophagectomy in the management of esophageal carcinoma. *Br J Surg* 1990, 77:815–819.

80. Hankins JR, Attar S, Coughlin TR, *et al.*: Carcinoma of the esophagus: a comparison of the results of transhiatal versus transthoracic resection. *Ann Thorac Surg* 1989, 47:700–705.

81. Shahian DM, Neptune WB, Ellis FH, *et al.*: Transthoracic versus extrathoracic esophagectomy: mortality, morbidity and long-term survival. *Ann Thorac Surg* 1986, 41:237–246.

82. Guili R, Sancho-Garnier H: Diagnostic, therapeutic and prognostic features of cancer of the esophagus: results of the international prospective study conducted by the OESO group. *Surgery* 1986, 5:614–622.

83. Muller JM, Erasmi H, Stelzner M, *et al.*: Surgical therapy of esophageal carcinoma. *Br J Surg* 1990, 77:845–857.

84. Cuschieri A, Shimi S, Banting S: Endoscopic esophagectomy through a right thoracoscopic approach. *J R Coll Surg Edinb* 1992, 37:7–11.

85. Collard JM, Lengele B, Otte JB, *et al.*: En bloc and standard esophagectomies by thoracoscopy. *Ann Thorac Surg* 1993, 56:675–679.

86. Gossot D, Fourquier P, Celerier M: Thoracoscopic esophagectomy: technique and initial results. *Ann Thorac Surg* 1993, 56:667–670.

87. Buess GF, Becker HD, Naruhn MB, *et al.*: Endoscopic esophagectomy without thoracotomy. *Curr Probl Surg* 1991, 8:478–486.

88. Bumm R, Holscher AH, Feussner H, *et al.*: Endodissection of the thoracic esophagus: technique and clinical results in transhiatal esophagectomy. *Ann Surg* 1993, 218:97–104.

89. Manncke K, Raestrup H, Walter D, *et al.*: Technique of endoscopic mediastinal dissection of the oesophagus. *Endosc Surg Allied Technol* 1994, 2:10–15.

90. Sadanaga N, Kuwano H, Watanabe M, *et al.*: Laparoscopy-assisted surgery: a new technique for transhiatal esophageal dissection. *Am J Surg* 1993, 168:355–357.

91. Yahata H, Sugino K, Takiguchi T, *et al.*: Laparoscopic transhiatal esophagectomy for advanced thoracic esophageal cancer. *Surg Laparosc Endosc* 1997, 7:13–16.

92. DePaula AL, Hashiba K, Ferreira AB, *et al.*: Laparoscopic transhiatal esophagectomy with esophagogastroplasty. *Surg Laparosc Endosc* 1995, 1:1–5.

93. Willson P, Montgomery P, Mochloulis G, *et al.*: Laparoscopically-assisted total pharyngolaryngo-oesophagectomy. *Br J Surg* 1997, 84:870–871.

94. Cuschieri A: Thoracoscopic subtotal oesophagectomy. *Endosc Surg Allied Technol* 1994, 2:21–25.

95. Becker HD, Buess GF, Mentges BR, *et al.*: Endoscopic esophagectomy. *Adv Surg* 1993, 26:397–410.

96. Bumm R, Siewert JR: Results of transmediastinal endoscopic oesophageal dissection. *Endosc Surg* 1994, 2:16–20.

Laparoscopic Appendectomy

John Morgan Cosgrove
George Gallos

The first reported case of appendicitis appeared in 1554, when Jean Fernel noted at autopsy the luminal obstruction, necrosis, and perforation of the appendix and cecum [1,2]. Although Fernel was the first to describe this disease state as "perityphlitis," the cause and treatment of the disease continued to be an enigma for more than 300 years. In 1886, Reginald Fitz conclusively demonstrated, in a study involving 25 patients, that the appendix was the primary site and source of inflammation in perityphlitis [3,4]. In his milestone paper, Fitz endorsed early surgical intervention and appendectomy as imperative for cure, and coined the term *appendicitis*. In 1889, McBurney presented his successful experience involving early removal of the appendix, and helped to improve the method of early clinical diagnosis with his description regarding McBurney's point [5,6]. Both Fitz and McBurney's work were instrumental in leading to the advocacy of early operative intervention, which by 1901 proved to reduce the mortality of acute appendicitis from 50% to 15% [2,7,8]. Subsequent advances in anesthesia, antibiotics, surgical techniques, and diagnostic modalities have further reduced the incidence of total morbidity and mortality associated with acute appendicitis to 10% to 20% and 0.18% to 0.8%, respectively [9,10–12].

One of the more recent trends in surgical therapy involves the use of minimally invasive laparoscopic procedures. The first major clinical use of laparoscopy dates to 1911, when Jacobacus [13] reported on 115 examinations of the chest and abdominal cavities in 72 patients. Using a rigid Nitze endoscope, Jacobaeus was able to report on completely varied cases and provide accurate diagnosis of such distinct pathologic entities as cirrhosis, tuberculosis, and syphilis [14]. Although Jacobaeus' work demonstrated the possibility of a great diagnostic modality, it would take several decades and numerous technical improvements before laparoscopy would attain a therapeutic role. The first great contributions toward this goal were pioneered by Kalk [15,16]. He was responsible for the modernization and improvement of several laparoscopic instruments (most notably his punch biopsy forceps, which are still in use today), and for advocating the second trocar approach, which allowed for enhanced hand-eye coordination and remote palpation of abdominal organs. Kalk and Bruhl [16], in their description of over 2000 laparoscopic liver biopsies without a single incidence of mortality, showed that laparoscopy could be considered a safe approach when performed by experienced individuals.

Another notable figure in the history of laparoscopy is George Berci. Berci and coworkers [18–21] advanced laparoscopy by being among the first to implement the development of the Hopkins rod-lens system of image transmission in laparoscopic procedures, and by pioneering the integration of television, the charge-coupling device, and endoscopy. These advances in instrumentation, optics, imaging, and television have helped propel laparoscopy as a medium for complex therapeutic procedures, and set the stage in 1983 for Semm [23] to perform the first laparoscopic appendectomy as a prophylactic measure during an ancillary procedure to a gynecologic operation [14,23].

Although the methods and the means were available, it would take some time for surgeons to begin using the laparoscopic approach for appendectomy. This is evident by the fact that it took until the early 1990s before any substantial and sizable series on laparoscopic appendectomies were published [24–26]. In fact, the controversy concerning

CHAPTER

5

whether laparoscopic appendectomy is better than a conventional open procedure still has not been completely resolved [27••].

INDICATIONS

There are several preoperative conditions that specifically indicate a laparoscopic approach to appendectomy. Laparoscopic appendectomy is indicated in obese patients because conventional appendectomy in the obese patient often requires larger incisions for standard exposure and has an associated increased wound infection rate [28,29].

Likewise, a laparoscopic approach is indicated for women of reproductive age. They typically represent a diagnostic dilemma because acute gynecologic conditions (*eg*, pelvic inflammatory disease, ovarian cyst) often present with signs and symptoms similar to those of acute appendicitis, and as a result there is a negative diagnostic rate of 35% to 46% in this patient group [4,28]. The advantages of diagnostic laparoscopy include a small incision, an enhanced view of the gynecologic and intra-abdominal structures, and a reduction in the incidence of unnecessary laparotomies [30]. In general, our policy has been to use laparoscopy in all women of child-bearing age who have a negative pregnancy test. If there is an obvious appendicitis, an appendectomy is performed. In cases in which florid pelvic inflammatory disease is present along with the absence of gross signs of appendiceal pathology, we do not recommend prophylactic appendectomy because the staple line would be at risk. However, in any equivocal case, a laparoscopic appendectomy is performed to avoid future ambiguity between the diagnosis of an acute appendicitis and a gynecologic condition.

CONTRAINDICATIONS

There are certain situations in which a laparoscopic appendectomy should not be performed. Although feasible, the safety of laparoscopic appendectomy in pregnant women has yet to be established [27••]. Therefore, until a consensus has been reached concerning its safety, pregnancy remains a contraindication. Several authors have demonstrated that laparoscopic appendectomy is associated with a longer operative time than conventional appendectomy [31,32]. In those patients in whom prolonged operative time is a serious issue (*ie*, those with coagulopathy or cardiorespiratory instability) a laparoscopic approach should not be taken. Another contraindication involves the presence of an ileus or small bowel obstruction [14]. These two conditions interfere with the establishment of a safe pneumoperitoneum, and additionally may result in enterotomy during trocar penetration. Finally, four-quadrant peritonitis is better approached with a midline incision.

Relative contraindications include signs of caput medusae and other evidence of portal hypertension (*ie*, ascites), because the presence of engorged periabdominal veins may increase the risk of damaging a blood vessel during trocar insertion [33]. Because of the increased probability of bowel injury in the presence of extensive adhesions, a history of previous right lower quadrant surgery or inflammatory bowel disease should also serve as a relative contraindication or an impetus for a more conservative approach [14].

EQUIPMENT

The equipment needed to perform laparoscopic appendectomy is listed as follows:

1. Video camera
2. Video monitor
3. CO$_2$ Insufflator
4. 10-mm telescope (0° or 10°)
5. Hasson trocar (blunt tipped)
6. 5- and 11.5-mm trocars (sharp tipped)
7. Endoscopic stapler with refill and vascular cartridge
8. Endoscopic needle-nose dissector
9. Endoscopic Babcock
10. Endoscopic bag (optional)
11. Harmonic stapler (Ethicon Endosurgery, Cincinnati, OH) and endoscopic loop (optional)

TECHNIQUE

Before beginning the operation, the patient is given a broad-spectrum antibiotic, usually a cephalosporin. Next, it is imperative that surgeon, assistant, and equipment positions be established. Although various combinations are possible, the optimal arrangement for viewing and manipulation requires that the surgeon and assistant be on the same side of the table with direct view of the monitor, so that the appendix will be in straight line with, and juxtaposed between, the laparoscope and the television (Fig. 5-1). This positioning allows for line of sight to be 90° from the camera to the television.

Because establishing a pneumoperitoneum is an essential and critical step in any laparoscopic procedure, the initial trocar placement is a very important procedure and should be undertaken with great care. The best method in gaining safe access to the peritoneum is by the open Hasson technique [34]. First, an infra- or supraumbilical incision, approximately 3 cm long, is made directly in the midline. Dissection through any subcutaneous fat is then performed with an electrocautery device until the linea alba is reached. At this point, a direct cut down on the linea alba provides entry into the abdominal cavity. Next, army-navy retractors are used for direct visualization of the peritoneal cavity. If after visualization no adhesions of the small bowel are seen near the umbilical site, an 0-Vicryl suture is placed through the fascia on both sides of the incision. The Hasson (blunt tipped) 10-mm trocar is then placed into the incision and an airtight seal is created by securing the trocar down with the 0-Vicryl sutures. Once the initial trocar is in place, a pneumoperitoneum can be created by insufflating the abdominal cavity to 15 mm Hg pressure.

While insufflating, the laparoscope is adjusted to correct color tones by allowing its camera to equilibrate to a sterile white gauze pad ("white balance"). The laparoscope is then inserted into the peritoneum through the umbilical port, and a general survey of all four quadrants is performed to rule out coexisting pathology. Next, incisions for the two left-sided ports are placed through the skin. The incision for the second (11/12 mm) port is positioned just superior to the anterior superior iliac spine, and the incision for the third (5 mm) port is situated to the left of the rectus muscles and superiorly lateral to the umbilicus (Fig. 5-2). After incising the skin and subcutaneous tissue, a hemostat is used to spread down to the fascia. This is done to avoid resistance when placing the trocar. The respective sharp-tipped trocar is placed into its incision site and is carefully pushed down (*without* activating its blade) until the puncture site can be internally visualized by the laparoscope (Fig. 5-3). It is important to note that the trocars are not inserted through the fascia until transillumination demonstrates that there are no vessels in the intended area of puncture.

Once trocar installation is complete, the patient is placed into Trendelenburg and left lateral decubitus positions. This allows the small bowel to roll off and away from the cecum, thereby allowing for better visualization and manipulation of the appendix. The major anatomic landmarks used for identifying the appendix are the taenia coli. The anterior taenia coli runs along the colon to the base of the appendix. This feature allows the operator to systematically trace the colon to the appendix. If adhesions should obscure this identification, then conversion to an open procedure should be considered. To avoid any pitfalls (such as injury to the small bowel), the mesoappendix and the appendix must be clearly identified and freed up prior to any stapling procedure.

In most cases, the appendix will be intraperitoneal and can be mobilized by freeing up any surrounding adhesions. The best way to accomplish this is by first passing an endoscopic Babcock through the 5-mm port and stabilizing the appendix by grasping it in its midsection. The needle nose dissector can then be introduced through the 11/12-mm port and, with careful teasing and blunt dissection, can be manipulated to successfully free up any appendiceal adhesions. When the appendix appears considerably suppurative or gangrenous, extreme caution should be used when grasping the appendix to avoid excessive tension on its walls and subsequent perforation. Further, if dissection of any adhesions should prove difficult, or if the appendiceal base is gangrenous, conversion to an open procedure should be considered. Following mobilization of the appendix, the needle-nose endoscopic dissector is then used to create a window between the mesoappendix and the base of the appendix (Fig. 5-4).

Once the window is created, the dissector is removed and the endoscopic stapler (with a vascular cartridge) is introduced into the peritoneal cavity through the 11/12-mm port. The stapler is opened intra-abdominally, and one leg is placed through the window. The stapler is closed under direct vision of both stapling legs. After assuring that only the mesoappendix is within the row of staples, the instrument is fired. Once the mesoappendix has been controlled, the stapler is withdrawn and it is loaded with a regular refill. The endoscopic stapler is then reintroduced through the 11/12-mm port, and the appendix is raised anteriorly with the endoscopic Babcock. Next, the stapler is opened and positioned (in the same manner as above) so that it lies around the base of the appendix and is not in contact with the cecum (Fig. 5-5). A small remaining stump is acceptable. It is not necessary to cauterize or invert the stump [29].

After firing, the stapler is taken out and a second endoscopic Babcock is transported through the 11/12-mm port. The detached appendix is transferred from the first endoscopic

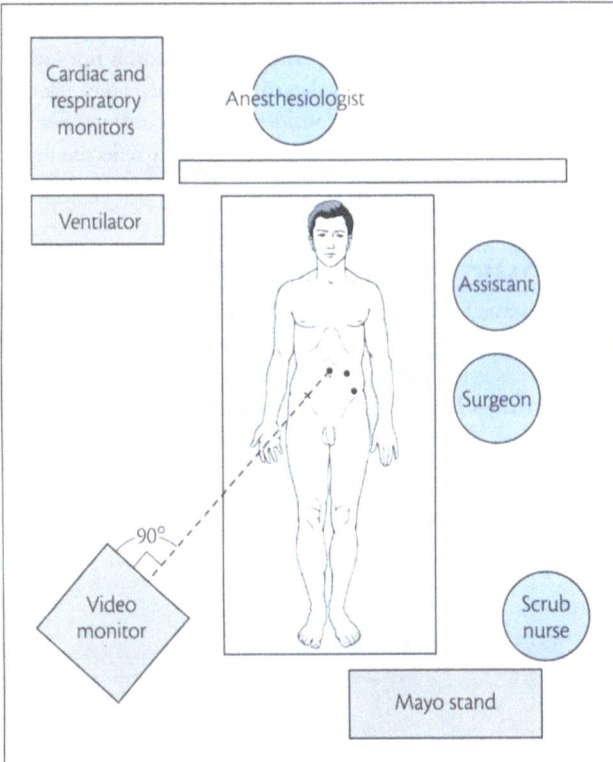

Figure 5-1 Operating room set-up for laparoscopic appendectomy.

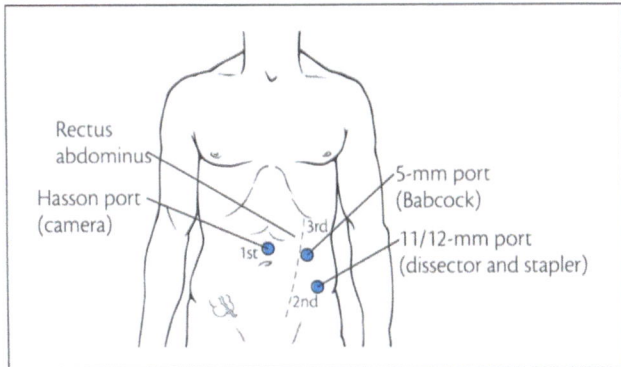

Figure 5-2 Port placement sites for laparoscopic appendectomy.

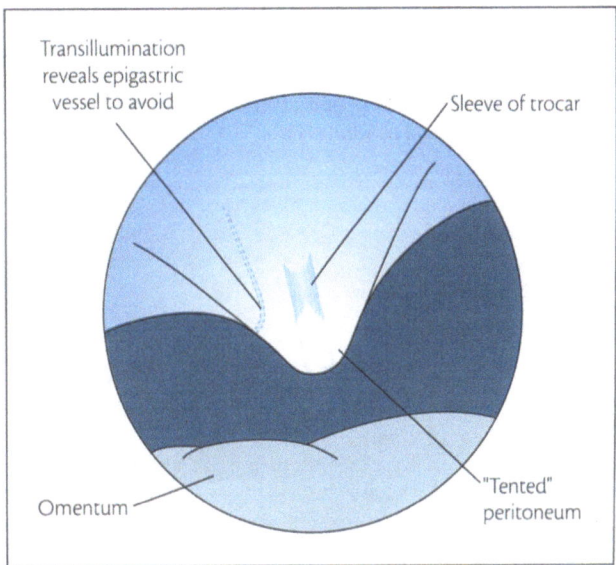

Figure 5-3 Internal visualization of puncture site.

Babcock (which is still grasping its midsection) to the second Babcock. The best method for removing the appendix involves completely withdrawing the second Babcock and appendix up into the sleeve of the 11/12-mm trocar, and then extracting the port with the appendix inside (Fig. 5-6). If the appendix is too large for the 11/12-mm port, or if perforation on removal is feared, the appendix can be transferred to an endoscopic bag prior to removal and then brought out through the umbilical port.

The same trocar is then placed back through the abdominal wall, and the stapled areas are examined for hemostasis. It is not necessary to use a pulse irrigator unless there was perforation and spillage of purulent contents into the peritoneal cavity. Once hemostasis has been established, all equipment is removed from the patient and the incisions that housed the ports are examined for bleeding. If subcutaneous bleeding is present at any of the incisions, cautery is used to achieve hemostasis and the incisions are closed. For closure, an 0-Vicryl "figure eight" stitch is used to close the fascia at the umbilical site. Port sites of 10 mm or larger require fascial closure, but it is not necessary to repair the fascia at the 11/12-mm (second) port site due to its unique location just above the anterior iliac spine. This area acts as a shutter mechanism closing over the defect.

An alternative method of controlling the mesoappendix is with the Harmonic scalpel. This instrument uses ultrasonic pulses to disrupt any protein bonds within tissue it is clamped on; thus it can effectively prevent any hemorrhage from vessels within the mesoappendix. The appendix can then be secured with an endoscopic loop.

The extraperitoneal retrocecal appendix is a more challenging technical exercise. In the majority of cases (approximately 65%), the appendix lies in a low retrocecal position, but is still considered to be in an intraperitoneal position [4,35]. This anatomic situation does not present a great difficulty and can be managed laparoscopically in the manner described previously. However, if the body of the appendix proves to be located behind the cecum or the ascending colon in an extraperitoneal retrocecal position (which occurs in approximately 5% of cases), then more extensive dissection is required (Fig. 5-7) [4,35]. First, it must be technically safe to mobilize the cecum off the retroperitoneum. This approach necessitates lysing the white line of Toldt (lateral peritoneal reflection). If the lateral peritoneal reflection is not readily identifiable or if there are extensive adhesions, then conversion to an open procedure should be considered. After cutting the white line of Toldt, the cecum is capable of being gently reflected medially to expose the appendix.

ANATOMIC HAZARDS

There are several anatomic hazards that one should be mindful of when performing a laparoscopic appendectomy. The first risk a surgeon faces is the potential for retroperitoneal injury on initial trocar insertion. Prior to pneumoperitoneum, the relatively close proximity of the intra-abdominal structures to the anterior abdominal wall can prove troublesome, especially if a blind nee-

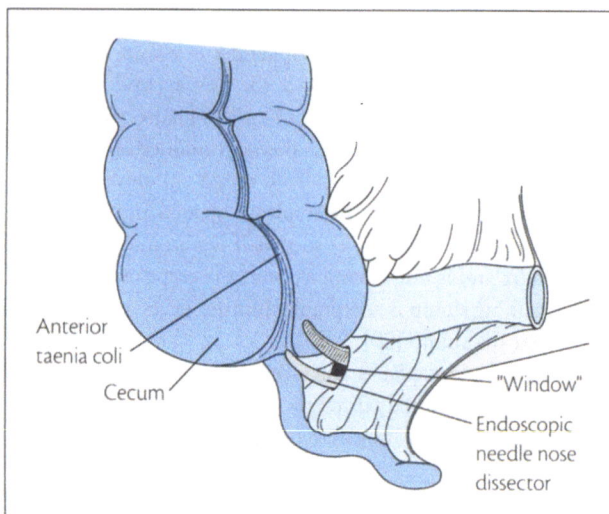

Figure 5-4 Use of the needle-nose endoscopic dissector to create window between the mesoappendix and the base of the appendix. (*Adapted from* Kelly and Hordon [7].)

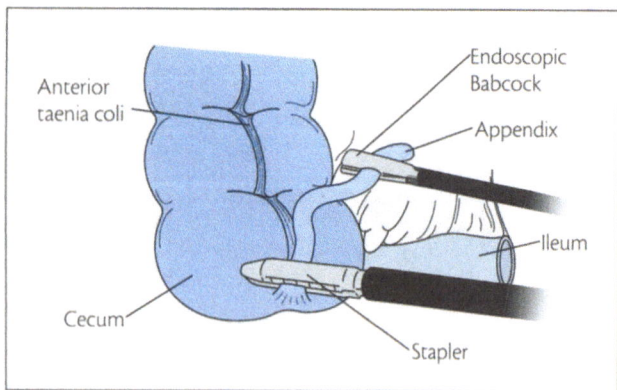

Figure 5-5 Stapling the base of the appendix.

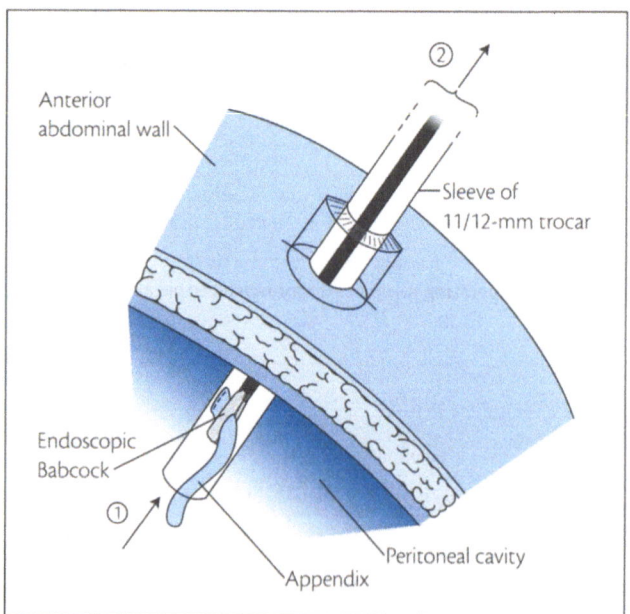

Figure 5-6 Removing the appendix. Second Babcock and appendix are drawn into the sleeve of the 11/12-mm trocar (*1*). Both are then completely extracted along with the port, thereby eliminating direct contact of the appendix with the incision and the risk of subsequent wound infection (*2*).

dle is passed into the peritoneum during the Veress technique [36]. The use of the open Hasson technique will almost always prevent catastrophic retroperitoneal injuries. Two additional methods used to prevent damage to the bladder include having the patient urinate just before admission to the operating room, or (rarely) the introduction of a Foley catheter before the surgery is undertaken.

Another concern is possible injury to vessels of the anterolateral abdominal wall. When performing a laparoscopic appendectomy, the main vessels to avoid in the region of the lower abdominal quadrants are the inferior epigastric and the ascending branch of the deep circumflex iliac vessels. The inferior epigastric artery typically begins just proximal to the inguinal ligament as a branch of the external iliac artery. It courses forward through extraperitoneal tissue to ascend obliquely along the medial margin of the deep inguinal ring, and continues up to pierce the transversalis fascia [37]. The inferior epigatric vessels then run superiorly in the transversalis fascia until they reach the arcuate line, where they enter the rectus sheath and arise between the rectus abdominus muscle and the posterior lamina of its sheath [37,38]. Once in the rectus sheath, the inferior epigastrics divide into numerous branches. To prevent lysing this artery or one of its main branches, the initial Hasson trocar should be placed directly in the midline, and the third trocar should be placed lateral to the left rectus abdominus muscle (Fig. 5-8A).

The deep circumflex iliac artery branches laterally from the external iliac at a point almost opposite to the inferior epigastric artery [37]. It ascends laterally in a sheath formed by the junction of the transversalis and iliac fascia until it reaches the anterior superior iliac spine. At this point, it gives off a large "ascending branch of the deep circumflex iliac artery," which runs superiorly between the internal oblique and transversus muscles to eventually anastomose with the lumbar and inferior epigastric arteries (Fig. 5-8B). Because of its close proximity to the anterior superior iliac spine, this artery or one of its main branches can present a hazard during the insertion of the second trocar. As a precau-

tion, the second trocar should be placed only about a finger breadth directly above the anterior superior iliac spine (Fig. 5-8B).

Another extremely important problem to avoid is injury to the bowel from electrocautery. The judicious use of cautery is essential in avoiding thermal injury to surrounding bowel and the subsequent development of coagulation necrosis (which may lead to a lethal fistula within 3 to 5 days postoperatively). Instead, most mobilization can be performed with blunt and sharp dissection.

POSTOPERATIVE MANAGEMENT

Patients with uncomplicated appendicitis following laparoscopic appendectomy are admitted overnight for precautionary observation, and are usually discharged within 24 hours. One perioperative dose of antibiotic therapy should be sufficient. For complicated appendicitis, intravenous therapy is suggested until enteral feedings resume, and nasogastric decompression is used if there is nausea or vomiting. A broad antibiotic regimen should also be maintained until the patient becomes afebrile and possesses a normal leukocyte count.

LAPAROSCOPIC VERSUS CONVENTIONAL APPENDECTOMY

Since its inception in 1983, laparoscopic appendectomy has been in the throes of controversy regarding its advantages over conventional appendectomy. This controversy largely persists today because the debate focuses on advantages that are not as clearly delineated as they have been for laparoscopic cholecystectomy. As a result, a very complex situation has emerged in which some authors have demonstrated laparoscopic appendectomy as a better approach, others have shown it to be worse, and yet others found no significant differences between the two [31,32,39,40]. Nevertheless, to gain an accurate assessment of laparoscopic appendectomy, it is necessary to examine the published results for each of these controversial topics.

Figure 5-7 Variation in position of appendix. (*Adapted from* Kelly and Hordon [7].)

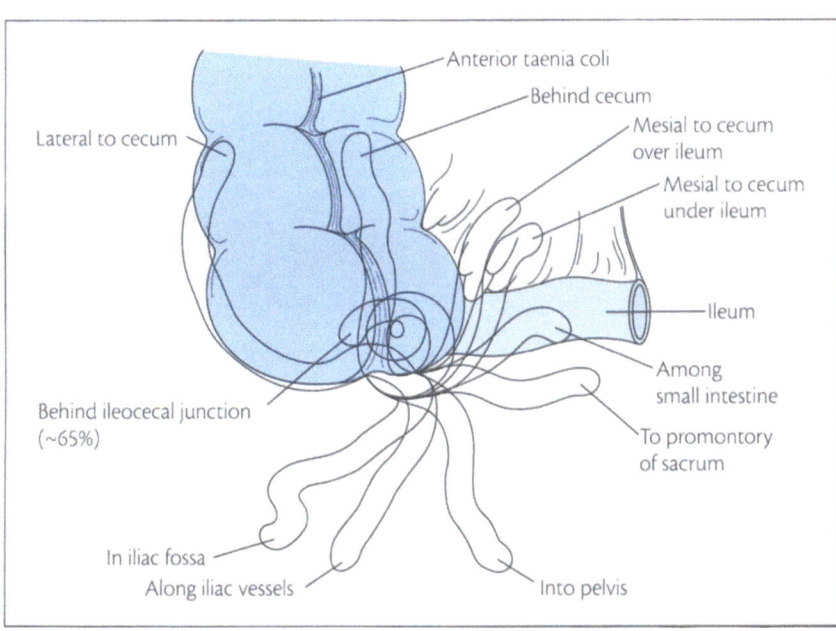

Managed care has created an increasing emphasis for decreased hospitalization, less postoperative pain, and a quicker return to normal activities. Therefore, it is not surprising to find these three elements at the crux of the laparoscopic appendectomy argument. In a retrospective analysis of 154 consecutive patients, Panton and coworkers [41] found the postoperative stay for laparoscopic appendectomy averaged 2.5 days; for open appendectomy, the average stay was 4.5 days ($P = 0.0049$). This same group also found that laparoscopic appendectomy patients had a considerably faster ($P < 0.00065$) return to work and normal activity than open appendectomy patients. Another study by Schroeder and coworkers [42] of 200 patients also demonstrated that postoperative length of stay was shorter (2.7 vs 3.8 days, $P < 0.001$) for laparoscopic appendectomy and that return to normal activity

was quicker (7.8 vs 13.2 days, $P < 0.016$) for laparoscopic appendectomy patients. Further, their study found that postoperative pain following laparoscopic appendectomy was significantly ($P < 0.003$) less than open appendectomy, and that amount of intramuscular pain medication was greater with traditional appendectomy ($P < 0.009$).

Vallina and coworkers [43] showed in a prospective study that although hospital stay was significantly shorter in their laparoscopic appendectomy group (81% discharged on first postoperative day, $P < 0.001$) and laparoscopic appendectomy patients required less narcotic analgesia ($P < 0.02$), the time it took to return to normal activity was not significantly different between the two groups. The advantages of the laparoscopic approach were also illustrated by Williams and coworkers [44] who found

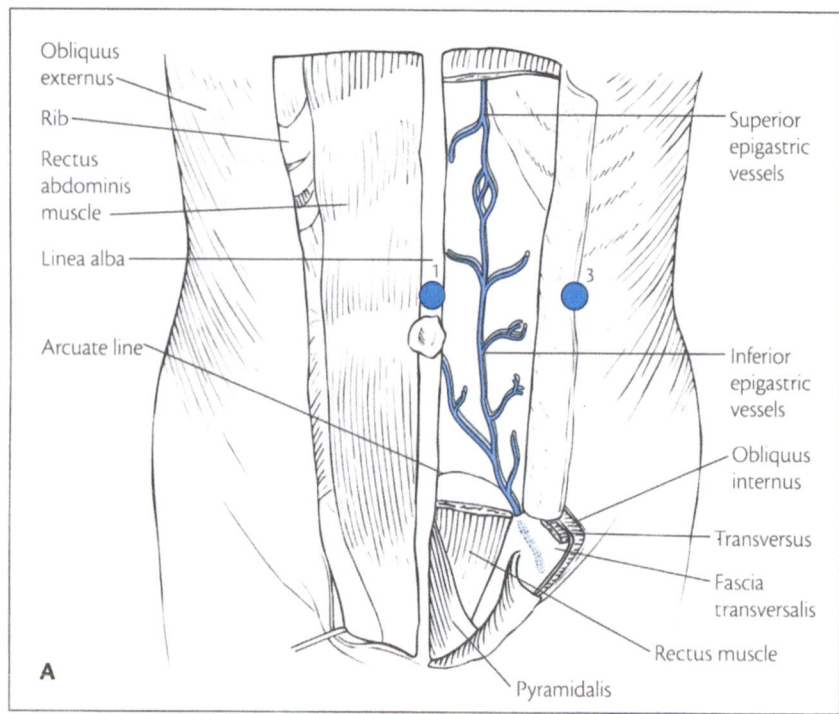

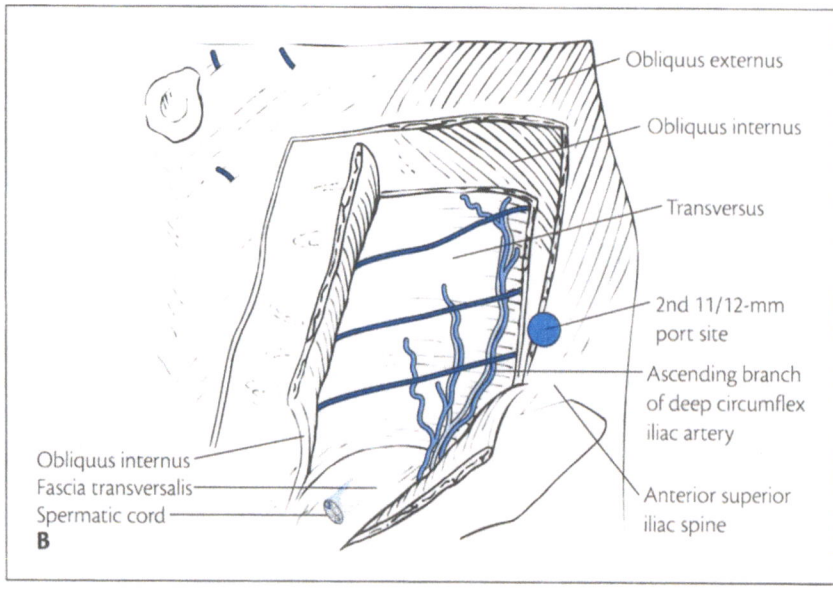

Figure 5-8 Anatomical hazards. **A**, To prevent lysing the inferior epigastric artery or one of its main branches, the initial Hasson trocar should be placed directly in the midline and the third trocar should be placed lateral to the left rectus abdominus muscle (*circles* indicate approximate port sites). **B**, To avoid the ascending branch of the deep circumflex artery or one of its main branches, the second trocar should be placed only about a finger's breadth directly above the anterior superior iliac spine. (*Adapted from* Williams *et al.* [37].)

that 69% of the laparoscopic appendectomy patients received less than 24 hours of postoperative analgesia compared with 44% of the open appendectomy patients. They also showed that 38% of the laparoscopic appendectomy patients were discharged within 24 hours versus 8% of the open appendectomy patients. In prospective analysis of 233 patients, Reiertsen and coworkers [45] reported that postoperative hospital stay and convalescence is longer ($P < 0.05$) with open appendectomy than with laparoscopic appendectomy. Another prospective randomized sampling of 62 patients by Attwood and coworkers [46] illustrated that their laparoscopic appendectomy patients were discharged earlier (2.5 vs 3.8 days, $P < 0.01$) and had a faster return to work. The benefits of laparoscopic appendectomy were also demonstrated in a prospective trial of 100 patients by Heinzelmann and coworkers [31], who also showed that hospital stay was shorter for their laparoscopic appendectomy group. However, Schirmer and coworkers [40] found that postoperative stay was not different for laparoscopic appendectomy (3.5 ± 0.5 days) compared with open appendectomy (5.9 ± 1.6 days). Similar results were published by Rosso and coworkers [47], who showed no difference between laparoscopic appendectomy and open appendectomy regarding hospital stay.

Interestingly, Clarkson and coworkers [48] reported no obvious difference for analgesia requirements or pain between laparoscopic appendectomy and open appendectomy patient groups, and they also found that postoperative stay averaged 6.7 days for laparoscopic appendectomy versus 5.6 days for open appendectomy. Another prospective randomized trial on 100 men by Mutter and coworkers [49•] demonstrated that postoperative pain measurements were not significantly different (4.7 vs 4.4) and length of hospital stay also proved insignificant (4.9 vs 5.3 days) between laparoscopic appendectomy and open appendectomy, respectively. Likewise, a prospective evaluation of 38 female patients by Zaninotto and coworkers [50] reported that no significant differences were observed in median postoperative stay (3 days for laparoscopic appendectomy vs 4 for open appendectomy) or in the number of days (15 for laparoscopic appendectomy vs 18 for open appendectomy) required to return to normal activity. Additionally, Minne and coworkers [51], in a prospective randomized analysis of 50 patients, found no statistical difference between laparoscopic appendectomy and open appendectomy groups for length of hospitalization (median 1.1 vs 1.2 days, respectively), recovery time (median 14 days for both groups), and postoperative pain. The Long Island Jewish Medical Center experience with 235 patients during the past 2 years showed that the average length of hospital stay for laparoscopic appendectomies was 2.4 days. The average length of hospital stay for the open appendectomies during the same period averaged 2.3 days.

Another issue is the cost differential between the two types of appendectomy. Approximately 250,000 case of appendicitis occur annually. If laparoscopic appendectomy is found to be significantly more expensive but becomes routinely performed, then it would be responsible for generating an even greater financial burden on our health care system [52]. In their analysis of 163 patients, McCahill and coworkers [53•] found that laparoscopic appendectomy performed for nonperforative appendicitis led to greater hospital charges ($7760 vs $5064, $P < 0.001$) and did not

reduce hospital stay. A statistical difference in cost between laparoscopic appendectomy and open appendectomy was also reported by Minne and coworkers [51] for operating room charges (median: $3191 laparoscopic appendectomy vs $1514 open appendectomy, $P < 0.001$) and for total hospital charges (median: $5430 laparoscopic appendectomy vs $3673 open appendectomy, $P < 0.001$). These results were also supported by the prospective study performed by Vallina and coworkers [43], who showed that the average cost of laparoscopic appendectomy was 30% greater than that of open appendectomy. Likewise, results ($5430 ± $1944 for open appendectomy vs $6838 ± $2572 for laparoscopic appendectomy) from a study by Apelgren and coworkers [32] also demonstrated that hospital costs for the laparoscopic approach proved to be significantly ($P < 0.05$) more expensive. However, Schirmer and coworkers [40] showed median hospital costs to be comparable ($5899 for laparoscopic appendectomy vs $5220 for open appendectomy). Schroeder and coworkers [42] also found that although the laparoscopic appendectomy approach was more expensive ($8683 vs $6213), the difference was not statistically significant. Interestingly, Gilchrist and coworkers [54] found that although laparoscopic appendectomy is approximately $1000 more expensive than open appendectomy, the total mean cost for each group was comparable because of the shorter hospital stay in the laparoscopic appendectomy group. Similar results were published on a retrospective analysis of 720 patients by Richards and coworkers [55•], who found overall hospital costs ($4800 for laparoscopic appendectomy vs $4950 for open appendectomy) to be comparable. The above results may in the future become reduced if several cost-cutting steps are taken. One of the more costly aspects of the procedure involves the use of the stapler. The stapler could be replaced by the cheaper ligatures, but the stapler's tendency to hasten the procedure and its proven efficacy in published results make the choice a difficult one [48,56•,57]. A more promising method to reduce the extra cost associated with the laparoscopic appendectomy approach is by using reusable instead of disposable instruments. This development proved to be more cost effective for laparoscopic cholecystectomy as reported by Apelgren and coworkers [32], and therefore should be applied to laparoscopic appendectomy (Apelgren and coworkers, Unpublished data).

Another controversial topic concerns the role of laparoscopic appendectomy in complicated cases of appendicitis. Various authors have advocated laparoscopic appendectomy regardless of the severity of the case. For example, Nowzaradan and coworkers [58] found that laparoscopic appendectomy resulted in less postoperative pain, shorter hospital stay, and faster return to normal activities compared with open appendectomy independent of the severity of appendicitis. Other authors claim that cases of suspected perforation are better managed laparoscopically [9,28]. These authors claim that the benefits afforded by the laparoscopic approach include better lavage of the affected area and limited wound exposure to infected tissue on removal of the appendix from the abdominal cavity. Although this theoretically may be true, other published results demonstrate otherwise. A study by Connor and coworkers [59] on 100 patients noted that involvement of the cecum or perforation at the base of the appendix put the appendiceal stump at increased risk for leak and abscess formation. Further, this group recommended conversion to an open procedure on finding intense inflammation or perforation at the base of the appendix. Bonanni and coworkers [60] reported that for complicated appendicitis (gangrenous, perforated, with abscess, or peritonitis), the laparoscopic technique required readmission in 45.5% of the patients compared with only 3% of the patients undergoing open appendectomy. However, Frazee and coworkers [61•] noted that although laparoscopic appendectomy was a good modality for dealing with gangrenous cases, laparoscopic appendectomy for perforative appendicitis was associated with prolonged hospitalization and an increased risk for infectious complications. Frazee and coworkers speculated that the problem in performing laparoscopic appendectomy in cases of severe inflammation is that the appendix tends to fragment by increased manipulation during dissection, which leads to increased contamination of the operative field.

CONCLUSIONS

As corroborated by the European Association for Endoscopic Surgery (EAES) Consensus Conference of 1995, it appears that in the majority of cases, laparoscopic appendectomy results in similar or shorter length of hospital stay, a similar or earlier return to normal activities, and less postoperative pain [27••]. Although these are clear advantages over open appendectomy, an updated literature review, personal experience, and the EAES consensus statement all attest that the current laparoscopic approach to appendectomy is not sufficiently better than the traditional open approach to be considered a gold standard. Laparoscopic appendectomy is particularly useful in cases of diagnostic uncertainty (especially in women of child-bearing age) and in the obese. However, in complicated cases of appendicitis, or in slim men, one cannot unequivocally say that laparoscopic appendectomy provides any substantial advantages over the open approach; therefore, especially because of its excessive costs, a laparoscopic procedure should be viewed with some skepticism in such situations.

REFERENCES AND RECOMMENDED READING

Recently published papers of particular interest have been highlighted as:

* Of interest
•• Of outstanding interest

1. Fernel J: Universa medicina. In *Classic Descriptions of Disease*, edn 3. Edited by Major RH. Springfield, IL: CC Thomas; 1945:646–648.

2. Graffeo CS, Counselman FL: Appendicitis. *Emerg Med Clin North Am* 1996, 14:653–671.

3. Fitz RH: Perforating inflammation of the vermiform appendix, with special reference to its early diagnosis and treatment. *Trans Assoc Am Physicians* 1886, 1:107–144.

4. Sabiston: *Textbook of Surgery*, edn 13 (vol 1). Philadelphia: WB Saunders Co.; 1986.

5. McBurney C: Experiences with early operative interference in cases of diseases of the vermiform appendix. *N Y Med J* 1986, 50:676.

6. Seal A: Appendicitis: a historical review. *Can J Surg* 1981, 24:427–433.

7. Kelly HA, Hordon E: *The Vermiform Appendix and Its Diseases*. Philadelphia: WB Saunders; 1905.

8. Parker W: An operation for abscess of the vermiform appendix caeci. *Med Record (NY)* 1867, 2:25.

9. Bailey RW, Flowers JL: *Complications of Laparoscopic Surgery*. St. Louis: Quality Medical Publishing; 1995:161–182.

10. Lewis FR, Holcroft JW, Boey J, Dunphy JE: Appendicitis: a critical review of diagnosis and treatment in 1,000 cases. *Arch Surg* 1975, 110:667–684.

11. Berry J, Malt RA: Appendicitis near its centenary. *Ann Surg* 1984, 200:567–575.

12. Kazarian KK, Roeder WJ, Mersheimer WL: Decreasing mortality and increasing morbidity from acute appendicitis. *Am J Surg* 1970, 119:681–685.

13. Jacobaeus HC: Kurze ubersicht uber meine erfahrungen mit der laparothorakoscopie. *Munch Med Wochenscher* 1911, 58:2017.

14. Cameron JL: *Current Surgical Therapy*. St. Louis: Mosby; 1995:1025–1028.

15. Kalk H: Erfahrungen mit der Laparoskopie. *Z Klin Med* 1929, 111:303–348.

16. Kalk H, Bruhl W: *Leitfaden der Laparoskopie*. Thieme: Stuttgart; 1951.

17. Berci G: Peritoneoscopy. *BMJ* 1962, 1:562.

18. Berci G: A new approach in optics: the Hopkins "rod lens" system. *Proceedings of the 15th American Symposium of the Society of Photo Optic Engineers*, 3:207.

19. Berci G, Davids J: Endoscopy and television. *BM J* 1962, 1:1610.

20. Berci G, Urban J: A miniature black and white TV camera for endoscopy and other medical applications. *Biomed Eng* 1972, 17:116–121.

21. Shulman AG, Berci G: Intraoperative biliary endoscopy (choledochoscopy) in California hospitals. *Am J Surg* 1985, 149:703–704.

22. Berci G, Brooks P, Paz-Partlow M: TV laparoscopy: a new dimension in visualization and documentation of pelvic pathology. *J Reprod Med* 1986, 31:585–588.

23. Semm K: Endoscopic appendectomy. *Endoscopy* 1983, 15:59–64.

24. Gotz F, Pier A, Bacher C: Modified laparoscopic appendectomy in surgery: a report on 388 operations. *Surg Endosc* 1990, 4:6–9.

25. Valla JS, Limone B, Valla V, *et al.*: Laparoscopic appendectomy in children: report of 465 cases. *Surg Laparosc Endosc* 1990, 1:166–172.

26. Pier A, Gotz F, Bacher: Laparoscopic appendectomy in 625 cases: from innovation to routine. *Surg Laparosc Endosc* 1991, 1:8–13.

27.•• Neugebauer E, Troidl H, Kum CK, *et al.*: The E.A.E.S. consensus development on laparoscopic cholicystectomy, appendectomy, and hernia repair. *Surg Endosc* 1995, 9:550–563.
As of September 1997, this is the only concensus published concerning the feasibility, efficacy, an economy of laparoscopic appendectomy versus the conventional open approach. Their results reflect an assessment of the evidence in previously published articles.

28. MacFayden BV, Ponsky JL: *Operative Laparoscopy & Thoracoscopy*. Philadelphia: Lippincott-Raven; 1996.

29. Calder JDF, Gajraj H: Recent advances in the diagnosis and treatment of acute appendicitis. *Br J Hosp Med* 1995, 54:129–133.

30. Laine S, Rantala A, Gullichsen R, Ovaska J: Laparoscopic appendectomy: is it worthwhile? A prospective randomized study in young women. *Surg Endosc* 1997, 11:95–97.

31. Heinzelman M, Simmen HP, Cummins AS, Largiarder F: Is laparoscopic appendectomy the new 'gold standard'? *Arch Surg* 1995, 130:782–785.

32. Apelgren KN, Molnar RG, Kisala JM: Laparoscopic appendectomy is not better than open appendectomy. *Am Surg* 1995, 61:240–243.

33. Ger R, Abrahams P, Olson TR: *Essentials of Clinical Anatomy*, edn 2. New York: Parthenon Publishing Group; 1996.

34. Hasson HM: Open laparoscopy: a report of 150 cases. *J Reprod Med* 1974, 12:234–238.

35. Wakely CPG: Position of vermiform appendix as ascertained by analysis of 10,000 cases. *J Anat* 1933, 67:277.

36. Veress J: Neves instrument zur ausfuhrung von brustoder bach-punktionen und pneumothoraxbehandlung. *Dtsch Med Wochenschr* 1938, 64:1480–1481.

37. Williams PL, Warwick R, Dyson M, Bannister LH: *Gray's Anatomy*, edn 37. Edinburgh: Churchill Livingstone; 1989.

38. Moore KL: *Clinical Oriented Anatomy*, edn 2. Baltimore: Williams & Wilkins; 1985.

39. Frazee RC, Roberts JW, Symmonds RE: A prospective randomized trial comparing open versus laparoscopic appendectomy. *Ann Surg* 1994, 219:725–731.

40. Schirmer BD, Schmieg RE, Dix J: Laparoscopic versus traditional appendectomy for suspected appendicitis. *Am J Surg* 1993, 165:670–675.

41. Panton ON, Samson C, Segal J, Panton R: A four year experience with laparoscopy in the management of appendicitis. *Am J Surg* 1996, 171:538–541.

42. Schroeder DM, Lathrop JC, Lloyd LR, *et al.*: Laparoscopic appendectomy for acute appendicitis: is there really any benefit? *Am Surg* 1993, 59:541–547.

43. Vallina VL, Velasco JM, McCulloch CS: Laparoscopic versus conventional appendectomy. *Ann Surg* 1993, 218:685–692.

44. Williams MD, Miller D, Graves ED, *et al.*: Laparoscopic appendectomy, is it worth it? *South Med J* 1994, 87:592–598.

45. Reiertsen O, Trondsen E, Bakka A, *et al.*: Prospective nonrandomized study of conventional versus laparoscopic appendectomy. *World J Surg* 1994, 18:411–415.

46. Attwood SE, Hill AD, Murphy PG, *et al.*: A prospective randomized trial of laparoscopic versus open appendectomy. *Surgery* 1992, 112:497–501.

47. Rosso R, Rothenbuhler JM, Linder P: Laparoskopische versus konventionelle Appendektomie: ein Vergleich. *Helv Chir Acta* 1993, 59:567–569.

48. Clarkson R, Waldner H, Siebeck M, Scheiberer L: Hat die laparoskopische Appendektomie Vorteile? Die Laparoskopische appendektomie im Vergleich zur konventionellen Appendektomie-Eine begleitende Untersuchung bei Einfuhrung der Laparoskopie. *Zentralblatt fur Chirurgie* 1995, 118:733–740.

49.• Mutter D, Vix M, Bui A, *et al.*: Laparoscopy not recommended for routine appendectomy in men: results of a prospective randomized study. *Surgery* 1996, 120:71–74.

An interesting study that examined the role of laparoscopic appendectomy in 100 men all with similar (very suggestive) clinical parameters, but of varying age distribution. They do, however, recommend the laparoscopic approach for those men presenting atypical pain of uncertain diagnosis and obese men. These two groups could comprise a significant portion of the male patient population.

50. Zaninotto G, Rossi M, Anselmino M, *et al.*: Laparoscopic versus conventional surgery for suspected appendicitis in women. *Surg Endosc* 1995, 9:337–340.

51. Minne L, Varner D, Burnell A, *et al.*: Laparoscopic vs. open appendectomy: prospective randomized study of outcomes. *Arch Surg* 1997, 132:708–712.

52. Addiss DG, Shaffer N, Fowler BS, Tauxe RV: The epidemiology of appendicitis and appendectomy in the United States. *Am J Epidemiol* 1990, 132:910–925.

53.• McCahill LE, Pellegrini CA, Wiggins T, Helton WS: A clinical outcome and cost analysis of laparoscopic versus open appendectomy. *J Surg* 1996, 171:533–537.

This paper presents an extensive cost analysis of laparoscopic appendectomy compared with the open procedure. However, it examines 163 appendectomies performed at the University of Washington Medical Center during a period of 4 years, and the laparoscopic sample only constitutes 17% of the total number of appendectomies performed.

54. Gilchrist BF, Lobe TE, Schropp KP, *et al.*: Is there a role for laparoscopic appendectomy in pediatric surgery? *J Pediatr Surg* 1992, 27:209–212.

55.• Richards KF, Fisher KS, Flores JH, Christensen BJ: Laparoscopic appendectomy: comparison with open appendectomy in 720 patients. *Surg Laparosc Endosc* 1996, 6:205–209.

This paper reported on a large review of both procedures over a 3-year period at the LDS Hospital in Salt Lake City. It surprisingly demonstrated comparable overall costs that are probably a reflection of the significantly reduced morbidity rates achieved by the laparoscopic approach in their study.

56.• Ortega AE, Hunter JG, Peters JH, *et al.*: A prospective randomized comparison of laparoscopic appendectomy to open appendectomy. *Am J Surg* 1995, 169:208–213.

This article presented evidence on 253 patients involved in a prospective, randomized study highlighting several of the benefits of laparoscopic over conventional appendectomy. Interestingly, they noticed a statistically significant number of patients with emesis following the laparoscopic procedure.

57. Wagner M, Aronsky D, Tschudi J, *et al.*: Laparoscopic stapler appendectomy: a prospective study of 267 consecutive cases. *Surg Endosc* 1996, 10:895–899.

58. Nowzaradan Y, Barnes JP, Westmoreland J, Hojabri M: Laparoscopic appendectomy: treatment of choice for suspected appendicitis. *Surg Laparosc Endosc* 1993, 3:411–416.

59. Connor TJ, Garcha IS, Ramshaw BJ, Mitchell CW, *et al.*: Diagnostic laparoscopy for suspected appendicitis. *Am Surg* 1995, 61:187–189.

60. Bonanni F, Reed J, Hartzell G, *et al.*: Laparoscopic versus conventional appendectomy. *J Am Coll Surg* 1995, 179:273–278.

61.• Frazee RC, Bohannon WT: Laparoscopic appendectomy for complicated appendicitis. *Arch Surg* 1996, 131:509–512.

This study found that laparoscopic appendectomy for perforative appendicitis was associated with prolonged hospitalization and an increased risk of infectious complications.

Laparoscopic Colon and Small Bowel Surgery

Morris E. Franklin, Jr.
Jorge Balli

Laparoscopic cholecystectomy and laparoscopic antireflux procedures have become the standard for treating gallbladder disease and refractory gastroesophageal reflux in the United States and virtually every developed nation. Relatively few other procedures in the overall scheme of surgery have been embraced with as much enthusiasm as these operations. The advantages to the patient, compared with standard open procedures, include less pain, quicker recovery, less hospitalization time, fewer complications (in the hands of skilled surgeons), and quicker return to full activity. Few surgeons, however, have adapted laparoscopic technology to other procedures.

Appendectomy appears to be the next gastrointestinal procedure to proceed from laparoscopic cholecystectomy. However, many surgeons still believe that the benefits of appendectomy are minimized by a laparoscopic approach, although the advantages of laparoscopic appendectomy are being reported in increasing numbers [1,2•], Glass and coworkers (Paper presented at the Society of Laparoscopic Surgeons Meeting, Orlando, 1996). These studies demonstrated a relatively clear advantage in cost as well as a lessening in postoperative pain and a quicker return to full function. Other series have indicated that the overall cost is virtually the same for laparoscopic versus open appendectomy, but that the complication rate for laparoscopy (particularly that of wound infections) is tremendously reduced in all patients considered and the recovery time is improved (Franklin and coworkers, Unpublished data).

Reports of small bowel obstructions being relieved laparoscopically, as well as Meckel's diverticulectomy and small bowel resections, are beginning to appear, but these are far from common practice in most surgical communities. Larger series of colon resections for benign and malignant diseases from authors such as Franklin, Jacobs, Wilson, Köckerling, Phillips, Groce, and Fowler also are beginning to appear; however, the great majority of colon resections and colon procedures (both resectional and nonresectional) for the most part are still performed with open techniques. Many surgeons have incorporated some form of laparoscopic bowel surgery into their practice, but a far greater number have not embraced laparoscopic surgery for a variety of reasons.

TECHNICAL ADVANCES

During the past year, few true technical advances have occurred in laparoscopy. However, there has been a gradual improvement in the currently available tools, particularly regarding the reliability and safety of these tools. Prominent among the technical advances is the introduction of 10-mm scissors as well as the incorporation of bipolar cautery into the realm of laparoscopic colon and small bowel surgery. Very little doubt exists that better functioning and more reliable laparoscopic stapling devices are now available than in the early 1990s. Endo-GIA and TA devices (US Surgical

Corporation, Norwalk, CT) provide a very secure method of controlling larger portions of mesentery as well as individual vessels (Fig. 6-1). Many authors incorporate both laparoscopically assisted as well as totally intracorporeal techniques for resection of bowel segments as well as anastomosis. This primarily resulted from more experience with these techniques, as well as improvement in stapling devices, vascular control devices, and bowel contents control devices, such as bags, clamps, and so forth. Nevertheless, laparoscopically assisted colon resection and small bowel surgery remain the most widely used and accepted form of laparoscopic bowel procedures. Laparoscopic Glassman Bulldog clamps (Klein Medical, San Antonio, TX) have also become available for control of large vessels followed by division and application of pretied loops for controlling bowel contents, and preventing spillage in those patients whose bowel is open intraperitoneally during a given procedure (Fig. 6-2). These devices obviate occupying a trocar site with an externally directed clamping device, and they have the advantage of being manipulable intra-abdominally during a given procedure.

Reports are appearing concerning gasless techniques for right and left colon resections, as well as a large series of laparoscopic cholecystectomy procedures performed with a nondisposable laparoscopic lift system by Speranza (Paper presented at the 4th Brazilian Conference of Endoscopy, Geonia, Brazil, 1994) from Argentina. A significant advance, for those surgeons who believe that the ability to handle a specimen or palpate vessels and intra-abdominal structures is vital, has been the pneumatic sleeve. This device incorporates a closed-sleeve mechanism that can be attached to the abdominal wall and form a seal around an incision large enough to accommodate the surgeon's hand. A hand then can be introduced through the pneumatic sleeve, maintaining pneumoperitoneum and allowing palpatory dissection of vessels, palpation of lymph nodes, and reportedly enhanced mobilization of a given segment of the colon compared with pure intracorporeal laparoscopic techniques. This device should be available commercially very shortly, and it certainly will

enhance the ability to feel the structures to be sure of the anatomy and aid in dissection. The importance of temperature regulation during laparoscopic surgery has become more prominent during the past year, and numerous devices are being introduced that heat irrigation fluids, heat intravenous fluids, and help maintain the hemostasis of a patient undergoing a laparoscopic bowel procedure. Several companies now have introduced carbon dioxide humidifying devices that will greatly aid in maintaining and preventing excessive heat loss during somewhat prolonged laparoscopic bowel procedures. The ultrasonic dissector (Ethicon Endosurgery Inc., Cincinnati, OH) is gaining wide acceptance as a time-saving and safe tool for dividing mesentery, once the main trunk of a parent vessel has been secured with either a suture tie or staples. The primary use of the device has been in the division of short gastric vessels as a part of the stomach mobilization for Nissen fundoplications and other procedures for the treatment of gastroesophageal reflux. Use of the device for divisions of colonic mesentery was initially described by Fowler and Geis and is now used extensively by others both in colonic disease as well as small bowel mesentery divisions. We have also used the device in creating enterotomies of the small bowel as well as gastrotomies for foreign body and benign tumor removal from the stomach.

A new and exciting technique using minisite laparoscopy instrumentation to aid in removal of benign lesions of the colon has been introduced in our institution. In this technique, benign polyps or other lesions that are at poor angles for removal with the colonoscope are approached with an intraluminal technique and are mobilized and maneuvered into positions to allow easy access with the colonoscopic snare. This technique, which may offer a method to handle extremely difficult or large sessile polyps without the need for formal colon resection, has been quite successful in our hands.

STATUS OF CURRENT PROCEDURES

Numerous procedures are now being performed laparoscopically for a variety of small bowel diseases. These include Meckel's

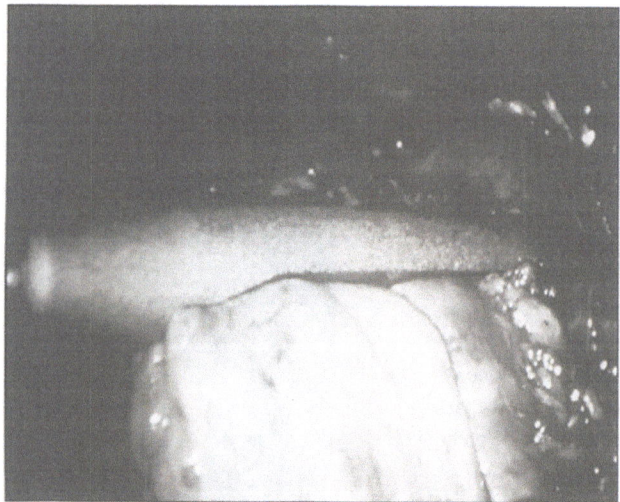

Figure 6-1 An Endo-GIA (US Surgical Corporation, Norwalk, CT) dividing the transverse colon in a right intracorporeal hemicolectomy. (*See* Color Plate.)

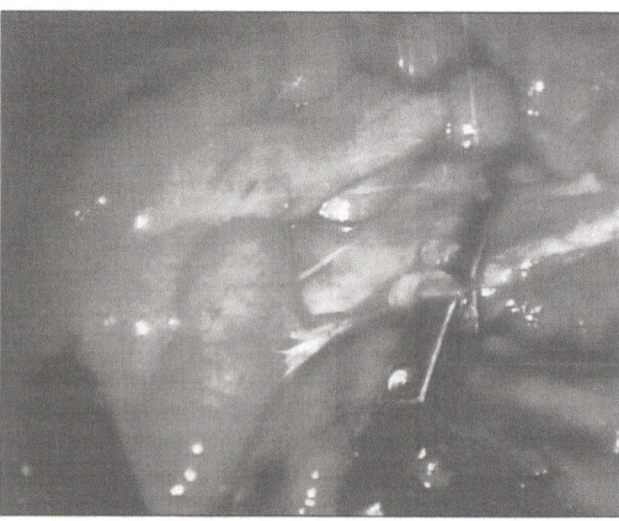

Figure 6-2 A laparoscopic Glassman Bulldog clamp (Klein Medical, San Antonio, TX) on a vessel for control. (*See* Color Plate.)

diverticulectomy, lysis of adhesions, and resection of bowel for intestinal obstruction and extensive resection for benign and malignant diseases. Reissman and coworkers [3] reported a large series of resections for Crohn's disease. Foreign body removal for problems such as gallstone ileus, perforation from objects (*eg,* fish bones or toothpicks), reduction of incarcerated hernia from inguinal and incisional hernia, and bypass procedures for malignancy all have been performed as well. Cuschieri (Paper presented at the World Congress of Endosurgery, Kyoto, 1994) reported a large series of bypass procedures for pancreatic malignancy complemented by ongoing studies in numerous centers, especially those by Conlon (Personal communication) from Memorial Sloan–Kettering in New York. One area that may have a great deal of applicability but rarely is used is laparoscopic resolution of intestinal obstruction. In a large series by Petelin (Paper presented at the World Congress of Endosurgery, Kyoto, 1994) as well as by Dorman and coworkers [4], the success rate of the laparoscopic approach has been exceptionally high. An additional series by a group in Belgium demonstrated similarly good results from a laparoscopic approach to intestinal obstruction (Vereecken and the Belgium Group for Endoscopic Surgery (BGES), Paper presented at the Society of American Gastroendoscopic Surgeons, Phoenix, 1993). Judicious use of laparoscopy in intestinal obstruction and also diagnosis in extremely ill patients seems to be an area of increased interest and enhanced use. The application of laparoscopic techniques for determination of bowel viability has been used in my hospital in the intensive care unit on several occasions (Franklin, Paper presented at the VIII Curso Internacional de Cirugia General, Monterrey, Mexico, 1997). Laparoscopy also has been used to demonstrate perforation and massive fecal contamination in patients whose disease has not been salvageable (Figs. 6-3 and 6-4). This has resulted in early diagnosis and greatly aided early decision-making for patients with viable disease or those with no chance of survival in the intensive care unit (Petelin, Personal communication; Franklin and coworkers, Unpublished data) [5].

Tremendous interest has been generated in the area of laparoscopic colon resection—varying from isolated reports of right and sigmoid colon resections to extensive subtotal and total colectomy, low anterior resection, transverse colon resections, and abdominoperineal resections—by a number of authors for a variety of lesions. Early series demonstrated the frustration that surgeons experienced with the new technique. These series exhibited a wide variety of complications and an extraordinarily high incidence of conversion to open surgery, and, by the authors' own admissions, the learning curve was very steep [6,7]. These series are compared with surgeons with previous experience performing laparoscopy and who adapted laparoscopic techniques to colon procedures; thus, in the setting of previously acquired laparoscopic skills, the conversion rate was very low [8••,9]. Laparoscopy for colonic diseases now is performed for a variety of both malignant and nonmalignant disease processes, varying from the mere diagnosis of disease to staging and frank therapeutic resections. Resections done laparoscopically include extensive resections for the attempted cure of malignant disease, as well as limited, segmental resections for palliation of advanced disease. In addition, laparoscopy is being used for colonic polypectomy, in which the procedure is performed with a colonoscope under laparoscopic monitoring (Franklin and Gayet, Unpublished data). Perforation can be readily detected and repaired immediately with this technique.

Laparoscopic procedures have been used for construction of colostomies, take-down of colostomies, and repair of Hartmann's pouch, and now have become the technique of choice for many groups who realize that even in the setting of prior multiple operations and extensive inflammation, colostomy repair and reconstruction of a preexistent Hartmann's pouch after a proper waiting time often is superior to standard open procedures. Many wound complications attendant to the open procedures are completely avoided with these techniques; thus there is a decrease in the duration of hospitalization and resultant costs [10]. Second-look procedures for suspected recurrent carcinoma also have been used in isolated instances by various authors (Greene, Personal communication).

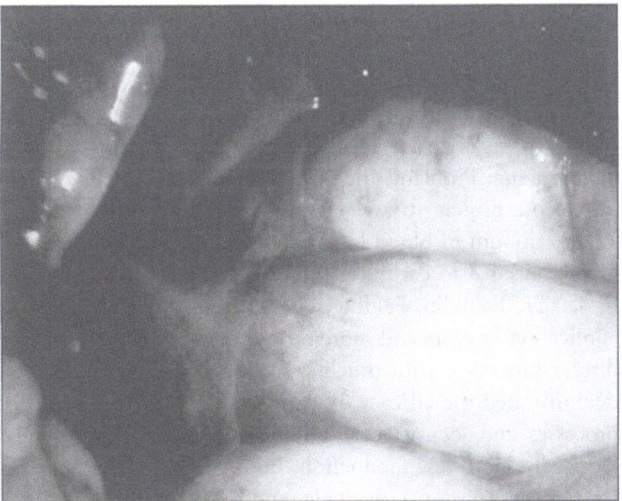

Figure 6-3 Dead bowel of a patient in an intensive care unit demonstrating extensive necrosis and no need for further treatment. (*See* Color Plate.)

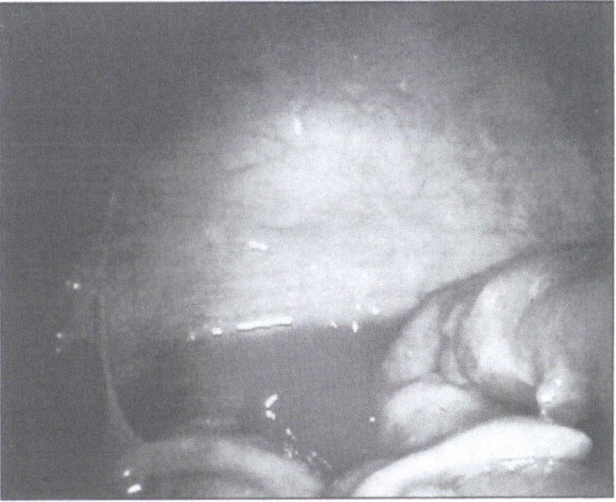

Figure 6-4 Diverticular perforation with peritonitis. (*See* Color Plate.)

CONDITIONS EASILY TREATED WITH LAPAROSCOPY

A number of indications for small bowel surgery can be accomplished easily with laparoscopy. Among these are intestinal obstruction, foreign body removal, perforation repair, and obstruction. There has been very little experience in resection of the small bowel for carcinoma. Reissman and coworkers [3] have extensive experience with small bowel resection for Crohn's disease.

Surgical treatment of intestinal obstruction presents problems in accessing the peritoneal cavity. Litwin has stated that after obtaining access with the Veress needle, the amount of gas insufflated in the peritoneum is proportional to the success in completing the surgery (Litwin, Paper presented at the Postgraduate Course in Society of American Gastrointestinal Endoscopic Surgeons, San Diego, 1997).

I have approached virtually 100% of intestinal obstructions laparoscopically during the past 4 years and have found few problems with insufflation or identification of the obstruction. In 87% of the patients, resolution of the small bowel obstruction was accomplished laparoscopically. Causes of these obstructions include adhesions, internal hernias, volvulus, and foreign bodies such as gallstones and gallstone ileus (Kwitko, Paper presented at the International Symposium on Minimal Access Surgery, Montreal, 1994). In all cases, the small bowel must be examined; retrograde examination from the cecum is the easiest method. I primarily use 5-mm laparoscopic Glassman clamps and handle the bowel atraumatically. I strongly urge avoiding routine graspers to hold the small bowel, because this injures the tissues much like a hemostat injures the bowel. If only 5-mm graspers are available, running the bowel using the mesentery prevents bowel injury. Obviously, this approach is unwise in patients who have had multiple prior operations. If a foreign body (*eg*, gallstone or toothpick) is in the bowel, it can be removed easily by performing an enterotomy. The enterotomy can be closed using either laparoscopic suturing techniques or with a stapling device, such as an Endo-GIA stapler. Resection of the small bowel also can be accomplished totally intracorporeally with either a hand-sewn anastomosis or a functional end-to-end, side-to-side, triple-stapled anastomosis, or extraperitoneally by a number of techniques.

CLINICAL APPLICATIONS

Today, laparoscopy is being applied to a number of small bowel and colonic procedures. Table 6-1 lists the currently used techniques for laparoscopic application to the small bowel. Laparoscopy currently is being used in many centers for evaluation of small bowel trauma where minimal injuries have been repaired primarily; this method is currently undergoing further evaluation. Because intestinal obstruction has a wide variety of causes, many surgeons use laparoscopy as their primary treatment option for intestinal obstruction. It results in lower cost, less hospitalization, and quicker rehabilitation of the patient. Laparoscopic evaluation of perforated viscus also is being evaluated, as are diagnostic modalities for determination of ischemic bowel.

Colonic procedures can be divided into resectional and nonresectional procedures. Nonresectional procedures include diagnostic laparoscopy for benign and malignant disease, diagnostic procedures for diverticulitis with possible therapeutic options including treatment of perforations, drainage of diverticular phlegmon, and lavage and drainage for peritonitis [11]. Other nonresectional therapies include the previously mentioned colotomy and laparoscopically monitored colostomy for polypectomy, colotomy for foreign body removal, and laparoscopically monitored colonoscopic polypectomy, in which large polyps are excised with a colonoscope while being monitored laparoscopically and the repair of perforations readily achieved. In the realm of carcinoma, many advanced laparoscopists now are using laparoscopy as one of several evaluation devices for staging and resection of colon cancer. There are several large series conducted in the United States, Brazil, Europe, and Australia in which resection and colectomy, resection with end-on-end colostomy, and resection and anastomosis have been performed. Evaluation of liver metastasis and frank resection of metastatic lesions have been performed by several authors using laparoscopic ultrasound techniques.

ADVANCES IN THE FIELD

Initial reports of laparoscopic colon procedures were somewhat discouraging. Problems included a steep learning curve (leading to an exorbitantly large rate of conversion to open surgery), a large amount of blood loss, and extraordinarily long periods of time needed to complete the procedure. More recent series by Jacobs, Franklin, Felding, and Geis have demonstrated an application of more and more procedures for a wider variety of disease processes, with much better results. These series have demonstrated the efficacy of colon resection for many disease processes and, consistently, an increase in cost-effectiveness, reduced blood loss, reduction in operating time, speedier recovery, less postoperative pain, and fewer complications, particularly wound complications. Currently several large multi-center studies are in progress regarding the efficacy of laparoscopic colon resection for carcinoma. A nationwide registry is

---

Table 6-1

Techniques for application of laparoscopy to the small bowel

Relief of small bowel obstruction secondary to adhesions or incarcerated hernias

Foreign body removal

Bypass procedure for malignant and benign disease

Bypass procedure for intestinal obstruction

Bypass procedure for ischemic bowel that includes resection of Meckel's diverticulum

Inflammatory bowel disease (*eg*, Crohn's disease) with evaluation and resection as indicated

available and a nationwide multicenter study for randomized case selection also is in progress. These data undoubtedly will help clarify the role of laparoscopic colon resection for cure and palliation of colon carcinoma. At present, patients should be informed of the investigational nature of laparoscopic colon resection for carcinoma, and that the data regarding the efficacy of this procedure for cancer cure are not conclusive.

Trocar site implantations have been the Achilles heel of laparoscopic colon resections for carcinoma. Numerous techniques for reducing the chance of this problem have been introduced and are being practiced by a number of surgeons worldwide. Among the instruments and techniques in progress, tumor-resistant trocars that will effectively resolve this problem. These devices are not on the market as yet, but are certainly on the drawing board.

ONGOING STUDIES AND DEVELOPMENTS

Among the new developments in laparoscopic surgery for colon and small bowel resection is that of very careful preoperative staging in the case of carcinoma, including CT, magnetic resonance imaging (MRI), and even diagnostic laparoscopy. Radioactive immunologic imaging with monoclonal antibodies and laparoscopic sensor probes are being used in several centers to help determine the efficacy of the laparoscopic approach to colon procedures. Various ultrasound devices, particularly for staging colon cancer, evaluation of potential liver metastasis, and for evaluation of para-aortic nodes in the process of these dissections, are being studied as well. There also is a wider acceptance of the importance of intraoperative colonoscopy, particularly for demonstrating nonvisible intraluminal lesions (especially those of adenomatous polyps) as well as using immediately preoperative colonoscopy with ink marking of polyps that are planned to be removed laparoscopically either by colotomy or by segmental bowel resection. There have been several attempts to use intraluminal devices for actual intraluminal surgery of the large and small bowel. The applicability of this technology is yet to be determined. This technique certainly should have some applicability, however, in resection of larger polyps and perhaps ligation of bleeding arteriovenous malformations in patients for whom resection is not feasible.

Reports are also appearing on the approach to metastatic liver disease, including hepatic artery catheterization for chemotherapy and resection of liver metastases (Vereecken and the BGES, Paper presented at the Society of American Gastroendoscopic Surgeons, Phoenix, 1993) [7,12]. Second-look procedures are becoming more popular for rising carcinoembryonic antigen titers or other indications of recurrent carcinoma. Investigations of cryosurgical techniques for treatment of liver metastases are also currently being conducted. In the realm of anastomotic technique, several descriptions of transanal anastomotic techniques—both suturing and application of a stapling device from a transanal standpoint—have appeared. The work of Buess and coworkers [13] with transanal resection of early carcinomas is well known, but has been very slow to receive acceptance in the United States.

NEW EQUIPMENT

Very little in the way of new equipment is available for laparoscopic bowel surgery. Several devices have been refined, however, and are now becoming commercially available. These devices can be adapted readily to laparoscopic colon and small bowel procedures. Among these is the ultrasound probe for evaluation of liver metastases, which will probably become a standard of care for laparoscopic colon resection for carcinoma. Improved camera optic systems and scopes with movement of the chip to the end of the scope will be a dramatic improvement. Future devices will include cordless laparoscopes that have radiotransmission of signals as well as the optical system. This certainly will help the laparoscopic surgeon to perform the surgery without the cumbersome addition of cords. Computer-controlled laparoscopic holding and manipulating devices are now available to decrease the number of assistants needed for a given procedure as well as provide a steady optical field.

Improved suturing and stapling techniques are arriving as well. The US Surgical Corporation has developed a new suturing device that does not require passage of a suture from the outside, but provides a suturing device loaded within the suture driver itself. Wound protectants for transabdominal extraction of carcinomatous lesions in particular are being used more often and should provide a valuable aid in preventing implantation of tumor cells when carcinoma is being approached laparoscopically.

Köckerling from Erlangen, Germany has designed and is currently using a laparoscopic purse-stringing device that secures the anvil during the performance of intracorporeal anastomoses. Although laparoscopically assisted colon resection techniques are the most common technique for completing laparoscopic colon resections and stapled anastomosis, there is a growing interest in totally intracorporeal techniques by a number of investigators.

The need for smaller Endo-GIA stapling and cutting devices has been met by US Surgical Corporation with the release of the Endo GIA-II. This 12-mm instrument will allow use of 30-, 45-, and 60-mm stapling techniques with the same nongasfired instrument. This instrument will allow an entire procedure to be performed without changing trocars or requiring changes in stapling instruments frequently during a procedure. New bags are arriving daily that will be impermeable to carcinoma cells as well as to bacteria and greatly reduce the chance of carcinoma implantation and fecal contamination as specimens are being removed.

The current generation of circular staplers is a vast improvement over the initial generation, and a low-profile anvil has made placement of the anvil in the proximal segment of bowel intracorporeally much easier. The reliability of the circular staplers is well documented. Improvement in these staplers is becoming evident. Consistent vascular control devices, such as clips and TA staplers, also have enhanced the laparoscopic surgeon's ability to complete colon and small bowel resection. Sixty-millimeter Endo-GIA stapling and cutting devices have revolutionized many of the procedures currently being performed. Very little known but nevertheless widely applicable laparoscopic surgical devices are the laparoscopic Glassman

Bulldog intestinal and vascular clamps produced by Klein Medical. These devices allow adequate control of open bowel contents as well as excellent control of larger vessels, where division and control with a pretied loop device is required.

CONCLUSIONS

Almost all small and large bowel disease processes, at least initially, can be approached laparoscopically with good resolution of a high percentage of the cases. My approach to all intestinal obstructions is in the routine manner over the first 24 hours, and if no improvement or worsening occurs in any parameter, a laparoscopy is immediately performed. Approximately 85% of intestinal obstructions have been resolved with laparoscopic technique, and determination of the disease process has been accurate in 100% of patients [14••].

All patients with diverticulitis now are initially treated conservatively with antibiotics and intravenous fluids. If the condition worsens or the patient does not improve significantly within the first 24 hours, a diagnostic laparoscopy is performed. If a perforation is recognized and fecal contamination is minimal, the perforation is closed, an appendices epiploica sutured over the hole, and the cavity is drained. If there is extensive contamination and the hole cannot be closed, or an abscess is present, a diverting colostomy or diversion with resection is performed along with drainage of the abscess. If the patient has gross fecal contamination or the phlegmon is so large that it cannot be handled laparoscopically, an open procedure is performed. Using this technique, I have now performed approximately 64 emergency procedures on patients with diverticulitis.

My approach to carcinoma of the colon is to inform the patient very carefully of the investigational nature of the laparoscopic colon resection. Second, I inform the patient that the case will be entered into a large study group to determine the efficacy of laparoscopic colon resection for cure of carcinoma. Third, if any doubt exists as to the adequacy of the resection for a given carcinoma, the procedure will be converted to open surgery. Fourth, an open procedure is offered to each and every patient for resection of the colon. In my practice, I find very few patients who will opt for an open procedure; thus, I have a large number of laparoscopic colon resections for carcinoma with results that are equal to or better than open procedures from a large group of patients operated on by standard open techniques.

At this time, the vast majority of small and large bowel procedures can be performed laparoscopically, at least in the hands of those surgeons who feel confident of handling these procedures with the laparoscope. It is imperative that each surgeon who deals with small and large bowel disease fully inform each and every patient about the pros and cons of open versus laparoscopic procedures, of both benign and malignant disease, and communicate in an objective, truthful, straightforward manner. Finally, each surgeon who opts to perform this type of surgery, both open and closed, should keep meticulous records and be willing to submit these records for close scrutiny and publication of results.

REFERENCES AND RECOMMENDED READING

Recently published papers of particular interest have been highlighted as:

• Of interest

•• Of outstanding interest

1. Frazee R, Roberts J, Symmonds R, *et al.*: A prospective randomized trial comparing open versus laparoscopic appendectomy. *Ann Surg* 1994, 219:725–731.

2.• Richards K, Fisher K, Flores J, Christensen B: Laparoscopic appendectomy: comparison with open appendectomy in 720 patients. *Surg Laparosc Endosc* 1996, 6:205–209.
The first large randomized study on laparoscopic appendectomy demonstrating diminished pain for the patient.

3. Reissman P, Salky BA, Pfeifer J, *et al.*: Laparoscopic surgery in the management of inflammatory bowel disease. *Am J Surg* 1996, 171:47–50.

4. Dorman J, Franklin M, Schuessler W: Laparoscopic treatment of gallstones ileus: a case report and review of the literature. *J Laparoendosc Surg* 1994, 4:165–171.

5. Bender J, Talamini M: Diagnostic laparoscopy in critically ill intensive care unit patients. *Surg Endosc* 1992, 6:302–304.

6. Wexner S, Johonsen O, Nagueras J, Jogelman D: Laparoscopic total abdominal colectomy: a prospective trial. *Rectum* 1992, 35:651–655.

7. Monson J, Darzi A., Carey P, Guillou P: Prospective evaluation of laparoscopic-assisted colectomy in an unselected group of patients. *Lancet* 1992, 324:831–833.

8.•• Franklin M, Ramos R, Rosenthal D, Schuessler W: Laparoscopic colonic procedures. *World J Surg* 1994, 17:51–56.
This paper reports that the conversion rate to open surgery during colon procedures was very low when the surgeons had previous experience performing laparoscopy.

9. Jacobs M, Vergeja G, Goldstein D: Minimally invasive colon resection. *Surg Laparosc Endosc* 1991, 1:144–150.

10. Franklin M, Rosenthal D, Norem R: Prospective evaluation of laparoscopic colonic resection versus open colon resection for adenocarcinoma: a multicenter study. *Surg Endosc* 1995, 9:811–816.

11. Franklin ME, Dorman JP, Jacobs M, Plasencia G: Is laparoscopic surgery applicable to complicated colonic diverticular disease? *Surg Endosc* 1997, 11:1021–1025.

12. Franklin M, Rosenthal D, Ramos R: Laparoscopic colectomy: utopia or reality? *Gastrointest Endosc Clin North Am* 1993, 3:353–365.

13. Buess G, Mentges B, Manncke K, *et al.*: Minimally invasive surgery in the treatment of rectal cancer. *Int J Colorectal Dis* 1991, 6:77–81.

14.•• Franklin ME, Dorman J: Laparoscopic surgery in acute small bowel obstruction. *Surg Laparosc Endosc* 1994, 4:1289–1296.
In this study the authors report that approximately 85% of intestinal obstructions were resolved with a laparoscopic technique.

Laparoscopy for Staging of Malignancy

Patrick G. Jackson
David W. Rattner

Accurate staging is a critical step in caring for patients with cancer: it dictates not only the possible therapeutic options at the time of diagnosis, but also provides important prognostic information. Clinical staging of abdominal malignancies requires a thorough history and physical examination and may require endoscopic examinations, imaging studies, and laparoscopy. These modalities are complimentary, and each should be selected so that any information gained from the examination will alter treatment options. Laparoscopy is useful in combination with imaging studies for staging esophageal, gastric, hepatic, biliary, and pancreatic neoplasms [1]. Laparoscopy is particularly useful and cost-effective in reducing the number of nontherapeutic laparotomies with their associated morbidity, cost, and convalescence.

With the advent of balloon dilation, endoscopic stenting, radiation therapy, and less radical palliative procedures, laparotomy is no longer the sole method available for palliating unresectable cancers. Although CT scans and magnetic resonance imaging provide excellent resolution and define anatomic proximity and even invasion into adjacent vital structures, they often fail to detect small metastases in the peritoneal cavity or on the surface of the liver (Fig. 7-1). Failure to detect these lesions understages disease and may lead to a laparotomy when another mode of therapy might be as effective and cause less morbidity. Not only is laparoscopy highly sensitive for the detection of small metastases, but when combined with intraoperative ultrasound, it provides the surgeon with a laparoscopic evaluation of both solid and hollow viscera.

ESOPHAGEAL AND GASTRIC CANCER

Over half the cases of gastric and lower esophageal carcinoma are incurable at the time of presentation [2]. The surgeon's first decision is to identify which patients have inoperable disease and then to determine which patients with potentially resectable disease would in fact benefit from resection. Although nearly half of all patients with cancer limited to the field of resection will die of disease within 2 years [3], radical resection is the only possibly curative procedure. Conversely, radical surgery does not change outcome in patients with proven preoperative metastatic disease [4]. Given these facts, it is logical to assume that if laparoscopy results in more accurate preoperative staging, it could alter the indications for surgery when alternative methods of treatment and palliation are available. O'Brien and coworkers [5•] looked at the sensitivity, specificity, and diagnostic accuracy of CT, ultrasound, and laparoscopy with and without biopsy in the staging of adenocarcinoma of the esophagogastric region. They found that the sensitivity of laparoscopy in detecting metastases was 97% versus 37% with ultrasound and CT together. Several additional studies in patients with gastric cancer have shown more accurate staging with the addition of laparoscopy to CT scanning and ultrasonography [6–10] because these imaging modalities are insensitive in detecting small superficial liver metastases. However, the laparoscope has a sensitivity of between 87% and 100%.

Historically, any patient with gastric cancer would undergo a palliative subtotal gastrectomy with proven metastatic disease, or a radical subtotal procedure for possible

CHAPTER

7

cure. Therefore, laparoscopic staging would not obviate the need for a laparotomy. Many surgeons have questioned whether laparoscopic staging actually avoids a laparotomy or simply postpones it so the patient can return for a late laparotomy secondary to a complication of the disease. However, van Dijkum and coworkers [8] found that none of the patients who were staged as incurable by laparoscopy required reoperation for their disease. Further, several effective palliative therapies are available, such as intraluminal stents, laser ablation, chemotherapy, or radiotherapy, that would avoid further surgical intervention [9].

Some cancer treatment centers disagree on timing and patient selection for laparoscopic staging of gastric cancers. Oncologic surgeons at MD Anderson hospital report using laparoscopic staging for any patient with gastric cancer who does not have proven evidence of metastatic disease and does not require urgent operation for bleeding or obstruction [10]. However, others at Memorial Sloan–Kettering hospital do not use laparoscopic staging for any patient with T1 or T2 lesions by endoscopic ultrasound, but take these patients directly to laparotomy [11]. Despite various differences in staging algorithms, many studies clearly show the improved accuracy and efficacy of laparoscopic staging of esophageal and gastric cancers, which translates into better-tailored treatment protocols [5•,6–11].

The laparoscopic approach to staging of esophagogastric cancers involves a systematic evaluation of the abdomen. After the umbilical trocar is placed, the entire peritoneal cavity is inspected for any suspicious masses or nodes. Next, a 10-mm port is placed in the right midclavicular line lateral to the umbilicus, and a 5-mm port placed in the left upper quadrant. Any peritoneal fluid is taken for cytologic evaluation. The instruments are then used to evaluate the esophagus and stomach. Following a division of the lesser omentum to the right of the gastroesophageal junction, the lesser curvature can be retracted to expose the celiac axis for possible biopsy of suspicious nodes. The lesser sac can thus be evaluated by the creation of an omental window. Alternatively, the lesser sac can be entered by division of the avascular window in the transverse mesocolon to the left of the middle colic vessels. Finally, an evaluation of the liver and biopsy of any suspicious lesions is performed.

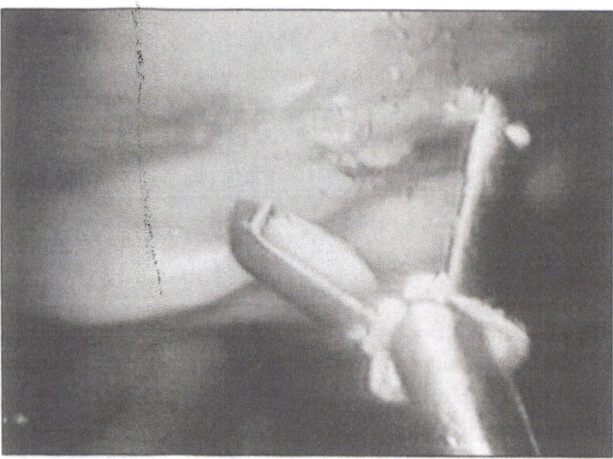

Figure 7-1 Laparoscopic detection of a 2-mm tumor implant on the peritoneal surface (between the jaws of the grasper) that was not detected by preoperative imaging studies.

HEPATIC MALIGNANCY

Although malignant tumors in the liver are common, few are appropriate for surgical resection. The most common hepatic malignancies are metastatic lesions. Although hepatic metastases can originate from nearly any primary site, the most frequent sites of the primary tumor are lung, prostate, colon, breast, pancreas, and stomach. Therefore, a standard evaluation involves a thorough physical examination, chest radiography, bone scan, prostate-specific antigen (PSA) screening or mammography, and upper and lower gastrointestinal studies. In cases in which the primary tumor was intra-abdominal, staging laparoscopy is less likely to be helpful than in primary hepatic tumors because there usually has been prior extensive intra-abdominal surgery, which precludes adequate laparoscopic examination of the entire peritoneal cavity. In rare instances in which resection of hepatic metastases is considered for tumors originating extra-abdominally, there are not enough data to comment on the utility of preresection laparoscopic staging. Based on experience with intraoperative ultrasound, laparoscopy combined with laparoscopic ultrasound may be beneficial in avoiding nontherapeutic laparotomies in these rare cases.

Patients with hepatocellular carcinoma deserve a careful staging evaluation because the prognosis is generally poor (depending on the subtype), and there are a variety of therapeutic options ranging from relatively noninvasive (eg, alcohol ablation and chemoembolization) to transplantation. Many hepatomas are multifocal or have satellite lesions that are not detected by preoperative imaging studies. The relationship of the tumor to major vascular structures may also be difficult to ascertain with certainty preoperatively. As with pancreatic cancer, a nontherapeutic laparotomy is not beneficial and should be avoided in these patients. Babineau and coworkers [12] showed that preoperative laparoscopy altered management in 48% of all patients whose hepatic malignancies were thought to be resectable by other staging modalities. The sensitivity of laparoscopy for detecting metastatic deposits was 78%, with specificity of 100%. In their study, a nontherapeutic laparotomy was avoided in 41% of patients. With the current availability of laparoscopic ultrasound, the impact of laparoscopic staging is potentially greater than that shown in the previous study [11] because one can anticipate identification of small lesions deep in the hepatic parenchyma that cannot be detected by other imaging modalities and that will serve as a contraindication to resection in some situations.

PANCREATIC CANCER

Like esophageal, gastric, and hepatocellular carcinoma, pancreatic cancer has a dismal prognosis. Currently, surgical resection provides the only chance for cure. For unknown reasons, the survival rate for resected patients in the past decade seems to be increasing, and therefore every effort should be made to identify the favorable subset of patients whose disease is resectable. Fewer than 10% of patients have potentially resectable disease. In the past, any patient with the diagnosis of pancreatic cancer underwent a laparotomy for tissue diagnosis and either palliative or curative procedure, depending on intraoperative findings. With the advent of endoscopic biliary stents, only patients with gastric outlet obstruction benefit from a purely palliative laparotomy. The addition of laparoscopy to the preoperative evaluation of patients with adenocarcinoma of the pancreas minimizes the number of nonessential laparotomies and increases the resectability rate of those patients who ultimately undergo a laparotomy.

The evaluation of any patient with a suspected pancreatic neoplasm initially involves ultrasound and CT. The ultrasound is a useful first test because it can demonstrate dilation of the common bile or pancreatic ducts, and the head of the pancreas can usually be seen. Compared with the normal pancreatic parenchyma, carcinomas are generally hypoechoic, and pancreatitis is commonly hyperechoic. A CT scan with intravenous bolus contrast and thin sections (2 mm) through the area of the head of the pancreas should be the next imaging study performed. This examination is particularly useful in delineating the relationship of the tumor to the portal and superior mesenteric veins, as well as identifying peripancreatic lymphadenopathy, the presence of ascites, contiguous organ involvement, and hepatic metastases. Unless the patient has evidence of severe mesenteric arterial vascular disease, this scan obviates the need for angiography in assessing resectability. Nonetheless, CT is at best only 70% sensitive in detecting metastases, and therefore overestimates the number of patients who should be considered for curative resection.

Many studies have shown the clear benefit of laparoscopy in reducing the number of palliative laparotomies in patients whose disease is thought to be resectable on the basis of CT and angiography [13–16]. Laparoscopy detects previously unrecognized peritoneal implants, suspicious lymph nodes, and small liver metastases. It can also be used to assess the primary tumor, obtain a tissue diagnosis, biopsy any suspicious lesions, and obtain washings for cytology. The laparoscope, when combined with laparoscopic ultrasound, is extremely accurate in assessing resectability. Conlon and coworkers [17••] have shown a 91% resectability rate among patients staged with the laparoscope in addition to traditional studies. Five of the six failures in accurate staging in their series were caused by intraparenchymal liver metastases. Other groups have demonstrated

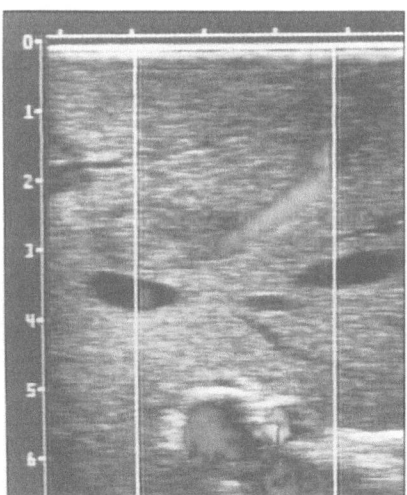

Figure 7-2
Intraparenchymal hepatic metastasis demonstrated by laparoscopic ultrasound. No hepatic surface abnormality was seen during laparoscopy.

the efficacy of laparoscopic ultrasound in detecting small hepatic metastases [18] (Fig. 7-2).

Warshaw [19] in 1991 showed a high correlation between positive peritoneal cytology and unresectability in patients whose disease was preoperatively determined to be resectable. Although many patients with malignant ascites will have peritoneal implants, as many as 15% of patients whose disease was deemed resectable by all criteria will have malignant cells found in peritoneal washings (despite the absence of visible peritoneal implants). As of 1995, that team had yet to find a patient with positive peritoneal cytology whose pancreatic cancer was resectable with clear margins [20]. Updating their experience through 1997, they found that even patients who underwent apparently successful Whipple resections but had positive peritoneal cytology failed to survive longer than 7 months and developed metastases within a median of 3 months. On the basis of these data, they now advocate no further surgical treatment for any patient with positive peritoneal cytology [21•].

Technique

After placement of the umbilical trocar and camera, a thorough visual inspection of the abdomen is begun. Five hundred mL of normal saline are instilled into the abdomen and the patient is rotated into left and right lateral positions as well as Trendelenburg and reverse Trendelenburg position to wash all surfaces of the peritoneum . The irrigant is collected for cytology and immunocytology. Attention is then directed to the right upper quadrant and the liver. Both the superior and inferior surfaces of the liver are inspected for any evidence of metastasis. The inferior surface of the diaphragm is examined, as well as the anterior peritoneal lining. Any suspicious nodules or masses are biopsied. The placement of a 5-mm trocar in the right upper quadrant is useful for this purpose, and can be used for exposure later in the procedure. The camera is then turned to the left upper quadrant where the stomach and inferior surfaces of the diaphragm are visualized and checked for any evidence of direct extension or implantation. Next, the small and large bowel are evaluated and the pelvis inspected for suspicious masses or implants.

An attempt is then made to examine the pancreas itself. This examination can be performed by a supragastric, infragastric, or infracolic approach. The supragastric approach is similar to the exposure of the celiac axis described earlier, by division of the lesser omentum to the right of the lesser curvature of the stomach (Fig. 7-3). This approach allows visualization of the head, body, and tail. It allows biopsy of any suspicious nodes. However, it is not as effective for inspection of the superior mesenteric vein. The infragastric approach involves the creation of access to the lesser sac through the avascular window in the greater omentum between the greater curvature of the stomach and the transverse colon. This is usually performed by retracting the greater curvature superiorly. The laparoscope is inserted into the lesser sac to evaluate the posterior body and tail of the pancreas (Fig. 7-4). Finally, the infracolic approach uses the plane to the left of the middle colic vessels to approach the inferior portion of the pancreas. This exposure gives the best evaluation of the inferior mesenteric vein and the inferior portion of the pancreas, which is important only if one is considering resecting a mass in the body or tail of the pancreas (Fig. 7-5). Although one can biopsy the pancreatic mass at time of laparoscopy, this should only be performed if the tumor is clearly unresectable and there has not been a prior tissue diagnosis. If there is no evidence of metastatic disease, the primary is considered resectable; if the patient is a good surgical candidate, the next step is a laparotomy with intent to cure. The pancreas is a highly vascular gland with substantial lymphatic drainage, and adenocarcinoma of the pancreas has a strong capacity for dissemination and vascular invasion. Warshaw [19] showed that among pancreatic masses thought to be resectable, those that were percutaneously

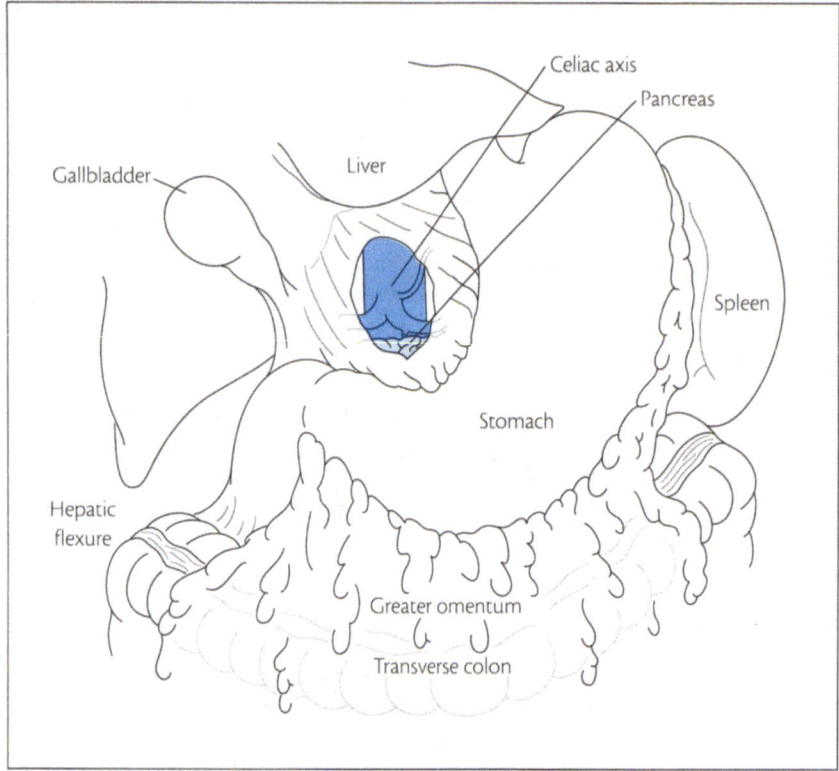

Figure 7-3 The supragastric approach to exposing the celiac axis and neck of the pancreas.

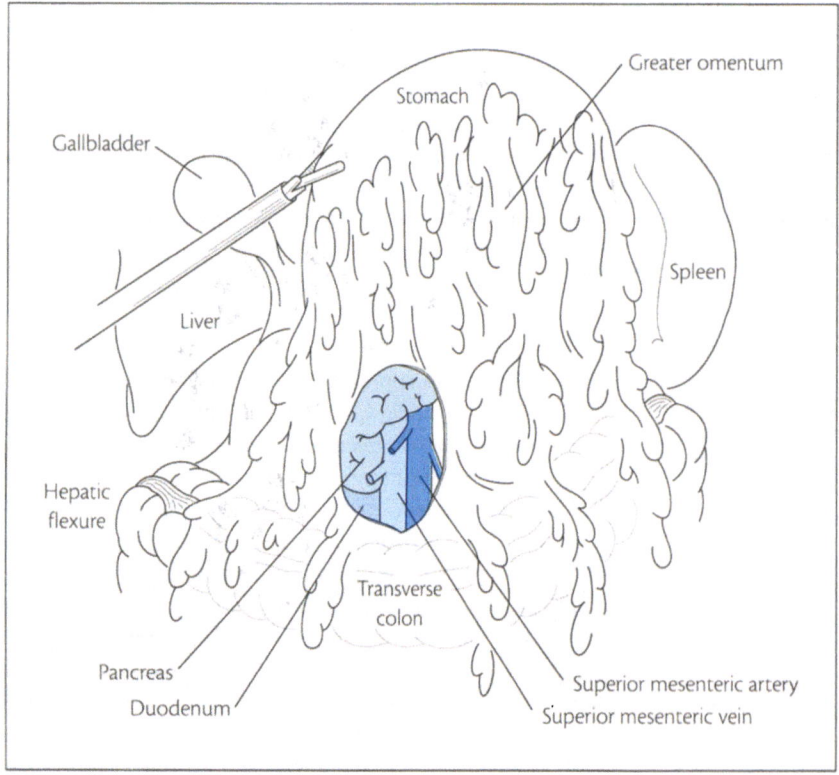

Figure 7-4 The infragastric approach to expose the mesenteric vessels and inferior border of the pancreas.

biopsied had a 75% rate of positive cytology, compared with only 19% among nonbiopsied patients [17••]. This finding suggests that the very act of diagnosis may eliminate the possibility for cure. Because a negative biopsy will not avert a laparotomy, it is generally unnecessary.

GALLBLADDER CARCINOMA

Cancer of the gallbladder occurs in approximately 1% of all cholecystectomy specimens and is usually an incidental finding [22]. The disease at the time of diagnosis frequently is limited to the wall of the gallbladder with no extension transmurally, and cholecystectomy is the only therapy required. Some have advocated re-excision of all port sites once the diagnosis becomes apparent, but some studies have shown a survival advantage conferred by extended lymphadenectomy or more radical resection of the liver bed for gallbladder cancer [23–25]. Survival in this disease is determined almost solely by the stage of disease at the time of presentation rather than the form of therapy.

When preoperative ultrasonography detects a polypoid mass in the gallbladder, the surgeon should be cautious about performing a laparoscopic cholecystectomy. Findings at laparoscopic cholecystectomy that should raise the suspicion of gallbladder cancer may also be consistent with acute cholecystitis, such as a thickened gallbladder wall, adherent omentum, or a swollen or large gallbladder. Direct invasion of the liver bed is an ominous sign. There is little use for laparoscopy in the routine evaluation or treatment of gallbladder cancer. In patients who have conflicting preoperative data regarding diagnosis, or who would not be considered for a radical resection, there may be a role for laparoscopic assessment and cholecystectomy. However, in most patients, the presumed diagnosis of gallbladder cancer without evidence for metastases necessitates an open cholecystectomy with a partial hepatic resection.

HODGKIN'S LYMPHOMA

The success of combination chemotherapy and radiation in the treatment of Hodgkin's lymphoma has significantly reduced the need for staging laparotomy. Staging laparotomy or laparoscopy is only indicated when it will change subsequent treatment. Surgeons with advanced laparoscopic skills can duplicate the standard staging laparotomy with a more rapid return to full functional status and hence more rapid institution of definitive therapy [26].

External-beam radiation therapy is the mainstay of treatment for stage I or IIA disease, and combination chemotherapy for stage III or IV. Therefore, the involvement of the spleen or intra-abdominal lymph nodes may change the stage, and therefore therapy, in some patients. Lymphangiography is highly accurate in assessing retroperitoneal and abdominal lymph nodes. However, it is an insensitive test for the evaluation of the portal, celiac, and splenic nodes, which are studied by CT. Neither lymphangiography nor CT is sensitive for detecting disease of the spleen [27]. Among patients with stage I, II, or IIIA disease, laparoscopy is useful in confirming splenic or nodal involvement, thus necessitating the addition of chemotherapy. Prior to staging laparoscopy, all patients should receive vaccines against *Haemophilus influenzae* and *Neisseria meningitidis*, and the polyvalent pneumococcal vaccine. Splenectomy is contraindicated in patients older than 40 years of age, or who have received MOPP (mechlorethamine, vincristine, procarbazine, and prednisone) chemotherapy, because it appears to be a risk factor for the development of acute myeloid leukemias.

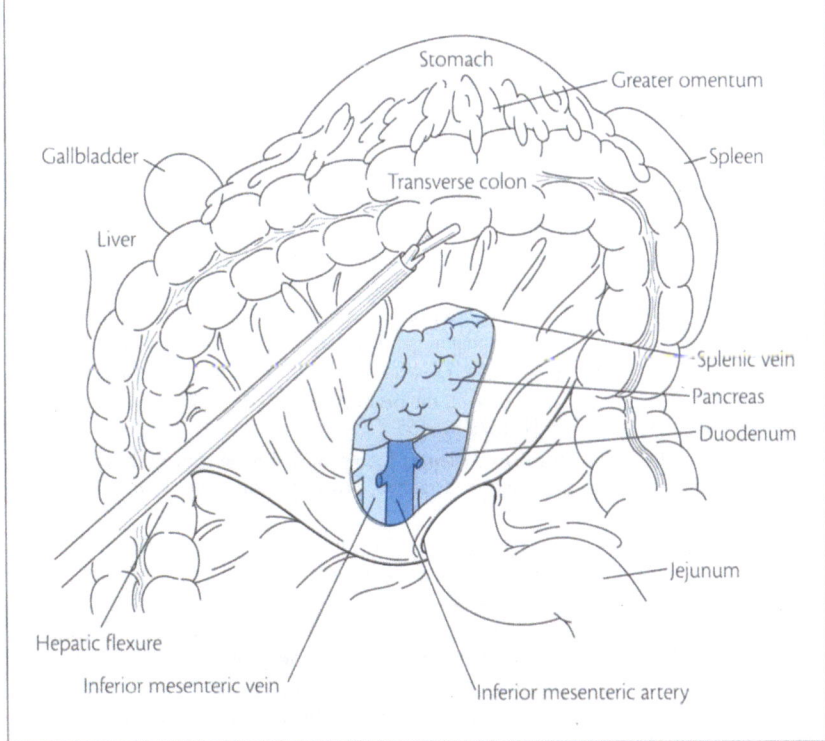

Figure 7-5 The infracolic approach for exposure of the body and tail of the pancreas as well as the inferior mesenteric vein.

The laparoscope can be used effectively in the evaluation and biopsy of portal lymph nodes, spleen, and liver. Evaluation begins in the right upper quadrant with examination of the liver and porta. Lymph node specimens are taken from the hilar, cystic, and common duct nodes. Any suspicious nodules can be biopsied and electrocautery used for hemostasis in the liver bed. If no obvious liver involvement is noted, a small wedge of the left lobe should be taken for pathologic confirmation. Attention is then turned to the spleen, where the short gastric arteries are identified and ligated. The splenic hilum is then carefully inspected for any suspicious nodules. Then, the splenic artery and vein are divided and the spleen freed from its remaining attachments and placed in the pelvis. After splenectomy, the lesser sac is entered as described earlier. The celiac node is exposed and removed. The mesocolon is inspected and nodal biopsy taken. An examination of the pelvis should be performed with the patient in the Trendelenburg position. Representative lymph node specimens are taken for pathologic confirmation. Unlike splenectomy for hepatologic disorders, the spleen must be removed intact. This is generally done through a low midline or Pfannenstiel's incision to minimize postoperative discomfort.

COMPLICATIONS

As with any surgical procedure, laparoscopy must be judged by its risks and benefits. The complication rate for laparoscopic staging is between 1% and 3%, and is usually a hematoma from a biopsy site, or a wound infection. An unusual complication that deserves mention is that of port site metastasis. It is unclear whether laparoscopic staging carries with it an increased risk for development of metastasis in the trocar sites in patients who subsequently undergo a potentially curative resection. The development of port site metastasis has been described in gastric, biliary, pancreatic, colonic, and gynecologic malignancies. The risk of tumor spread is small, and it is not a contraindication to the use of the laparoscope for staging. However, after a curative resection in which the laparoscope was used preoperatively, the surgeon must be aware of this complication when following up a patient for recurrence.

The absolute contraindication to laparoscopic staging is when there is no information to gain from the procedure. For example, once the diagnosis of metastatic pancreatic cancer is made, an attempt should be made to palliate the patient, which might involve endoscopic biliary or duodenal stenting. Other relative contraindications for the procedure are poor preoperative cardiac or pulmonary function, such that the patient would not tolerate the physiologic insult of pneumoperitoneum. Another contraindication is in cases in which the improved staging will not prevent a palliative laparotomy. An example of this is a patient with pancreatic cancer and evidence of duodenal obstruction who will require a gastrojejunostomy for palliation regardless of the primary tumor's resectability.

CONCLUSIONS

The use of the laparoscope for staging must be viewed in a critical light. It is neither useful nor necessary for the evaluation of all intra-abdominal malignancies. However, for malignancies with a poor prognosis in which alternative therapies and modes of palliation exist, laparoscopic staging optimizes resource utilization, minimizes nonessential laparotomies, and reduces pain and morbidity by tailoring therapy appropriately to the stage of disease. Laparoscopy has the unique ability to identify small foci of intra-abdominal disease that are below the threshold of detection of other imaging modalities, and may combine the ability to provide staging information with therapy.

REFERENCES AND RECOMMENDED READING

Recently published papers of particular interest have been highlighted as:

•   Of interest

••   Of outstanding interest

1. Cushieri A. Laparoscopy in general surgery and gastroenterology. *J Appl Med* 1981, 7:555–558.

2. Stone R, Rangel D, Gordon H, *et al.*: Carcinoma of the gastroesophageal junction. *Am J Surg* 1977, 134:70–75.

3. Morita M, Kuwano H, Ohno S, *et al.*: Characteristics and sequence of recurrence patterns after curative esophagogastrectomy for squamous cell carcinoma. *Surgery* 1994, 116:1–7.

4. Macdonald J, Gohmann J: Chemotherapy of advanced gastric cancer: present status, future prospects. *Semin Oncol* 1988, 15:42–49.

5.• O'Brien M, Fitzgerald E, Lee G, *et al.*: A prospective comparison of laparoscopy and imaging in the staging of esophagogastric cancer before surgery. *Am J Gastroenterol* 1995, 90:2191–2194.
This study demonstrates that laparoscopy detects more than twice as many metastases as conventional imaging studies in patients with gastric and esophageal cancer.

6. Possik R, Franco E, Pires D, *et al.*: Sensitivity, specificity, and predictive value of laparoscopy for the staging of gastric cancer and for the detection of liver metastases. *Cancer* 1986, 58:1–6.

7. Stell D, Carter C, Stewart I, *et al.*: Prospective comparison of laparoscopy, ultrasonography and computed tomography in the staging of gastric cancer. *Br J Surg* 1996, 83:1260–1262.

8. van Dijkum E, de Wit L, van Delden O, *et al.*: The efficacy of laparoscopic staging in patients with upper gastrointestinal tumors. *Cancer* 1997, 79:1315–1319.

9. Fuchs C, Mayer R: Gastric carcinoma. *N Engl J Med* 1995, 333:32–41.

10. Lowy A, Mansfield P, Leach S, *et al.*: Laparoscopic staging for gastric cancer. *Surgery* 1996, 119:611–614.

11. Conlon K, Karpeh M: Laparoscopy and laparoscopic ultrasound in the staging of gastric cancer. *Semin Oncol* 1996, 23:347–351.

12. Babineau T, Lewis D, Jenkins R, *et al.*: Role of staging laparoscopy in the treatment of hepatic malignancy. *Am J Surg* 1994, 167:151–155.

13. Warshaw A, Tepper J, Shipley W: Laparoscopy in the staging and planning of therapy for pancreatic cancer. *Am J Surg* 1986, 151:76–80.

14. Warshaw A, Gu Z, Wittenberg J, *et al.*: Preoperative staging and assessment of resectability of pancreatic cancer. *Arch Surg* 1990, 125:230–233.

15. John T, Greig J, Carter D, *et al.*: Carcinoma of the pancreatic head and periampullary region. *Ann Surg* 1995, 221:156–164.

16. Bemelman W, deWit L, vanDelden O, *et al.*: Diagnostic laparoscopy combined with laparoscopic ultrasonography in staging of cancer of the pancreatic head region. *Br J Surg* 1995, 82:820–824.

17.•• Conlon K, Dougherty E, Klimstra D, *et al.*: The value of minimal access surgery in the staging of patients with potentially resectable peripancreatic malignancy. *Ann Surg* 1996, 223:1341140.
An excellent series of patients subjected to a thorough laparoscopic staging examination including the use of laparoscopic ultrasound. This paper reports the highest resectability rate yet for patients with pancreatic cancer, which is attributable to the meticulous laparoscopic examination performed by the authors.

18. Murugiah M, Patterson-Brown S, Windsor J, *et al.*: Early experience of laparoscopic ultrasonography in the management of pancreatic carcinoma. *Surg Endosc* 1993, 7:119–124.

19. Warshaw A: Implications of peritoneal cytology for staging of early pancreatic cancer. *Am J Surg* 1991, 161:26–30.

20. Fernandez del-Castillo C, Rattner D, Warshaw A: Further experience with laparoscopy and peritoneal cytology in the staging of pancreatic cancer. *Br J Surg* 1995, 82:1127–1129.

21.• Makary M, Warshaw A, Centeno B, *et al.*: Influence of peritoneal cytology on treatment of patients with pancreatic cancer. *Arch Surg* 1998, in press.
This important paper documents that patients with positive peritoneal cytology are unlikely to be resectable even if other imaging studies are favorable, and that the few patients with positive cytology whose disease is resected do not live longer than patients treated with palliative means only.

22. Beltz W, Condon R: Primary carcinoma of the gallbladder. *Ann Surg* 1974, 180:180–184.

23. Evander A, Ihse I: Evaluation of intended radical surgery in carcinoma of the gallbladder. *Br J Surg* 1981, 68:158–160.

24. Wannebo H, Castle W, Fechner R: Is carcinoma of the gallbladder a curable lesion? *Ann Surg* 1982, 195:624–631.

25. Donahue J, Nagorney D, Grant C, *et al.*: Carcinoma of the gallbladder: does radical resection improve outcome? *Arch Surg* 1990, 125:237–241.

26. Rhodes M, Rudd M, O'Rourke N, *et al.*: Laparoscopic splenectomy and lymph node biopsy for hematologic disorders. *Ann Surg* 1995, 222:43–46.

27. Jandl J: *Blood: Textbook of Hematology*. Boston: Little, Brown & Co., 1987.

Laparoscopic Inguinal Hernia Repair

Robert L. Soares, Jr.
Joseph F. Amaral

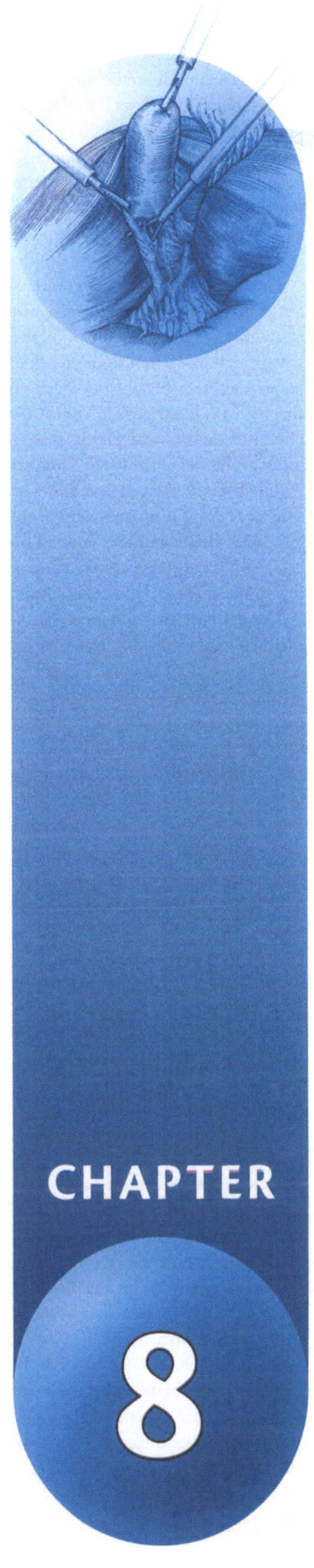

Inguinal hernia repair is the most common general surgical operation in the United States, with 710,000 inguinal and femoral herniorrhaphies performed in 1994 [1]. Given the long history and success with conventional inguinal surgery, why consider a laparoscopic approach? First, it is estimated that the 3- to 8-week recovery period allotted to most patients after hernia repair results in 10 to 15 million workdays lost each year. Patients have come to accept, and usually demand, this time off. Second, although specialized centers report recurrence rates of less than 1% [2,3], most long-term studies of hernia repair in general surgical practices as well as those reporting results of the repair of recurrent hernias suggest that a recurrence rate of 7% to 21% is more typical [4–6]. Finally, significant pain and immobilization are associated with conventional inguinal hernia repair, as manifest in the limp that most patients exhibit during the first postoperative week. Cunningham and coworkers [7] recently documented a 62.9% incidence of inguinal groin pain syndromes at 1 year after open hernia repair and 53.6% at 2 years. Further, in 11% of the patients studied, the pain was considered severe. Thus, it is reasonable to consider laparoscopic approaches to the repair of inguinal hernias if one can demonstrate improved or equivalent recurrence rates, less postoperative pain and immobilization, and earlier return to work.

HISTORICAL ASPECTS OF INGUINAL HERNIA REPAIR
Open herniorrhaphy

The following brief overview of the history of inguinal hernia repair focuses on development of the surgical principles now considered fundamental to successful herniorrhaphy. Before the late nineteenth century, the status of hernia repair was chaotic. Although general agreement existed that castration was unnecessary in repairing groin hernias, most surgeons believed that infection encouraged scarring and led to low rates of recurrence [8]. Most surgeons who used an inguinal approach excised the sac and left the wound open to heal by secondary intention (*ie*, the McBurney procedure) [8]. Lister and his first American pupil, Marcy, advocated antiseptic herniorrhaphy using carbolized catgut suture. In this procedure, the sac was pulled through the external ring and external oblique aponeurosis, and the internal ring was tightened [8,9]. Thus, three of the modern principles of inguinal herniorrhaphy were established: antisepsis, high ligation of the sac, and tightening of the internal ring. Unfortunately, their technique was not generally accepted. Sepsis rates remained high, and 4-year recurrence rates were almost 100% [8,9].

Bassini's epoch-making report in 1890 changed the way that hernias were managed. Bassini believed that inguinal repairs failed because of reliance on the external oblique aponeurosis (a single layer of scar weakened by passage of the cord) [8,9]. He advocated reconstruction of the inguinal floor using silk. Bassini sutured the transversalis fascia with the transversus aponeurosis and internal oblique to the ilioinguinal ligament after anterolateral transposition of the cord. Thus, the fourth principle of modern inguinal herniorrhaphy was established: reconstruction of the inguinal floor using transversalis fascia.

Precise anatomic studies of the inguinal floor were performed by Anson and coworkers [10] in the late 1940s. These dissections proved that the transversalis fascia inserts on the iliopectineal (Cooper's) ligament, not the inguinal ligament. The iliopectineal ligament was first used by Lotheissen of Vienna for hernia repair but thereafter was ignored until popularized by McVay [8]. The McVay repair established the importance of the iliopectineal ligament in the secure repair of both inguinal and femoral hernias.

The importance of tension on the repair as a contributing factor in hernia recurrence was recognized by Halsted and coworkers, and led to the development of the relaxing incision [8]. Even when the repair is not under tension, however, the transversalis fascia may be generally weakened and inadequate for herniorrhaphy. This knowledge led to the use of fascial grafts, silver-filigree prosthetics, and plastic materials such as polypropylene mesh for hernia repair [8,9]. Thus, the fifth principle of modern inguinal herniorrhaphy—tensionless repair—was established. This concept is ultimately represented in the modern, tensionless, mesh hernia repair advocated by Lichtenstein and coworkers [3,4]. Using this repair, these authors reported a 0.13% recurrence rate for 3125 consecutive primary repairs [11].

There has been controversy about the proper approach to inguinal herniorrhaphy: transabdominal, anterior inguinal, or extraperitoneal. The origin of the extraperitoneal approach is attributed to Cheatle [8]. Despite its use by Henry in the 1930s, the extraperitoneal iliopubic tract repair was not popularized until the late 1950s by Nyhus [12]. This approach does not violate the inguinal canal; thus it is for Nyhus the procedure of choice for femoral and recurrent hernias. Nyhus does not recommend this approach for primary direct defects because of the poor view of Hesselbach's triangle from the lateral border of the rectus muscle and the inability to perform a relaxing incision when excessive tension exists on the repair. Stoppa [13] obviated the visual- and tension-related problems of the Nyhus repair for direct hernias by locating the incision in the midline and using prosthetic mesh. Stoppa realized that early recurrences reported by Nyhus resulted from using inadequately sized mesh. This led Stoppa to develop the giant mesh repair, which has reported recurrence rates of less than 1% [13].

Laparoscopic herniorrhaphy

Credit for the first laparoscopic hernia repair predates the revolution started by laparoscopic cholecystectomy. In 1982, Ger and coworkers [14,15] reported a series of 12 patients whose internal ring defects were closed using Michel clips at laparoscopy, and one patient was treated laparoscopically using a specially designed stapler. Bogojavalensky recently introduced laparoscopic treatment of inguinal and femoral hernias by means of a preperitoneal patch repair (Paper presented at the 18th Annual Meeting of the American Association of Gynecological Laparoscopists, Washington, DC, 1989). In 1990, Popp [16] reported a laparoscopic inguinal hernia repair that was accomplished by suturing dehydrated dura mater over the inguinal area.

The first series of laparoscopic hernia repairs was published in 1990 by Schultz and coworkers [17]. Twenty patients were treated by a laparoscopic approach in which the peritoneum was opened and a plug of polypropylene mesh inserted in the internal ring.

The inguinal area was covered with an additional piece of mesh that was not sutured in place. The peritoneum then was reapproximated using titanium clips that had been developed for cystic duct and artery ligation during laparoscopic cholecystectomy. Follow-up ranged from 3 to 11 months. One recurrence was reported, and the average return to unrestricted activity was 3.3 days, with return to the workplace in 3.9 days. Schultz and coworkers thus documented their ability to perform outpatient laparoscopic herniorrhaphy with minimal discomfort, insignificant complications, and early return to productive activity.

Many of the initial attempts at laparoscopic herniorrhaphy did not adhere to the recognized principles of hernia repair. In fairness to these early pioneers, limitations in instrumentation rather than ignorance of the principles of hernia surgery may have been responsible for these initial laparoscopic approaches. Subsequent improvements in technology allowed a return to established principles. For example, both Schultz and coworkers [17] and Corbitt [18] noted a 2-year recurrence rate of 25% with the nonstapled plug and patch technique. This technique subsequently was modified by eliminating the plug, increasing the mesh size, and stapling the mesh in place. Similarly, in early experience using a transabdominal intraperitoneal onlay polypropylene mesh in 50 patients reported by Filipi and coworkers [19] and Redmond and coworkers [20], the first three patients with direct hernias experienced recurrence. Also, four other patients developed extensive adhesions to the mesh. These results led the investigators to abandon this technique in favor of a transabdominal preperitoneal approach.

Evidence also exists that some early practitioners of laparoscopic hernia repair had a limited understanding of the anatomic structures of the inguinal region when viewed posteriorly. This is particularly true for nerves that run through the groin, and is reflected in reports of nerve entrapment syndromes such as meralgia paresthetica [21–24]. Such syndromes are caused by injuries to the lateral femoral cutaneous nerve or the femoral branch of the genitofemoral nerve.

By the end of the early evolutionary period, transabdominal preperitoneal mesh repair and the extraperitoneal approach had emerged as the preferred methods. The success of these two techniques is based on fixation of prosthetic mesh to the classically defined structures in open herniorrhaphy: the transversus abdominus aponeurotic arch, pubic tubercle, iliopectineal ligament, and iliopubic tract. Indeed, these preferred laparoscopic approaches adhere to the basic principles of hernia repair.

LAPAROSCOPIC HERNIA REPAIR
Inguinal anatomy

The important anatomic structures are easily found via a transabdominal approach. The inferior epigastric vessels, obliterated umbilical artery, spermatic vessels, and vas deferens are visible through the peritoneum. The inferior epigastric vessels travel across the transversalis fascia medial to the internal ring as they enter or exit the rectus muscle. The obliterated umbilical ligament, identifiable by its variable mesentery, is located midway between Cooper's ligament and the internal ring. Although it may be confused with the epigastric vessels, careful inspection will show the umbilical ligament traveling to the umbilicus rather than the rectus muscle. The spermatic vessels run lateral to the internal inguinal ring and join the vas deferens near the ring. The vas deferens always travels from the medial to lateral. The space between the spermatic vessels and vas deferens has been named the "triangle of doom" because the external iliac vessels lie behind the peritoneum in this space.

A transverse incision in the peritoneum allows identification of the deeper structures after minimal dissection. These structures include the internal inguinal ring and transversalis sling, iliopubic tract, pubic tubercle, Cooper's ligament, transverses aponeurotic arch and the external iliac vessels and femoral space. Cooper's ligament is a firm white structure that usually has a vein running on its surface. The iliopubic tract is visible lateral to the internal ring as a groove in the tissues and medial to the internal ring as a band running to the pubic tubercle. The transverse abdominus arch is visible superior to the iliopubic tract near the pubic tubercle. Finally, the external iliac vessels and the femoral space are easily found inferior to the iliopubic tract by observing the pulsation of the external iliac artery.

The femoral branch of the genitofemoral nerve and the lateral cutaneous nerve of the thigh are located inferior to the iliopubic tract and lateral to the femoral artery [25]. They are not seen unless searched for by reflection of the peritoneum and careful dissection in this area (Fig. 8-1). The femoral nerve lies deep to the iliopsoas muscle and is not visible during the dissection. Recent reports of nerve entrapment and injury by staples have focused attention on this part of the anatomy [22,24].

The anatomy of the inguinal region when viewed via the extra peritoneal approach is the same as seen with the transabdominal transperitoneal approach, except that the obliterated umbilical artery is not seen. All structures are visible with only minimal dissection because no peritoneal incisions are required.

General features

We perform all laparoscopic herniorrhaphies under general anesthesia, although epidural anesthesia is also an option, especially with extraperitoneal repairs. All patients receive a prophylactic

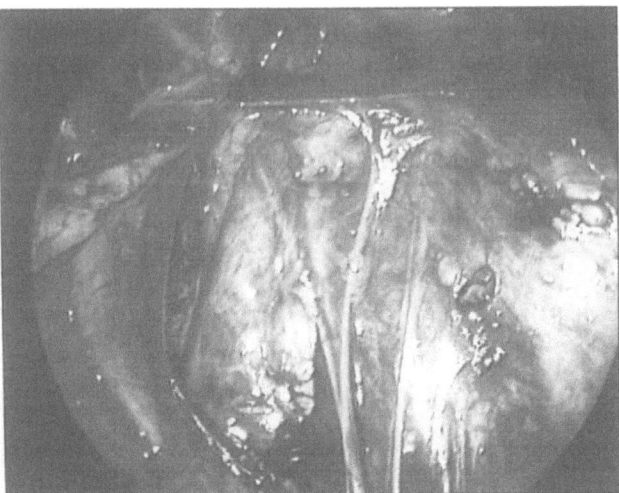

Figure 8-1 Various nerves that can be trapped or injured by staples. (*See* Color Plate.)

preoperative antibiotic, lower extremity compression stockings, an orogastric tube, and urethral catheter. The abdomen and external genitalia are not shaved but are prepared with povidone-iodine solution. The external genitalia are not draped into the operative field. The procedure is performed with the patient in Trendelenburg position.

Absolute contraindications to laparoscopic herniorrhaphy include inability to tolerate general anesthesia, uncorrected coagulopathy, and strangulated hernias. Relative contraindications to the procedure include large scrotal hernias, because the sac usually cannot be reduced, the procedure is time-consuming, and large defects are difficult to cover adequately by laparoscopy.

Transabdominal preperitoneal procedure

Laparoscopy is initiated either with a closed (Veress needle) or an open (Hasson) technique. In the closed technique, a 12-mm skin incision is made at the umbilicus and is carried down to the anterior rectus fascia by blunt dissection. The anterior abdominal wall is grasped and elevated away from the viscera. A Veress needle is inserted toward the pelvis at a 45° angle to the abdominal wall. Gentle pressure is applied until two "pops" are felt, indicating entry into the peritoneal cavity. Appropriate placement is checked first by aspiration to ensure that no blood, urine, or intestinal contents returns, then by instillation of air followed by inability to aspirate the air, and finally by instillation of saline to assure free flow into the peritoneal cavity (which is at or below atmospheric pressure). Carbon dioxide is then insulated via the needle to create a 15 mm Hg capnoperitoneum. The initial pressure should be less than 5 mm Hg. The needle is then replaced by a 10 mm port. A 0° laparoscope is inserted via the umbilical port and the abdominal cavity is inspected for visceral or vascular injury.

We prefer the open laparoscopic technique for all laparoscopic procedures including herniorrhaphy because of the reduced incidence of vascular and intestinal injuries. The open technique is initiated by making a 12-mm umbilical skin incision, which is then carried down to the anterior fascia by blunt dissection. The fascia is grasped with Kocher clamps and incised vertically in the midline. Traction sutures of 0-polyglycolic acid are placed through the anterior fascia on either side of the midline, and are used to close the wound at the end of the procedure. Under direct vision, the posterior sheath and peritoneum are incised and entry into the peritoneal cavity is confirmed by free passage of a blunt instrument. A blunt trocar-cannula system is advanced into the umbilical wound and secured with the traction sutures. Before insufflation, the peritoneal cavity is inspected with the laparoscope to reconfirm intraperitoneal placement.

Following insufflation, the abdomen is visually explored for pathology other than hernia. A cannula is then placed under laparoscopic guidance lateral to each rectus abdominus muscle at the level of the umbilicus. A 5-mm cannula is placed on the left side and an 11-mm cannula, suitable for stapler use, is placed on the right side. Because most surgeons are right-hand dominant, stapling is facilitated by placement of the larger cannula on the right, regardless of the side of the hernia.

An alternative approach is to use two 5-mm cannulas instead of a 5-mm and 10- and 11-mm cannulas. In this technique, the stapler is placed down the midline 10- and 12-mm umbilical Hasson-type cannula for stapling and a 5-mm scope is used at that time through one of the 5-mm cannulas. Although changing the scope does add a little time to the procedure, this time difference is more than made up for by the lack of fascial closure needed for the 5-mm cannula sites and by the better cosmetic result.

Differentiating direct from indirect inguinal hernias is accomplished by inspection of the peritoneum. An indirect defect generally has well-defined edges, travels from lateral to medial, and is always located lateral to the spermatic cord and epigastric vessels. In contrast, direct hernias are bulges in the floor of the inguinal region and are located medial to the cord and epigastric vessels.

The peritoneum lining the hernia defect is grasped and everted into the abdomen. The peritoneum is incised transversely from the umbilical ligament to a point several centimeters lateral to the internal inguinal ring. The incision is made superior to the defect and parallel to the iliopubic tract. The ultrasonically activated scalpel (Harmonic scalpel, Ethicon Endosurgery, Cincinnati, OH) is particularly useful in making this incision because the cavitation produced elevates the peritoneum from the underlying tissues. Superior and inferior peritoneal flaps are then raised by blunt dissection, allowing identification of underlying structures and subsequent peritoneal closure over the mesh repair (Fig. 8-2A–D).

With an indirect hernia, the sac is found superior to the cord and should be completely reduced to eliminate the possibility of postoperative hydrocele formation. The sac is dissected free from the cord structures, and large sacs are transacted after reduction. Small reduced sacs are preserved and used in subsequent closure of the peritoneum. In women, the sac and round ligament may be transacted with an endoscopic linear stapler. In direct hernias, no further dissection is required after the peritoneal flaps have been raised.

After the cord structures have been freed from the hernia sac, the defect is covered with polypropylene mesh. A 10 x 15 cm piece of mesh is trimmed to an oval shape, rolled into a tight cylinder, delivered into the abdomen via the 11-mm cannula, and unrolled over the hernia defect. The mesh is secured in position with staples, starting medially at the iliopectineal ligament and progressing superiorly and laterally along the transversus aponeurotic arch and transversalis fascia. No staples are

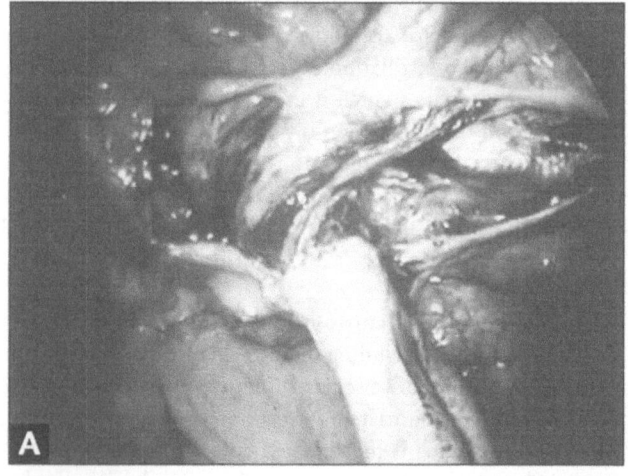
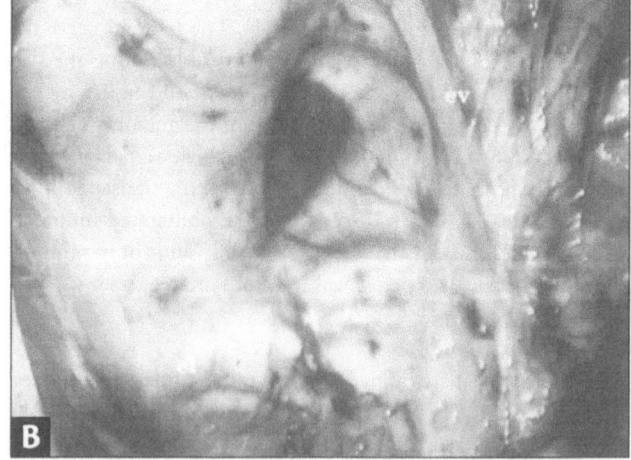
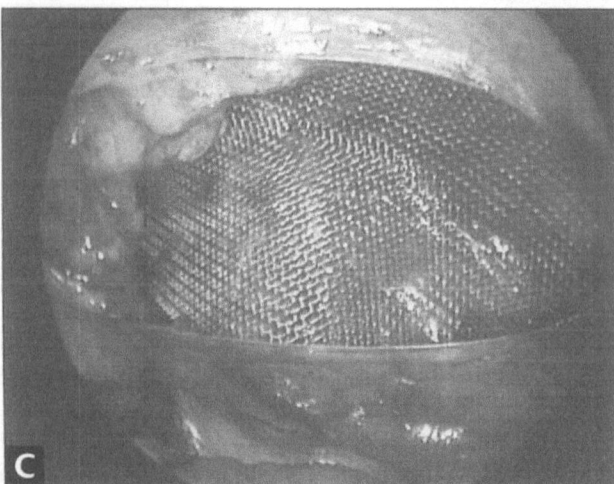
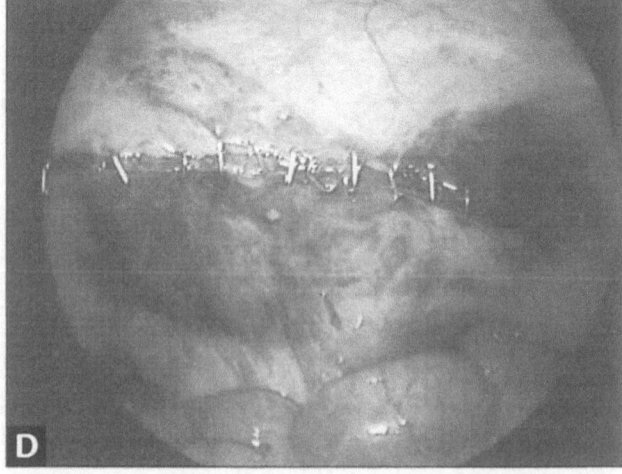

Figure 8-2 Transabdominal inguinal hernioplasty. **A,** The sac is dissected off the spermatic cord in an indirect and direct repair. **B,** In a direct herina, the defect is seen medial to epigastric vessels. **C,** Mesh is placed over the cord and is stapled to Cooper's ligament and the transversus abdominus arch. **D,** The peritonium is closed. cl—Cooper's ligament; ev—epigastric vessels. (*See* Color Plates.)

placed over the epigastric vessels, nor is the mesh stapled over the area inferior to the iliopubic tract and lateral to the internal ring in the vicinity of the lateral femoral cutaneous nerve and the femoral branch of the genitofemoral nerve. The pitfalls of stapling in these areas, with ensuing complications of vascular injury and neuralgias, have been described in several recent reports [26•,27].

Some surgeons prefer to cut a keyhole in the mesh and wrap the mesh around the spermatic cord. To date no study has shown any advantage of this technique over that involving a mesh without a keyhole. Our concern with creating a keyhole is that the cut in the mesh is a potential site for later failure of the repair.

Following mesh repair of the hernia defect, the peritoneum is reapproximated over the mesh with staples. Peritoneal closure is accomplished with closely spaced staples to prevent bowel herniation between the peritoneum and mesh, a complication that has been reported in recent case series [28]. Interestingly, two animal studies of adhesion formation after laparoscopic herniorrhaphy have demonstrated significantly fewer adhesions with exposed mesh than with peritoneal reapproximation [29,30], whereas a third study demonstrated a significant reduction in adhesion formation when the peritoneum was closed over the mesh [31]. Incidentally, we have seen no adhesions to the peritoneal closure in approximately 10 patients who have undergone laparoscopy after laparoscopic inguinal hernia repair.

The extraperitoneal approach

The extraperitoneal approach involves creation of an extraperitoneal space for insufflation and surgery. The advantages of this approach over the transperitoneal method derive from having an intact peritoneum in the extraperitoneal approach. Because this procedure is performed completely outside the peritoneal cavity, the risk of visceral injury is negligible, and there is no interference from bowel during dissection. The urinary bladder also is seen more clearly and is therefore less likely to be injured. Postoperative shoulder pain is virtually absent with the extraperitoneal approach because there is no gas in the peritoneal cavity. Anatomic structures are more recognizable during dissection because they are not covered with peritoneum. Finally, creation of the extraperitoneal space results in complete dissection of direct inguinal hernias and facilitates the dissection of indirect hernia sacs.

The extraperitoneal space can be created by blunt, manual dissection or by use of a disposable balloon dissector. A 12-mm transverse umbilical incision is made, exposing the anterior rectus sheath, which is then divided transversely to reveal the rectus musculature and posterior sheath. The balloon dilator is inserted along the posterior rectus sheath and advanced to the pubic tubercle. Incorrect balloon placement above the anterior sheath will result in creation of a subcutaneous space, whereas placement below the posterior sheath will result in peritoneal rupture. After proper placement, the balloon is filled with saline or air, then is deflated and removed. At this point, an open laparoscopy cannula is placed in the umbilical incision and the extraperitoneal space is insufflated to 15 mm Hg. Two cannulas are placed in the extraperitoneal space lateral to each rectus muscle and at the level of the umbilicus, with a 5-mm cannula on the left and an 11-mm cannula on the right.

Anatomic structures for repair are now identified, with repair proceeding as previously described for the transabdominal approach. With direct hernias, dissection is essentially completed by the balloon. Indirect hernias are managed by complete reduction of the sac, exercising extreme care not to perforate the sac. Peritoneal rupture will result in limited exposure, which may be overcome by venting the pneumoperitoneum with a large-bore angiocatheter. Once the sac has been completely reduced, a pretied ligature is placed at the base of the sac. If the sac contains adherent omentum, it is reduced intraperitoneally and not transected. The polypropylene mesh is secured over the hernia defect with staples as described for the transabdominal approach (Fig. 8-3).

Results

Numerous reports exist detailing the experiences of individual surgeons with either the transabdominal preperitoneal [32–39] or totally extraperitoneal [40–46] techniques of laparoscopic hernia repair. In almost all cases these authors have reported excellent results with few complications (Tables 8-1 and 8-2). Major complications included bowel and bladder injuries and small bowel obstruction with the transabdominal approaches as well as the previously mentioned nerve entrapment syndromes. The totally extraperitoneal approach has not been associated with these complications nor with any other unusual complications. However, this is more likely the result of experience gained in avoiding complications from the laparoscopic transabdominal approach than it is likely to be from the approach itself. The only truly negative study reported to date is that of Cooper and McAlhaney [47]. These authors reported a 21.3% morbidity and a 13.8% recurrence rate in 61 patients undergoing 72 laparoscopic hernia repairs with a mean follow-up of 21 months.

Phillips and coworkers [48] explored the issue of laparoscopic hernia recurrence. In their multicenter study of 3229 repairs with 54 recurrences, the most common cause of recurrence was use of too small a piece of mesh (60%). Other reasons included no staples present to anchor the mesh (32%) and failure of the staples (8%). Most remarkable in this study was the finding that

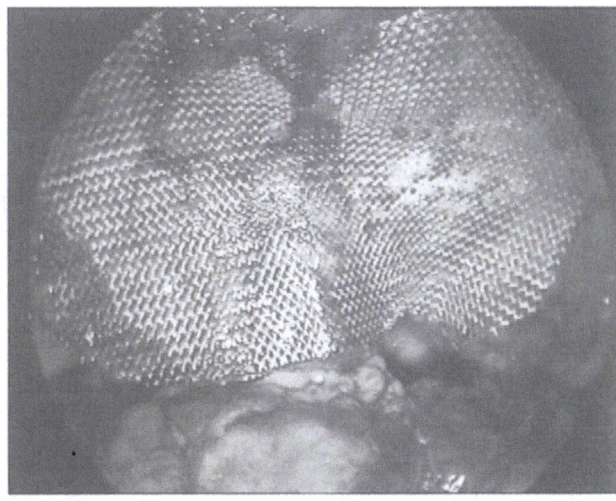

Figure 8-3 Total extraperitoneal hernioplasty. (*See* Color Plate.)

Table 8-1

Transabdominal preperitoneal hernia repair series with over 100 repairs

Study	Patients, n	Follow-up, mo	Major complications, %	Minor complications, %	Recurrence, %
Geis et al. [32]	450	< 24	0	4.0	0.6
Newman et al. [33]	102	< 12	2.2	21.0	1
Wheeler [34]	135	< 18	3.6	5.5	0
Felix et al. [35]	326	< 18	4.4	14.2	0
Paget [36]	222	< 18	1.0	9.0	1.8
Panton and Panton [37]	106	< 12	0	15.2	0
Kavic [38]	224	< 36	0	3.7	0.9
Quilici et al. [39]	509	< 36	0	16.4	0.2

Table 8-2

Totally extraperitoneal laparoscopic hernia repair series with more than 50 repairs

Study	Patients, n	Follow-up, mo	Major complications, %	Minor complications, %	Recurrence, %
McKernan and Laws [40]	51	< 12	3.0	6.0	0
Ferzli et al. [41]	122	< 20	1.0	5.9	0
Kieturakis et al. [42]	150	< 36	0.8	6.0	2
Ferzli and Kiel [43]	326	< 22	2.0	11	1.6
Ramshaw et al. [44]	247	Not stated	1.6	6.4	0.4
Vanclooster et al. [45]	195	> 6	0.5	4.1	0
Heithold et al. [46]	503	< 36	1.2	2.9	0.4

20% of the hernias "recurred" because they were not repaired at the initial operation. Although one might suspect that direct hernias would be more likely to recur because of the larger defects typically present in direct hernias, this was not the case in Phillips and coworkers study, with 39 recurrences occurring in direct hernias and 42 occurring in indirect hernias.

One large study has been reported comparing the totally extraperitoneal (TEP) approach to the transabdominal preperitoneal (TAPP) approach. In this study, Rainshaw and coworkers [49] compared 290 TAPP repairs with 210 TEP repairs. Although complications and recurrences were significantly less in the TEP group, the results do not support the superiority of the TEP over the TAPP repair. In this study, patients were evaluated in a prospective continuous fashion. There is little doubt that because the TEP repairs represented the last 210 repairs performed, these authors would have better results in that group and that the first 290 TAPP repairs represented the early portions of their learning curves.

Unfortunately, large trials by a small group of highly skilled individuals who are very experienced in the procedure fail to provide us with a good overall status of these operations. These types of reports tend to favor the publication of the best results.

Fortunately, laparoscopic herniorrhaphy has been evaluated in an ever-increasing number of prospective, comparative [50–54] (Table 8-3) and prospective, randomized trials [55–63] (Table 8-4). Unfortunately, even the gold standard randomized trial has significant limitations in evaluating open versus laparoscopic approaches. Generally, these trials have small numbers of patients with short periods of follow-up. The surgeons have significantly less experience with the laparoscopic approach in comparison with the open approach and there are numerous types of open repairs that can be compared with a few laparoscopic types of repairs. Further, debate continues regarding which is the best open repair. Finally, there are uncontrolled biases that cannot be accounted for because the study cannot be blinded.

Although follow-up is necessarily of short duration in trials of this new procedure, several benefits are apparent for laparoscopic procedures when compared with various open hernia repair techniques. Analgesic requirements are generally less in patients undergoing laparoscopic repairs. Those patients receiving laparoscopic hernia repairs also return to work in a shorter time, a benefit that is particularly apparent in patients undergoing bilateral repairs. Disadvantages of the laparoscopic technique include significantly greater operative costs and the risks

Table 8-3

Results of prospective, nonrandomized comparisons of laparoscopic transabdominal preperitoneal versus open hernia repairs

Study	Laparo-scopies, n	Open, n	OR time	Pain	Work	Complications	Cost	Recurrence
Cornell and Kerlakian [50]	24	60 (S)	20% greater	50% less	7 d less	Same	50% greater	Same
Millikan et al. [51]	51	75 (V)	Same	Less	39 d less	43% less	90% greater	Same
Brooks [52]	43	57 (M)	20% greater	Same	5 d less	Same	40% greater	Greater
Wilson et al. [53]	121	121 (M)	Same	Same	11 d less	Same	Not stated	Same
Barkun et al. [54]	43	49 (V)	Same	Less	Same	Same	40% greater	Same

M—mesh repair; OR—operating room; S—shouldice-type repair; V—variable open repair.

Table 8-4

Results of prospective, randomized trials of laparoscopic versus open hernia repairs

Study	Follow-up, mo	Laparo-scopies, n	Open, n	OR time	Pain	Work	Compli-cations	Cost	Recurrence
Stoker et al. [55]	7	75 (TA)	75 (D)	15 min less	70% less	14 d less	3 times less	Not stated	Same
Payne et al. [56]	10	48 (TA)	52 (M)	12 min more	Not stated	8 d less	Same	20% more	Same
Maddern et al. [57]*	8	42 (TA)	44 (D)	Same	Same	Same	Same	Not stated	Greater
Lawrence et al. [58]	Not stated	58 (TA)	66 (D)	Not stated	Less	Same	10%	320% more	Same
Vogt et al. [59]	8	30 (IP)	31 (V)	18 min less	3 times less	11 d less	Same	Not stated	Same
Wright et al. [62]	Not stated	60 (TE)	60 (M)	13 min more	80% less	Not stated	Same	Not stated	Not stated
Filipi et al. [60]	11	24 (TA)	29 (M)	22 min more	Same	Same	Same	Not stated	Not stated
Tschudi et al. [61]	6	44 (TA)	43 (S)	28 min more	3 times less	23 d less	Same	Not stated	Less
Liem et al. [63]	20	487 (TE)	507 (V)	5 min less	Less	Less	Same	Not stated	Less

*Used local anesthesia.

D—darn; IP—intraperitoneal onlay mesh; M—mesh; S—shouldice; TA—transabdominal preperitoneal; TE—totally extraperitoneal; V—variable.

inherent in general anesthesia. The ultimate measure of any herniorrhaphy technique is recurrence; here the data are inconclusive. Clearly, studies with longer follow-up are needed before definitive conclusions can be drawn regarding recurrence rates.

CONTROVERSIES

Laparoscopic inguinal herniorrhaphy has generated considerable argument and controversy within the surgical community, and several prominent opponents of the procedure have expressed their opinions in the surgical literature. The Lichtenstein Hernia Institute has pronounced that "laparoscopic hernia repair cannot equal the safety, simplicity, and cost-effectiveness of open, tension-free hernioplasty, nor can it surpass its postoperative durability;" its workers have supported this statement with their own data [11,64]. The tension-free Lichtenstein repair has a recurrence rate of 0.12% in 3125 herniorrhaphies followed from 1 to 8 years, with a 1-week return to work rate of 51.7% for laborers and 75% for office workers.

For some opponents of laparoscopic inguinal herniorrhaphy, the campaign against the procedure becomes a crusade against the medical-industrial complex. Rutkow [65] exposes the apparent evils of the instrument makers in a screed against the "socioeconomic tyranny of surgical technology." Dent [66] derides laparoscopic hernia repair as "technology in search of justification," and cites the words of St. Jerome in warning us that "the scars of others should teach us caution."

The most recent surgeon-skeptic regarding laparoscopic herniorrhaphy is Wantz [67], who complains that "the media and laparoscopic surgeons have oversold the idea that patients could expect less discomfort but have ignored the associated liabilities." He opines that "the continued use of the technique by some is amusing, it might be explained by selfish desire to gain experience, stubborn refusal to believe that tension-free hernioplasties produce superb results, or more likely, inability to do tension-free hernioplasties skillfully and expediently with local anesthesia." Wantz concludes his editorial by declaring that "if, as the laparoscopists regularly claim, they are unable to get the superb outcomes other surgeons obtain with open procedures, they have no one to blame but themselves."

Although these passages of purple prose, often dripping with sarcasm, are entertaining additions to the literature, they shed more heat than light on the subject of laparoscopic herniorrhaphy. What is needed is a dispassionate dissertation on the state of the laparoscopic art as applied to hernia repair. A recent review by Memon *et al.* [68•] comes close to satisfying this requirement. These authors expose the two key factors that have combined to make laparoscopic herniorrhaphy such a controversial technique: "first, there is resistance to changing a time-honored procedure, irrespective of the potential benefits; second, novices practicing a new procedure without proper training cause an increase in morbidity and mortality, giving the new operation a bad reputation."

One study that does shed some light on the debate over the effectiveness of the laparoscopic repair is a prospective, randomized study of the tensile strength of hernia repairs in a porcine model by Horgan and coworkers [69••]. These authors found that both open mesh repairs and laparoscopic repairs are significantly stronger than the normal, nonherniated inguinal region at 4 weeks after operation. Further, the laparoscopic repair is significantly stronger than the open mesh repair.

CONCLUSIONS

Very few of the arguments for or against laparoscopic herniorrhaphy are based on strong, objective data. Although it would be difficult to find anyone on either side of the argument who would contest the contention that the laparoscopic procedure is more costly, no prospective studies exist to support or refute this assertion, especially when the possible savings to society of earlier return to work are considered. Bilateral or recurrent hernias are often put forward as indications for the laparoscopic operation, but here also prospective, randomized trials are lacking. The conventional wisdom is that local anesthesia is preferable to general anesthesia, but in this era of balanced anesthesia and such innovations as laryngeal mask airways, no

objective data have been generated to support this opinion, especially in a relatively healthy patient population undergoing an elective procedure such as inguinal herniorrhaphy. The ultimate indicator of success for the hernia surgeon is rate of recurrence; however, no well-designed, prospective, randomized trials with long-term follow-up exist to determine the best type of open herniorrhaphy. Until this question is answered, it will be difficult to design a prospective, randomized trial of sufficient power to settle the issue of the safety and utility of laparoscopic inguinal hernia repair.

REFERENCES AND RECOMMENDED READING

Recently published papers of particular interest have been highlighted as:

•   Of interest

••   Of outstanding interest

1. Rutkow IM: Surgical operations in the United States. *Arch Surg* 1997, 132:983–990.

2. Glassow F: Short stay surgery (Shouldice technique) for repair of inguinal hernia. *Ann R Coll Surg Engl* 1976, 58:133–139.

3. Lichtenstein IL, Shulman AG, Amid PK, *et al.*: The tension free hernioplasty. *Am J Surg* 1989, 157:188–192.

4. Lichtenstein IL, Shore JM: Exploding the myths of hernia repair. *Am J Surg* 1976, 132:307–315.

5. Nyhus LM: The recurrence of the groin hernia: therapeutic solutions. *World J Surg* 1989, 13:541–544.

6. Thieme ET: Recurrent inguinal hernia. *Arch Surg* 1971, 103:238–241.

7. Cunningham J, Walley JT, Mitchell P, *et al.*: Cooperative hernia study: pain in the postrepair patient. *Ann Surg* 1996, 224:598–602.

8. Read RC: Historical survey of the treatment of hernia. In *Hernia.* Edited by Nyhus LM, Condon RE. Philadelphia: JB Lippincott; 1989:1–17.

9. Ponka JL: Significant contributions toward understanding and sound treatment of hernias. In *Hernias of the Abdominal Wall.* Philadelphia: WB Saunders; 1980:1–17.

10. Anson BJ, Morgan EH, McVay CB: Surgical anatomy of the inguinal region based upon a study of 500 body halves. *Surg Gynecol Obstet* 1960, 11:707–725.

11 Amid PK, Shulman AG, Lichtenstein IL: Current state of the Lichtenstein open tension-free hernioplasty: does laparoscopic hernia repair measure up? *Contemp Surg* 1993, 43:229–233.

12. Nyhus LM: The preperitoneal approach and iliopubic tract repair of inguinal hernias. In *Hernia.* Edited by Nyhus LM, Condon RE. Philadelphia: JB Lippincott; 1995:153–177.

13. Stoppa R:J The preperitoneal approach and prosthetic repair of groin hernias. In *Hernia.* Edited by Nyhus LM, Condon RE. Philadelphia: JB Lippincott; 1995:188–210.

14. Ger R: The management of certain abdominal hernias by intra-abdominal closure of the neck. *Ann R Coll Surg Engl* 1982, 64:342–344.

15. Ger R, Monroe K, Duvivier R, *et al.*: Management of indirect inguinal hernias by laparoscopic closure of the neck of the sac. *Am J Surg* 1990, 159:370–373.

16. Popp LW. Improvement in endoscopic hernioplasty: transcutaneous aquadissection of the musculofascial defect and preperitoneal endoscopic patch repair. *J Laparoendosc Surg* 1991, 1:83–90.

17. Schultz L, Graber J, Peitrafitta J, *et al.*: Laser laparoscopic herniorrhaphy: a clinical trial preliminary results. *J Laparoendosc Surg* 1990, 1:41–45.

18. Corbitt JD: Transabdominal preperitoneal herniorrhaphy. *Surg Laparosc Endosc* 1993, 3:328–333.

19. Filipi CJ, Fitzgibbons RJ, Salerno GM, *et al.*: Laparoscopic herniorrhaphy. *Surg Clin North Am* 1992, 72:1109–1124.

20. Redmond EJ, Salerno GM, Annabali R, *et al.*: Laparoscopic herniorrhaphy. In *Current Techniques in Laparoscopy*. Edited by Brooks DC. Philadelphia: Current Medicine; 1993:18.1–18.11.

21. Keating JP, Morgan A: Femoral nerve palsy following laparoscopic inguinal herniorrhaphy. *J Laparoendosc Surg* 1993, 3:557–559.

22. Eubanks S, Newman L, Goehring L, *et al.*: Meralgia paresthetica: a complication of laparoscopic herniorrhaphy. *Surg Laparosc Endosc* 1993, 3:381–385.

23. Krause MA: Nerve injury during laparoscopic inguinal hernia repair. *Surg Laparosc Endosc* 1993, 3:342–345.

24. Seid AS, Deutsch H, Jacobson A. Laparoscopic herniorrhaphy. *Surg Laparosc Endosc* 1992, 2:59–60.

25. Spaw AT, Ennis BW, Spaw LP. Laparoscopic hernia repair: the anatomic basis. *J Laparoendosc Surg* 1991, 1:269–77.

26.• Brick WG, Colbom GL, Gadacz TR, *et al.*: Crucial anatomic lessons for laparoscopic herniorrhaphy. *Am Surg* 1995, 61:172–177.
Cadaveric demonstrations of the variability of nerves and vessels in the inguinal area when viewed transabdominally.

27. Sampath P, Yeo CJ, Campbell JN: Nerve injury associated with laparoscopic inguinal herniorrhaphy. *Surgery* 1995, 118:829–833.

28. Phillips EH, Arregui M, Carroll BJ, *et al.*: Incidence of complications following laparoscopic hernioplasty. *Surg Endosc* 1995, 9:16–21.

29. Eller R, Twaddell C, Poulos E, *et al.*: Abdominal adhesions in laparoscopic hernia repair. *Surg Endosc* 1994, 8:181–184.

30. Durstein-Decker C, Brick WG, Gadacz TR, *et al.*: Comparison of adhesion formation in transperitoneal laparoscopic herniorrhaphy techniques. *Am Surg* 1994, 60:157–159.

31. Vader VL, Vogt DM, Zucker KA, *et al.*: Adhesion formation in laparoscopic hernia repair. *Surg Endosc* 1997, 11:825–829.

32. Geis WP, Crafton WB, Novak MJ, *et al.*: Laparoscopic herniorrhaphy: results and technical aspects in 450 consecutive procedures. *Surgery* 1993, 114:765–774.

33. Newman L, Eubanks S, Mason E, *et al.*: Is laparoscopic herniorrhaphy an effective alternative to open hernia repair? *J Laparoendosc Surg* 1993, 3:121–128.

34. Wheeler KH: Laparoscopic inguinal herniorrhaphy with mesh: an 18-month experience. *J Laparoendosc Surg* 1993, 3:345–350.

35. Felix EL, Michas CA, McKnight RL: Laparoscopic herniorrhaphy transabdominal preperitoneal floor repair. *Surg Endosc* 1994, 8:100–104.

36. Paget GW: Laparoscopic inguinal herniorrhaphy: a personal audit of 222 hernia repairs. *Med J Aust* 1994, 161:249–252.

37. Panton ON, Panton RJ: Laparoscopic hernia repair. *Am J Surg* 1994, 167:535–537.

38. Kavic MS: Laparoscopic hernia repair. *Surg Endosc* 1995, 9:12–15.

39. Quilici PJ, Greaney EM, Quilici J, *et al.*: Transabdominal preperitoneal laparoscopic inguinal herniorrhaphy: results of 509 repairs. *Am Surg* 1996, 62:849–852.

40. McKeman JB, Laws HL: Laparoscopic repair of inguinal hernias using a totally extraperitoneal prosthetic approach. *Surg Endosc* 1993, 7:26–28.

41. Ferzli GS, Massaad A, Dysarz FA, *et al.*: A study of 101 patients treated with extraperitoneal endoscopic laparoscopic herniorrhaphy. *Am Surg* 1993, 59:707–708.

42. Kieturakis MJ, Nguyen DT, Vargas H, *et al.*: Balloon dissection facilitated laparoscopic extraperitoneal hernioplasty. *Am J Surg* 1994, 168:603–607.

43. Ferzli G, Kiel T: Evolving techniques in endoscopic extraperitoneal herniorrhaphy. *Surg Endosc* 1995, 9:928–930.

44. Ramshaw BJ, Tucker J, Duncan T, *et al.*: The effect of previous lower abdominal surgery on performing the total extraperitoneal approach to laparoscopic herniorrhaphy. *Am Surg* 1996, 62:292–294.

45. Vanclooster P, Meersman AL, de Gheldere CA, *et al.*: The totally extraperitoneal laparoscopic hernia repair: preliminary results. *Surg Endosc* 1996, 10:332–335.

46. Heithold DL, Ramshaw BJ, Mason EM, *et al.*: 500 total extraperitoneal approach laparoscopic herniorrhaphies: a single-institution review. *Am Surg* 1997, 63:299–301.

47. Cooper SS, McAlhaney JC: Laparoscopic inguinal hernia repair: is the enthusiasm justified? *Am Surg* 1997, 63:103–105.

48. Phillips EH, Rosenthal R, Fallas M, *et al.*: Reasons for early recurrence following laparoscopic hernioplasty. *Surg Endosc* 1995, 9:140–145.

49. Rainshaw BJ, Tucker JG, Duncan TD, *et al.*: Technical considerations of the different approaches to laparoscopic herniorrhaphy: an analysis of 500 cases. *Am Surg* 1996, 62:69–72.

50. Cornell RB, Kerlakian GM: Early complications and outcomes of the current technique of transperitoneal laparoscopic herniorrhaphy and a comparison to the traditional open approach. *Am J Surg* 1994, 168:275–279.

51. Millikan KW, Kosik ML, Doolas A: A prospective comparison of transabdominal preperitoneal laparoscopic hernia repair versus traditional open hernia repair in a university setting. *Surg Laparosc Endosc* 1994, 4:247–253.

52. Brooks DC: A prospective comparison of laparoscopic and tension-free open herniorrhaphy. *Arch Surg* 1994, 129:361–366.

53. Wilson MS, Deans GT, Brough WA: Prospective trial comparing Lichtenstein with laparoscopic tension-free mesh repair of inguinal hernia. *Br J Surg* 1995, 82:274–277.

54. Barkun JS, Wexler MJ, Hinchey EJ, *et al.*: Laparoscopic versus open inguinal herniorrhaphy: preliminary results of a randomized controlled trial. *Surgery* 1995, 118:703–710.

55. Stoker DL, Spiegelhalter DJ, Singh R, *et al.*: Laparoscopic versus open inguinal hernia repair: randomised prospective trial. *Lancet* 1994, 343:1243–1245.

56. Payne JH, Grininger LM, Izawa MT, *et al.*: Laparoscopic or open inguinal herniorrhaphy? A randomized prospective trial. *Arch Surg* 1994, 129:973–979.

57. Maddern GJ, Rudkin G, Bessell JR, *et al.*: A comparison of laparoscopic and open hernia repair as a day surgical procedure. *Surg Endosc* 1994, 8:1404–1408.

58. Lawrence K, McWhinnie D, Goodwin A, *et al.*: Randomised controlled trial of laparoscopic versus open repair of inguinal hernia: early results. *BMJ* 1995, 311:981–985.

59. Vogt DM, Curet MJ, Pitcher DE, *et al.*: Preliminary results of a prospective randomized trial of laparoscopic onlay versus conventional inguinal herniorrhaphy. *Am J Surg* 1995, 169:84–89.

60. Filipi CJ, Gaston-Johansson F, McBride PJ, *et al.*: An assessment of pain and return to normal activity: laparoscopic herniorrhaphy vs open tension-free Lichtenstein repair. *Surg Endosc* 1996, 10:983–986.

61. Tschudi J, Wagner M, Klaiber C, *et al.*: Controlled multicenter trial of laparoscopic transabdominal preperitoneal hernioplasty vs shouldice herniorrhaphy: early results. *Surg Endosc* 1996, 10:845–847.

62. Wright DM, Kennedy A, Baxter JN, *et al.*: Early outcome after open versus extraperitoneal endoscopic tension-free hernioplasty: a randomized clinical trial. *Surgery* 1996, 119:552–557.

63. Liem MS, van der Graaf Y, Steensel CJ, *et al.*: Comparison of conventional anterior surgery and laparoscopic surgery for inguinal-hernia repair. *N Engl J Med* 1997, 336:1541–1547.

64. Lichtenstein IL, Shulman AG, Amid PK: Laparoscopic hernioplasty. *Arch Surg* 1991, 126:1449.

65. Rutkow IM: Laparoscopic hernia repair: the socioeconomic tyranny of surgical technology. *Arch Surg* 1992, 127:1271.

66. Dent TL: Laparoscopic herniorrhaphy: technology in search of justification. *Laparosc Surg* 1994, 2:111–113.

67. Wantz GE: Laparoscopic herniorrhaphy. *J Am Coll Surg* 1997, 184:521–522.

68.• Memon MA, Rice D, Donohue JH: Laparoscopic herniorrhaphy. *J Am Coll Surg* 1997, 184:325–335.

A comprehensive review of the various controversies associated with laparoscopic herniorrhaphy.

69•• Horgan LF, Shelton JC, O'Riordan DC, *et al.*: Strengths and weaknesses of laparoscopic and open mesh inguinal hernia repair: a randomized controlled experimental study. *Br J Surg* 1996, 83:1463–1467.

An excellent animal surgery study providing a standardized method for mechanically testing inguinal hernia repairs in pigs.

Laparoscopic Surgery of the Spleen, Adrenal, and Pancreas

D.E.M. Litwin

John J. Kelly

Mark P. Callery

CHAPTER

9

The advances in laparoscopic instrumentation and technique that have taken place during the past several years have made the performance of solid organ surgery more feasible. Laparoscopic management of disease processes involving the spleen, adrenal, and especially the pancreas were initially considered to be impractical. Through careful planning, leading members of the laparoscopic community have overcome significant barriers to perform safe surgery while maintaining sound medical and surgical principles.

MANAGEMENT OF THE SPLEEN

The spleen is located posteriorly in the left upper abdomen in close approximation with the diaphragm, stomach, pancreas, colon, kidney, and ribs nine through eleven. It is anchored to surrounding structures by ligamentous attachments in a suspensory fashion. These attachments are the result of peritoneal reflections formed and refashioned during intra-abdominal embryologic development. The ligaments, depending on their location, have a variable degree of additional fatty tissue and vascularity. Their identification and management have always been key elements to safe, open splenectomy. For laparoscopic splenectomy, this is equally (if not more) true. Proper positioning and meticulous dissection under direct view allows for safe and hemostatic lapararoscopic splenectomy.

The spleen functions as a component of the reticuloendothelial system and the body's immune system. These functions can occasionally recruit the spleen into playing significant roles in disease processes that are either primary or secondary. Although many of these disease processes may be managed medically, surgical removal is indicated for some conditions (Table 9-1).

Laparoscopic removal of the spleen has become increasingly accepted. For some conditions like idiopathic thrombocytopenic purpura (ITP) (which comprises the majority of elective splenectomies), others and we consider it to be the gold standard [1,2•]. Initially, studies involving laparoscopic splenectomy (LS) consisted of small series or case reports [3–5]. These studies have demonstrated that LS is technically feasible and also suggest that less pain, quicker recovery, and shorter hospital stays are possible. Larger series followed [2•,6•,7•]. These studies confirmed safe, technically feasible removal with low conversion rates (5% to 10%) of even moderate to large-sized spleens of variable pathology.

Hospital stay was dramatically reduced by 2 to 4 days in most studies [1,2•,8], as was postoperative pain and time until return to full activity. Operating times were found to be generally longer by about 20 to 40 minutes. However, we believe that this difference narrows with experience. Friedman and coworkers [2•] series included data on their last ten ITP splenectomies. For their group, laparoscopic operative time of 94 minutes compared most favorably with their hospital's experience with open splenectomies

Table 9-1

Potential indications for splenectomy

Trauma

Hemolytic anemia
  Hereditary spherocytosis
  Elliptocytosis
  Enzyme deficiency
  Idiopathic autoimmune
  Thalassemia
  Sickle cell disease

Thrombocytopenia
  Idiopathic thrombocytopenic purpura
  Thrombotic thrombocytopenic purpura
  Felty's syndrome
  Lupus

Myeloproliferative or lymphoproliferative disease
  Non-Hodgkins lymphoma
  Staging for Hodgkins lymphoma
  Secondary hypersplenism resulting in cytopenia or physical
    symptoms from size
  Hairy cell leukemia
  Angiogenic myeloid metaplasia

Hypersplenism
  Associated with neoplastic process as above, splenic vein
    thrombosis, and portal hypertension

Splenic artery aneurysm

Storage disease
  Gaucher's

Other
  Sarcoidosis
  Cyst
  Infarct
  Abscess
  Tumors

(103 minutes). Total hospital costs in many large series were also comparable [2•,6•]. Still additional savings from a quicker return of patients to productive status are postulated.

Experience gained with splenic resection has allowed us and other investigators to safely manage some splenic salvage techniques laparoscopically. These techniques include partial splenectomy or splenorrhaphy for the fragmented spleen [9,10], and even a case of partial splenectomy for congenital spherocytosis in an infant (actually done twice in the same infant) (Rossi and Litwin, Abstract presented at the Society of American Gastrointestinal Surgeons [SAGES], Philadelphia, March 15–17, 1996). This was done to reduce the need for blood transfusion while theoretically preserving additional time for maturation of immune function. Laparoscopic splenic salvage has also been performed for posttraumatic splenic cyst management [11–13].

Techniques

Splenic resection

The indication for splenectomy must be thoroughly reviewed in conjunction with the hematologist. Candidates receive vaccinations (generally against *Pneumococcus* species, but may also

receive *Haemophilus influenzae* type b and meningococcus vaccine) more than 2 weeks prior to the day of surgery. Candidates have their blood typed and held unless significant platelet or hemoglobin abnormalities require cross-matching for potential emergent intraoperative use. We do not routinely transfuse platelets in the immediate preoperative setting for ITP and have safely removed spleens with platelet counts as low as 3000. In such extreme thrombocytopenic patients, we do transfuse at the end of the case in order to lower the potential perioperative morbidity from hematoma formation either intra-abdominally or subcutaneously. A bowel preparation is not routinely used.

Patients are positioned with the aid of a beanbag mattress in the full lateral approach and careful attention is made to the padding of pressure points. The operating table is slightly flexed at the level of the patient's kidney, and the table placed in slight reverse Trendelenburg position. A three-port technique is now used for most spleens with ITP, as they are of normal size. A fourth port is added for more difficult (usually the larger) spleens. Placement of the initial port is chosen at the left anterior axillary line and just below the costal margin. The abdomen is entered here with a Veress needle and insufflated to 15 mm Hg (Fig. 9-1). A 10-cm trocar is placed here as the camera port and a 30° laparoscope is used. A second port of 5 mm is placed in the epigastrium for blunt retraction or for dissection. A 12-mm port is placed in the left midaxillary line for similar use, and for introduction of the linear stapler or ultrasonic scalpel. To safely place this port, frequently the splenic flexure of the colon must be released from its most superior and lateral retroperitoneal attachments (reflection). This is done with the use of scissors introduced from the epigastric port. A fourth port of 5 mm can be placed if necessary in the left flank. The surgeon and camera operator are positioned on the patient's abdominal side. An assistant may be necessary on the opposite side to manage the fourth port. A surgeon of smaller to average height is usually more comfortable operating from a small step. An exploration of the left upper quadrant is initiated and continues throughout the dissection in order to identify the presence of accessory spleens.

The removal of the spleen consists of a series of maneuvers that safely and progressively mobilizes it on its hilum. This mobilization is initiated by the careful division to the splenocolic ligament with electrocautery. As the most inferior section of the spleen is freed, the most inferior segmental branch or branches to the spleen can be exposed, clipped, and divided. The inferior margin of hilum begins to come into view. At this point it is important that the surgeon be able to rotate the spleen medially and laterally over the hilum of the spleen. Next, electrocautery is used along the avascular posteriolateral attachments of the spleen (splenorenal ligament) while bluntly rotating the spleen medially through the epigastric port (Fig. 9-2). This is divided up to the level of the phrenic attachments (ligament). Some of the phrenic attachment will be left until near completion of the entire dissection to serve as superior suspension.

The short gastric vessels and stomach should come into view as the superior pole is reached. Care must be taken not to injure the stomach with the electrocautery. A variable amount of progress toward the hilar vessels may be made from this posterior approach. During any parts of the dissection, small vessels may

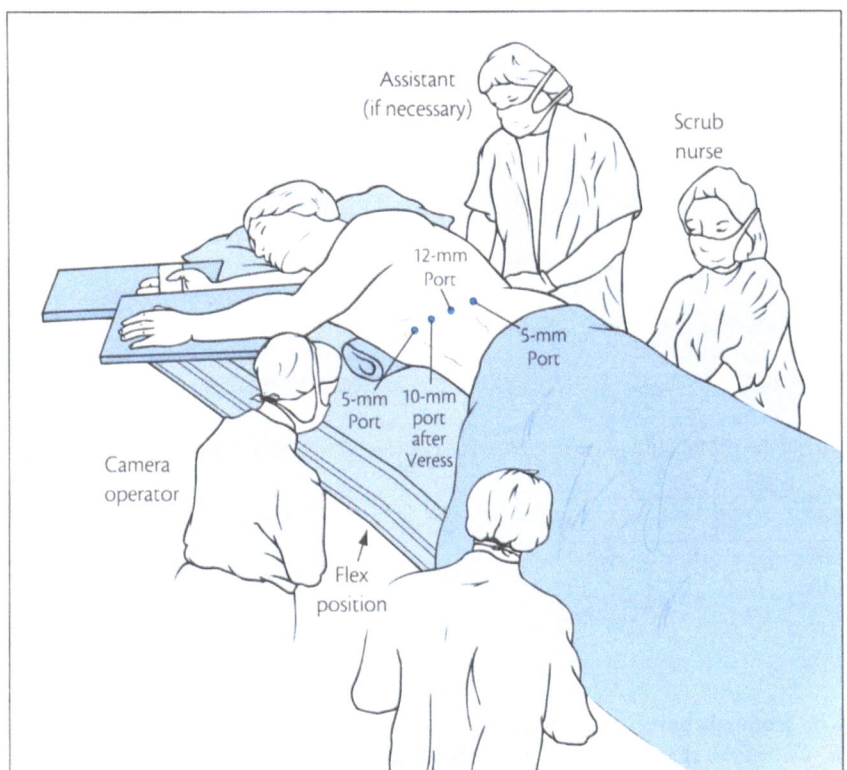

Figure 9-1 Laparoscopic splenectomy. Positioning of patient and operating personnel. Port placement is standard three ports with optional fourth (5-mm) port.

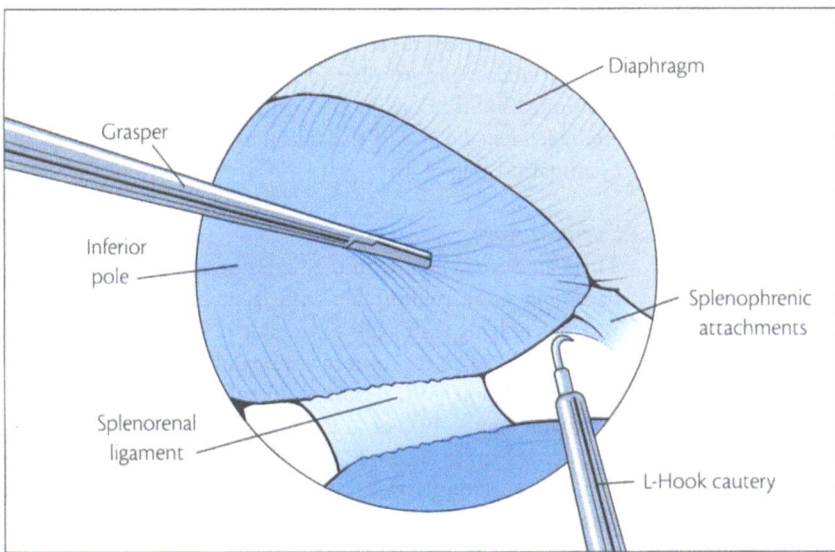

Figure 9-2 Division of the splenorenal ligament. A 5-mm grasper through the epigastric port maintains medial rotation of the spleen to expose the splenorenal ligament, which will be divided with electrocautery. Several vessels to the inferior pole are shown divided here.

be disrupted and cause bleeding that locally obscures and stains the tissues. Irrigation techniques can be frustrating, either because the area cannot be aspirated with complete satisfaction, or aggressive aspiration changes the pneumoperitonium conditions. Irrigation can also spread the staining of tissues and can create an annoying moist reflection to the tissues. We prefer to use laparoscopic sponges for the same purpose one would use sponges in an open technique: to blot and identify vessels in need of control, or to temporarily tamponade an oozing site so that dissection may be carried out in another location while hemostasis develops. (We use a vaginal pack or throat pack sponge, which contains a radiopaque marker. The sponge is cut into strips of approximately 5 cm and entered as a formal count on the surgical field.

Sponges may be introduced into ports 10 mm in size or larger.) The spleen can then be laterally rotated.

An opening into the lesser sac at the level of the hilum is created. This is accomplished by the division with electrocautery or ultrasonic scalpel of the inferior splenogastric attachments. At this point, the spleen can be well elevated and hilum identified. Fine dissection in the area of the hilum is generally not required, but can be carried out if necessary. The tail of pancreas, if present, is generally identified as it approaches the hilum. If needed, additional distance between tail of pancreas and hilum of spleen can be obtained by careful dissection to provide more "release" of the hilar vessels and "retraction" of the pancreas. The splenic artery and vein are then divided en bloc with a 30-mm endoscopic stapler (Fig. 9-3).

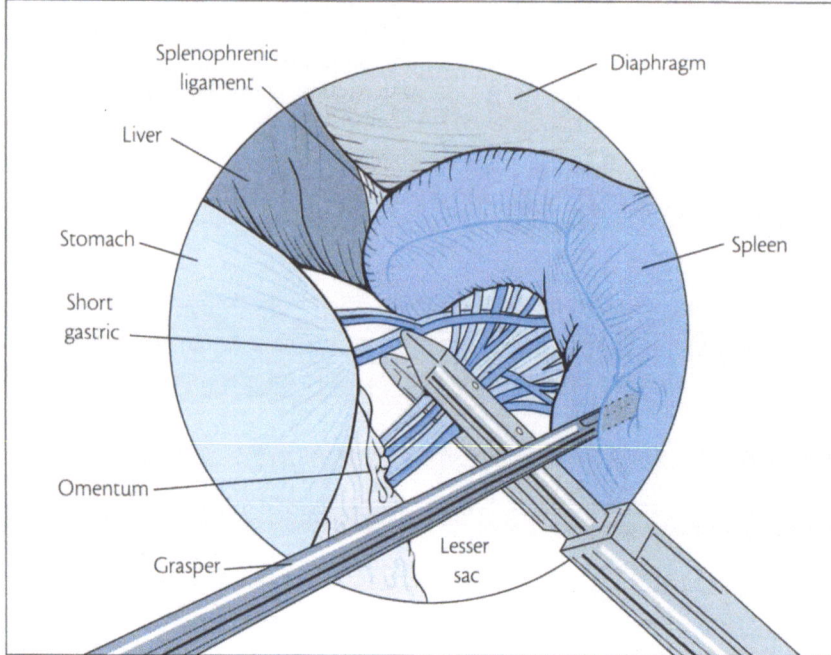

Figure 9-3 Division of hilar vessels. An endoscopic stapling device is introduced through the 12-mm midaxillary port. The spleen has been rotated laterally, and some inferior pole elevation is created with the grasper.

Several firings of the stapling device may be required, but are usually not necessary, to divide the hilum. We believe that the complication of an arteriovenous malformation will not occur if the vessels are stapled across. The splenic dissection is completed with division of the short gastric vessels approached anteriorly or posteriorly (clips, electrocautery, or ultrasonic scalpel) and finally the remainder of phrenic ligament to allow placement into a bag. A large, sturdy specimen bag, *eg*, the 15-mm Endo Bag (US Surgical Corporation, Norwalk, CT), is introduced through the 12-mm port site. We prefer a bag with a stiff outer rim that allows retrieval with a scoop-type technique. Digital enlargement of the port site is all that is required to accept this 15-mm instrument (avoiding the cost for an additional 15-mm trocar). The edges of the bag are delivered through this port site. A ring forcep is used to bluntly separate the spleen into sections that may be withdrawn through the trocar site. Suction is used to aspirate released blood or splenic tissue. Extreme care must be taken to avoid tearing the bag. Patience is usually all that is required, but upward lift on the edges of the bag will avoid the formation of folds at the base of the bag that might inadvertently be grabbed and torn. Once the spleen is removed, this port site is temporarily occluded for reinsufflation and a final hemostatic look.

In the author's (DL) experience, this technique has been successfully used in an ongoing series of elective splenectomies now exceeding 50 patients. ITP was the indication for splenectomy in more than 70% of cases. In our early series of 30 patients, there were five conversions (17%) for reasons including bleeding (*n* = 2), size (*n* = 2), and unsure diagnosis of splenic cyst (*n* = 1) after an intraoperative aspiration of the cyst produced blood. Operating times averaged 155 minutes and length of hospital stay was just under 5 days. The average weight of the nonconverted splenectomies was 165 g. For ITP splenectomy, operative time is around 90 minutes and patients

generally go home on postoperative day 2. There were three postoperative complications: fever (*n* = 1), pneumonia (*n* = 1), and postoperative bleeding requiring angiographic embolization of the splenic artery (*n* = 1). Currently, our approach is to recommend laparoscopic splenectomy for all spleens that are normal in size, and we plan to do all of these in a full lateral position. Modifications in laparoscopic technique and success are dependent on size of the spleen as evident by the physical examination (Fig. 9-4).

Splenic salvage

There are several reports in the literature from authors who are becoming more comfortable with laparoscopic spleen surgery and are applying their skills to the role of splenic salvage. These reports have taken the form of segmental resection for traumatic fragmentation [10], dexon mesh splenorrhaphy for grade 3 traumatic injury [9], or use of fibrin glue [14]. Rossi and Litwin's (Abstract presented at SAGES, 1996) experience with partial splenectomy consists of the infant previously mentioned with congenital spherocystosis.

This procedure took the form of a splenic "debulking" procedure, which is possible due to the segmental blood supply of the spleen. The short gastric vessels were taken early on between clips. The superior pole vessels were subsequently identified and divided between clips. Once devascularization of 75% of the splenic parenchyma was carried out, the parenchyma was fractured with a blunt laparoscopic instrument leaving a 1-cm cuff of devascularized splenic tissue. Hemostasis was excellent.

Splenic cyst unroofing

Many splenic cysts are formed as a result of trauma, but some may be epidermoid in origin. Intervention for splenic cysts is generally indicated on the basis of the pain they produce due to their size. Because of size, the cysts are easily found. Large cysts

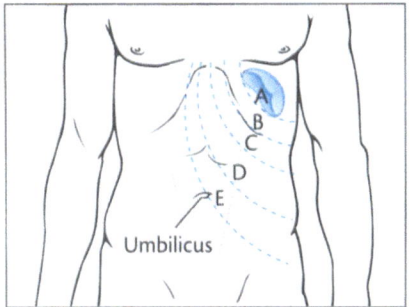

Figure 9-4 Laparoscopic operative planning by splenic size. Normal-sized spleen (*A*). There is a high laparoscopic success rate with low conversion; approach in full lateral position. Slight enlargement of spleen (*B*); same conditions as in *A*. Spleen just palpable at costal margin (*C*). Likely high success rate; still approach in full lateral position, but supine with 30° rotation might be considered. Very large spleens (*D*) may be preferably approached supine with 30° rotation. There is a significant conversion rate; consider splenic artery ligation first; might be consideration for HandPort technique. Extremely large spleen (to umbilicus) (*E*). Although successful laparoscopic approach is reported by most surgeons, an open technique is prudent.

are thin-walled and a significant portion of the wall does not contain any overlying splenic parenchyma.

The cyst may be entered with the use of electrocautery. Once entered and the cyst fluid aspirated, the cystotomy is extended with the use of the hook electrode or scissors. The thin portion of the cyst is widely unroofed until normal splenic parenchyma is reached. Once significant overlying parenchyma is reached, the excision of the cyst wall is terminated. We would not advise extending the unroofing into the splenic parenchyma. Occasionally, opening the cyst wall requires the use of 10-mm Mayo-type scissors.

We also recommend suturing or stapling omentum into the cyst to prevent coaptation of the walls and cyst recurrence. In our experience, however, the cyst will frequently recur, but will be small and asymptomatic. We believe that this recurrence is caused by the softness of the spleen, which allows for some degree of cyst wall coaptation.

The approach to splenic cysts with the aid of laparoscopic ultrasound has been described [11]. Again, we find that cysts large enough to generate symptoms requiring operative intervention will easily be found. Entirely intraparenchymal cysts are likely to be small, asymptomatic, and not require operative therapy.

MANAGEMENT OF THE ADRENALS

The adrenal glands are found in a retroperitoneal location just above and slightly medial to the kidney. The adrenal, as an organ of the neuroendocrine system, is responsible for production of the steroid hormones (androgens, cortisol, aldosterone) from its cortex, and the catecholamines (epinephrine and norepinephrine) from its medulla. The surgical removal of the adrenal gland or glands may become necessary for the primary treatment of adrenal masses achieving significant size or hormonal function. Resection has traditionally been indicated for any hormonally active neoplasm, and for any nonfunctioning lesion greater than 5 or 6 cm [15,16]. Controversy still exists

over the operative versus conservative management of nonfunctioning lesions between 3 to 5 cm. Some authors favor resection [17,18,19•] for the following reasons: 1) potential for malignancy, 2) potential for unrecognized hormonal activity, or 3) underestimation of size by CT scan. As less-invasive techniques become more widely practiced, it may be prudent for this population of tumors to be resected.

Familiarity and recognition of anatomic relationships between the adrenal gland and surrounding structures is key to successful open or laparoscopic adrenal surgery. Understanding of the adrenal's rich blood supply is also important to both approaches, but meticulous control is even more important in laparoscopic surgery. Numerous small arterial branches are derived from the renal artery, phrenic artery, and directly from the aorta. The adrenal vein is frequently a single central vein on either side. The length of the left adrenal vein (approximately 2 cm) is longer than its counterpart on the right (0.5 to 1 cm), in part due to the right gland's tight relationship to the inferior vena cava (IVC). The left adrenal vein empties into the left renal vein, and is usually joined by the left phrenic vein at or near this connection. The right adrenal vein directly enters the IVC somewhat posteriorly. Rarely, a second right adrenal vein may be present that separately enters the IVC or the right hepatic vein.

Indications for adrenalectomy include 1) functioning cortical adenoma (Cushing's syndrome); 2) aldosteronoma (Conn's syndrome); 3) adrenocortical carcinoma; 4) pheochromocytoma; 5) nonfunctioning cortical adenoma (> 5 cm, controversy for > 3 cm); 6) isolated metastatic lesion (most commonly from lung, breast, stomach, and melanoma); and 7) other, including myelolipoma and adrenal cysts. (The diagnosis of each is beyond the scope of this chapter.)

Laparoscopic adrenalectomy has now been described in the literature to treat all of these indications. It may be argued, however, that in preoperatively diagnosed adrenocortical carcinoma with invasion of surrounding structures, the open approach may be preferred. Gagner and coworkers [20,21] were the first to publish a significant series on laparoscopic adrenalectomy. In 18 patients, 21 adrenalectomies were attempted. Indications included functional cortical adenoma (three patients); nonfunctioning cortical adenoma (five patients); aldosteronoma (two patients); pheochromocytoma (three patients, one with multiple endocrine neoplasia 2B); bilateral adrenal hyperplasia from pituitary Cushing's disease (two patients); and angiomyolipoma (one patient, who required conversion due to difficulty with dissection of this 15-cm mass).

Postoperative complications were relatively minor and few in number. Operating time was reasonable (average 2.3 hours) as was mean discharge date (4 days). Gagner and coworkers [22••] have now performed well over 100 adrenalectomies with similar success. Similar series confirm these results [23–27]. Several have retrospectively compared laparoscopic versus open adrenalectomy in their institutions [23,24,26]. These findings suggest that the laparoscopic technique takes longer (30 to 80 minutes), but there is significant advantage in blood loss, transfusion use, pain control, length of stay (as much as 4 days difference), and return to activity. Most advanced laparoscopic surgeons now consider the laparoscopic approach the standard for adrenalectomy, at least with respect to benign disease. Questions are still asked as to what size is safe for the laparoscopic approach, the management of malignant or potentially malignant (*ie*, pheochromocytoma) adrenal disease, and the optimal minimally invasive approach.

Many experienced adrenal surgeons, including us, do not set size criteria limitations. We also feel that preoperative studies and laparoscopic exploration (± ultrasound) are adequate for most lesions including pheochromocytoma [28]. We consider invasive adrenal malignancy, however, to be a relative contraindication. The author (DL) has gained significant experience in over 50 consecutive laparoscopic adrenalectomies (Unpublished data). In these patients, there were no conversions, and operating time averaged less than 2 hours. The largest tumor resected was over 11 cm. There were no significant complications, no transfusions required, and the average length of stay was 3 days.

Techniques

Laparoscopic adrenalectomy

Minimally invasive surgery of the adrenal gland appears to consist of three main approaches: transabdominal flank (lateral), anterior transabdominal (supine), and retroperitoneal (lateral). Most larger series have been published using the flank approach, and this is the approach we now favor. We credit Gagner and coworkers [21] with the original description of the lateral approach to the spleen and adrenal, and adopted his approach after our earlier experience with the supine approach. The supine approach might initially offer some advantage to the operator's ease of orientation and access to bilateral processes, but generally results in a more difficult laparoscopic exposure, and is more time-consuming. Additionally, more retraction of internal organs is required. The retroperitoneal approach may show promise for small, unilateral, benign tumors, especially with the introduction of balloon dissectors [29], but the experience is still limited and it appears to have little advantage over the lateral approach.

Left adrenalectomy

The patient and operating personnel are positioned as described for splenectomy. The ports are also positioned in a similar fashion, with the only exception being a 10-mm port substituted for the 12-mm port at the midaxillary line. If necessary, the camera may alternate between the two larger ports. Access to the anterior surface of the adrenal is accomplished by initial division of the posterior peritoneal attachments of the spleen. Progressive medial rotation of the spleen is carried out by further division of the splenorenal attachments. The tail of the pancreas frequently comes into view, which signifies an adequate dissection (Fig. 9-5). By this stage the adrenal gland is almost always identified because of its unique position and color. For continued exposure, the spleen may need to be bluntly retracted medially. In such case the optional 5-mm port may be placed in the left flank. A laparoscopic sponge is placed on a 5-mm grasper similar to a sponge stick configuration, and the spleen is "pushed" and held medially by the assistant. Dissection can now continue through the more comfortably positioned epigastric and midaxillary ports.

Rarely, Gerota's fascia must be incised and the perinephric fat pad bluntly dissected to appreciate the gland. In the most difficult cases, the upper pole of the kidney must be identified through the perinephric fat, and the adrenal gland found in its superior-medial position. Much of the remainder of the dissection essentially consists of meticulous identification and hemostatic control of multiple small vessels.

Dissection is initiated by division of the inferior and lateral margins of gland with the use of electrocautery. Countertraction of the gland is accomplished by blunt retraction or by grasping the surrounding connective tissue of the gland. Grasping the gland itself will result in tearing of the gland, which is friable, and obscurative bleeding will occur. At the upper lateral aspect of the adrenal gland, there is often a sizeable vein that may need additional cautery coaptation or even require clips.

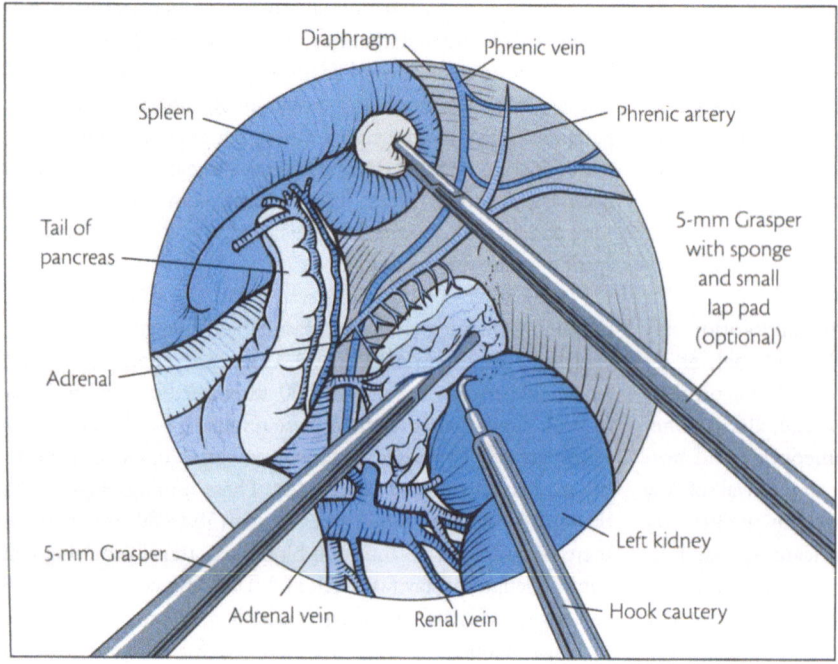

Figure 9-5 Left adrenal gland. The spleen has been medially displaced, exposing hilum and tail of the pancreas. The adrenal gland and surrounding anatomy are exposed.

Diaphragm

Phrenic vein

Spleen

Phrenic artery

Tail of pancreas

5-mm Grasper with sponge and small lap pad (optional)

Adrenal

Left kidney

5-mm Grasper

Adrenal vein   Renal vein   Hook cautery

At the most inferior and somewhat medial margin of the gland, the left adrenal vein will most universally be found. Unless immediate control is necessary, such as for a pheochromocytoma, its division is left until later. Next, division of the medial to superior margin is made with L-hook electrocautery. This region contains multiple small vessels representing mainly arterial arcades from the phrenic artery. If small bleeding or oozing is encountered, we like to control the field with laparoscopic sponges as we described previously for laparoscopic splenectomy. The adrenal vein can then be dissected out bluntly and divided between multiple clips. The posterior attachment to the adrenal is generally avascular and can easily be developed. The adrenal gland is placed in a small laparoscopic specimen bag for removal.

Right adrenalectomy

Patient position and port set up is similar as that described for left adrenalectomy. However, the fourth port (5 mm), optional on previous descriptions, is now placed in the right flank as a requirement to bluntly retract the right lobe of the liver. Frequently it is more comfortable during right adrenalectomy for the camera operator to stand opposite the operator. The camera operator may also serve as the assistant from this side while manipulating the liver retraction. The operator will again work out of the epigastric (5 mm) port and the right midaxillary port (10 mm).

Exposure of the right adrenal gland will be initiated by mobilization of the right lobe of the liver through division of the triangular ligament. The right lobe is medially retracted and additional mobilization carried out to the level of the IVC (Fig. 9-6). Again, liver retraction is accomplished through the 5-mm flank port with the technique described to retract the spleen for the left adrenalectomy.

Meticulous dissection is similar to that performed for the left adrenal gland. Lateral and medial margins can be again mobilized with primary use of electrocautery. The right adrenal vein will be found along the midpoint of the gland's medial margin. Two areas that may require extra care due to unnamed vessels include locations in the inferior and superior poles. Clips are frequently required for adequate hemostasis.

MANAGEMENT OF THE PANCREAS

The laparoscopic management of pancreatic disease is one of the most challenging in laparoscopic surgery. This is especially true when considering that of pancreatic resection. Well-trained laparoscopic surgeons have found that operating on the pancreas, like virtually all intra-abdominal procedures, is technically feasible. Laparoscopic principles suggest that the patient will probably benefit from less postoperative pain, improved wound cosmetics, quicker return to routine activities, and shorter hospital stay. Ultimately the acceptance of many laparoscopic operations will be determined by their degree of difficulty, the operating time, the cost (both hospital and societal), and patient outcomes. In comparison with the literature available on other laparoscopic operations, the information available on pancreatic resection is too scant to draw firm conclusions. However, leaders in the field have demonstrated that pancreatic resection is feasible, and are carefully examining their outcomes to further elucidate the role of this technically demanding procedure.

Laparoscopic procedures for the pancreas fall into four main categories: 1) laparoscopic staging of pancreatic malignancy, 2) bilioenteric or gastroenteric bypass, 3) pancreatic resection, and 4) management of pancreatic pseudocysts.

Anatomic considerations

The majority of the pancreas lies in a retroperitoneal position, transversely oriented from the second and third portions of the duodenum to the hilum of the spleen. Anterior access to the gland (body and tail) is readily obtained by division of the gastrocolic omentum. This division may be performed by electrocautery (mono- or bipolar), multiple individual clip application or vascular stapling device, or ultrasonic scalpel dissection. Access may also be obtained through the gastrohepatic ligament,

Figure 9-6 Exposure to right adrenal.

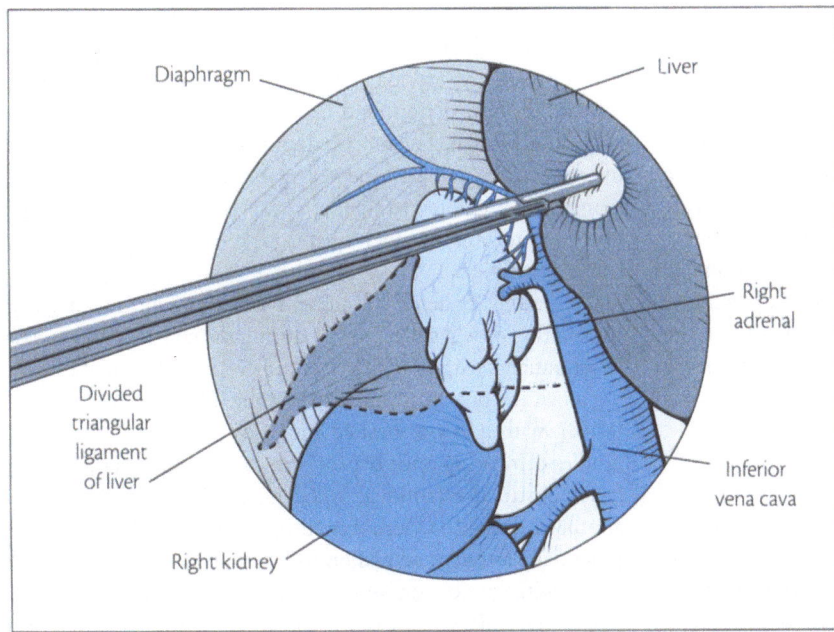

Diaphragm

Liver

Right adrenal

Divided triangular ligament of liver

Inferior vena cava

Right kidney

although the exposure is usually less adequate. The patient is positioned in a slight head-up position to allow gravity retraction of the viscera. An oblique angle (30° or 45°) telescope is necessary for adequate visualization. Laparoscopic ultrasound is proving to be an essential tool for many aspects of pancreatic surgery.

Laparoscopic staging of pancreatic malignancy

Patients with pancreatic malignancy generally present at later stages of disease. Frequently the disease is unresectable due to tumor size or tumor metastases by the time symptoms occur.

Surgical resection for pancreatic cancer still offers the only reasonable chance at a cure. Historically, many patients underwent unnecessary laparotomy in an effort to assess resectability. CT scans have helped many patients avoid the morbidity of a nontherapeutic laparotomy. However, even with this modality, unresectability rates at laparotomy can approach 60% [30]. This is most often due to the presence of unrecognized peritoneal metastases (< 1 cm) and tumor invasion not appreciated on CT scan. Spiral CT and magnetic resonance imaging (MRI) are more reliable for predicting unresectability, but are still not adequate in our opinion. In a large multicenter study, Megibow and coworkers [31] reported a sensitivity of 77%, a specificity of 50%, and an overall accuracy of 73% for dynamic CT scanning. Also in their study, they found no additional benefit from MRI.

Diagnostic laparoscopy further narrows patient selection for therapeutic laparotomy. Warshaw and coworkers [32,33] found that an additional 35% of patients could avoid laparotomy with the use of diagnostic laparoscopy. Despite improving noninvasive imaging methods since Warshaw and coworker's early reports, more recent studies [34,35••] confirm Warshaw and coworker's initial findings that a significant number of patients (22% to 35%) can avoid laparotomy with the use of staging laparoscopy.

Further, the sensitivity for evaluation of unresectable disease appears further enhanced with the addition of the laparoscopic ultrasound to the laparoscopic staging procedure. Callery and coworkers [34] use a multifrequency laparoscopic ultrasound probe to search for occult metastases and assess posterior invasion into vascular structures like the portal vein. Tumors other than pancreatic were included. Fifty patients were referred for staging laparoscopy after interpretation of conventional noninvasive imaging modalities had determined the tumor to be resectable. Laparoscopic ultrasound established unresectability in 11 patients (22%) in whom staging laparoscopy alone was negative. In another study by John and coworkers [35••] involving 40 consecutive patients with pancreatic cancer presenting for diagnostic laparoscopy, laparoscopic ultrasound found an additional 25% (10 patients) whose disease was unresectable when compared with laparoscopy alone. They found the use of ultrasound significantly improved specificity and accuracy as compared with laparoscopy alone (88% and 81% vs 50% and 60%, respectively).

Staging laparoscopy technique

Patients generally undergo staging laparoscopy on the same day they are scheduled for resection. Patients are placed in the supine position on an electrically equipped bed (preferably). A 10-mm trocar is placed in the infraumbilical position to serve as the camera port. The abdomen is insufflated to 15 mm Hg. A 30° laparoscope is used. A second port of 5 mm is placed in the right midclavicular line several centimeters from the subcostal margin. A four-quadrant exploration is then carried out. Grasping devices, biopsy forceps, or electrocautery instruments may be alternatively introduced through the 5-mm port. Important peritoneal surfaces to visualize for areas of metastases include the undersurface of abdomen including falciform, diaphragm, and liver. The omentum must be examined thoroughly and when possible retracted superiorly to evaluate the base of the transverse colon, its mesentery, and the ligament of Treitz (this may require an additional port).

If there is evidence of unresectability, the procedure is terminated. Otherwise laparoscopic ultrasound is carried out. A second 10-mm port is placed in the right midclavicular line at the level of the umbilicus. Laparoscopic ultrasound is then performed using a 9-mm in diameter linear array 7.5-MHz contact ultrasound probe with Doppler flow capability (B & K Medical, North Billerica, MA). The liver is systematically scanned (anterior, lateral, inferior) at penetration depths of 7 cm for evidence of metastatic spread or extent of primary tumor invasion. Frequently, biliary and pancreatic metastases to the liver have a characteristic bulls-eye appearance with an echoic rim encircling a mixed-echo tumor center. If found, biopsy for such lesions may be attempted percutaneously with laparoscopic ultrasound guidance.

Attention is then turned to ultrasonic evaluation of the portahepatic, peripancreatic, para-aortic, and celiac axis for evidence of nodal disease. Lymph nodes greater than 10 mm may be biopsied. Laparoscopic ultrasound with Doppler flow capability is then used to help locate and assess the potential for tumor extension to surrounding peripancreatic vascular structures (primarily portal vein, but also superior mesenteric vein and artery, and celiac axis). We do not routinely perform cytology as part of our staging procedure.

Bilioenteric or gastroenteric anastamosis for pancreatic malignancy

Unresectable patients might be candidates for biliary or enteric bypass. The risk and benefits of bypass must be weighed against existing palliative options, the patient's condition, existing or impending obstruction, and expected length of survival based on tumor burden. For most patients with unresectable disease, life expectancy can be expected to be less than 1 year. Proper management tailored to the individual patient's needs is important as to offer as much quality of life free from hospitalization as possible.

Commonly, patients will present with some degree of biliary obstruction or will suffer from it during the course of the disease. Most patients with obstructive jaundice are best treated by placing an endoscopic or percutaneous stent. The success rate is high (85%), with a low associated mortality (1% to 2%) [36,37]. Studies comparing open bypass with those stented endoscopically for obstructive jaundice found no advantage to the surgical approach [38,39]. Morbidity from stent placement includes potentially frequent admission to hospital (occlusion, infection) and significant cost for endoscopic retrograde cholangiopancreatography (ERCP) and stent. However, repeat placement has become less necessary with the use of improved techniques and stent design [40]. Patients may present or develop distorted duodenal anatomy that makes initial or subsequent stent placement impossible. This finding may be coupled with gastric outlet obstruction. In these patients, bypass procedures may be offered after evaluation of surgical risk or life expectancy.

The morbidity of open surgical bypass is substantial (19%) [39]. Laparoscopic biliary (cholecystojejunostomy) or gastric bypass (gastrojejunostomy) is feasible. There is potential for shorter recovery, shorter return to activity, and low morbidity, as evident in several small studies [40]. We favor an approach, as suggested by Nathanson [41], that the bypass should be reserved for a later date from the diagnostic laparoscopy at such time when duodenal obstruction precludes repeat stent or there is stent failure (blockage, recurrent sepsis). For the stomach, failure would include when symptoms of gastric outlet arise. Conditions at initial laparoscopy that might argue for immediate bypass include inability to stent the biliary system in the preoperative setting, endoscopic or radiologic evidence of impending duodenal obstruction, or laparoscopic impression of large locally advanced mass with minimal to no evidence of metastatic spread.

Biliary and gastric bypass

Cholecystojejunostomy may be carried out if the gallbladder is present and suitable for anastomosis, and the cystic duct is patent and its junction to the common bile duct (CBD) is far from the tumor. Frequently this information is available by preoperative imaging studies (ERCP or percutaneous transluminal cholangiography). If not, patency of cystic duct and its relation to primary tumor location may be obtained by performing a cholangiogram after cannulation of the gallbladder. Similarly, laparoscopic ultrasound may be used for such an assessment.

For either anastomosis, patients are positioned supine and the port placement is the same. A 10-mm trocar is placed at the inferior umbilical region and a 30° laparoscope is used. Additional ports and operating room personnel are positioned as seen in Figure 9-7.

The omentum and transverse colon are elevated with instruments introduced through the epigastric and either 12-mm port. The small bowel is traced back to the ligament of Treitz. A loop of small bowel is then chosen that will comfortably reach stomach and gallbladder without tension (note that this is true once the transverse colon and omentum are allowed to return to normal position). For the biliary bypass, a cholecystotomy is performed with electrocautery on the gallbladder fundus. The biliary contents are then aspirated. An enterotomy is performed on the antimesenteric surface of the chosen small bowel loop. A 30-mm endoscopic stapler is introduced through the right 12-mm port. The jaws of the stapler are opened and one arm of the stapler is inserted into the enterotomy. The jaws of the stapler are then closed to function as a large grasper. The stapler and small bowel contained within are then maneuvered adjacent to the cholecystotomy. The jaws of the stapler are opened again and the free arm of the stapler maneuvered into the cholecystotomy. Assistance is provide by a blunt grasping instrument inserted through the additional ports (epigastric). After proper alignment is assured, the stapler is fired to complete the anastomosis. The

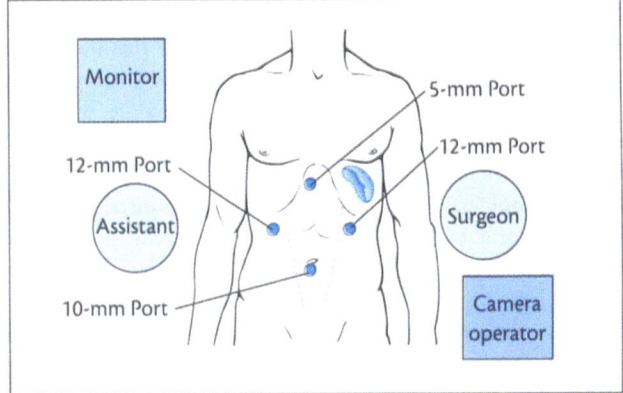

Figure 9-7 Port and personnel placement for biliary and gastric bypass.

original -otomy sites may be closed with additional firings of the stapler. At this point the endoscopic stapler will be introduced through the left 12-mm port. Care must be taken not to narrow the anastomosis or the lumen of the small bowel significantly. We generally reserve suturing in cases where closure of the initial -otomy sites is technically difficult to align for staple closure or when we feel staple closure will create narrowing.

To fashion the gastric bypass, a dependent site is chosen along the greater curvature. The gastrocolic omentum is divided close to the greater curve within the gastroepiploic arcade for a distance of approximately 3 to 4 cm with the ultrasonic scalpel or by electrocautery. A gastrotomy is made on the greater curvature. The anastomosis will be formed along the greater curve but will extend into the posterior wall of the stomach. Typically, the stapled anastomosis will be created by introducing the stapler through the right 12-mm port. The anastomosis should consist of two firings of the 30-mm endoscopic linear cutter. The original -otomy sites are closed through the left 12-mm port.

Ideally, the stapled anastomosis should be aligned to cross the greater curvature to the posterior surface (ie, through the area of divided gastrocolic omentum). If fashioned in this way, the original -otomy sites will be easier to close and the anastomosis more dependent.

We have had experience with 15 patients (six cholecystojejunostomies, seven gastrojejunostomies, and two doublebypasses). The hospital stay has ranged from 5 to 20 days. Patients have had a mean survival of just over 4.5 months. In general, patients have been palliated well up until their death.

Laparoscopic pancreatic resection

Indications for complete or partial pancreatic resection include adenocarcinoma, insulinoma (neuroendocrine), and chronic pancreatitis. Improved technique and postoperative care have rendered morbidity and mortality for pancreatic resection, including Whipple's procedure, to less than 5%. Laparoscopic techniques could potentially lower this rate even more or at least afford less pain and a more rapid recovery.

Laparoscopic Whipple's procedure was first carried out by Gagner (Personal communication) in 1992 in a small series of three patients with various diseases (pancreatitis, ampullary cancer, adenocarcinoma). He subsequently has reported on a pylorus-preserving technique performed in one patient with pancreatitis [43]. The initial experience indicates that it is technically feasible, but because of its operative time, complexity, and as yet no demonstrated improvement in outcome, this procedure must be considered investigational. Hand-assist devices may make pancreatic resection more practical.

Laparoscopic pancreatic procedures involving distal pancreatectomy appear to hold more promise at present. Soper and coworkers [43] reported success with his technique in the pig model. Gagner and coworkers [44] successfully performed distal pancreatectomy for a variety of disease processes including islet cell tumors, cystadenocarcinoma, and pseudocyst. The spleen was preserved in all cases and operating times ranged from 2.5 to 5 hours. Cases were managed with the patient in the left lateral position, with pancreatic division carried out with a 60-mm linear cutter. Others are reporting initial success with distal resection [45,46].

Laparoscopic management of pancreatic pseudocyst

Pancreatic psuedocysts may be defined as a collection of pancreatic secretions, serous fluid, or necrotic debris surrounded by a nonepithelialized wall made up of granulation tissue and variable degrees of fibrous tissue. Pancreatic pseudocysts must be distinguished from true cysts of the pancreas, which are characterized histologically by the presence of an epithelial lining. Pseudocyst formation is the result of a postinflammatory process arising from patients with acute or chronic pancreatitis. An understanding of the natural history of pancreatic pseudocyst is important when deciding on invasive therapy versus expectant management. Studies like those by Bradley and coworkers [47] had a great influence in the management of pseudocystic disease. Bradley and coworkers suggested the likelihood of regression diminished and the likelihood of complications rose dramatically after a 6-week period. More recent data [48,49] suggest that this patient population may be watched safely for longer periods. Yeo and coworkers [49] followed asymptomatic patients with pseudocysts by CT scanning for 1 year (48% were successfully observed with only a 2.7% complication rate). The only predictor for intervention was size greater than 7.4 ± 0.6 cm.

General asymptomatic patients with pancreatic pseudocyst may be followed up for extended periods of time. This conservative approach is more likely to be successful in patients with small (< 6 cm) pseudocysts. Other options are available for drainage procedures (eg, percutaneous transgastric, ERCP). We favor the surgical approach as the more reliable method.

Laparoscopic pseudocyst drainage

Preoperative decision making and subsequent laparoscopic operative approach should mimic that of open operative planning. The selection of procedure will depend on the anatomic location of the pseudocyst, pseudocyst size [50], and associated pancreatic duct or distal common bile duct abnormalities.

Reports by Newell and coworkers [51] document that pseudocyst-gastrostomy is technically easier than pseudocyst-jejunostomy, while remaining equally efficacious. Laparoscopic pseudocyst-gastrostomy is technically easier, but cyst-jejunostomy is also

technically feasible for the cyst not amenable to gastric drainage by standard surgical principles.

Laparoscopic pseudocyst-gastrostomy was first performed by Petelin (Personal communication) in 1991. Principles of operative drainage include biopsy of cyst wall to rule out neoplasm, dependent drainage, and precise hemostatic technique to avoid hemorrhage. We describe the technique we have used to perform pseudocyst-gastrostomy.

The patient position and port placement are the same as described for the bypass procedure. The pseudocyst may often be seen pushing the stomach forward. A small gastrotomy is established with cautery over the most prominent portion of the pseudocyst. Ultrasound may be helpful in locating the pseudocyst and the site of the initial gastrotomy. The gastrotomy is then extended for several centimeters with electrocautery.

A small window is developed through the posterior wall of the stomach with electrocautery. One must remember that the posterior wall of stomach and cyst capsule will be fused and that this requires a deeper dissection with cautery than may feel comfortable for the surgeon. Ultrasound may be helpful in identifying the location of the pseudocyst, and in some cases to plan dissection where the stomach wall or cyst is thinnest. The window is made large enough to accommodate the endoscopic stapler. A biopsy of the wall may be carried out at this time. Two firings of the stapler are used to create a substantial anastomosis (stapler insertion through the more comfortable 12-mm port, usually the right). Hemostasis at the staple line should be assured. The gastrotomy is closed with either sutures or staples.

CONCLUSIONS

The laparoscopic approach to solid organ surgery has rapidly been shown to be of considerable value. For splenectomy and adrenalectomy, it has become the procedure of choice for most elective surgery. The laparoscopic approach to the pancreas has value with respect to staging, bypass procedures, and pseudocyst drainage. Pancreatic resection is feasible, but must still be considered investigational.

REFERENCES AND RECOMMENDED READING

Recently published papers of particular interest have been highlighted as:
* •   Of interest
* ••   Of outstanding interest

1. Brunt LM, Langer JC, Quasebarth MA, Whitman ED: Comparative analysis of laparoscopic versus open splenectomy. *Am J Surg* 1996, 172:596–601.

2.• Friedman RL, Fallas MJ, Carroll BJ, *et al.*: Laparoscopic splenectomy for ITP: the gold standard. *Surg Endosc* 1996, 10:991–995.
This study reports on a significant single institute series of laparoscopic ITP splenectomy. Laparoscopic exceeded open splenectomy in virtually every outcome measured.

3. Carroll BJ, Phillips EH, Semel CJ, *et al.*: Laparoscopic splenectomy. *Surg Endosc* 1992, 6:183–185.

4. Delaitre B, Maignien B: Laparoscopic splenectomy: technical aspects. *Surg Endosc* 1992, 6:305–388.

5. Thibault C, Mamazza J, Letourneau R, Poulin E: Laparoscopic splenectomy: operative technique and preliminary report. *Surg Laparosc Endosc* 1992, 2:248–253.

6.• Glasgow RE, Yee LF, Mulvihill SJ: Laparoscopic splenectomy: the emerging standard. *Surg Endosc* 1997, 11:108–112.
Large series of consecutive laparoscopic splenectomies compared with concurrent open cases. Major outcomes including costs significantly improved.

7.• Park A, Gagner M, Pomp A: The lateral approach to laparoscopic splenectomy. *Am J Surg* 1997, 173:126–130.
This paper is an excellent description and review of laparoscopic splenectomy and the group's reasoning for favoring the lateral approach. The authors have had significant experience with alternative techniques.

8. Diaz J, Eisenstat M, Chung R: A case-controlled study of laparoscopic splenectomy. *Am J Surg* 1997, 173:348–350.

9. Koehler RH, Smith RS, Fry WR: Successful laparoscopic splenorrhaphy using absorbable mesh for grade III splenic injury: report of a case. *Surg Laparosc Endosc* 1994, 4:311–315.

10. Poulin EC, Thibault C, DesCoteaux JG, Cote G: Partial laparoscopic splenectomy for trauma: technique and case report. *Surg Laparosc Endosc* 1995, 5:306–310.

11. Feliciotti F, Sottili M, Guerrieri M, *et al.*: Conservative ultrasound-guided laparoscopic treatment of posttraumatic splenic cysts: report of two cases. *Surg Laparosc Endosc* 1996, 6:322–325.

12. Targarona EM, Martinez J, Ramos C, *et al.*: Conservative laparoscopic treatment of a posttraumatic splenic cyst. *Surg Endosc* 1995, 9:71–72.

13. de Melo VA, Alves Junior A, Andrade LC, *et al.*: Splenic cyst: review of the literature and report of 2 cases. *Rev Hosp Clin Fac Med Sao Paulo* 1995, 50:289–293.

14. Tricarico A, Tartaglia A, Taddeo F, *et al.*: Videolaparoscopic treatment of spleen injuries: report of two cases. *Surg Endosc* 1994, 8:910–912.

15. Siren JE, Haapiainen RK, Huikuri KT, Sivula AH: Incidentalomas of the adrenal gland: 36 operated patients and review of literature. *World J Surg* 1993, 17:634–639.

16. Copeland PM: The incidentally discovered adrenal mass. *Ann Surg* 1984, 199:116–122.

17. Prinz RA, Brooks MH, Churchill R, *et al.*: Incidental asymptomatic adrenal masses detected by computed tomographic scanning: is operation required? *JAMA* 1982, 248:701–704.

18. Belldegrun A, Hussain S, Seltzer SE, *et al*: Incidentally discovered mass of the adrenal gland. *Surg Gynecol Obstet* 1986, 163:203–208.

19.• Linos DA, Stylopoulos N, Raptis SA: Adrenaloma: a call for more aggressive management. *World J Surg* 1996, 20:788–793.
Reintroduces the issue and the reasoning for favoring adrenalectomy for incidental (3 to 6 cm) masses, especially in the era of laparoscopy. Series of patients chosen to emphasize their position could suffer from selection bias.

20. Gagner M, Lacroix A, Bolte E: Laparoscopic adrenalectomy in Cushing's syndrome and pheochromocytoma [letter]. *N Engl J Med* 1992, 327:1033.

21. Gagner M, Lacroix A, Bolte E, Pomp A: Laparoscopic adrenalectomy: the importance of a flank approach in the lateral decubitus position. *Surg Endosc* 1994, 8:135–138.

22.•• Gagner M, Pomp A, Heniford BT, *et al.*: Laparoscopic adrenalectomy: lessons learned from 100 consecutive procedures [in process citation]. *Ann Surg* 1997, 226:238–247.
The largest published series (low morbidity, three conversions, and significantly favorable short- and long-term outcomes). Certainly helps to establish laparoscopic adrenalectomy as the gold standard for the vast majority of adrenal masses.

23. Prinz RA. A comparison of laparoscopic and open adrenalectomies. *Arch Surg* 1995, 130:489–494.

24. Brunt LM, Doherty GM, Norton JA, *et al.*: Laparoscopic adrenalectomy compared to open adrenalectomy for benign adrenal neoplasms [see comments]. *J Am Coll Surg* 1996, 183:1–10.

25. Marescaux J, Mutter D, Wheeler MH: Laparoscopic right and left adrenalectomies: surgical procedures. *Surg Endosc* 1996, 10:912–915.

26. MacGillivray DC, Shichman SJ, Ferrer FA, Malchoff CD: A comparison of open vs laparoscopic adrenalectomy. *Surg Endosc* 1996, 10:987–990.

27. Horgan S, Sinanan M, Helton WS, Pellegrini CA: Use of laparoscopic techniques improves outcome from adrenalectomy. *Am J Surg* 1997, 173:371–374.

28. Gagner M, Breton G, Pharand D, Pomp A: Is laparoscopic adrenalectomy indicated for pheochromocytomas? *Surgery* 1996, 120:1076–1080.

29. Walz MK, Peitgen K, Hoermann R, *et al.*: Posterior retroperitoneoscopy as a new minimally invasive approach for adrenalectomy: results of 30 adrenalectomies in 27 patients. *World J Surg* 1996, 20:769–774.

30. Fernandez-del Castillo C, Warshaw AL: Laparoscopy for staging in pancreatic carcinoma. *Surg Oncol* 1993, 2(suppl 1):25–29.

31. Megibow AJ, Zhou XH, Rotterdam H, *et al.*: Pancreatic adenocarcinoma: CT versus MR imaging in the evaluation of resectability. Report of the Radiology Diagnostic Oncology Group. *Radiology* 1995, 195:327–332.

32. Warshaw AL, Gu ZY, Wittenberg J, Waltman AC: Preoperative staging and assessment of resectability of pancreatic cancer. *Arch Surg* 1990, 125:230–233.

33. Warshaw AL, Tepper JE, Shipley WU: Laparoscopy in the staging and planning of therapy for pancreatic cancer. *Am J Surg* 1986, 151:76–80.

34. Callery MP, Strasberg SM, Doherty GM, *et al.*: Staging laparoscopy with laparoscopic ultrasonography: optimizing resectability in hepatobiliary and pancreatic malignancy. *J Am Coll Surg* 1997, 185:33–39.

35.•• John TG, Greig JD, Carter DC, Garden OJ: Carcinoma of the pancreatic head and periampullary region: tumor staging with laparoscopy and laparoscopic ultrasonography. *Ann Surg* 1995, 221:156–164.
This series as well as that by Callery and coworkers [34] suggest the standard for staging laparoscopy should include laparoscopic ultrasound to avoid unnecessary laparotomy.

36. Soehendra N, Grimm H, Berger B, Nam VC: Malignant jaundice: results of diagnostic and therapeutic endoscopy. *World J Surg* 1989, 13:171–177.

37. Huibregtse K, Katon RM, Coene PP, Tytgat GN: Endoscopic palliative treatment in pancreatic cancer. *Gastrointest Endosc* 1986, 32:334–338.

38. Andersen JR, Sorensen SM, Kruse A, *et al.*: Randomised trial of endoscopic endoprosthesis versus operative bypass in malignant obstructive jaundice. *Gut* 1989, 30:1132–1135.

39. Sarr MG, Cameron JL: Surgical management of unresectable carcinoma of the pancreas. *Surgery* 1982, 91:123–133.

40. Rhodes M, Nathanson L, Fielding G: Laparoscopic biliary and gastric bypass: a useful adjunct in the treatment of carcinoma of the pancreas. *Gut* 1995, 36:778–780.

41. Nathanson LK: Laparoscopic cholecyst-jejunostomy and gastroenterostomy for malignant disease. *Surg Oncol* 1993, 2(suppl 1):19–24.

42. Gagner M, Pomp A: Laparoscopic pylorus-preserving pancreatoduodenectomy. *Surg Endosc* 1994, 8:408–410.

43. Soper NJ, Brunt LM, Dunnegan DL, Meininger TA: Laparoscopic distal pancreatectomy in the porcine model. *Surg Endosc* 1994, 8:57–61.

44. Gagner M, Pomp A, Herrera MF: Early experience with laparoscopic resections of islet cell tumors. *Surgery* 1996, 120:1051–1054.

45. Cuschieri A, Jakimowicz JJ, van Spreeuwel J: Laparoscopic distal 70% pancreatectomy and splenectomy for chronic pancreatitis. *Ann Surg* 1996, 223:280–285.

46. Salky BA, Edye M: Laparoscopic pancreatectomy. *Surg Clin North Am* 1996, 76:539–545.

47. Bradley EL, Clements JL Jr., Gonzalez AC: The natural history of pancreatic pseudocysts: a unified concept of management. *Am J Surg* 1979, 137:135–141.

48. Yeo CJ, Sarr MG: Cystic and pseudocystic diseases of the pancreas. *Curr Probl Surg* 1994, 31:165–243.

49. Yeo CJ, Bastidas JA, Lynch-Nyhan A, *et al.*: The natural history of pancreatic pseudocysts documented by computed tomography. *Surg Gynecol Obstet* 1990, 170:411–417.

50. Johnson LB, Rattner DW, Warshaw AL: The effect of size of giant pancreatic pseudocysts on the outcome of internal drainage procedures. *Surg Gynecol Obstet* 1991, 173:171–174.

51. Newell KA, Liu T, Aranha GV, Prinz RA: Are cystgastrostomy and cystjejunostomy equivalent operations for pancreatic pseudocysts? *Surgery* 1990, 108:635–640.

Laparoscopy for Acute and Chronic Abdominal Pain

Mary E. Klingensmith
David C. Brooks

One of the premier strengths of laparoscopy has been its usefulness as a diagnostic modality that can minimize morbidity and shorten the postoperative recovery period. Laparoscopy is increasingly being applied in clinical situations in which the diagnosis is uncertain, or in patients in whom a traditional laparotomy might impose significant morbidity.

Patients presenting to the surgeon with an acute or chronic abdominal process may benefit from interventional laparoscopy. Applications in patients with either acute or chronic syndromes are discussed in this chapter, including the utility of laparoscopy in treating patients with small bowel obstruction (SBO) and in the trauma and intensive care unit (ICU) settings.

GENERAL TECHNIQUE
Acute and chronic abdominal disorders

As a general rule, the majority of laparoscopies for evaluating an abdominal condition should be performed under general anesthesia. Patient positioning and manipulation are most easily accomplished under general anesthesia, and a rapid conversion to laparotomy can be performed if necessary. Limited diagnostic evaluations can be performed under local anesthetic with sedation [1], and this approach may be advantageous in an ICU or trauma setting, as discussed later.

The operating room set-up should afford the surgeon the greatest degree of flexibility in positioning. A mobile television monitor and a flexible scrub nurse and first assistant will allow optimal positioning such that the case may be assisted in the most efficient manner possible. The patient's arms should be placed at his or her side to further allow for flexibility in equipment and operating room personnel positioning. A naso- or orogastric tube should be inserted to decompress the stomach, and a Foley catheter should be considered to decompress the bladder and diminish the possibility of inadvertent injury.

An open approach is the preferred method for establishing access to the abdomen, to avoid potential injury to viscera. Once initial pneumoperitoneum is established, the surface anatomy of the abdomen is methodically inspected. Any free fluid that is encountered should be sampled for culture. Routine inspection of all four quadrants, done in a manner to exclude specific pathology in each area, often will allow early identification of the site of the problem. It should be remembered that early identification of pathology does not relieve the surgeon of the responsibility of examining the entire abdomen [2].

After initial inspection, a centrally placed probe can be used to expose deeper aspects of the abdominal cavity. For suspected upper abdominal disease, a 10-mm trocar and probe can be placed in the subxiphoid or right upper quadrant position; for lower abdominal or pelvic pathology, the trocar and probe should be placed in the lower midline, just above the bladder (Fig. 10-1).

Modifications for the intensive care unit or trauma setting

Laparoscopy in the ICU or emergency ward may be accomplished with use of a local anesthetic and sedation. Support from anesthesiologists who are familiar with laparoscopic procedures can facilitate patient comfort. The intubated patient will be easier to manage in these situations, and it would be reasonable to consider elective intubation for laparoscopy, according to the severity and nature of the patient's injuries or illness.

Ideally, all equipment necessary for bedside laparoscopy (*eg*, monitor, light source) should be dedicated for ICU or emergency ward use and kept on a portable cart that is readily accessible. Additionally, a complete set of disposable trocars and cannulas should be available, as well as a limited selection of laparoscopic instruments (*eg*, grasping forceps, blunt probes, biopsy forceps). In general, disposable instrumentation is easier to maintain and store despite the fact that it may be slightly more costly. Similarly, dedicated personnel, including anesthetists and scrub personnel familiar with laparoscopic instruments and set-up of the portable laparoscopy cart, should be available to assist for efficient completion of bedside laparoscopy.

Prior to commencing, the patient should be moved to a narrow bed or gurney, as the regular-width ICU bed can lead to significant back strain on the operating team while trying to lean over the patient. The bed must be readily adjustable so that Trendelenburg and reverse Trendelenburg positions can be easily accommodated.

In the trauma or ICU setting, when local anesthetics are being used, a 2-mm scope should be considered. In addition, low insufflation pressures should be selected to minimize patient discomfort. Initial flows should be less than 2 L/min, with insufflation pressures between 7 and 10 mm Hg.

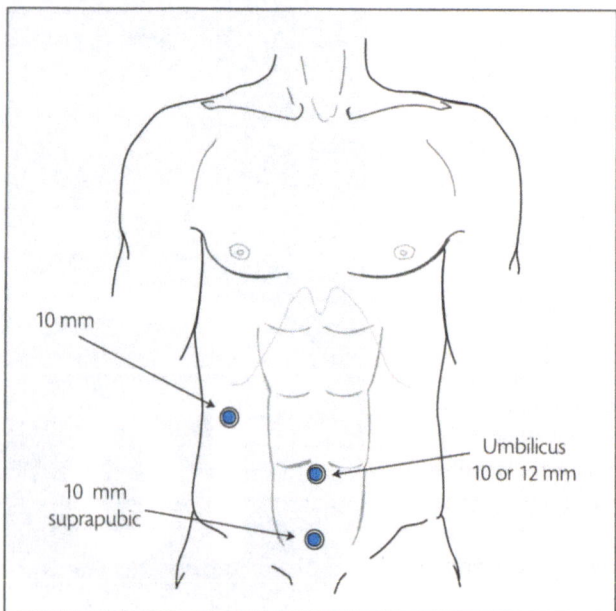

Figure 10-1 Ports for laparoscopic evaluation of acute abdomen.

THE ACUTE ABDOMEN
Differential diagnoses

The list of differential diagnoses for patients presenting with an acute abdomen is quite extensive. The astute physician will narrow the diagnostic possibilities to include those that might be expected to occur in a given patient, with careful consideration to a patient's past medical and surgical history as well as active disease processes.

For example, the premenopausal female patient who presents to the emergency ward with lower abdominal pain might be considered to have appendicitis, pelvic inflammatory disease (PID), or ruptured ectopic or ovarian cyst. It has been well-documented that laparoscopy in such patients allows diagnostic accuracy, as well as providing therapeutic options [3,4].

The elderly diabetic patient in an ICU might be considered to have acute calculous or acalculous cholecystitis, ischemic bowel disease (embolic or low-flow), pancreatitis, diverticulitis (Meckel's or colonic), perforation (duodenal or gastric ulcer, diverticulum), or even appendicitis or typhlitis [3]. Further, the victim of blunt or penetrating trauma presents with a third set of possible diagnoses, including those that might lead to hemoperitoneum such as liver or splenic injuries.

Indications and contraindications

There are several settings in which diagnostic laparoscopy is favored over conventional laparotomy.

- Patients in whom the most likely diagnosis can easily be handled laparoscopically, even by those surgeons with fairly basic laparoscopic skills. Such patients might be those in whom appendicitis or adnexal pathology is suspected but not confirmed.
- Critically ill patients in an ICU setting may benefit from bedside laparoscopy, and the timely manner in which crucial diagnostic information can be gathered. The therapy can be tailored without wasting valuable time transporting the patient to a variety of radiology sites where monitoring is suboptimal and crises seem to inevitably occur. Bedside laparoscopy may avoid an unnecessary trip to the operating room in patients who cannot afford the rigors of transport. It follows that a timely diagnosis will allow care to be delivered in the most expeditious and cost-effective manner.
- Patients in whom the most likely diagnosis would not be managed primarily by operative means, *ie*, patients in whom a diagnosis of PID, pancreatitis, or some ischemic or low-flow visceral injuries can be made. In these patients, adequate uncertainty of the diagnosis would have to be present to lead to the decision to proceed with diagnostic laparoscopy.
- Trauma settings in which the "triage" of injuries is critical: the diagnosis or exclusion of intra-abdominal catastrophe aids in timely attention to other potentially life-threatening injuries, such as intracranial or intrathoracic trauma or long-bone injuries.

Relative contraindications include trauma patients in whom hypovolemia or blunt myocardial injury is confirmed or suspected, who might not tolerate the additional cardiac stress of pneumoperitoneum [5••]. Diagnostic laparoscopy should be used with caution in trauma patients with closed head injuries unless intracranial pressure (ICP) monitoring can be easily performed, because it has been reported that pneumoperitoneum can cause a rise in mean ICP in experimental situations [5••]. Additionally, an ICU patient in whom an easily correctable lesion is highly suspected may benefit from transport to an operating room (as opposed to being investigated by bedside laparoscopy) and, in some cases, may be better served by conventional laparotomy for the most efficient and thorough attention to a given disease process.

Evaluation

As with any patient with an acute abdominal process, thorough preoperative evaluation is mandatory, including complete history and physical, routine blood work (including complete blood count, electrolytes, liver chemistries, amylase, and lipase), and urinalysis. Imaging studies may provide further information, and should be used as indicated, including supine and upright plain radiographs, ultrasound, and CT.

Prior to operative intervention, adequate hydration and, in some cases, antibiotic administration should be delivered. Attention to comorbid diseases is imperative. Finally, a thorough anesthesia evaluation should complete the preoperative assessment, with close communication between surgeon and anesthesiologist imperative for expeditious patient care [2].

Technique for management of specific diagnoses

Suspected appendicitis or gynecologic abdominal disease

Readers are referred to Chapter 5 for the description of techniques for laparoscopic appendectomy.

Benign adnexal disease can mimic acute appendicitis on presentation. Ruptured ovarian cysts and adnexal torsion both can present with pain, localized abdominal findings, leukocytosis, and fever. Ruptured cysts most often present 2 to 6 days after ovulation; at laparoscopy, blood or blood-tinged fluid may be recovered, and one ovary typically appears enlarged, often with a recognizable fracture or bleeding site. Treatment is supportive; if no further bleeding is identified, no further surgical intervention is needed. If indicated, an ovarian cystectomy can be performed to control hemorrhage, with careful attention to avoid simply "unroofing" the cyst—cystectomy with removal of the entire cyst wall is required [6••].

If adnexal torsion is identified, and found to be complete, including necrosis, adnexectomy should be performed, with division of the vascular pedicle. In all cases of torsion, the underlying cause should be identified (adhesions, intraovarian tumor) and corrected [6••].

Pelvic inflammatory disease can also mimic appendicitis in some cases. Symptoms of localized pain, fever, and leukocytosis typically occur 2 to 3 days after menstruation, and when a tubal infection is established, symptoms begin. On laparoscopy, the fallopian tubes appear indurated, hyperemic, and edematous. A leukocytic discharge can be seen from the distal end of the tube in some cases, resulting in a mucopurulent collection in the cul-de-sac. Fibrinous adhesions can often be seen around the tube and ovary. Treatment is always supportive, with intravenous

antibiotics, except in the case of the ruptured tubovarian abscess, in which removal of the abscess and drainage has been found to decrease overall morbidity [6••].

Abdominal sepsis

Treatment by laparoscopy of the patient with presumed abdominal sepsis of unknown cause has been accomplished successfully by some surgeons [7]. Using a systematic method of inspection, which involves manipulation of the patient's position (supine, Trendelenburg, reverse Trendelenburg, right-side up, left-side up), and a meticulous inspection of the entire bowel using atraumatic bowel graspers, a diagnosis can be made in the vast majority of patients; in fact, most can be treated successfully by a laparoscopic approach. Diagnoses in one recent series included perforated viscous (colon, appendix), gangrenous cholecystitis, ischemic bowel disease, and closed loop small bowel obstruction [7].

Suspected intestinal ischemia

The diagnosis of intestinal ischemia by laparoscopic means can be difficult. Intraluminal blood or feces or suboptimal imaging can result in dark-colored bowels. A recent study from Germany describes the use of Doppler ultrasound, laser Doppler, pulse oximetry, and spectrophotometry to provide a technical measurement of blood flow or oxygenation. These tools served as adjuncts to the sometimes misleading visual impression gained from laparoscopy [8].

Trauma

The use of laparoscopy in the trauma setting must be carefully applied to a select group of patients. Review of the literature reveals a variety of opinions as to which patients are candidates for laparoscopy in the trauma setting. Ultimately, each surgeon will select patients according to his or her experience and degree of comfort in any given situation.

Some authors exclude all gunshot wound victims from diagnostic laparoscopy but encourage its use in stabbing victims [9,10]. It has been suggested that patients who might best benefit from diagnostic laparoscopy include those with small stab wounds to the abdomen, back or flanks, or with tangential gunshot wounds to the abdomen. Others who might benefit include patients with blunt torso injuries and equivocal abdominal findings, and patients who will be unavailable for serial abdominal exams (ie, those undergoing anesthesia for other injuries) [5••]. A recent study from France reported that laparoscopy is a safe and accurate method for evaluating abdominal stab wounds. When compared retrospectively with laparotomy, it was associated with less morbidity and a shorter hospital stay than laparotomy [10]. Laparoscopy can be performed under local anesthesia, in the emergency department, preferably with dedicated equipment and staff. However, if done in the operating room, rapid conversion to laparotomy, if deemed necessary, is possible.

Upon laparoscopy, methodical inspection for traumatic intra-abdominal penetration must be performed. An assessment of the amount of hemoperitoneum (minimal to severe) and its location (ie, left paracolic gutter) can suggest diagnosis (ie, ruptured spleen) and dictate further courses of action, including conversion to laparotomy if a persistent source of bleeding is suspected but cannot be identified. A systematic evaluation of intra-abdominal contents is imperative. If a penetrating wound is discovered, careful inspection of the liver, diaphragm, and spleen should be undertaken first, followed by the stomach, small bowel, colon, omentum, and mesentery. Finally, the retroperitoneum should be inspected for the presence of hematoma [10]. The presence of succus in the abdominal cavity indicates a visceral injury, and should be acted on immediately because missed hollow visceral injuries are common in patients treated by laparoscopy alone [5••]. Superficial liver lacerations can be managed laparoscopically by the application of fibrin glue [11]. The ability to manage injuries by laparoscopic means will depend both on the nature of the injury and the ability of the surgeon to perform advanced laparoscopic techniques [10]. However, in the carefully chosen patient, laparoscopy offers an effective means to timely diagnosis with little comorbidity.

Small bowel obstruction
The utility of laparoscopy in management of acute symptoms of SBO is somewhat novel. A recent report suggests that a laparoscopic approach to treatment of SBO is advantageous in selected patients [12]. In a series of 40 patients with symptoms of complete or partial SBO, laparoscopic or laparoscopically assisted treatment was successful in identifying and treating the cause of the SBO in a majority of patients, with the most common cause being adhesions. Central to the approach is a systematic inspection of the entire small bowel from the ligament of Treitz to the ileocecal valve. It was concluded that laparoscopic treatment of SBO is effective, led to decreased length of hospital stay, and provided good long-term results. Laparoscopy was deemed most effective in patients with recurrent partial SBO.

CHRONIC ABDOMINAL PAIN
Laparoscopy is being used with increasing frequency in evaluating chronic abdominal complaints. Long recognized by gynecologists as an important diagnostic and therapeutic tool, laparoscopy is seeing increased use by general surgeons in the investigation of causes of chronic and recurrent abdominal pain.

It is not uncommon for patients with chronic abdominal pain to be evaluated by many different physicians, with surgeons becoming involved in the care of these patients by consultation, increasingly as a "last resort" referral to seek a resolution of the chronic abdominal pain.

Several recent studies have demonstrated that laparoscopy can result in improvement of chronic abdominal pain [13,14•,15,16]. One proposed advantage to diagnostic (and therapeutic) laparoscopy over conventional laparotomy is that optimal visualization of the entire abdomen and pelvis is possible, with less trauma to the abdomen than in open surgery. Experimental evidence suggests that laparoscopy is associated with a lesser extent of adhesion recurrence than conventional laparotomy [17].

Patient selection and preoperative evaluation
Most authors agree that careful patient selection is critical in determining a favorable outcome in the difficult patient group with chronic abdominal pain. The definition of "chronic" pain varies from series to series, with the range being described as chronic or recurrent abdominal pain of 2 to 6 months' duration. The majority of patients studied have been women [14•,15,16], although smaller numbers of men with chronic pain have also been studied [13]. All patients typically undergo thorough physical examinations as well as laboratory tests and various imaging studies, and are often referred to the general surgeon when the chronic pain is deemed of unclear cause.

Note should be made of failed diagnostic and therapeutic measures. Specifically, patients who have undergone prior surgery (for a different or identical complaint) should not be excluded from consideration. These patients, particularly those in whom reproducible tenderness is found, have been demonstrated to benefit from laparoscopy, because a successful laparoscopic adhesiolysis can often be performed [13].

Common findings
In a variety of series, laparoscopy has been shown to provide a diagnosis to which the chronic pain could be attributed. The majority of studies report finding adhesions in most of the patients studied (Fig. 10-2) [13,14•,15], with appendicitis (chronic or acute), hernias (inguinal or umbilical) (Fig. 10-3),

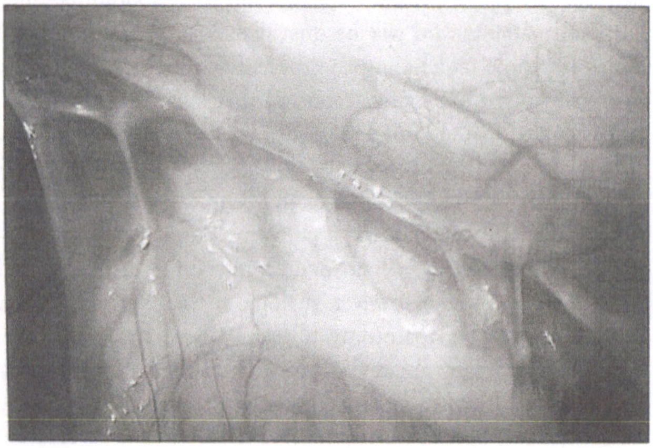

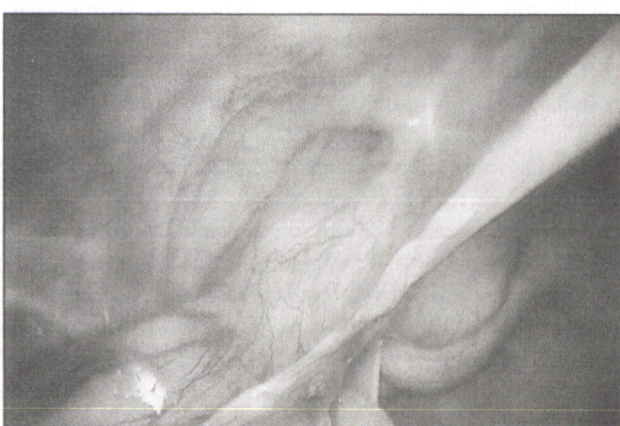

Figure 10-2 Typical appearance of intra-abdominal adhesions. (*See* Color Plate.)

Figure 10-3 Appearance of an indirect inguinal hernia as viewed through a laparoscope. (*See* Color Plate.)

and endometriosis also commonly noted. Each of these findings can be managed via a laparoscopic approach in the vast majority of patients, with the conversion rate to open laparotomy being zero in three recent studies [13,14•,15].

Interestingly, it has also been noted that even in the absence of definitive findings at laparoscopy, many patients report an improvement in their chronic pain postoperatively [13,14•,16]. Whether this is the result of the reassurance provided to the patient from the results of the laparoscopy [16] or by other factors is often unknown.

Technique

An open technique is preferred for trocar insertion, particularly in those patients who have undergone prior surgery. A 10- or 12-mm trocar is inserted in the umbilical position and the abdomen is inspected in a systematic fashion. Other trocars can be inserted under direct vision according to anatomic concerns, in which suspected or confirmed pathology has been visualized. All four quadrants of the abdomen should be inspected, with patient position manipulated (*eg*, Trendelenburg, left-side down) to afford the best visualization. The surgeon should be prepared to run the bowel with atraumatic graspers if inspection fails to reveal obvious pathology. Whether adhesions or other pathology are noted, a laparoscopic approach at therapy should be attempted.

CONCLUSIONS

Abdominal pain has multifactorial causes, depending on the acuity of the onset, comorbid medical processes, and the past surgical history. Traditionally, acute inflammatory or vascular causes are the primary causes of acute abdominal pain. Many of these processes can be dealt with both diagnostically and therapeutically via the laparoscope. At present, controlled randomized studies have failed to demonstrate a significant advantage to laparoscopy, but experienced laparoscopic surgeons have found that in certain situations, diagnostic and therapeutic laparoscopy for acute abdominal pain can immeasurably assist in the management of these patients.

In chronic abdominal pain, the role of laparoscopy to both diagnose and treat chronic conditions appears to be salutary. When appropriately selected using specific criteria, and after thorough work-up to rule out other, nonsurgical causes, patients with chronic abdominal pain, who have had prior abdominal surgery and in whom the pain can be localized to a specific area of the abdomen, will frequently be provided with a diagnosis and a therapeutic intervention. The available data suggest that in over 70% of patients followed up in the early postprocedural period, objective and subjective relief of pain can be achieved. Whether or not long-term relief, or the absence of recurrent pain, will be maintained is unclear. Nevertheless, in this difficult group of patients laparoscopy may prove beneficial.

REFERENCES AND RECOMMENDED READING

Recently published papers of particular interest have been highlighted as:

• Of interest

•• Of outstanding interest

1. Allen PD: Anesthesia for minimally invasive surgery. In *Principles of Endosurgery*. Edited by Loughlin KR, Brooks DC. Cambridge, MA: Blackwell Science; 1996:65–69.

2. Brooks DC: Laparoscopy in the acute abdomen. In *Principles of Endosurgery*. Edited by Loughlin KR, Brooks DC. Cambridge, MA: Blackwell Science; 1996:192–193.

3. MacFayden BV, Wolfe BM, McKernan JB: Laparoscopic management of the acute abdomen, appendix, and small and large bowel. *Surg Clin North Am* 1992, 72:1169–1183.

4. Taylor EW, Kennedy CA, Dunham RH, *et al.*: Diagnostic laparoscopy in women with acute abdominal pain. *Surg Laparosc Endosc* 1995, 5:125–128.

5.•• Poole GV, Thomae KR, Hauser CJ: Laparoscopy in trauma. *Surg Clin North Am* 1996, 76:547–556.
A concise review of an underutilized technique, with helpful algorithms for various trauma situations.

6.•• Applegren KN, Cowan BD, Metcalf AM, *et al.*: Laparoscopic appendectomy and the management of gynecologic pathologic conditions found at laparoscopy for presumed appendicitis. *Surg Clin North Am* 1996, 76:469–482.
Provides practical information for the general surgeon who may unexpectedly encounter gynecologic conditions upon laparoscopy.

7. Geis WO, Kim HC: Use of laparoscopy in the diagnosis and treatment of patients with surgical abdominal sepsis. *Surg Endosc* 1995, 9:178–182.

8. Matern U, Haberstroh J, El Saman A, *et al.*: Emergency laparoscopy: technical support for the laparoscopic diagnosis of intestinal ischemia. *Surg Endosc* 1996, 10:883–887.

9. Berci G, Sackier JM, Paz-Partlow M: Emergency laparoscopy. *Am J Surg* 1991, 161:332–335.

10. Mutter D, Nord M, Vix M, *et al.*: Laparoscopy in the evaluation of abdominal stab wounds. *Dig Surg* 1997, 14:39–42.

11. Schrenk P, Woisetschlager R, Wayand WU, *et al.*: Diagnostic laparoscopy: a survey of 92 patients. *Am J Surg* 1994, 168:348–351.

12. Metzger A, Luque-de Leon E, Tsiostos GG, *et al.*: Laparoscopic management of SBO (small bowel obstruction): indications and outcome [abstract]. *Gastroenterology* 1997, 112:A1459.

13. Klingensmith ME, Soybel DI, Brooks DC: Laparoscopy for chronic abdominal pain. *Surg Endosc* 1996, 10:1085–1087.

14.• Miller K, Mayber E, Moritz E: The role of laparoscopy in chronic and recurrent abdominal pain. *Am J Surg* 1996, 172:353–357.
A good review of the current literature on laparoscopy for chronic abdominal pain.

15. Steege JF, Stout AL: Resolution of chronic pelvic pain after laparoscopic lysis of adhesions. *Am J Obstet Gynecol* 1991, 165:278–283.

16. Baker PN, Symonds EM: The resolution of chronic pelvic pain after normal laparoscopy findings. *Am J Obstet Gynecol* 1992, 166:835–836.

17. Luciano AA, Maier DB, Koch EI, *et al.*: A comparative study of postoperative adhesions following laser surgery by laparoscopy versus laparotomy in the rabbit model. *Obstet Gynecol* 1989, 74:220–224.

Gastric Surgery and Bariatric Procedures

Frank H. Chae
Robert C. McIntyre, Jr.
Gregory V. Stiegmann

The primary therapy for peptic ulcer disease is the protection of mucosal lining from the effects of luminal acid. The use of antacids, sulcrafate, H_2-receptor blockers, and proton pump inhibitors is associated with healing in 90% of diseased patients. Furthermore, the eradication of *Helicobacter pylori* with a regimen of bismuth, tetracycline, and metronidazole is associated with even higher cure rates with a significant reduction in recurrence. Overall, less than 10% of peptic ulcer patients require surgical management for failure of medical therapy [1–3].

PEPTIC ULCER DISEASE
Duodenal ulcer
After optimal medical therapy intractable duodenal ulcers require surgical intervention. Highly selective vagotomy is a popular procedure for the treatment of duodenal ulcer. The laparotomy method is associated with 4% to 15% ulcer recurrence rates with virtually no complications (<1%) such as dumping, diarrhea, and gastric atony [4–6]. The laparoscopic approach can duplicate these results while adding the advantages of minimally invasive surgery. Although various approaches to laparoscopic vagotomy have been described, the laparoscopic highly selective vagotomy offers the best features of minimally invasive surgery without compromising on established standard outcome [6,7••,8••,9]. On the other hand, if prepyloric ulcers are discovered, the highly selective vagotomy is associated with high recurrence rates of 30% or more. In this setting, a truncal vagotomy with a drainage procedure should be considered.

Highly selective vagotomy
Endoscopic evaluation is performed preoperatively to detect pyloric narrowing or the presence of prepyloric ulcers. Endoscopic pyloric dilatation should be performed if narrowing is found. The patient is placed in the supine position with legs spread apart. A Foley catheter and nasogastric tube are inserted prior to positioning. Pneumoperitoneum is created by insufflation of CO_2 through the Veress needle and an intra-abdominal pressure of 15 mm Hg is maintained. Five trocars are then introduced into the abdomen, one for the 30° laparoscope, one for the operating instruments, two for the grasping forceps, and one for the retractor or irrigator. The operating surgeon stands between the patient's legs with the patient in a 30° reverse Trendelenburg.

The left lobe of the liver is retracted using an expandable retractor. The gastrohepatic omentum is incised and the lesser sac is entered above the hepatic branch of the anterior vagus nerve. An atraumatic grasper or a Babcock clamp is used in the surgeon's left hand, and a dissecting scissor such as the Harmonic scalpel (Ethicon Endosurgery Inc., Cincinnati, OH) is used in the right hand. The dissection is continued to the level of the right crus of the diaphragm, dividing the phrenoesophageal ligament and the gastrophrenic peritoneum (Fig. 11-1). The anterior vagus is identified by its vertical orientation under the preesophageal peritoneum and dissected off the esophageal surface. For the posterior vagus, the right crus is seized with the right grasper and retracted to the patient's right to expose the preesophageal peritoneum. The peritoneum is incised along the length of the border of the right crus, allowing the separation of the abdominal esophagus outward and permitting access to its posterior wall and mesoesophagus. Located within this angle is the posterior vagus characterized by its white cord appearance. A Penrose drain is passed around the esophagus without including the vagus nerves in the bundle. The vagi dissection is then extended 6 cm above the gastroesophageal junction for division of all small vagal branches innervating the stomach.

The anterior surface of the stomach is stretched with the right and left grasping forceps. A point about 6 cm from the pylorus is selected along the lesser curvature and the dissection is carried in a cephalad direction with the Harmonic scalpel. The nerve branches are divided with their associated vessels up to the phrenoesophageal bundle (Fig. 11-2). If the crow's foot is visible, an attempt should be made to identify and preserve at least one antral branch.

The posterior layer of the lesser sac at the crow's foot is divided and the lesser sac entered. The cephalad dissection is carried out along the lesser curvature to the gastroesophageal junction (Fig. 11-2). The posterior vagus should be elevated off the gastroesophageal junction to check for the criminal nerve of Grassi. With the use of traction forceps, the esophagus can be rolled gently to the right so that the left edge is exposed to reveal any hidden criminal nerves.

Blood is evacuated from the subphrenic areas and all port sites injected preperitoneally with 0.25% to 0.5% marcaine. Once the ports are removed, the fascial defects in each trocar wound should be closed. Nasogastric decompression is continued until the next morning and oral feeding is rapidly advanced to soft diet as tolerated. Meals taken in small portions are recommended in the early postoperative period to accommodate temporary delayed gastric emptying. Prokinetic agents such as Propulsid

(Janssen Pharmaceutical, Titusville, NJ) may alleviate this symptom for the first few weeks.

Discussion

Highly selective vagotomy represents an ideal operation that delivers maximal benefit with minimal side effects. Acid production is reduced, and by preserving the antropyloric nerve branches, the motility of the distal stomach is maintained. Thus, pylorospasm is minimized to promote physiologic emptying of the stomach, making drainage procedures unnecessary. However, highly selective vagotomy is not effective for ulcers in the pyloric region, and hence truncal vagotomy with gastrojejunostomy may be required.

Results to date are extremely promising for laparoscopic highly selective vagotomy. Awad and coworkers [7••] reported on a series involving 119 patients undergoing the procedure with a mean follow-up of 16 months and found that 94% of the patients had a Visick I or II grading and 6% had a Visick III or IV grading. These results are comparable with the laparotomy data. No deaths occurred with the following complications: 3% gastric perforation, 2% bleeding, and 1% reoperation. The intraoperative conversion rate was only 3% and mean hospital stay was 3 days. Cadiere and coworkers [10] report on a series of 33 patients with no mortality, morbidity, or conversions despite 21% presenting with perforated ulcer. Mean hospital stay for elective patients was 2 days. Follow-up was possible in 76% of the original group. Analysis revealed 88% of patients with Visick I or II grades and 12% of patients with Visick III or IV grades.

Other successful laparoscopic approaches that await long-term follow-up evaluation include the posterior truncal vagotomy and anterior seromyotomy (Taylor procedure) as employed by Katkhouda and coworkers [11]. In a study of 90 patients, the reported follow-up ranged from 2 to 41 months and revealed an approximate 4% recurrence rate with minor complications: mild diarrhea, decreased gastric emptying, and worsened gastroesophageal reflux disease.

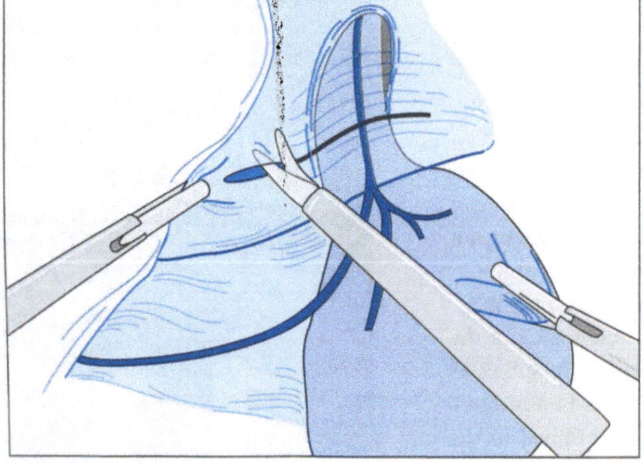

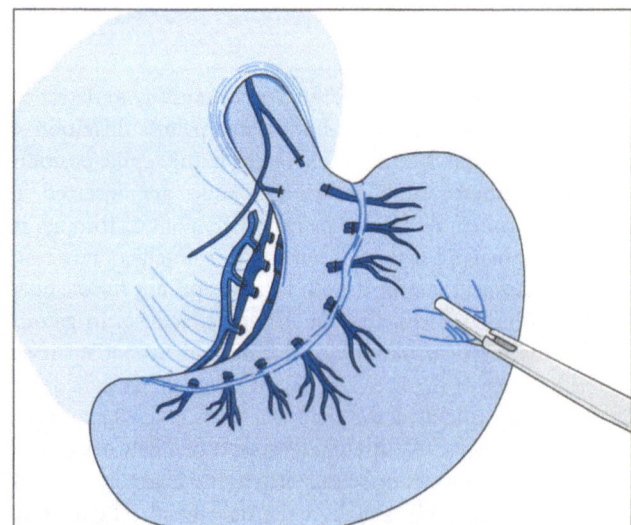

Figure 11-1 Division of the gastrohepatic omentum above the hepatic branch of the vagus nerve. Dissection is extended to the left to divide the phrenoesophageal ligament.

Figure 11-2 Completed dissection and denervation of the lesser curve of the stomach.

An alternative procedure is the laparoscopic posterior truncal vagotomy with anterior linear gastrectomy as reported by Gomez-Ferrer and coworkers [12]. One hundred thirty-six patients with chronic duodenal ulcer underwent this procedure while some had also received an antireflux procedure (17%) or a cholecystectomy (10%). Postoperative morbidity was 3% with zero mortality. Mean hospital stay was 3.1 days (range, 2 to 13 days). Follow-up was at a mean of 25 months (range, 6 to 33 months) in 131 patients and resulted in 96.2% falling in the Visick I or II category while 3.8 % fell in the Visick III or IV category.

Other promising procedures that can be applied laparoscopically for the treatment of ulcer disease include the total truncal vagotomy with endoscopic pyloric dilatation, the total truncal vagotomy by thoracoscopy, and the posterior truncal vagotomy with anterior highly selective vagotomy (Hill-Barker procedure) [13–15]. More prospective trials are underway to evaluate these procedures.

Highly selective vagotomy adapts well to laparoscopic surgery and promises even more popularity for peptic ulcer disease therapy. An acceptable alternative may be the posterior truncal vagotomy with anterior seromyotomy as modified by Katkhouda and coworkers [11]. On the other hand, despite good initial results reported for the posterior truncal vagotomy with anterior linear gastrectomy, the value of this rather invasive gastric resection over the less invasive vagotomy remains questionable.

Gastric ulcer

Giant gastric ulcers (> 3 cm) and gastric ulcers failing medical therapy are best treated by surgery. Although the highly selective vagotomy may be applied to type I gastric ulcer disease, the inflammation usually present in the lesser curvature can result in a very difficult dissection. There is also a high recurrence rate for type II or III gastric ulcers, making the highly selective vagotomy undesirable for gastric ulcer disease. Thus, unlike duodenal ulcer, the best surgical approach for gastric ulcer is either a distal gastrectomy incorporating the ulcer, or truncal vagotomy with a drainage procedure and ulcer biopsy. Certainly, both methods have been adapted to laparoscopy but there is not enough data to conclude the efficacy of either approach for the treatment of gastric ulcer. Laparoscopic truncal vagotomy with gastrojejunostomy has been studied for the treatment of gastric outlet obstruction in peptic ulcer disease and offers the best promise, but the results are too preliminary to adequately address its role in the treatment of benign gastric ulcer disease.

Repair of perforated peptic ulcer

Patients with an acute duodenal ulcer perforation who are clinically stable and have no prior history of duodenal ulcer disease may be treated with laparoscopic closure and omental patch repair. Late presentation usually entails extensive peritonitis, contamination with gastric contents, and fibrinous reaction that may preclude a safe laparoscopic repair. Iatrogenic injury with laparoscopic instruments is highly probable in the hostile abdomen with a distended and edematous bowel. On the other hand, gastric perforation from ulcer erosion usually entails a definitive distal gastrectomy if the patient is stable enough, but for moribund patients, a patch or primary closure of anterior gastric wall perforation may be appropriate.

Patient positioning and trocar placements previously described for highly selective vagotomy can be employed, but only three trocar ports may be necessary. Most of the duodenal perforations should be located on the anterior duodenal wall within 1 cm of the pylorus. An intraoperative endoscopic examination may be necessary if the perforation is not visualized on initial examination. The duodenum can be submerged in saline irrigation as the stomach is insufflated to create air bubbles through the defect. After a simple intracorporeal suture closure with an omental patch, the peritoneum is irrigated with saline (4 to 8 liters). Nasogastric decompression should continue for 3 to 6 days until bowel function returns. H_2-blockers or proton pump inhibitors should be continued postoperatively [8••].

Siu and coworkers [16] employed only three ports to execute a single laparoscopic omental patch repair for perforated peptic ulcer. Of 33 patients, there was a 15% intraoperative conversion rate and 3% postoperative failure rate due to leakage of repair. Return to daily activity was usually within 10 days and mortality rate was zero. Matsuda and coworkers [17] reported slightly better success rates in 11 patients. The next logical step would be to add highly selective vagotomy to the omental patch repair in the setting of chronic ulcer disease history. Although no large trials examining this issue have been reported, there are isolated reports of successful laparoscopic vagotomy and Graham patch repair for a perforated peptic ulcer [6,18].

Repair of gastric outlet obstruction

Patients presenting with gastric outlet obstruction due to ulcer disease require endoscopy to evaluate the distensibility of the pylorus and to exclude neoplasm or Crohn's disease. In poor risk patients, it is reasonable to attempt balloon dilatation of the pylorus, but surgical treatment is usually required in most obstructed patients. The standard operation is truncal vagotomy with a drainage procedure by laparotomy, but laparoscopic adaptations have been successfully executed.

Laparoscopic truncal vagotomy with gastrojejunostomy may be applied to treat pyloric stenosis due to benign peptic ulcer disease. The dissection for total truncal vagotomy is similar to the approach described in highly selective vagotomy. Once the anterior and posterior vagi are identified and isolated from the esophagus, each of the nerves are transected between two clips and a 1-cm section is removed for histologic confirmation. The gastrojejunostomy should be 8 cm long on the greater curvature and close to the pylorus, about 6 cm away. A window in the transverse mesocolon is created just behind the colic arcade by using a Harmonic scalpel. The loop of jejunum is then brought through the window and approximated against the stomach. The Harmonic scalpel is then used to establish a gastrotomy and a jejunotomy so that the tips of the linear Endo-GIA stapler (US Surgical Corporation, Norwalk, CT) (60 mm) can be inserted through the openings for application. The luminal staple line is then inspected for hemostasis and the remaining enterotomy is closed either by firing a second Endo-GIA stapler or by intracorporeal suturing.

Wyman and coworkers [19] report an intraoperative conversion rate of 8% with a median operative time of 210 minutes in 12 patients with pyloric stenosis secondary to duodenal ulceration. At a median postoperative follow-up of 6 months, all patients had good symptomatic outcomes (Visick grades I or II). Alternatively, laparoscopic truncal vagotomy with Jaboulay gastroduodenostomy to relieve gastric outlet obstruction has been described [20].

Repair of bleeding peptic ulcer

Only experimental studies exist for laparoscopic management of bleeding benign gastric ulcers [21,22]. Laparoscopic Billroth II gastrectomy has been performed for bleeding gastric ulcer after endoscopic failure, but its long-term outcome remains preliminary [23]. Theoretically, in hemodynamically stable patients, laparoscopic repair of duodenal ulcer hemorrhage with a definitive acid-reducing procedure is feasible. The duodenotomy required to expose the bleeding vessel in the ulcer crater, the technique to reclose the duodenotomy, and the execution of truncal vagotomy with a gastrojejunostomy are all within the capabilities of advanced laparoscopic surgery. However, the actual benefit gained from this approach remains to be explored.

GASTRIC NEOPLASM

Most of the work involving laparoscopic gastrectomy focuses on benign disease. Its role in gastric carcinoma is still under scrutiny. Current data are uncontrolled and incomplete to accurately assess the role of laparoscopic gastrectomy in carcinoma therapy; however, the role of laparoscopy in tumor staging is very encouraging.

Wedge resection for benign tumors

Wedge resections of the stomach employing the laparoscopic approach may be performed for leiomyomas with success [24,25]. For posterior wall lesions, a transgastric approach may be employed to resect the tumor. The patient positioning and trocar placements are as described previously for highly selective vagotomy, but only four trocar ports are necessary. Both the endoscope and the laparoscope are employed to locate the tumor and help delineate the area of resection. An Endo-GIA 30-mm stapler may be fired multiple times in sequence for the wedge resection of the tumor, leaving behind a resealed and patent stomach. The specimen should be placed in an endoscopic retrieval bag prior to removal and sent for frozen section. The stomach is then immersed in saline irrigation and distended with air through the endoscope to check for staple line leakage. Intracorporeal suturing can reinforce any point along the staple line that is bleeding or leaking air.

Transgastric wedge resection

For tumors located in the posterior wall near the greater or lesser curvatures, the Harmonic scalpel is used to dissect either the short gastric vessels, the gastrocolic omentum, or the gastrohepatic ligament to obtain optimal operative exposure. Gentle stomach manipulation with Babcock or noncrushing clamps aided by endoscopic direction may be necessary to expose the tumor location. A wedge resection may be attempted if easy access to the tumor is available, if not, a transgastric resection should be employed. An anterior gastrotomy is made directly over the tumor site initially with electrosurgery or a Harmonic scalpel and extended with an Endo-GIA 30-mm stapler. Working through the gastrotomy, the posterior wall tumor is resected in the same manner as described previously. The anterior gastrotomy is then reapproximated either with interrupted sutures or Babcock clamps for the Endo-GIA 60-mm stapler closure.

Intragastric wedge resection

An interesting approach for small-sized tumors located in the cardia or the posterior wall is laparoscopic intragastric surgery [24]. In this technique, a nasogastric tube with a balloon is endoscopically inserted into the duodenum to prevent air loss and then three trocars are inserted into the stomach wall through the anterior abdominal wall. Visualization is coordinated by the use of both the endoscope and the laparoscope. The tumor is enucleated using a dissector and electrosurgery, after which it is removed in a retrieval bag and brought out through the esophagus by the gastroscope. Unfortunately, wedge resection with a free margin for large-sized tumors and obtaining control of bleeding may prove to be unnecessarily challenging for this approach.

Malignant tumors

Despite the numerous data regarding minimally invasive gastrectomy for gastric carcinoma therapy, no definitive conclusion can be drawn. Gastrectomy by way of laparoscopy, whether total or assisted, remains an experimental management of gastric malignancy. There is still the unresolved issue of trocar site tumor seeding reported in various cancer operations. On the other hand, staging laparoscopy for gastric cancer has a beneficial role in patient management [26••,27•].

Staging laparoscopy

Burke and coworkers [26••] performed staging laparoscopy in 110 patients with nonobstructed and nonbleeding gastric cancer whose preoperative evaluation revealed no evidence of metastatic disease. Thirty-seven percent of these patients were found to have unsuspected metastatic disease by laparoscopy (84% sensitivity, 100% specificity). The average time of discharge was 1.4 days for laparoscopy and 6.5 days for staging laparotomy ($P < 0.05$). Lowy and coworkers [27•] also demonstrated similar findings in 71 patients. Thus, laparoscopy can accurately identify occult metastasis and avoid unnecessary laparotomy.

Staging laparoscopy may be performed with either two or three ports (5 or 10 mm) using a 30° scope and Babcock instruments. Since the majority (72%) of the metastatic lesions found by Burke and coworkers were peritoneal implants, one- or two-port placement for examination of the peritoneum may be all that is necessary [26••]. If the peritoneum is free from lesions, the liver, the diaphragm, the serosal surfaces, the omentum, the bowel and its mesentery, and the pelvic organs should be examined and biopsied if necessary. The regions of ligament of

Treitz and porta hepatis should be also examined for nodal involvement. Laparoscopic ultrasonography for examination of the liver may enhance the staging capacity of the tumor [28]. In symptomatic patients or those free from metastatic disease, an open exploration should be considered in the same setting for either palliative or curative resection.

Gastric resection

Although there have been feasibility reports of totally laparoscopic gastrectomy (Billroth II) for carcinoma, the extended operative times required, along with the lack of tactile ability for tumor localization, lymph node, and liver metastases, make laparoscopic surgery extremely unattractive [29,30]. Hand-assisted laparoscopic resection using the Dexterity Pneumo Sleeve (Dexterity, Research Triangle Park, NC) device has been reported, but its advantage over open gastrectomy remains to be proven [31].

Certainly, for selected early-stage gastric adenocarcinoma, leiomyosarcoma, or lymphoma, laparoscopic extended wedge resections with endoscopic staplers may be considered [23]; however, this is not recommended for stage II and stage III gastric adenocarcinomas.

Palliation: gastric bypass

Palliative laparoscopic procedures should benefit patients who have limited life expectancy. For patients with incurable malignant gastric outlet obstruction and cholestasis, laparoscopic gastrojejunostomy combined with endoscopic biliary stent placement should provide good functional results with minimal operative morbidity [32•].

Four trocars (10 mm and one 12 mm for the endoscopic stapler) are placed. After the table is tilted 30° Trendelenburg, the transverse colon and the omentum are swept cephalad to identify the ligament of Treitz. The jejunal loop is then brought up antecolic to the stomach and fixed to the antrum with two stay sutures. A Harmonic scalpel may be used to create openings for the stapler jaws in the stomach and the jejunum. A 30-mm Endo-GIA stapler is then introduced and fired in two consecutive applications for a wide gastrojejunostomy. The remaining opening can be closed by an intracorporeal running suture. A diverting jejuno-jejunostomy may then be created in the same manner approximately 25 cm distal to the gastrojejunostomy to avoid exposure of bile acids to the anastomosis. Biliary decompression should be performed preoperatively either by endoscopic or transhepatic stenting. If this is not possible, a bilioenteric bypass may be performed with an open gastrojejunostomy instead of laparoscopy.

GASTROSTOMY

Although percutaneous endoscopic gastrostomy (PEG) is the preferred method for providing long-term gastric decompression or enteral nutrition in patients who are unable to swallow, there are certain limitations. Ascites, previous upper abdominal surgery, and subtotal or total stenosis of the hypopharynx or esophagus secondary to tumor usually mandates the performance of surgical gastrostomy. Either the open Stamm gastrostomy using local anesthesia or laparoscopic-assisted gastrostomy may be employed. Stiegmann and coworkers [33] demonstrated no difference between the PEG and the open Stamm gastrostomy using local anesthesia with regard to morbidity, mortality, or tube function.

Laparoscopic gastrostomy

An advantage of laparoscopic gastrostomy over PEG—coupled with the advantages of minimally invasive surgery—is that a feeding catheter with a larger diameter may be placed. Thus, mashed normal food can be used for nutrition rather than expensive liquid formula. Laparoscopy also allows the securing of stomach and tube to the abdominal wall for a tighter seal, a step not available with endoscopy. However, the advantage of laparoscopic gastrostomy over the open Stamm gastrostomy under local anesthesia is less clear.

Laparoscopically assisted gastrostomy as described by Peitgen and coworkers [34] may be performed with two 10-mm trocars and one 5-mm trocar. The 30° laparoscope should be panning from the left lower quadrant port for optimal view of the stomach. Three intracorporeal full-thickness stitches using 2-0 absorbable sutures are placed in triangular fashion on the anterior stomach wall (Fig. 11-3). Both ends of each suture are then pulled through the abdominal wall for anchoring by using a special awl (No. 26173 AK; Storz, Germany) beneath the left costal margin. An incision of 1 cm is made through the abdominal wall in the center of the suture triangulation. Then, an 18-gauge needle is inserted into the center of the triangle on the stomach wall, where a guidewire is threaded into the lumen. A 26-F dilator with a peel-away sheath (Cpli-2638; Cook, Germany) is introduced into the stomach over the guidewire and then the inner dilator is removed. A 24-F Foley catheter is placed through the peel-away sheath and the balloon tip inflated. The stomach is then fixed to the abdominal wall by tying the traction sutures placed previously. Checking for leakage from the gastrostomy may be accomplished by a contrast study. Feeding may commence the next day as tolerated. The Foley catheter is exchanged as needed in an outpatient setting.

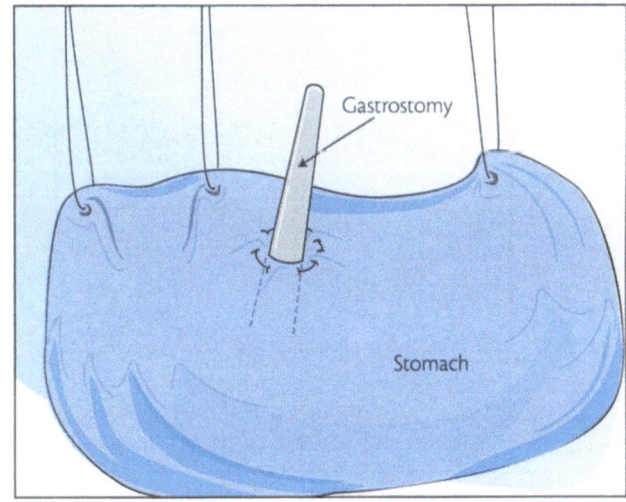

Figure 11-3 Three stay sutures are placed for gastropexy surrounding the gastrostomy.

Of 42 patients with laparoscopic gastrostomy, Peitgen and coworkers [34] reported a mean operative time of 38 ± 11 minutes. No procedure-related mortality is claimed, although one patient died of myocardial infarct 3 days after surgery and another patient died 2 days later of pneumonia from an esophagopulmonary fistula. Gastric perforation occurred in one patient due to grasping forceps. The incidence of stomal infection was 0.11% per 100 days of use.

Gastric surgery: conclusions

With the growth of enhanced dexterity skills in laparoscopy coupled with improved operative hardware, more conventional procedures are being adapted to minimally invasive surgery. The ease of the laparoscopic procedure should no longer dictate the type of operation chosen. The past multicenter studies of open conventional procedures should not be ignored but adapted to assess the most appropriate laparoscopic approach.

BARIATRIC SURGERY

Since 1960 the National Center for Health Statistics has conducted surveys of the prevalence of obesity every 10 years. These surveys have revealed that unhealthy weight has increased at record levels over the past decade from 25% of adults in 1980 to 34% of the American population as of 1990. As a result, an estimated 58 million American adults, or a third of the adult population, is overweight [35]. This incidence of obesity is highest in minority populations, low-income groups, and women. The prevalence of obesity is increasing despite an expenditure of over 30 billion dollars annually on commercial weight loss products [36]. Increasing rates of obesity are a major public health threat. One third of all cases of hypertension can be attributed to obesity. Eighty-eight percent to 97% of all cases of type II (noninsulin-dependent) diabetes, 57% to 70% of coronary artery diseases, 11% of breast cancers, and 10% of colon cancers are attributable to obesity. Furthermore, 30%

of obese patients have gallstones compared with only 10% of nonobese patients. Other obesity related conditions include osteoarthritis, gout, dyslipidemia, sleep apnea, obesity hypoventilation syndrome, deep venous thrombosis, pulmonary embolus, venous stasis disease, and pseudotumor cerebrii. Furthermore, obese patients have a higher mortality for malignancies that include colorectal, prostate, endometrial, and ovarian carcinomas [36–38].

It is now clear that overweight patients die at a younger age and that weight loss and maintenance of healthy weight returns life expectancy to that of the general population. Risk for morbidity and mortality accompanying severe obesity is proportional to the degree of excess weight (Fig. 11-4). The mortality rate associated with obesity rises from normal at a body mass index (BMI) of 20 to 25 kg/m² [BMI = weight (kg)/height (m²)] to three times normal with a BMI ≥ 40 kg/m² (Fig. 11-4) [39]. Approximately 4 million Americans have a BMI between 35 and 40 kg/m². An additional 4 million Americans have a BMI over 40 kg/m², which is roughly equivalent to 100 pounds of excess body weight. These patients at highest risk for morbidity and mortality are categorized as having "clinically severe obesity" [40,41].

As important as the severity of obesity is the distribution of body fat. Patients with central, or android, fat deposition are at a much higher risk for developing complications of obesity than are those with peripheral, or gynoid, fat deposition. The distribution of body fat is often measured by the waist-hip ratio. Upper body obesity is defined as a ratio of 1.0 or higher in men and 0.8 or higher in women. However, the waist circumference and sagittal diameter may be more accurate measures of the body fat distribution that the waist-hip ratio [42,43]. CT-calibrated anthropometry is a technique based on a model of obesity composed of three body compartments: lean body mass, visceral adipose tissue (AT), and subcutaneous AT. The visceral AT may be calculated using the weight, height, and sagittal trunk diameter. Using the Swedish Obese Subjects (SOS) database, Sjostrom [44] has demonstrated that the visceral AT is more closely related to metabolic aberrations and disease than the waist hip ratio. Collectively, these studies have shown that AT distribution may be more important than absolute weight in predicting obesity comorbidity.

Data from the SOS intervention study have defined the prevalence of several risk factors and diseases related to obesity. The SOS project consists of two parts, one a register and one an intervention study. The aims of the study are to examine if long-term weight reduction decreases total morbidity and mortality of specific diseases. Depending on sex and age, various symptoms and diseases seem to be 1.2 to 105 times more common among obese individuals (Table 11-1). Large prospective studies have found that severe obesity (BMI > 35 kg/m²) is associated with an approximate twofold increase in total mortality and a sevenfold increase in mortality due to diabetes, cerebrovascular and cardiovascular disease, as well as cancer [45].

Indications for surgery

Treatment options for the obese patient include behavior therapy, low-calorie diets, medication, and surgery [36,40,41]. The aim of treatment should be to reduce morbidity rather than attain

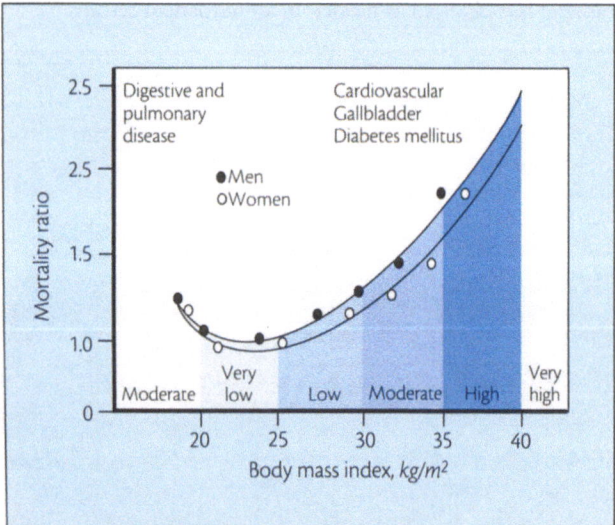

Figure 11-4 Relationship of body mass index (BMI) to risk (all cause mortality). The curvilinear plot is adapted from data derived from the American Cancer Society. (*Adapted from* Bray [39].)

Table 11-1

Prevalence ratios (obese:control) for various symptoms and diseases in men and women

Symptom or disease	Prevalence ratios	
	Men	Women
Dyspnea	4.3	4.7–6.4
Angina	15	6.8–37
History of myocardial infarction	4.5–5.4	0.7:0
Hypertension	2.1	2.4–11
Diabetes	5.2	6.6–24
Stroke		0.7:0
Claudication	4.6	26–105
Gallbladder disease	1.7	1.8–2.8
Back pain	2.1	1.6–1.9

Data from Sjostrom [44].

the cosmetic standard of ideal weight. Patients seeking initial therapy for obesity should be considered for a nonsurgical program including diet, exercise, behavior modification, and perhaps medical therapy. However, these treatments have a high rate of recidivism [36,40], making surgery the treatment of choice for clinically severe obesity (BMI ≥ 40 kg/m²). Patients may also be considered candidates for surgical treatment with lesser degrees of obesity (BMI 35 to 40 kg/m²) if they suffer from significant comorbidity including cardiopulmonary conditions, severe diabetes, or obesity related physical problems that cause significant lifestyle limitations [40,41].

Third party payers often require a long history of obesity (> 5 years), failure of a physician-supervised program for control of weight (longer than 1 year), and no history of substance abuse, psychoses, or uncontrolled depression [46]. Other contraindications to surgery for obesity include active hepatitis or cirrhosis, Crohn's disease, renal failure, malignancy, or a specific endocrine disorder as the cause of obesity.

Preoperative assessment

The morbidly obese patient is at an increased risk for numerous complications that include wound infection and dehiscence, thrombophlebitis and pulmonary embolus, postoperative apnea and airway obstruction, respiratory failure, and cardiac failure. In a series of over 1500 gastric procedures for morbid obesity, Sugerman [47] reported a total adverse event rate of only 16.1% with an operative mortality of only 0.4%. The majority of these complications were minor wound infections and seromas (10% of patients). Thus, proper preoperative evaluation and preparation may lead to a low perioperative morbidity and mortality.

Our preoperative assessment includes a careful history and physical exam. The history should include a detailed review of the patient's history of obesity, previous therapy and results, and usual dietary habits. A multidisciplinary approach using clinical

dietitians is extremely helpful in evaluation and postoperative counseling of the patient. All patients should be screened for those conditions listed above. We routinely perform a chest radiograph, electrocardiogram, complete blood count, and urine analysis. We also perform fasting glucose, glycosylated hemoglobin, insulin level, and a lipid panel (total and low-density lipoprotein [LDL]/high-density lipoprotein [HDL] cholesterol) in all patients. Patients without clinically evident diabetes undergo an oral glucose tolerance test to screen for glucose intolerance. Other tests are done on the basis of the history and physical exam. These may include electrolyte and renal function studies in patients with hypertension and on diuretics. If malnutrition-induced cirrhosis is suspected or the patient has a history suggestive of coagulopathy, liver function studies and coagulation tests are obtained. Patients with moderate to severe gastroesophageal reflux symptoms should have an upper gastrointestinal contrast study.

Additional conditions that should be screened for include undiagnosed obstructive sleep apnea (OSA). OSA refers to the occurrence of episodes of complete or partial pharyngeal obstruction during sleep. The related symptoms and signs include multiple episodes of apnea, sleep fragmentation, oxygen desaturations, disruptive snoring, and excessive daytime somnolence [48]. The constellation of symptoms and signs is called *sleep apnea syndrome* (SAS). The 1993 community based study by Young and coworkers [49] found that OSA (defined as an apnea-hypopnea index [AHI] > 5) occurred in 9% of women and 24% of men. Adults with symptoms of sleepiness and an AHI > 5 accounted for 2% of women and 4% of men [49]. A BMI > 28 kg/m² is present in 60% to 90% of patients with OSA evaluated in a sleep center [48]. Patients with suspected SAS should undergo a preoperative polysomnography at a sleep center to confirm or exclude the diagnosis [48,50,51]. Patients found to have significant disease are treated with nasal continuous positive airway pressure (CPAP). A tracheostomy may be necessary to treat patients who do not respond to nasal CPAP or cannot tolerate it. An extra long tracheostomy tube is necessary in these patients. Patients with SAS are at an increased risk of acute upper airway obstruction after operation. They are also at an increased risk for ventricular arrhythmias and sinus arrest during these apneic episodes and must be observed very closely for this problem.

Obesity hypoventilation syndrome (OHS) is suspected in patients who present with severe shortness of breath or congestive heart failure. Spirometry reveals a decrease in forced vital capacity, residual lung volume, expiratory reserve volume, functional residual capacity, and maximal minute volume ventilation. The syndrome is confirmed by arterial blood gases revealing arterial hypoxemia ($PaO_2 < 55$ torr) and hypercarbia ($PaCO_2 > 47$ torr). These patients have severe pulmonary hypertension and polycythemia (Hg > 16 g/dL). In patients with OHS, a Swann-Ganz catheter should be inserted the day before surgery. If a pulmonary artery wedge pressure of > 18 mm kg is found, diuresis should be performed. Polycythemia should be treated by phlebotomy to an Hg of ≤ 15 g/dL. Some patients require a markedly elevated pulmonary capillary wedge pressure to maintain cardiac output. Excessive diuresis may lead to hypotension and should be avoided. The optimal pulmonary capillary wedge pressure in the morbidly obese patient should be determined by the relative change in cardiac output with either volume challenge or diuresis. If pulmonary hypertension is suspected, an echocardiogram may be done. Because of an increased risk of fatal pulmonary embolus in a patient with severe pulmonary hypertension, patients with a mean pulmonary artery pressure > 40 mm Hg should receive a preoperative caval filter [52].

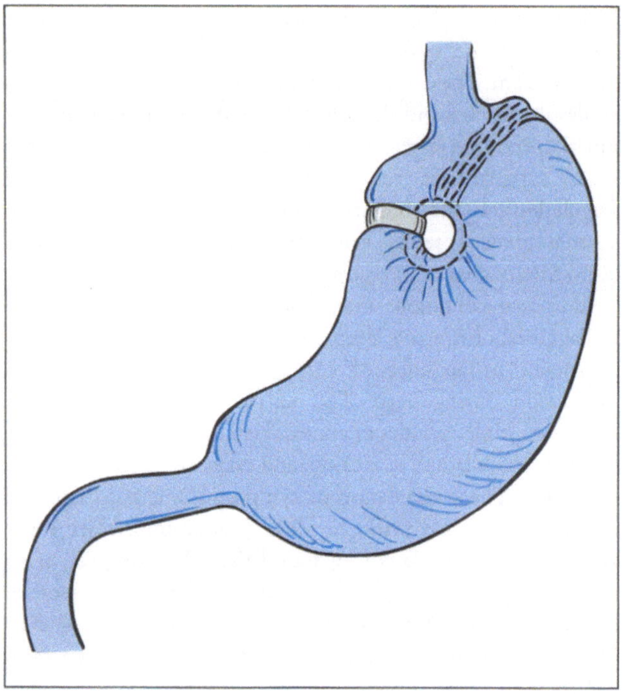

Surgical treatment for weight control

The most frequently performed gastric procedures for morbid obesity today include the Roux-en-Y gastric bypass (RYGB) and vertical banded gastroplasty; however, four basic approaches have been traditionally used for the treatment of obesity [46].

The first operation done for obesity was the jejunoileal bypass. This operation was done by bypassing 90% of the jejunum and ileum to induce a global malabsorption. This operation was abandoned due to a high incidence of severe complications such as hepatic failure, cirrhosis, nephropathy, and numerous other metabolic complications. The gastroplasty was developed to limit the amount of oral intake per meal. This operation involves partitioning the stomach into a small upper pouch that empties through a restricted stoma. The vertical banded gastroplasty (VBG) as championed by Mason [53], is the most popular version of the gastroplasty (Fig. 11-5). The third approach to obesity is the RYGB. This operation also involves formation of a small upper gastric pouch that is anastamosed to a Roux-en-Y jejunal limb (Fig. 11-6). The operation both limits oral intake per meal as well as induces dumping syndrome. Lastly, the partial biliopancreatic bypass induces a selective maldigestion and malabsorption. This operation involves a partial gastrectomy and diversion of the biliary and pancreatic secretions to the distal 50 cm of ileum; it is primarily performed in the "super" obese population (BMI > 60 kg/m²).

There have been numerous modifications to the above procedures. However, these modifications follow the principles outlined above. One modification of the RYGB is to separate the stapled stomach rather than to staple it in continuity [54].

Figure 11-5 Vertical banded gastroplasty. (*Adapted from* Sugerman *et al.* [56].)

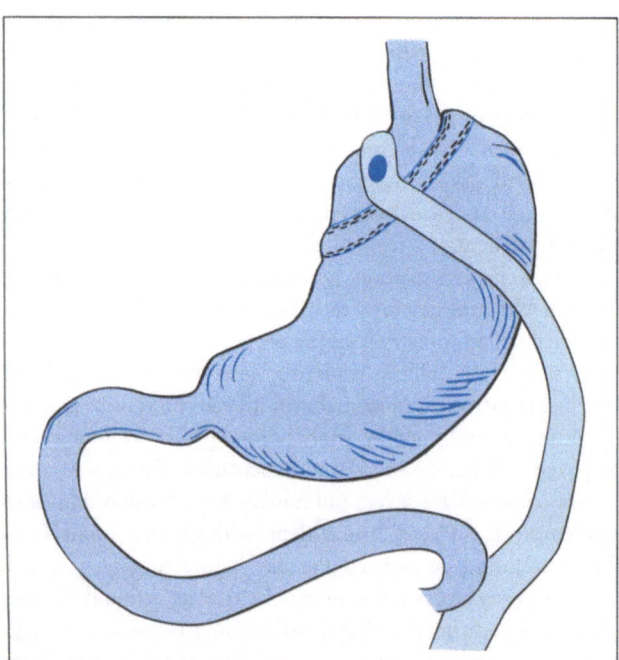

Figure 11-6 Roux-en-Y gastric bypass. (*Adapted from* Sugerman *et al.* [56].)

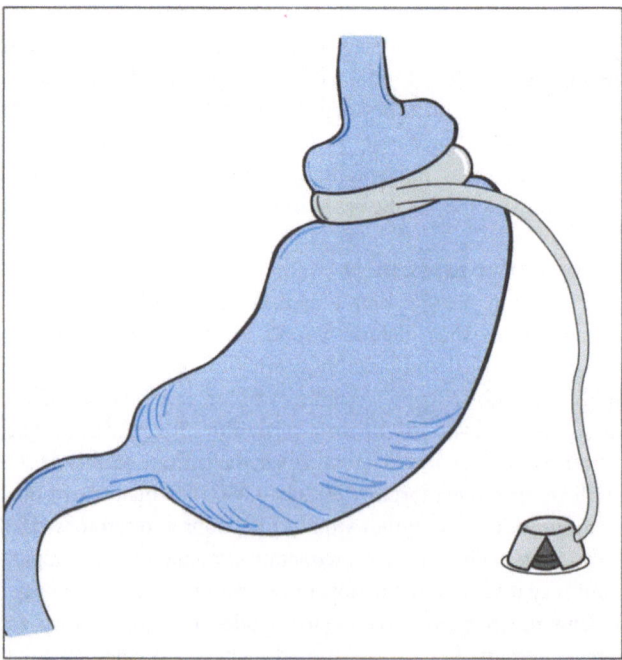

Figure 11-7 Laparoscopic adjustable silicone gastric band (Lap Band; Bioenterics Corporation, Carpinteria, CA).

This modification is aimed at reducing staple line disruption. To this aim, some surgeons have advocated using four rows of staples. Another variation of the gastric bypass involves placement of a silastic ring to restrict the size of the outlet to prevent dilation of the stoma. The most recent development has been the modification of the adjustable silicone gastric band developed by Kuzmak [55]. This gastric banding device has been modified for laparoscopic placement and is a form of gastric restriction or gastroplasty (Fig. 11-7).

Results of surgery

The goals of surgery are to induce and maintain weight loss. Additionally, surgical treatment of obesity should be to reverse or ameliorate obesity comorbidity. The goal of surgery is not to achieve some "ideal" body weight. Outcome from surgery is usually expressed as the amount or percent of excess weight lost.

Several trials have compared the effect of gastric restriction versus gastric bypass. Sugerman and coworkers [56] compared VBG with RYGB in a randomized, prospective trial that included preoperative dietary separation of patients based on consumption of "sweets." Twenty patients were randomized into each group and followed for up to 3 years. Patients having VBG lost 37% of excess weight compared with 64% for patients undergoing RYGB. There was no significant difference in weight loss from RGYB between sweets eaters and non–sweets eaters, (69% vs 67%). However, patients who consumed sweets had less weight loss following VBG (36% vs 57%). Interestingly, non–sweets eaters had similar weight loss following VBG and RYGB (57% vs 67%).

Subsequently several trials have confirmed that RYGB results in more weight loss compared with VBG. The Adelaide study [57] also found that RYGB resulted in significantly greater weight loss compared with VBG. In this study, success was defined as loss of ≥ 50% of excess weight or a current pregnancy. RYGB had a success rate of 67% compared with 48% for VBG at 3 years [57]. MacLean and coworkers [54] also found a higher success rate with RYGB when defined as a BMI ≤ 35 kg/m². RYGB had a success of 77% versus 57% for VBG. The study by Brolin and coworkers [58] may explain the greater weight loss with RYGB. In this trial, patients were prospectively selected for RYGB or VBG based on their preoperative eating habits. Thirty patients underwent VBG and the remaining 108 were found to be sweets eaters and had RYGB. Weight loss peaked at 74 ± 23 lbs at 12 months after VBG versus 99 ± 24 lbs at 16 months following RYGB. Twelve of 30 VBG patients lost ≥ 50% excess weight compared with 100 of 108 after RYGB. Evaluation of dietary intake after surgery revealed that there was a significantly higher milk/ice cream and nonliquid sweets intake in the VBG group compared with those patients having RYGB. Thus, problematic postoperative weight loss after VBG may result from an adverse effect on postoperative eating habits.

Early complications following operations for obesity include subphrenic abscess or leak from an anastamosis or staple line. This complication (2% to 3%) is usually amenable to percutaneous aspiration and drainage, however, a small number of patients will require reoperation. The majority of early postoperative complications are minor wound infections and seromas

(10% of patients). Late complications of the RYGB include vitamin B12 and iron-deficiency anemia (up to 50% of patients) [59]. On the other hand, vitamin B12 and iron-deficiency anemia is uncommon after VBG (less than 10%). Incisional hernia occurs in up to 20% of morbidly obese patients undergoing laparotomy [60]. Other late complications include failure to lose weight, late weight regain, erosion of foreign material, and outlet stenosis. Staple line disruption has been a common problem and has prompted the use of four rows of staples instead of two. Another approach has been to divide the stomach to produce an isolated gastric pouch [54].

Surgery induced weight loss results in a significant reduction in comorbidity. In the above series by Brolin and coworkers [58] there were 32 medical problems in 23 patients (77% of patients) who underwent VBG and 146 problems in 72 RYGB patients (69% of patients). Problems included hypertension, hyperlipidemia, arthritis, diabetes, angina, venous stasis, and sleep apnea. VBG resulted in resolution or improvement in comorbidity in 66% of patients. RYGB resulted in resolution or improvement in 96% of patients. Data from Pories and coworkers [61] demonstrate that RYGB leads to resolution of diabetes in the vast majority of patients. In his series of 608 patients, Pories and coworkers found that 27% of patients had noninsulin-dependent diabetes and another 27% had impaired glucose tolerance. Following RYGB, 82.9% of patients with noninsulin-dependent diabetes mellitus and 98.7% of patients with impaired glucose tolerance had normal glucose, glycosylated hemoglobin, and insulin [61]. Obese patients report significant impairment in quality of life above and beyond the impact of medical complications of the disease. This impaired quality of life results from poor physical health, mental well-being, and psychosocial function. Operated patients with significant weight loss demonstrate dramatic improvement in quality of life [62].

Laparoscopic vertical banded gastroplasty

The primary aim of laparoscopic surgery has been to perform the same operation using the laparoscope as during an open operation. Two series of laparoscopic VBG confirm that the same operation can be performed with the laparoscope as with open technique. Chua and Mendiola [63] reported 11 cases of laparoscopic VBG in 1995. The mean operating time was 202 minutes. The average length of hospital stay was 3.9 days and the average hospital charge was $12,800 (compared with a mean operating time of 105 minutes, 9.3-day stay, and $14,100 hospital charge in the preceding 11 open gastric bypass patients). Lonroth and coworkers [64] reported on 38 consecutive laparoscopic VBG operations. Three patients had to be converted to an open procedure and an additional three patients had to be reoperated on due to early postoperative complications. Compared with the reference group of 17 open VBG procedures, the laparoscopic technique resulted in less postoperative pain, earlier mobilization, and an improved respiratory status. Neither of these series contained data on weight loss. However, Catona and coworkers [65] reported weight loss comparable with open VBG in a series of 25 patients undergoing laparoscopic VBG (40% excess weight loss at 9 months).

The patient is placed in reverse Trendelenburg position with the legs separated in low stirrups. The surgeon stands between the patient's legs. An alternative approach is to place the patient supine with a footrest in the reverse Trendelenburg position. The surgeon stands on the patient's right side with an assistant on the left. Five trocars are placed in the standard manner for gastric surgery. The laparoscope (30°) is placed through the 10-mm midepigastric port, and the liver retractor is placed through a right subcostal port. There are two operating ports, one in each paramedian position (right, 10 mm to 33 mm; left, 15 mm). A window is created at the lesser curve of the stomach in an avascular plane using shears. The posterior stomach wall is freed of any adhesions. An alternative approach to the lesser sac is made by dividing the gastroepiploic vessels along the greater curvature. A 32-F dilator is placed via the mouth into the stomach. A site on the anterior stomach 4 to 5 cm from the gastroesophageal junction and 3 cm from the lesser curve is marked with the electrocautery. This site will be the center of the circular stapler. The right paramedian port is upsized to a 33-mm port to allow introduction of the circular stapling device. The anvil of the circular stapler is then placed posterior to the stomach. The pointed trocar is inserted through the stomach at the site previously marked with the cautery. The stapler is then connected and fired.

The attachments from the diaphragm to the fundus of the stomach are divided, and the fundus is dissected inferiorly using blunt technique. A linear 60-mm, four-row, noncutting stapler is introduced through the left paramedian port. The stapler is inserted through the circular window along the dilator and fired. A linear cutter is applied lateral to the previously placed rows of staples. At the circular window a strip of polypropylene or polytetrafluoroethylene (1.5 x 5 cm) is brought around the stoma. The band is sutured into place around the dilator. A nasogastric tube is not mandatory with this procedure.

Laparoscopic Roux-en-Y gastric bypass

Wittgrove and Clark [66] have reported on over 27 cases of laparoscopic gastric bypass with 3 to 18 months follow-up time. The laparoscopic RYGB results in a shorter hospital stay, diminished recovery time, and a rapid return to full activity. Weight loss results have been comparable with open operation. Additionally, 98 of 101 comorbidities were relieved in their series. These early data suggest that laparoscopic RYGB is a suitable alternative to the open operation.

Patient positioning and port placement is as for other gastric procedures. The dissection starts at the fundus of the stomach with division of the phrenicogastric ligament. The fundus is mobilized in an inferior direction by blunt dissection. On the anterior wall of the stomach, an electrocautery mark is made 4 to 5 cm distal to the angle of His to serve as a landmark for the size of the gastric pouch. The lesser omentum is then opened adjacent to the mark at 4 to 5 cm inside the nerve of Laterjet. Dissection is carried through the lesser sac to an opening near the angle of His. The medial subcostal port is changed to an 18-mm port and a straight four-row cutting 60-mm stapler is used to divide the stomach. A standard 60-mm Roux limb is fashioned by dividing the proximal jejunum with a 60-mm linear stapler. The limb is brought up in a retrocolic, retrogastric path to the small (15 mL) proximal gastric pouch. A circular stapler is used for the gastrojejunostomy. The anvil is inserted via the oral cavity by endoscopy and using a percutaneous pull wire technique. An anastamosis is fashioned by connecting the anvil to the stapler introduced through the 18-mm port. A stapled side-to-side enteroenterostomy is then done to restore gastrointestinal continuity.

Laparoscopic adjustable gastric banding

An alternative gastric restrictive operation is the adjustable silicone gastric banding (ASGB) procedure. ASGB was first introduced for placement through laparotomy by Kuzmak [55] in 1986. This operation has the advantage of being the least invasive operation as it is completely reversible and allows for adjustment of the gastric pouch outlet. When compared with VBG, the ASGB placed by laparotomy produced comparable weight loss in one series of 149 patients [67]. Eighty-three patients underwent VBG and 66 underwent ASGB. The preoperative mean BMI was 45 kg/m^2 in the VBG group versus 42 kg/m^2 in the ASGB group. At 6 months, the mean BMI in both groups was 32 kg/m^2. The band has been modified for laparoscopic placement (Lap Band; Bioenterics Corporation, Carpinteria, CA) and there are now several series in the literature [68,69]. Mean operative time for placement is 2 to 2.5 hours. Conversion rates are approximately 5%. A large omentum and left hepatic lobe hypertrophy are the main technical difficulties. Recovery is comparable with a laparoscopic cholecystectomy. Patients are able to take liquids several hours after the operation. Hospital stay is 1 to 2 days, and return to normal activity occurs within 7 to 10 days. Results of laparoscopic placement are comparable to the open procedure; however, the follow-up has been short to date. In one series of 30 patients, percent excess weight loss was 41.9% at 6 months and 70.6% at 12 months, however, there were only four patients at 1 year [69]. Another series of 283 patients from France revealed 43% excess weight loss at 6 months and 59% at 1 year. Again, only 18 patients were evaluated at 1 year. Pooled results from 10 surgical centers in Belgium involving 795 patients revealed mean excess weight loss of 60% [70]. Early complications are rare and include gastric perforation (< 1%) and access port leakage, infection, and rotation (4%) [70–74]. Delayed complications include band slippage (5%) and upper gastric pouch dilatation (5%) [70–74]. These complications can be minimized by reducing pouch size to 15 cc, positioning the band above the omental bursa, and placing at least four gastrogastric sutures to fix the band into position [71–73]. The laparoscopic ASGB is currently undergoing a multicenter Food and Drug Administration–moderated trial in North America [75].

The main steps of laparoscopic ASGB are as follows. The patient is placed in a lithotomy position and in reverse Trendelenburg as for most gastric operations. A total of six ports are placed. The liver retractor is placed through a right subcostal one, the camera (0°) is inserted through a subxiphoid positioned port. The main operating ports are in the right and left paramedian positions. The assistant uses a left subcostal and an epigastric port. The left paramedian port is 15 mm for introduction of the band device. All of the other ports are 10 mm.

A gastric calibration tube is placed via the mouth into the stomach. The balloon is inflated to 15 cc and pulled up through the gastroesophageal junction. A site on the lesser curve is chosen to begin dissection that corresponds to the widest circumference of the balloon. The balloon is deflated and the tube withdrawn into the esophagus. A retrogastric tunnel is then created using blunt dissection, staying close to the gastric wall. The posterior gastric wall should be easily recognized to prevent injury. Next, a small opening in the phrenogastric ligament is made with electrocautery. A grasping instrument is then placed through the retrogastric tunnel. The band is then introduced into the abdomen and grasped with the instrument. The band is pulled into position around the stomach. The calibration tube is then reinserted into the proper position and the band closed around the tube. The calibration tube allows for proper stoma calibration. At least four sutures are then placed in the seromuscular layer of the stomach just proximal and distal to the band to keep it in the proper position. The injection port is then connected to the band tubing and implanted into the left rectus sheath at the paramedian port site.

Bariatric surgery: conclusions

Obesity is a major national health crisis. It is clear that morbidly obese patients suffer from significant comorbidity and die at a younger age than healthy weight individuals. Weight loss to, and maintenance of normal weight corrects the majority of weight-related morbidity and returns life expectancy to that of the general population. Morbidly obese patients are at an increased risk of significant morbidity and mortality with operation. However, strict attention to detail allows for proper selection of patients for surgery with reduction in the perioperative risk. The most common operative approaches are either gastric restriction or gastric restriction along with induction of the dumping syndrome. Current techniques allow the laparoscopic surgeon to apply the VBG or the RYGB to the obese patient. The newer laparoscopic gastric banding procedure appears to result in favorable outcomes, however, long-term data are needed before the technique can be universally advocated.

REFERENCES AND RECOMMENDED READING

Recently published papers of particular interest have been highlighted as:

- • Of interest
- •• Of outstanding interest

1. Hunt RH: Peptic ulcer disease: defining the treatment strategies in the era of *Helicobacter pylori*. *Am J Gastroenterol* 1997, 92 (4 suppl):36s–40s.

2. Huang JQ, Hunt RH: Review: eradication of *Helicobacter pylori*: problems and recommendations. *J Gastroenterol Hepatol* 1997, 12(8):590–598.

3. Peek RM, Blaser MJ: Pathophysiology of *Helicobacter pylori*-induced gastritis and peptic ulcer disease. *Am J Med* 1997, 102(2):200–207.

4. Donahue PE, Griffith C, Richter HM: A 50-year perspective upon selective gastric vagotomy. *Am J Surg* 1996, 172(1):9–12.

5. Jordan PH, Thornby J: Twenty years after parietal cell vagotomy or selective vagotomy antrectomy for treatement of duodenal ulcer: final report. *Ann Surg* 1994, 220(3):283–293.

6. Laws HL, McKernan JB: Endoscopic management of peptic ulcer disease. *Ann Surg* 1993, 217(5):548–555.

7.•• Awad W, Csendes A, Braghetto I, *et al*: Laparoscopic highly selective vagotomy: technical considerations and preliminary results in 119 patients with duodenal ulcer or gastroesophageal reflux disease. *World J Surg* 1997, 21(3):261–268.
The most extensive study on laparoscopic highly selective vagotomy to date.

8.•• Trus TL, Hunter JG: Minimally invasive surgery of the esophagus and stomach. *Am J Surg* 1997, 173:242–255.
A good overview article on minimally invasive surgery of the esophagus and stomach.

9. Casa AT, Gadacz TR: Laparoscopic management of peptic ulcer disease. *Surg Clin North Am* 1996, 76(3):515–522.

10. Cadiere GB, Himpens J, Bruyns J: Laparoscopic proximal gastric vagotomy. *Endosc Surg Allied Technol* 1994, 2(2):105–108.

11. Katkhouda N, Heimbucher J, Mouiel J: Laparoscopic posterior vagotomy and anterior seromyotomy. *Endosc Surg* 1994, 2:95–99.

12. Gomez-Ferrer F, Balique JG, Azagra S, *et al*: Laparoscopic surgery for duodenal ulcer: first results of a multicenter study applying a personal procedure. *Br J Surg* 1996, 83(4):547–550.

13. Katkhouda N, Mouiel J: Laparoscopic treatment of peptic ulcer disease. In *Minimal Invasive Surgery*. Edited by Hunter J, Sackier J. New York: McGraw Hill; 1993:123–130.

14. Kathoulda N, Mouiel J: Laparoscopic treatment of peptic ulcer disease. In *Current Techniques in Laparoscopy*. Edited by Brooks DC. Philadelphia: Current Medicine; 1994:9.1–9.9.

15. Bailey RW, Flowers JL, Graham SM, *et al*: Combined laparoscopic cholecystectomy and selective vagotomy. *Surg Laparosc Endosc* 1991, 1:45–49.

16. Siu WT, Leong HT, Li MK: Single stitch laparoscopic omental patch repair of perforated peptic ulcer. *J R Coll Surg Edinb* 1997, 42(2):92–94.

17. Matsuda M, Nishiyama M, Hanai T, *et al*: Laparoscopic omental patch repair for perforated peptic ulcer. *Ann Surg* 1995, 221(3):236–240.

18. Champagne LP, O'Leary JP: Laparoendoscopic approach to perforated peptic ulcer: case report and discussion. *Am Surg* 1996, 62(12):1003–1006.

19. Wyman A, Stuart RC, Ng EK, *et al*: Laparoscopic truncal vagotomy and gastroenterostomy for pyloric stenosis. *Am J Surg* 1996, 171(6):600–603.

20. Frantzides CT, Carlson MA: Laparoscopic jaboulay gastroduodenostomy for gastric outlet obstruction: a case report. *J Laparoendosc Surg* 1996, 6(5):341–344.

21. Potvin M, Gagner M, Pomp A: Laparoscopic transgastric suturing for bleeding peptic ulcers. *Surg Endosc* 1996, 10(4):400–402.

22. Bloechle C, Emmerman A, Strate T, *et al*: Laparoscopic versus conventional suture and abdominal lavage in stomach perforation with peritonitis of various durations. *Langenbecks Arch Chir Suppl Kongressbd* 1997, 114:813–819.

23. Goh PM, Alponat A, Mak K, Kum CK: Early international results of laparoscopic gastrectomies. *Surg Endosc* 1997, 11:650–652.

24. Taniguchi E, Kamiike W, Yamanishi H, *et al*: Laparoscopic intragastric surgery for gastric leiomyoma. *Surg Endosc* 1997, 11(3):287–289.

25. Ibrahim IM, Silvestri F, Zingler B: Laparoscopic resection of posterior gastric leiomyoma. *Surg Endosc* 1997, 11(3):277–279.

26.•• Burke EC, Karpeh MS, Conlon KC, Brennan MF: Laparoscopy in the management of gastric adenocarcinoma. *Ann Surg* 1997, 225(3):262–267.
A definitive study on the relevance of laparoscopy in the management of gastric carcinoma.

27.• Lowy AM, Mansfield PF, Leach SD, Ajani J: Laparoscopic staging for gastric cancer. *Surg* 1996, 119(6):611–614.
An earlier study advocating the need for staging laparoscopy.

28. Anderson DN, Campbell S, Park KG: Accuracy of laparoscopic ultrasonography in the staging of upper gastrointestinal malignancy. *Br J Surg* 1996, 83(10):1424–1428.

29. Goh P, Tekant Y, Isaac J, *et al.*: The technique of laparoscopic Billroth II gastrectomy. *Surg Laparosc Endosc* 1992, 2:258–260.

30. Watson DI, Devitt PG, Game PA: Laparoscopic Billroth II gastrectomy for early gastric cancer. *Br J Surg* 1995, 6(4):239–244.

31. Naitoh T, Gagner M: Laparoscopically assisted gastric surgery using dexterity pneumo sleeve. *Surg Endosc* 1997, 11:830–833.

32.• Brune IB, Feussner H, Neuhaus H, *et al.*: Laparoscopic gastrojejunostomy and endoscopic biliary stent placement for palliation of incurable gastric outlet obstruction with cholestasis. *Surg Endosc* 1997, 11:834–837.
A study that shows promise for palliative laparoscopic bypass.

33. Stiegmann GV, Goff JS, Silas D, *et al.*: Endoscopic versus operative gastrostomy: final results of a prospective randomized trial. *Gastrointest Endosc* 1990, 36(1):1–5.

34. Peitgen K, Walz MK, Krause U, *et al.*: First results of laparoscopic gastrostomy. *Surg Endosc* 1997, 11:658–662.

35. Kuczmarski RJ, Flegal KM, Campbell SM, Johnson CL: Increasing prevalence of overweight among US adults. *JAMA* 1994, 272:205–211.

36. National Task Force on the Prevention and Treatment of Obesity: Long term pharmacotherapy in the management of obesity. *JAMA* 1996, 276:1907–1915.

37. Rosenbaum M, Leibel RL, Hirsch J: Obesity. *N Engl J Med* 1997, 337:396–407.

38. Stunkard AJ: Current views on obesity. *Am J Med* 1996, 100:230–236.

39. Bray GA: Pathophysiology of obesity. *Am J Clin Nutr* 1992, 55:488S–494S.

40. NIH Technology Assessment Conference Panel: Consensus Development Conference: Methods for voluntary weight loss and control. *Ann Intern Med* 1993, 119:764–770.

41. Hubbard VS, Hall WH: National Institutes of Health Consensus Development Conference Draft Statement on Gastrointestinal Surgery for Severe Obesity, 25-27 March 1991. *Obesity Surg* 1991, 1:257–265.

42. Seidell JC, Andres R, Sorkin JD, Muller DC: The sagittal waist diameter and mortality in men: the Baltimore longitudinal study on aging. *Int J Obesity* 1994, 18:61–67.

43. Kvist H, Chowdhury B, Grangard U, *et al.*: Total and visceral adipose-tissue volumes derived from measurements with computed tomography in adult men and women: predictive equations. *Am J Clin Nutr* 1988, 48:1351.

44. Sjostrom LV: Morbidity of severely obese subjects. *Am J Clin Nutr* 1992, 55:508S–515S.

45. Sjostrom LV: Mortality of severely obese subjects. *Am J Clin Nutr* 1992, 55:516S–523S.

46. Balsiger BM, Luque-De Leon E, Sarr MG: Surgical treatment of obesity: who is an appropriate candidate? *Mayo Clin Proc* 1997, 72:551–558.

47. Sugerman HJ: Obesity. In *Care of the Surgical Patient.* Edited by Wilmore DW, Brennan MF, Harken AH, *et al.* New York: Scientific American; 1994:4-1–4-13.

48. Strohl KP, Redline S: Recognition of obstructive sleep apnea. *Am J Resp Crit Care Med* 1996, 154:279–289.

49. Young T, Palta M, Dempsey J, *et al.*: The occurrence of sleep disordered breathing among middle-aged adults. *N Engl J Med* 1993, 328:1230.

50. Douglas NJ, Thomas S, Jan MA: Clinical value of polysomnography. *Lancet* 1992, 339:347–350.

51. Pack AI: Simplifying the diagnosis of obstructive sleep apnea. *Ann Intern Med* 1993, 119:528–529.

52. Greenfield LJ, Scher LA, Elkins RC: KMA-Greenfield filter placement for chronic pulmonary hypertension. *Ann Surg* 1979, 189:560.

53. Mason EE: Gastric surgery for morbid obesity. *Surg Clin North Am* 1992, 72:501–513.

54. MacLean LD, Rhode BM, Samplais J, Forse RA: Results of the surgical treatment of obesity. *Am J Surg* 1993, 165:155–162.

55. Kuzmak LI: Gastric banding. In *Surgery for the Morbidly Obese Patient.* Edited by Deitei M. Philiadelphia: Lea & Febiger; 1989:225–259.

56. Sugerman HJ, Starkey JV, Birkenhauer R: A randomized, prospective trial of gastric bypass vs. vertical banded gastroplasty for morbid obesity and their effects on sweets vs. non-sweets eaters. *Ann Surg* 1987, 205:613–624.

57. Hall JC, Watts JM, Dunstan RE, *et al.*: Gastric surgery for morbid obesity. *Ann Surg* 1990, 311:419–427.

58. Brolin RE, Robertson LB, Kenier HA, Cody RP: Weight loss and dietary intake after vertical banded gastroplasty and Roux-en-Y gastric bypass. *Ann Surg* 1994, 220:782–790.

59. Brolin RE, Gorman JH, Gorman RC, *et al.*: Iron deficiency and anemia after Roux-en-Y gastric bypass: a prospective outcome study. *Obesity Surg* 1997, 7:101A.

60. Sugerman HJ, Kellum JM, Reines HD, *et al.*: Greater risk of incisional hernia with morbidly obese than steroid dependent patients and low recurrence with prefascial polypropylene mesh. *Am J Surg* 1996, 171:80–84.

61. Pories WJ, Swanson MS, MacDonald KG, *et al.*: Who would have thought it? An operation proves to be the most effective therapy for adult onset diabetes mellitus. *Ann Surg* 1995, 222:339–352.

62. Kral JG, Sjostrom LV, Sullivan MBE: Assessment of quality of life before and after surgery for severe obesity. *Am J Clin Nutr* 1992, 55:611S–614S.

63. Chua TY, Mendiola RM: Laparoscopic vertical banded gastroplasty: the Milwaukee experience. *Obesity Surg* 1995, 5:77–80.

64. Lonroth H, Dalenback J, Haglind JK, *et al.*: Vertical banded gastroplasty by laparoscopic technique in the treatment of morbid obesity. *Surg Lap Endosc* 1996, 6:102–107.

65. Catona A, Gossenberg M, Mussini G, *et al.*: Videolaparoscopic vertical banded gastroplasty. *Obesity Surg* 1995, 5:323–326.

66. Wittgrove AC, Clark GW: Laparoscopic gastric bypass, Roux-en-Y: experience of 27 cases, with 3-18 months follow-up. *Obesity Surg* 1996, 6:54–57.

67. Belachew M, Jacquet P, Lardinois F, Karler C: Vertical banded gastroplasty vs. adjustable silicone gastric banding in the treatment of morbid obesity: a preliminary report. *Obesity Surg* 1993, 3:275–278.

68. Belachew M, Legrand MJ, Defechereux TH, *et al.*: Laparoscopic adjustable silicone gastric banding in the treatment of morbid obesity. *Surg Endosc* 1994, 8:1354–1356.

69. Favretti F, Cadiere GB, Segato G, *et al.*: Laparoscopic adjustable silicone gastric banding: technique and results. *Obesity Surg* 1995, 5:364–371.

70. Belva P, Takieddine M, Lefebvre JC, Vaneukem P: Laparoscopic gastric banding with Lap-Band, results and complications (Belgium and European data). XI International Symposium on Obesity Surgery and The II Congress of the International Federation for the Surgery of Obesity. *Obesity Surg* 1997, 7:298A.

71. Belachew M: Management of complications of laparoscopic adjustable gastric banding (LAGB). XI International Symposium on Obesity Surgery and The II Congress of the International Federation for the Surgery of Obesity. *Obesity Surg* 1997, 7:304A.

72. Belachew M: An initially small pouch and more gastrogastric sutures will reduce the rate of pouch dilatation and/or stomach slippage after laparoscopic adjustable gastric banding. *Obesity Surg* 1997, 7:110A.

73. Favretti F, Cadiere GB, Segato G, *et al.*: Laparoscopic adjustable gastric banding (LapBand): how to avoid complications. *Obesity Surg* 1997, 7:110A.

74. Chelala E, Cadiere GB, Favretti F: Conversions and complications in 185 laparoscopic adjustable silicone gastric banding cases. *Surg Endosc* 1997, 11:268–271.

75. Wittgrove AC, Greenstein R, Martin L, *et al.*: Multicenter study of laparoscopic gastric band: 100 patients with 3 to 18 month follow-up. *Surg Endosc* 1997, 11:177A.

Endoscopic Parathyroid and Thyroid Surgery

L. Michael Brunt

General surgery has undergone a revolutionary change in the past several years due to the widespread introduction of laparoscopic surgery into clinical practice. Many open abdominal operations have now been largely replaced by laparoscopic procedures, which result in less morbidity and postoperative pain, produce less scarring, and lead to a faster recovery [1]. Because of this change, surgeons have been seeking less invasive or minimally invasive methods for performing a variety of procedures, either by endoscopic techniques or with smaller open incisions. In the field of endocrine surgery, laparoscopic adrenalectomy has already supplanted open adrenalectomy at many institutions [2–5], and laparoscopic techniques have been used in patients with pancreatic islet cell tumors [6].

One of the newest frontiers is in minimally invasive soft tissue surgery performed outside an established body cavity. The neck has been one of the soft tissue spaces of considerable interest, and endoscopic or endoscopic-assisted techniques have recently been used to perform both thyroidectomy and parathyroidectomy in humans. Several technical advances have facilitated the development of these new procedures, including the availability of balloon space makers, external lifts, ultrasonic coagulators, and smaller 2- to 3-mm diameter endoscopic instrumentation. This chapter describes some of these recent developments and highlights the possibilities that endoscopic surgery in closed or virtual soft tissue spaces may hold.

BACKGROUND

Thyroidectomy and parathyroidectomy are the two most commonly performed endocrine surgical procedures. The most frequent indication for thyroidectomy is a solitary nodule that is not clearly benign on fine-needle biopsy. Parathyroidectomy is most commonly performed for primary hyperparathyroidism, in which a single enlarged gland or adenoma accounts for 85% or more of cases. The principles of neck exploration for these two disorders are well established, and the morbidity of operation is low when carried out by an experienced surgeon. Unlike many open abdominal operations, recovery is also rapid and most patients are discharged from the hospital the day after surgery and return to unlimited physical activity within 10 to 14 days. However, surgical neck exploration as currently performed leaves patients with a readily visible scar that may be exaggerated by tissue injury from dissecting the neck flaps, and it is still an invasive procedure with associated risks, discomfort, and complications. Moreover, little has changed technically in thyroid and parathyroid surgery in the past three decades despite numerous technologic advances and an embracement of minimally invasive surgical approaches for a variety of disease processes affecting other organ systems.

The question that must be addressed is whether a need exists for any improvement in current surgical methods for treating patients with these conditions. Already many surgeons are attempting to perform thyroidectomy and parathyroidectomy through smaller and smaller open incisions to achieve better cosmetic results. However, as open

CHAPTER

12

incisions become smaller, surgical exposure, access, ease of dissection, and even safety may be compromised. Further evidence that parathyroidectomy, for example, is viewed as an invasive procedure by patients and by referring endocrinologists is the reluctance of many individuals with asymptomatic or minimally symptomatic disease to undergo a definitive and curative operation despite the cumulative risks of hyperparathyroidism over time, including osteoporosis and other metabolic sequelae.

In parathyroid surgery, there has also been renewed interest in a focused, unilateral exploration of the neck rather than the accepted gold standard of bilateral neck exploration with identification and biopsy of all four parathyroids. Exploration of both sides of the neck avoids the problem of missed multiple adenomas or asymmetric hyperplasia, which can occur in up to 5% to 15% of cases [7] and eliminates the need for preoperative localization studies. However, the advantages of unilateral neck exploration are that it results in less dissection, operative times are shorter, and costs may be lower [8–10,11•]. There may also be fewer injuries to the recurrent laryngeal nerve and the other parathyroid glands from leaving the contralateral neck undisturbed. Improvements in the accuracy of parathyroid imaging, such as ^{99m}Tc sestamibi scanning [10,11•,12] and intraoperative assessment of curative resection with the quick parathyroid hormone assay [8] have led to better outcomes from and wider application of the unilateral approach. These considerations become increasingly important in the current economic environment in health care.

Under these circumstances, an endoscopic or endoscopic-assisted approach to neck exploration may offer certain possible benefits, including improved visualization due to optical magnification, better cosmesis, less trauma to the neck musculature, less pain, and a more rapid recovery. Potential disadvantages of this approach might include longer operative times, increased hospital costs, possible risk of injury to the recurrent laryngeal nerve, potential tumor spillage, inability to localize the parathyroids, and adverse effects of neck insufflation. Consideration of an endoscopic approach to neck exploration, at the least, presents several challenges from an anatomic standpoint. Unlike the abdominal cavity, in which there is an easily distensible space for laparoscopy, the area that must be expanded and maintained to allow endoscopic access in the neck is composed of only potential spaces between soft tissue and muscle planes and the trachea. The thyroid and parathyroid glands are situated within the pretracheal space and are covered by the strap muscles anteriorly and laterally, which also limits exposure and access. The absence of a discrete anatomic compartmental boundary in the neck may pose further problems if insufflation with CO_2 gas is used because of the potential for gaseous diffusion subcutaneously and into the mediastinum. The thyroid and parathyroids are also highly vascular structures and are intimately related to the recurrent laryngeal nerve and inferior thyroid artery. Further, the location of the parathyroids, especially the inferior glands, is often variable.

Because of these demanding technical features, several technologic advances have been necessary to facilitate the development of endoscopic neck exploration. Miniature 2- to 3-mm endoscopic instruments have been constructed that are more suitable for smaller working spaces and the more delicate structures in the neck. Balloon space maker devices, first used in laparoscopic hernia repair, could be adapted to create a working space. Gasless laparoscopy has been used with mechanical lifts and retractors to maintain the working space and thus eliminate the need for insufflation of the neck. Ultrasonic coagulators and small clip appliers may be more appropriate for obtaining hemostasis in the neck rather than monopolar cautery. Laparoscopic ultrasound could also aid in intraoperative localization of the parathyroid adenoma, which is localized preoperatively by sestamibi scanning. These considerations led our group to first explore the possibility of an endoscopic approach to neck exploration in an experimental animal model [13•].

EXPERIMENTAL DEVELOPMENT

A canine model was chosen for the development of endoscopic neck exploration experimentally because dogs have four parathyroids of relatively constant location [14]. The two external parathyroid glands are found at the superior-lateral aspect of the thyroid, and the internal parathyroids are small (2 to 3 mm) glands that are partially embedded within the medial surface of the thyroid. Dogs also have an elongated neck with elastic soft tissue that should simplify the logistics of surgical exposure. Initial access to the neck was obtained with a 2-cm transverse incision placed at the sternal notch. The pretracheal space was then entered under direct vision by dividing the strap muscles in the midline. A balloon space maker device (General Surgical Innovations Inc., Cupertino, CA) was inserted into the pretracheal space and was inflated to 300-mL volume with saline in order to expand this working space (Fig. 12-1).

Both CO_2 insufflation and mechanical lifts were evaluated as methods to expose and maintain this space for the endoscopic dissection. The use of CO_2 insufflation at 15 mm Hg^{2+} insufflation pressure in one of our early experiments resulted in extensive subcutaneous emphysema in the neck and upper chest and bilateral pneumothoraces. An experiment was carried out subsequently in a porcine model in which the effects of increasing CO_2 insufflation pressure in the neck were evaluated hemody-

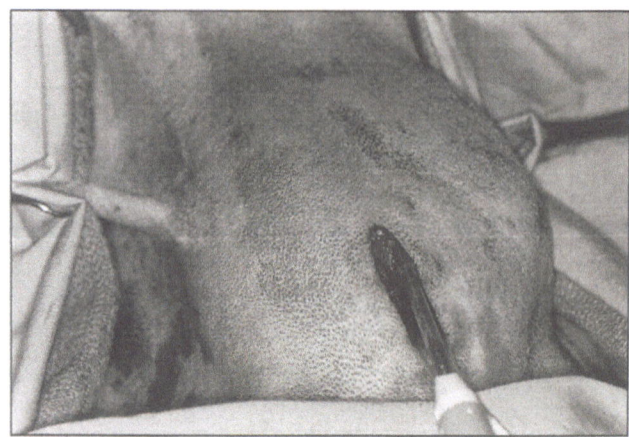

Figure 12-1 Expansion of the pretracheal space in a canine experimental model. A modified hernia balloon filled with saline is used to expand this space. (*From* Brunt *et al.* [13•]; with permission.).

namically and radiographically. Carbon dioxide insufflation was titrated at 3-mm Hg pressure increments from 0 to 20 mm Hg^{2+}. Oxygen saturation and ventilatory pressures were stable throughout the procedure. However, beginning at 9 to 12 mm Hg^{2+} insufflation pressure, pneumomediastinum was observed radiographically (Fig. 12-2), and at 15 and 20 mm Hg^{2+} pressure, both pneumomediastinum and subcutaneous emphysema in the neck were present. Although no adverse effects were noted at lower insufflation pressures, the results of these experiments together with the likely need for prolonged periods of insufflation during neck exploration in humans, led us to focus exclusively on techniques for gasless retraction.

A mechanical lift device consisting of a coiled metal ring attached to a lift bar was used to elevate the neck soft tissues. This device was inserted beneath the strap muscles in the pretracheal space and provided adequate surgical access to both sides of the neck. Endoscopic visualization was achieved with a 5-mm–angled 30° laparoscope inserted at the access site for the lift ring. Endoscopic 5- to 7-mm ports or trocar threads were then inserted under direct endoscopic vision into the lateral neck anterior to the sternocleidomastoid muscle on either side. Endoscopic dissection was carried out with pediatric 5-mm dissecting instruments and graspers. The initial endoscopic view of the expanded pretracheal space can be seen in Figure 12-3. Anatomic structures visualized endoscopically included the right and left thyroid lobes, external and internal parathyroids, laryngeal nerves, carotid artery, and jugular vein. A variety of methods of hemostasis were evaluated for endoscopic excision of the parathyroids and for thyroid lobectomy. Monopolar cautery was effective in controlling bleeding, but resulted in repetitive visual impairment due to smoke generation and fogging of the endoscope lens within this small space. Ultrasonic coagulation with the Harmonic scalpel (Ultracision; Ethicon Endosurgery Inc., Cincinnati, OH) produced some aerosolization but resulted in less fogging and better visualization and provided adequate hemostasis for parathyroidectomy. Endoscopic 5-mm clips were necessary for hemostasis involving the major thyroid arteries.

After the initial technical development phase, two sets of experiments were performed to evaluate the efficacy and safety of this technique [13•]. Four-gland parathyroidectomy was attempted in three dogs. The procedure was completed in an average of 136 ± 8.5 minutes without complications. Ten of 12 parathyroids were excised endoscopically, but two small internal parathyroids were not found in one animal. We next carried out a long-term survival study of endoscopic bilateral neck exploration and two gland external parathyroidectomy in six dogs. In one animal the procedure was unsuccessful because of an oversized mechanical lift device that resulted in inadequate exposure. Two-gland parathyroidectomy was successfully completed in each of the remaining five animals in an average of 130 minutes. There were no intraoperative complications, serum calcium levels were stable over 1 week of observation, and parathyroid tissue was identified histologically in all resected specimens. At autopsy, approximately 20 mL of seroma fluid was present in the pretracheal space of these animals and the vagus and laryngeal nerves and other structures were uninjured. In a series of related experiments, videoscopic thyroidectomy has also been successfully carried out in this canine model (Brunt, Unpublished data).

Experimental studies to evaluate the feasibility of endoscopic neck exploration have been reported by others as well. Gagner and Breton [15] performed endoscopic parathyroidectomy and thyroidectomy in a porcine model. Initial access to the neck was accomplished by insufflating the subplatysmal space with CO_2 at 30-mm Hg^{2+} insufflation pressure. Exposure was maintained with CO_2 throughout the procedure and the dissection was carried out with laparoscopic scissors. Access to the mediastinum for performing other procedures was possible as well. Norman and Albrink [16] recently evaluated videoscopic techniques for parathyroidectomy and thyroidectomy in dogs. The primary method of exposure was with CO_2 insufflation at 15 to 18 mm Hg^{2+} pressure. However, CO_2 insufflation alone did not provide adequate exposure or maintain the working space, and a conventional thyroid retractor had to be placed through a 1.5-cm neck incision to retract the strap muscles. Blunt dissection and

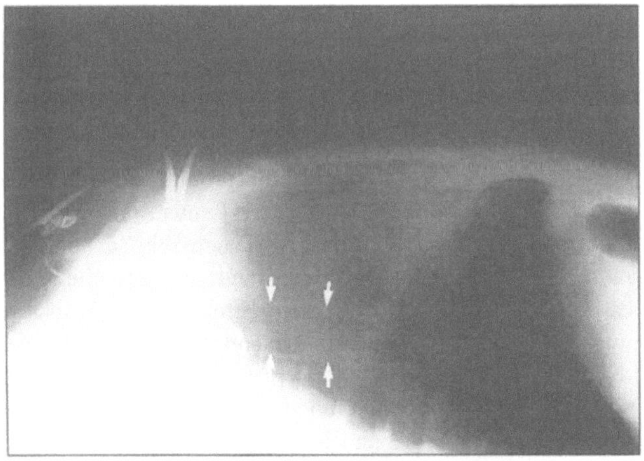

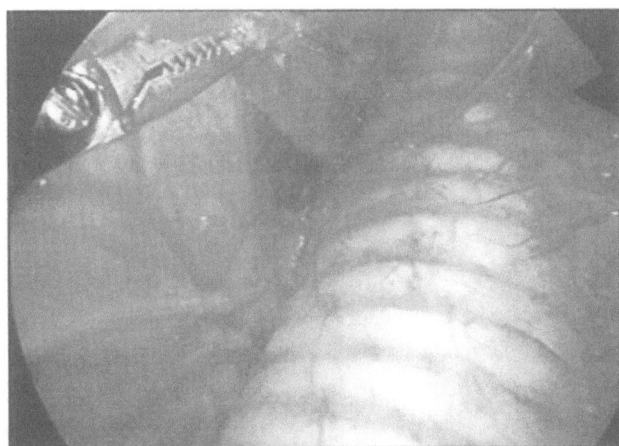

Figure 12-2 Pneumomediastinum following CO_2 insufflation of the pretracheal space (porcine model). A lateral chest radiograph shows extensive pneumomediastinum (*arrows*) at 15 mm Hg^{2+} insufflation pressure. (*From* Brunt *et al.* [13•]; with permission.)

Figure 12-3 Endoscopic view of the expanded pretracheal space in an experimental canine model. (*See* Color Plate.)

cautery were used for dissection and hemostasis. Insufflation was associated with mild to moderate degrees of subcutaneous emphysema in the neck and upper chest, but potential complications of pneumothorax and pneumomediastinum were not evaluated.

Prior to initiating clinical trials, we extended our experimental studies to human cadavers in order to prepare for some of the anticipated differences in neck anatomy. Some technical modifications were necessary because of these anatomic differences and the greater rigidity of human tissues. A smaller lift ring was used because of less flexibility in retracting the strap muscles. Medial retraction of the thyroid lobes, which was accomplished easily in the dog, required placement of a conventional Babcock clamp inserted via the open midline access site. Two 5-mm lateral ports were placed on each side of the neck, and pediatric dissecting instruments were used because these studies were carried out prior to the availability of 2- to 3-mm instrumentation. In five human cadavers undergoing endoscopic neck exploration, an attempt was made to identify and remove all four parathyroids. Operative time ranged from 45 to 135 minutes. All four glands were identified and removed endoscopically in two cases. In one case, three parathyroids were excised but the left superior gland was missed and in another case three glands were removed endoscopically but a fourth gland could not be found, even at open exploration. Only two upper glands were found in one case in which both inferior parathyroids had been displaced laterally, apparently from the initial balloon dissection of the pretracheal space. The endoscopic view of both the superior and inferior glands in one cadaver is shown in Figure 12-4 .

CLINICAL APPLICATION
Endoscopic parathyroidectomy
Endoscopic parathyroidectomy in humans was first performed successfully by Gagner [17] in 1995. The patient had familial hyperparathyroidism and initially presented with acute pancreatitis for which he required laparoscopic pancreaticojejunostomy with stone extraction as well as laparoscopic cholecystectomy. A preoperative sestamibi scan showed four-gland uptake

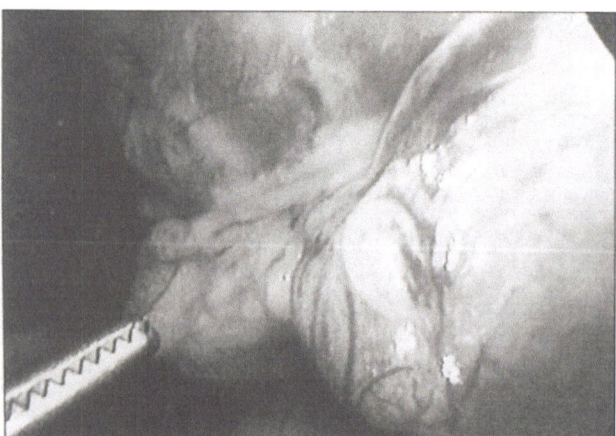

Figure 12-4 Endoscopic view of normal superior and inferior parathyroid glands in a human cadaver. (*See* Color Plate.) (*From* Brunt *et al.* [13•]; with permission.)

consistent with generalized parathyroid hyperplasia, and a subtotal (3.5-gland) parathyroidectomy was performed endoscopically. Access to the neck was obtained with four 5-mm ports placed 1 cm above the clavicle and sternal notch. Exposure was achieved by insufflation of the subplatysmal space with 15 mm Hg^{2+} pressure, which was maintained throughout the operation. Operative time was 5 hours and intraoperatively the patient experienced tachycardia and hypercarbia. Postoperatively, he had subcutaneous emphysema from the eyelids to the scrotum. He recovered uneventfully, however, and was discharged on the fourth postoperative day with a normal serum calcium level.

Since this initial report, endoscopic parathyroidectomy has been carried out by a small number of surgeons using either low-level gas insufflation of the neck or external retractors without CO_2 gas. Gagner (Personal communication) has excised parathyroid adenomas in several cases, but uses a lower CO_2 insufflation pressure (7 to 10 mm Hg^{2+}) to reduce the adverse effects of this technique. Duluq (Paper presented at the First International Conference of Endocrine Tele-Surgery, Strasbourg, France, 1997) has also successfully performed endoscopic parathyroidectomy in several patients with low-level (7 mm Hg^{2+}) CO_2 insufflation for exposure, but published details regarding these cases are lacking. Norman and Albrink [16] attempted parathyroidectomy in four patients after preoperative localization with sestamibi imaging. Initial access to the pretracheal space was achieved via a 1.5-cm incision, but CO_2 at a low insufflation pressure (8 mm Hg^{2+}) was used to maintain a working space. Although the parathyroid adenoma was visualized in three of the four cases, endoscopic excision was successful in only two patients, and only one normal parathyroid was identified out of these four explorations. At the conclusion of the endoscopic procedure, all patients were converted to open exploration via a 3.5-cm incision, through which the ipsilateral remaining parathyroids, both normal and adenomatous, were identified and either biopsied or removed. Postoperatively, there was subcutaneous air in the anterior neck, but no other sequela of CO_2 insufflation were noted.

We recently performed endoscopic parathyroidectomy in two patients with primary hyperparathyroidism using a gasless technique. Preoperative localization of the parathyroid adenoma was carried out with ^{99m}Tc sestamibi scanning, which identified abnormal uptake in the left neck of both patients. Patients consented for endoscopic parathyroidectomy under an investigational protocol approved by the Human Studies Committee at the Washington University Medical Center. Following the induction of general anesthesia, the parathyroid adenoma was more precisely localized with transcutaneous ultrasound and in each case was posterior to the thyroid lobe. A 1.5-cm incision was then made at the sternal notch, and the strap muscles were divided in the midline to enter the pretracheal space under direct vision. In the first patient, a modified space maker balloon was inserted into this space and inflated to 60-mL volume. After removal of the balloon, a working space was maintained with a hand-held S-shaped retractor. The strap muscles were further separated from the left lobe of the thyroid and the thyroid was retracted medially with a Babcock clamp placed through the open insertion site. Endoscopic visualization was achieved with a 3-mm 30° arthroscope. Two 4-mm ports were placed in the left neck anterior to the sternocleidomastoid muscle.

A normal inferior parathyroid was identified and biopsied, and the adenoma was localized to the superior position with the aid of laparoscopic ultrasound. The enlarged gland was posterior to the thyroid lobe and wedged between two branches of the inferior thyroid artery and the recurrent laryngeal nerve, which led to a lengthy and tedious dissection. Excision was accomplished by blunt dissection with 3-mm endoscopic instruments and the ultrasonic scalpel. Small Ligaclips (Ethicon Inc., Somerville, NJ) placed through the open insertion site were used to ligate the vascular pedicle. The second patient was approached in a similar fashion, but a small lift ring attached to a mechanical retractor was used to maintain exposure (Fig. 12-5). A left superior adenoma was removed that weighed 1.7 g. The recurrent laryngeal nerve and inferior thyroid artery (Fig. 12-6) were identified during the dissection, but we were unable to locate the inferior parathyroid despite careful examination of the region of the thyrothymic ligament. Total operative time in our two patients has averaged approximately 4 hours. There are several reasons for the long operative times in our cases. To some extent this reflects the learning curve for this procedure. Exposure was suboptimal at times due to the small space, and there was difficulty in retracting the strap muscles laterally and the thyroid gland medially. Very small amounts of bleeding or fluid accumulation obscured the operative field and required frequent sponging through the open insertion site. Manipulation and retraction of the parathyroid with the small instruments was sometimes difficult as well. Nonetheless, both our patients did well and were discharged on the first postoperative day in good condition. Parathyroid tissue was confirmed in all specimens and serum calcium levels have been normal postoperatively.

Miccoli [18] used an endoscopic-assisted approach similar to ours in approximately 20 patients. Hand-held retractors are used to maintain exposure, and the dissection has been carried out with one or two lateral ports. A brief period of insufflation is used initially to aid in expanding the pretracheal space, but the remainder of the operation is carried out with gasless retraction. Preliminary results have been favorable, but not all patients have had a normal ipsilateral parathyroid identified. Confirmation of successful excision of the parathyroid adenoma was made intraoperatively with use of the quick parathyroid hormone assay.

Alternatives to endoscopic parathyroidectomy

Minimally invasive or less invasive approaches to parathyroidectomy have been described recently that do not require endoscopic techniques or instrumentation. Norman and Chheda [19••] performed parathyroidectomy through a minimal 2- to 3-cm open incision after precise preoperative localization of the adenoma with sestamibi imaging. The technique used for parathyroid localization is analogous to that used for sentinel node mapping with radiolymphoscintigraphy. ^{99m}Tc sestamibi scanning is carried out 3 hours prior to surgical exploration. The operation is then directed with an 11-mm Neoprobe (Neoprobe Corporation, Dublin, OH), which is used to scan and quantitate radioactivity in all four quadrants of the neck. A 2- to 3-cm incision is made over the site of maximal gamma activity, and the adenoma is excised through this minimal incision. The authors have used this technique in 14 patients, 13 of whom had adenomas and one who was correctly predicted to have parathyroid hyperplasia. The adenomas were located operatively on average in just 19 ± 1.6 minutes. Nine cases were carried out under local anesthesia, and 11 (79%) patients were discharged the same day as surgery. Serum calcium levels were normal postoperatively and there were no operative complications.

This approach is potentially very attractive because it requires minimal dissection and can be carried out under local anesthesia as strictly an outpatient procedure. Both operative and recovery times should be short, which may result in lower hospital costs despite the use of preoperative scintigraphic localization. Frozen section examination by pathology may also become

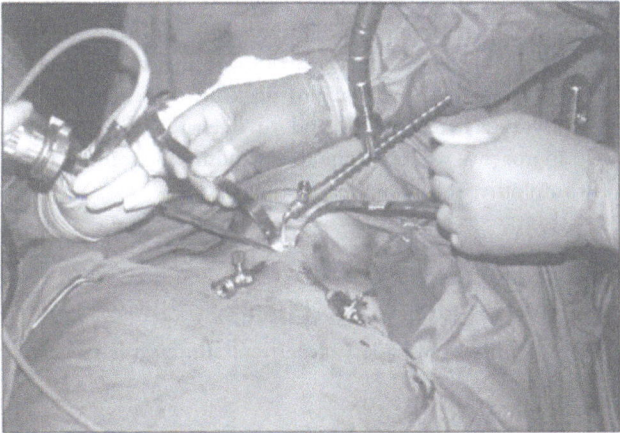

Figure 12-5 External view of the neck in a patient undergoing endoscopic parathyroidectomy. A lift ring attached to a flexible Bookwalter arm (Codman/Johnson & Johnson Professional Inc., Raynham, MA) is used to maintain the working space. Four-mm ports are placed above the clavicles and the endoscope is positioned at the open insertion site.

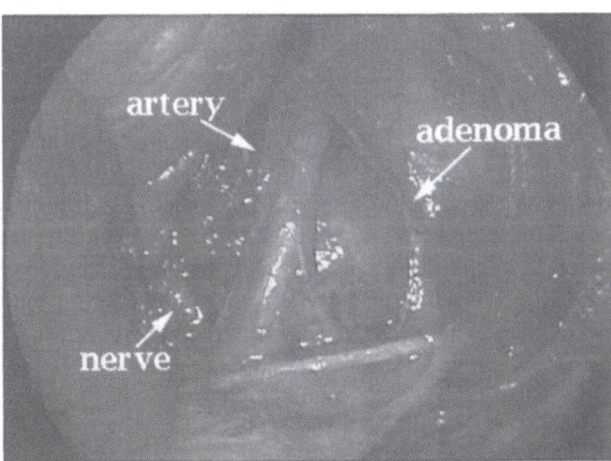

Figure 12-6 Endoscopic view of a left superior parathyroid adenoma. The recurrent laryngeal nerve courses to the left of the adenoma and the inferior thyroid artery overlies it. (*See* Color Plate.)

unnecessary if, after excision, all radioactivity is confined to the resected specimen. The limitations of this approach currently are that neither the ipsilateral parathyroid nor the recurrent laryngeal nerve have been routinely identified in these dissections. Further, the accuracy of "sentinel" mapping of the parathyroid adenoma must be confirmed by other investigators.

Thoracoscopic parathyroidectomy

Video-assisted thoracoscopy should be considered as an alternative to median sternotomy in patients with ectopic mediastinal parathyroid adenomas. Prinz and coworkers [20•] reported the use of thoracoscopic techniques to successfully excise mediastinal parathyroids in four patients with persistent hyperparathyroidism after failed cervical exploration. All glands were localized preoperatively by a combination of radionuclide scintigraphy and CT scans. The location of the abnormal glands in these four cases included the aortopulmonary window, near the ascending aorta, the aortic arch, and the region of the main pulmonary artery. Three thoracoscopic ports were used, including a 10-mm initial access port placed in the midaxillary line at the sixth intercostal space. Operative times averaged 3.25 hours and all patients became normocalcemic postoperatively, although one patient with secondary hyperparathyroidism developed recurrent hypercalcemia 9 months after surgery. A subxiphoid laparoscopic approach has also been used to excise a mediastinal parathyroid adenoma [21], but this technique would appear to provide access to glands in the anterior mediastinum only.

Endoscopic thyroidectomy

Clinical experience with endoscopic thyroidectomy has been very limited. Endoscopic excision of the thyroid is more technically demanding because of the more complex blood supply and the intimate relationship of the thyroid gland to the recurrent laryngeal nerve. Huscher and coworkers [22] recently reported successful endoscopic excision of the right thyroid lobe in a patient with a 4-mm nodule. A lateral approach was used in which three laparoscopic trocars were placed in the subplatysmal space along the anterior border of the sternocleidomastoid muscle from the jugular notch to the angle of the mandible. Both low-pressure CO_2 and a wall-lifter inserted at the jugular trocar site were used to maintain a working space. Division of the strap muscles was necessary to access the thyroid. The thyroid vessels were divided with clips, and an ultrasonic dissector was used to dissect the thyroid from the recurrent laryngeal nerve. In addition, both parathyroids were identified and preserved, as was the external branch of the superior laryngeal nerve. Operative time was 4.75 hours and the specimen was extracted through a 10-mm access site. The patient did well and was discharged on the second postoperative day. Pathologic examination showed a 3-mm papillary carcinoma with focal capsular invasion.

CONCLUSIONS

The limited early experience with endoscopic neck exploration prevents any definitive conclusions about its role in the management of patients with either hyperparathyroidism or thyroid disorders. Published experiences have to date been limited to small case reports, and results and outcomes have not been reported in detail. The minimally invasive open approach of "sentinel" parathyroidectomy reported by Norman and Chheda [19••] has much to commend it, including accurate localization, rapid operative times, and improved cosmesis, and it is an outpatient operation that can be performed under local anesthesia. From this brief review, it is apparent that considerable refinements in operative technique and instrumentation must yet occur if endoscopic neck exploration is to become applicable to significant numbers of patients. Although the laparoscope provides optical magnification of important neurovascular structures, including the recurrent laryngeal nerve, better methods for exposure and retraction of the strap muscles and thyroid would greatly facilitate visualization and dissection. Improved instruments are needed that allow safe manipulation of the parathyroid to lower the risk of parathyroid rupture as well as to speed the operative dissection. Suction and irrigation devices designed specifically for small spaces such as the neck would help maintain a dry operative field, which was problematic in our early cases because small amounts of fluid or blood obscure the anatomy. Surgeons will also need flexibility in the exposure and operative approach to deal successfully with variations in parathyroid anatomy.

Currently, endoscopic neck exploration should be considered experimental and should be limited to centers with expertise in both endocrine surgery and advanced laparoscopy. In addition, patients must be carefully selected for this approach until there is further experience and improved operative technique. Individuals who are obese, have a nodular goiter, have had previous neck surgery, or who are likely to have generalized parathyroid hyperplasia should not be considered for an endoscopic exploration. Despite these limitations and challenges, the search for less invasive means for performing neck exploration will undoubtedly continue, and has already led to renewed interest in a unilateral operative approach in patients with primary hyperparathyroidism. Cost concerns will continue to be an issue in this era of managed care and increasing fiscal constraints. Nonetheless, it remains difficult to predict the future based on today's technology, and it is likely that minimally invasive approaches will continue to expand not only into the neck but into other soft tissue spaces as well.

REFERENCES AND RECOMMENDED READING

Recently published papers of particular interest have been highlighted as:

• Of interest

•• Of outstanding interest

1. Soper NJ, Brunt LM, Kerbl K: Laparoscopic general surgery. *N Engl J Med* 1994, 330:409–419.

2. Duh Q-Y, Siperstein AE, Clark OH, *et al.*: Laparoscopic adrenalectomy: comparison of the lateral and posterior approaches. *Arch Surg* 1996, 131:870–876.

3.   Brunt LM, Doherty GM, Norton JA, *et al.*: Laparoscopic adrena-
     lectomy compared to open adrenalectomy for benign neoplasms.
     J Am Coll Surg 1996, 183:1–10.

4.   Gagner M, Lacroix A, Bolte E, Pomp A: Laparoscopic adrenalecto-
     my: the importance of a flank approach in the lateral position.
     Surg Endosc 1994, 8:135–138.

5.   Prinz RA: A comparison of laparoscopic and open adrenalec-
     tomies. *Arch Surg* 1995, 130:489–494.

6.   Gagner M, Pomp A, Herrera MF: Early experience with laparo-
     scopic resections of islet cell tumors. *Surgery* 1996,
     120:1051–1054.

7.   Habener JF, Potts JT, Jr.: Primary hyperparathyroidism. In
     Endocrinology, edn 2. Edited by DeGRoot LJ, Besser GM, Cahill
     GF, *et al.* Philadelphia: WB Saunders; 1989:954–966.

8.   Irvin GL, Prudhomme BS, Deriso GT, *et al.*: A new approach to
     parathyroidectomy. *Ann Surg* 1994, 219:574–581.

9.   Chapuis Y, Icard PH, Fulla Y, *et al.*: Parathyroid adenomectomy
     under local anesthesia with intraoperative monitoring of UcAMP
     and/or PTH. *World J Surg* 1992, 16:570–575.

10. Arkles LB, Jones T, Hicks RJ, *et al.*: Impact of complementary
     parathyroid scintigraphy and ultrasonography on the surgical
     management of hyperparathyroidism. *Surgery* 1996, 120:845–851.

11.• Wei JP, Burke GJ: Analysis of savings in operative time for prima-
     ry hyperparathyroidism using localization with technetium 99m
     sestamibi scan . *Am J Surg* 1995, 170:488–491.

This study evaluates the impact of localization studies on the surgical
treatment of patients with primary hyperparathyroidism. The authors
show that by using a strategy of preoperative localization based on scanning with ^{99m}Tc sestamibi, operative time for neck exploration can be
reduced by about 30 minutes. This study provides a framework for considering unilateral neck exploration in patients undergoing minimally
invasive or endoscopic approaches.

12. Johnston LB, Carroll MJ, Britton KE, *et al.*: The accuracy of
     parathyroid gland localization in primary hyperparathyroidism
     using sestamibi radionuclide imaging. *J Clin Endocrinol Metab*
     1996, 81:346–352.

13.• Brunt LM, Jones DB, Wu JS, *et al.*: Experimental development of
     an endoscopic approach to neck exploration and parathyroidecto-
     my. Surgery 1997, 122:893–901.

This paper describes experimental techniques developed in animals and
human cadavers for approaching neck exploration and parathyroidectomy endoscopically. The use of a gasless retraction system is described
that eliminates potential complications from using CO_2 insufflation
within the neck soft tissues.

14. Hullinger RL. The endocrine system. In *Miller's Anatomy of the
     Dog*, edn 2. Edited by Evans HE, Christensen GC. Philadelphia:
     WB Saunders; 1979:602–631.

15. Gagner M, Breton G: Endoscopic parathyroidectomy, thyroidecto-
     my, esophageal myotomy, and cervical lymph node dissection:
     technical aspects. *Surg Endosc* 1996, 10:230.

16. Norman J, Albrink MH: Minimally invasive parathyroidectomy: a
     feasibility study in dogs and humans. *J Laparoendosc Adv Surg Tech*
     1997, 7:301–306.

17. Gagner M: Endoscopic parathyroidectomy. *Br J Surg* 1996,
     83:875.

18. Miccoli P: Video-assisted parathyroidectomy. *J Endocrinol Invest*
     1997, 20:429–430.

19.•• Norman JG, Chheda H: Minimally invasive parathyroidectomy
     facilitated by intraoperative nuclear mapping. *Surgery* 1997,
     122:998–1004.

The authors describe a technique for minimally invasive parathyroidectomy performed through a 2- to 3-cm open incision after precise preoperative localization of the adenoma with sestamibi imaging. The
operation is directed by ^{99m}Tc sestamibi scanning and intraoperative
scanning with a Neoprobe. This operation can be carried out under
local anesthesia as an outpatient procedure with a short operative time.

20.• Prinz RA, Lonchyna V, Carnaille B, *et al.*: Thoracoscopic excision
     of enlarged mediastinal parathyroid glands. *Surgery* 1994,
     116:999–1005.

This paper provides the first description of thoracoscopic techniques
used to excise mediastinal parathyroids in four patients with persistent
hyperparathyroidism after failed cervical exploration.

21. Wei JP, Gadacz TR, Weisner LF, Burke GJ: The subxiphoid
     laparoscopic approach for resection of mediastinal parathyroid
     adenoma after successful localization with TC-99m-sestamibi
     radionuclide scan. *Surg Laparosc Endosc* 1995, 5:402–406.

22. Huscher CSG, Chiodini S, Napolitano C, Recher A: Endoscopic
     right thyroidectomy lobectomy. *Surg Endosc* 1997, 11:877.

Minimally Invasive Vascular Surgery

Takao Ohki
Frank J. Veith

During the past several decades, the operative mortality rate for elective repair of aortic aneurysms has markedly decreased, declining from 21% in surgical series carried out in the l950s to under 5% as reported in modern studies [1–5]. Lower extremity occlusive disease with ischemic tissue loss, which once mandated limb amputation, can now be treated with either interventional techniques or bypass surgery, resulting in favorable limb salvage rates [6]. Finally, despite advances in intensive care and resuscitation, severe, acute arterial injury from penetrating or blunt vascular trauma has remained a challenging problem, especially when central vascular injuries of the aortoiliac or subclavian arteries are involved [7–9].

Despite the improvements in the management of these vascular lesions, significant perioperative morbidity and mortality still occur in those cases with severe comorbid medical illnesses, scarring from previous operations, and multiorgan trauma [10–13]. In addition, even in a good-risk patient, standard vascular repair is not perfect and the quality of life following this treatment may be impaired because of postoperative pain, sexual dysfunction, and a lengthy hospital stay, resulting in high health care costs. All of these negative effects are related to the large incision and extensive tissue dissection required for access to the diseased area.

Endovascular grafting is an alternative treatment to standard open vascular repair. This procedure is a blend of intravascular stent and prosthetic graft technologies [14–17,18••,19,20,21•,22••,23–27,28•,29•,30,31•,32–35]. These devices may be inserted through remote arterial access sites to treat vascular lesions without the need to directly expose the diseased artery through an extensive incision or dissection. To date, endovascular grafts have been successfully used to treat aortic and peripheral artery aneurysms, long segment arterial occlusive disease, and vascular trauma.

This chapter describes some of the fundamental techniques and issues of endovascular grafting for aortoiliac occlusive disease and aneurysms. In addition, we describe some of the major endovascular graft types that are currently under investigation as well as strategies for their use.

REQUIRED EQUIPMENT AND OPERATING ROOM SET-UP

The vast majority of endovascular grafting procedures are currently performed in the operating room using a portable fluoroscope with road-mapping capabilities (model BV-212, Philips, the Netherlands; model 9600, OEC Medical Systems, Salt Lake City, UT). The rationale for performing procedures in the operating room includes 1) the need to be able to convert to an open surgical procedure when necessary without any time lag; 2) the mandatory need for a clean environment, because most of the devices require a surgical cut-down and, also, the risk of graft infection must be reduced; and 3) the possible need to perform a simultaneous open procedure such as a femoropopliteal bypass in conjunction with an endovascular graft insertion.

CHAPTER

13

In the basic operating room set-up, the operator usually stands on the right side of the patient and the screen of the fluoroscope is placed so that it faces the operator. The operating table must be radiolucent and have the ability to be controlled (height, rotation, and longitude) by the surgeon using a foot switch. An extension table is attached caudal to the operating table so that the lengthy guidewires and catheters do not fall on the floor. This table has wheels so that it can simultaneously move with the operating table. The cranial end of the operating table is placed toward the caudal end of the patient. This setting enables the C-arm to scan the patient from the head to the knee simply by moving the operating table. This ability is especially important when one is performing an abdominal aortic aneurysm (AAA) repair because of the frequent necessity of having to place a brachial wire (see the following paragraph for details). For this same reason, the patient's left upper extremity is kept sterile.

TECHNIQUES TO OBTAIN VASCULAR ACCESS

For devices that require sheaths larger than 12 to 14 F (outer diameter) for insertion, it is preferable to obtain a surgical cutdown rather than to insert the device through a percutaneous puncture. In most of the aortoiliac cases, an incision is made over the common femoral artery. If an AAA repair is being performed, a higher incision and a partial division of the inguinal ligament may be necessary in order to dissect the entire external iliac artery. This technique is helpful in straightening a tortuous external iliac artery, which is not an uncommon finding in complex AAA cases. In cases in which the common femoral artery is occluded and the endovascular graft must be anastomosed to more distal vessels, the incision should be made lower. Following arterial exposure, vessel loops are placed around the artery proximal and distal to the puncture site. An 18-gauge,

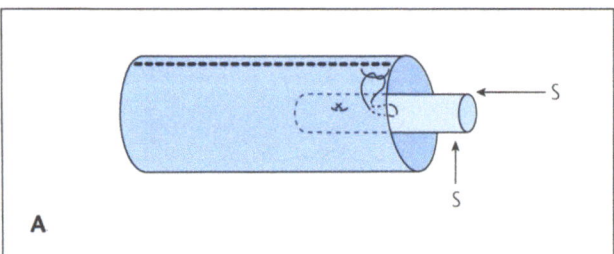

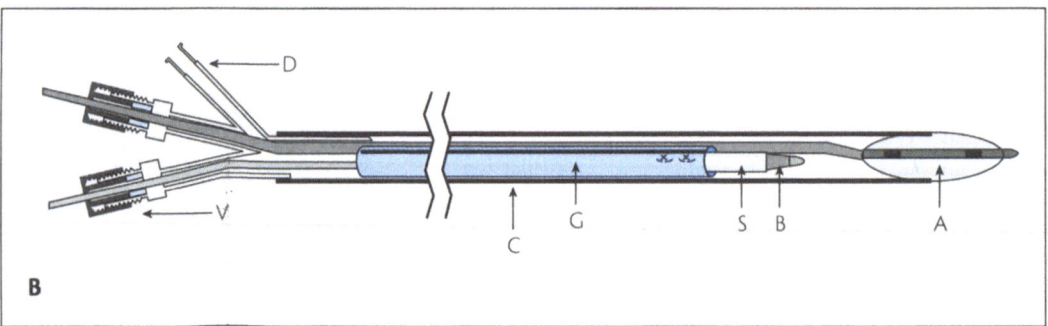

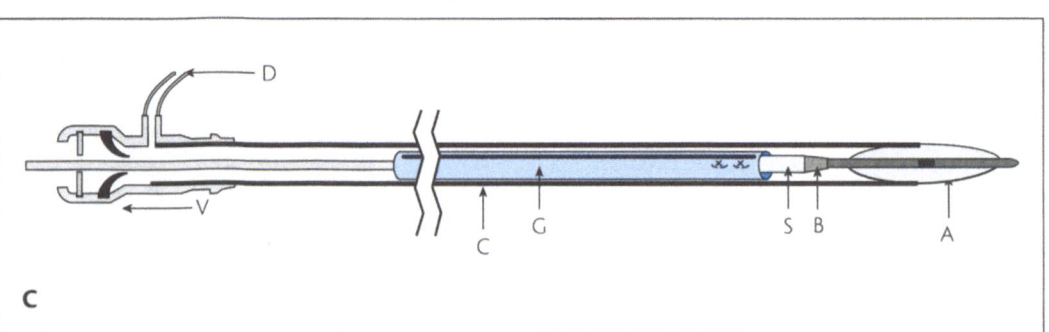

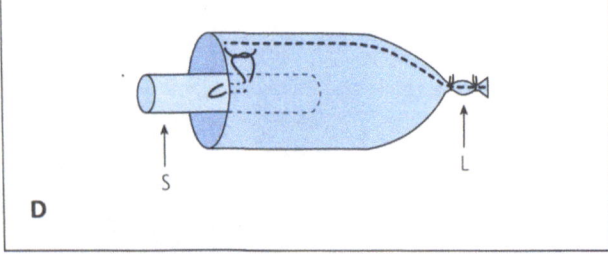

Figure 13-1 The Montefiore endovascular graft and delivery system. **A,** A Palmaz balloon-expandable stent (S) is sutured to the graft using four diametrically opposed "U" sutures (two on each side), which permit one half of the stent to protrude from the graft. **B,** Double-balloon catheter introducer and delivery system used for the delivery and deployment of endovascular stented grafts. In this system the introducer catheter is equipped with two separate balloon catheters. Balloon *A* forms a tapered tip to the catheter system and also allows pressurization of the flexible sheath (C) after saline is injected from port *D*. The second balloon (B) functions to deploy the overlying Palmaz stent (S). With expansion of balloon *B*, the endovascular graft (G) becomes firmly fixed to the underlying arterial wall. **C,** An alternative delivery system consisting of a single balloon catheter that has two balloons on a single shaft. The first balloon serves as a tip balloon (A), while the stent-graft complex is mounted onto the independent deploying balloon (B). **D,** Occluder device for the Montefiore graft. An occluder device consisting of a Palmaz stent (S) (P-308 and P-4014) attached to a polytetrafluoroethylene graft. Two ligatures (L) are applied to the other end of the occluder device. (*Adapted from* Ohki *et al.* [29•].)

one-wall needle is used to puncture the artery, and a 0.035-inch guidewire is inserted through the needle. The needle is then removed and an introducer sheath (7 to 9 F, 10 to 25 cm long) is inserted over the guidewire. The technique following this step depends on the vascular pathology and the anatomy (see separate discussions).

ENDOVASCULAR REPAIR OF AORTOILIAC OCCLUSIVE DISEASE

Endovascular graft

Two endovascular grafts are currently undergoing clinical trials for the treatment of aortoiliac occlusive disease: the Passager (Meadox Medical, Oakland, NJ) and the Montefiore graft. The Montefiore endovascular graft used for this purpose is composed of Palmaz balloon-expandable stents (P-294; Cordis/Johnson & Johnson Interventional Systems, Warren, NJ) and 6-mm thin-walled polytetrafluoroethylene (PTFE) grafts. Each stent is attached to the proximal end of the PTFE graft by four sutures so that one half of the stent protrudes from the end of the graft (Fig. 13-1A). After suturing the graft to the stent, the stent-graft complex is mounted onto an angioplasty balloon by manually crimping the stent over the balloon surface. The delivery system consists of a 6- to 8-mm × 4-cm angioplasty balloon (Diamond; Medi-tech Inc., Watertown, MA; OPTA; Cordis/Johnson & Johnson Interventional Systems) and a second balloon catheter (tip balloon). The entire stent, graft, and balloon complex is then wrapped around the shaft of the tip balloon and inserted into a delivery sheath so that the stent portion of the device is 2 cm distal from the delivery sheath tip (Fig. 13-1B). The 6-mm × 4-cm tip balloon is adjusted so that one third of the tapered portion of the balloon protrudes from the distal portion of the delivery sheath. A modified form of this delivery system consists of a dual balloon catheter (tip balloon and stent-deploying balloon) on a single shaft (Fig. 13-1C). In both delivery system configurations, the tip balloon functions to create a smooth transition zone at the distal end of the delivery sheath as well as to occlude the sheath, which permits pressurization of the sheath when saline is injected from the flush port. The pressurization provides variable pushability and flexibility of the sheath, depending on the amount of pressure applied. This feature facilitates the insertion of the delivery sheath through diseased and tortuous iliac arteries.

Bilateral iliac disease

In cases in which the iliac artery is occluded or diffusely stenosed bilaterally, a bilateral stent-graft repair can be performed. We initially preferred this procedure. However, because bilateral reconstructions were technically more difficult and often resulted in compromised outcomes, and because long intravascular maneuvering resulted in complications such as distal embolization, we now prefer to perform a unilateral repair followed by a femorofemoral bypass [29•]. The iliac artery in which the endovascular graft is deployed and the positioning of the proximal stent are determined by preoperative angiographic findings. Deployment of the endovascular graft will likely result in occlusion of the internal iliac artery and all the small branches along the vessel

that are covered by the graft. The presence and quality of the internal iliac artery will, therefore, influence the side of endovascular graft access and deployment. Similarly, the length and degree of disease of the common or external iliac artery will often determine the technical difficulty associated with vessel recanalization. Generally, it is easier and safer to recanalize through a stenotic rather than an occluded lesion. In addition, shorter lesions are easier to recanalize. The classification of disease patterns, the side to be used for endovascular graft insertion, and the location of the proximal stent can be determined using the algorithm outlined in Figure 13-2.

Operative technique

Following sheath placement in the femoral artery, either a Benson wire (Cook Inc., Bloomington, IN) or a Glidewire (Terumo, Tokyo, Japan) is used for recanalizing the occluded iliac artery. Under fluoroscopic control, a directional catheter (5-F Berenstein, Medi-tech Inc.) is used to direct and control the guidewire through the occluded or stenosed iliac artery [29•]. Care must be taken not to perforate the artery. One must keep in mind that although these guidewires have floppy tips, it can be very traumatic if only a short segment of the wire emerges from the catheter. It is of paramount importance to return to the true lumen at the proximal end of the occluded segment, because the guidewire has a tendency to traverse the dissection plane (between the adventitia and the media) through the occluded segment. This can be ascertained by feeling for the resistance of the guidewire at the proximal end (there is less resistance when the guidewire returns to the true lumen) or by gently injecting contrast through the catheter. In cases in which the contralateral iliac artery is patent, recanalization may be performed with a catheter placed through a percutaneous puncture of the contralateral side (Fig. 13-3A,B). This technique, termed *up and over*, has the advantage of assuring that the recanalized lumen will always join the true lumen at the proximal site. In addition, the contralateral catheter is useful for determining the exact location in which the stent should be placed relative to the aortic bifurcation or to the orifice of the internal iliac artery, while the stent-graft is inserted from the occluded side.

After successful wire passage, a 6- to 8-mm diameter angioplasty balloon is passed over the wire and the iliac artery is dilated along its entire length. The previously prepared endovascular graft device is then inserted into the newly created tract within the arterial wall over the same guidewire. Once the fixation stent is fluoroscopically located at the appropriate predetermined site, the tip balloon is deflated and the sheath is partially retracted while holding the balloon catheter in place. This will allow proximal stent exposure and deployment. The introducer sheath is then completely withdrawn, permitting the redundant portion of the distal end of the endovascular graft to emerge from the arteriotomy in the access vessel. The distal, redundant portion of the graft is then cut to an appropriate length and endoluminally hand sewn into the patent, distal runoff vessel (Fig. 13-3C,D). Combined infrainguinal occlusive disease can be managed by various anastomotic techniques. For bilateral occlusions, a 6-mm, externally supported, thin-walled PTFE graft is used for the femorofemoral bypass. The arteriotomy site used for insertion of the endovascular graft serves as the proximal anastomotic site of the femorofemoral bypass. The graft is then subcutaneously tunneled to the contralateral side and the recipient anastomosis is performed in a standard fashion to the patent distal runoff vessel.

ENDOVASCULAR REPAIR OF ABDOMINAL AORTIC ANEURYSMS
Endovascular grafts with self-expanding stents versus balloon-expandable stents

All endovascular grafts are basically a combination of vascular stents and prosthetic grafts, with the stents serving as fixation devices. Depending on the type of stent that is used, endovascular grafts can be categorized into two distinct types: self-expanding and balloon-expandable. The advantages of self-expanding devices include ease of deployment and the ability to accommodate to a

certain extent some degree of aortic neck enlargement. The balloon-expandable stent used for endovascular grafts has predominantly been the large Palmaz stent. Although this stent may be technically more demanding to accurately deploy at the desired location, it has a stronger radial (hoop) strength than any of the self-expanding stents. This may be important if one considers the high aortic pressure that these endovascular grafts have to withstand. In addition, this feature is also helpful in treating an aneurysm with severe angulation of the proximal neck—a condition for which most of the self-expanding devices are contraindicated. Most manufactured grafts, including the Endovascular Technologies graft (Menlo Park, CA), the Talent graft (World Medical Manufacturing Corp., Sunrise, FL), the Vanguard graft (Meadox Medical, Oakland, NJ), the Corvita graft (Corvita Corp., Miami, FL), and the AneuRx graft (Medtronics, Eden Prairie, MN), use a self-expanding stent (Fig. 13-4). An example of a "surgeon-made" device with self-expanding stents is the Chuter graft. The Palmaz stent has been used for many surgeon-made devices,

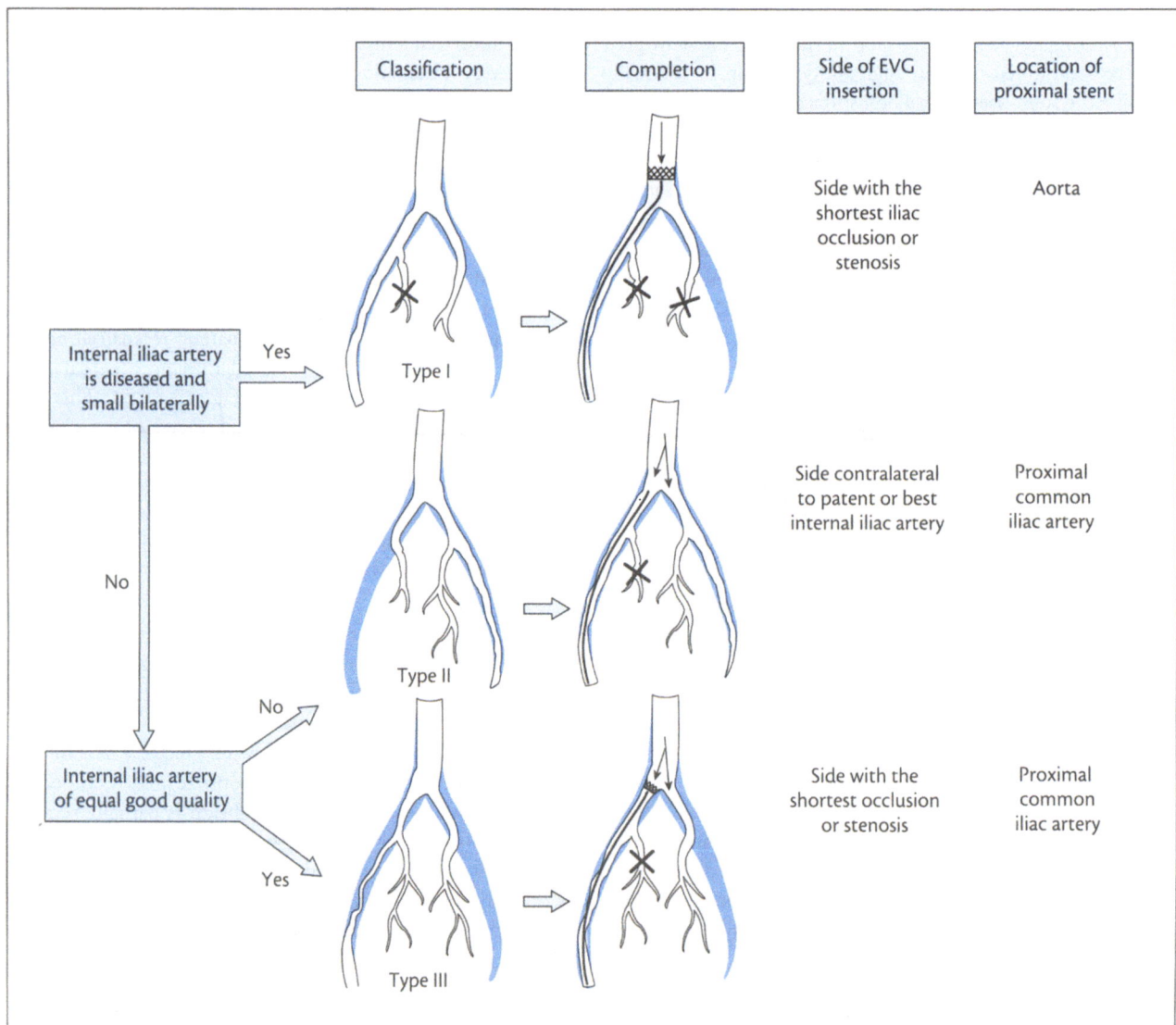

Figure 13-2 Algorithm and classification of endovascular grafting for bilateral aortoiliac occlusive disease. The classification of the distribution of disease, the determination of the appropriate side for graft insertion, and the identification of the location for proximal stent deployment may be approached using this algorithmic outline. EVG—endovascular graft. (*Adapted from Ohki et al.* [29•].)

including the Parodi (Barone Manufacturers, Buenos Aires, Argentina) [14], the Montefiore (Fig. 13-4), and the Leicester [25,26] grafts. The White-Yu endovascular graft attachment device (GAD) is a specially made, self-expanding stent [17,18••].

Most manufactured grafts have a stent that supports the entire length of the graft. This feature has several advantages. First, when endovascular grafts are deployed in tortuous arteries, this fully supported framework will prevent compression or kinking of the graft, phenomena that have been encountered in grafts that lack this support [21•]. Second, this full support gives additional column (longitudinal) strength to withstand distortion or displacement from the aortic flow. This is essential for keeping the graft in position during deployment. In addition, this feature may prevent distal migration of the graft even if the proximal stent lacks secure fixation.

Single component versus multiple component (modular) devices

Because the anatomy, length, and diameter of the aneurysm vary significantly from patient to patient, it is advantageous for an endovascular graft to have a certain dimensional adaptability to accommodate this variability. Variability in length between the proximal and the distal landing points can be managed by changing the amount of overlap between each component of the modular device. This concept was first described by the Sydney group and was called the "trombone" technique [17]. In the bifurcated grafts, the additional limb of a modular bifurcated graft and extenders will achieve longitudinal adaptability. The distal landing zone of the limb can be adjusted by chang-

ing the amount of overlap between the main body and the limb. In addition, the length of the main limb can be extended with an extender stent-graft. These types of endovascular grafts include the Vanguard, the Talent, the Corvita, and the AneuRx. Another approach to achieve adaptability is demonstrated by the Montefiore [36•] and the Leicester grafts [25]. These grafts have enough length so that the distal end of the graft will always emerge from the insertion arteriotomy site, thereby allowing the surgeon to customize the length of the graft during the procedure (Fig. 13-5). In addition, the use of a compliant proximal balloon (Maxi, Cordis/Johnson & Johnson Interventional Systems) will give adaptability in proximal stent diameter, because these balloons have a range of diameters, depending on the inflation pressure applied.

Endovascular grafts without such versatility include the Chuter and the Endovascular Technologies grafts (Fig. 13-4). Preoperative measurement of the length of the graft is crucial when using this type of graft [15,21•].

General selection criteria for endovascular repair

Certain anatomic features must be present prior to attempting endovascular graft placement for AAAs. The procedure is generally contraindicated if the following features are not present: 1) a segment of normal aorta greater than 1.5 to 2 cm long (proximal neck) distal to the renal ostia and proximal to the aneurysm; 2) a distal aortic neck of greater than 1.5 to 2 cm in length proximal to the aortic bifurcation (must be present if a tube graft is to be used); 3) adequate morphology for seating an attachment system if the site selected for distal implantation is

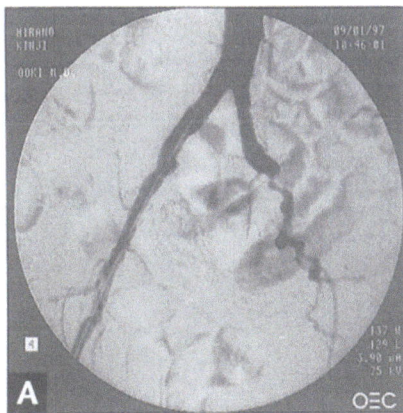

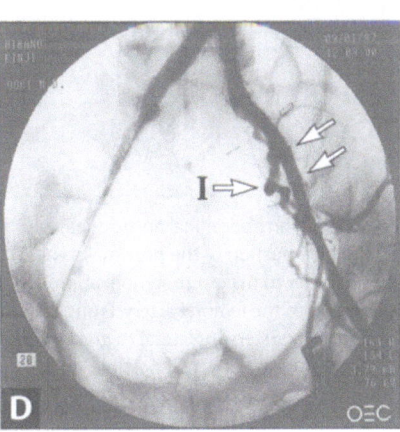

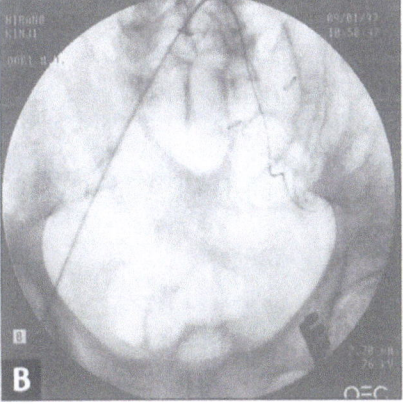

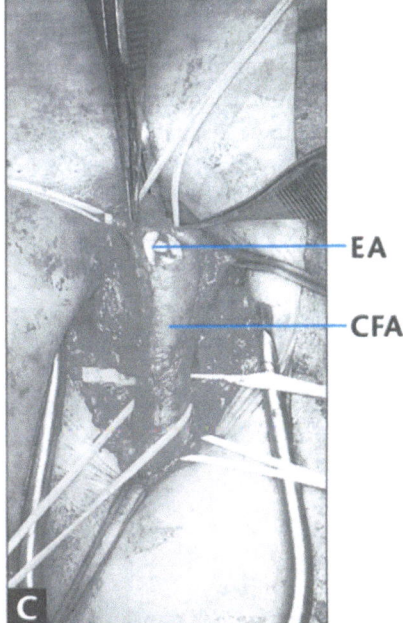

Figure 13-3 Procedure for recanalization. **A,** Intraoperative angiogram of an iliac artery with occlusive disease demonstrating complete occlusion of the left external iliac artery. The left internal iliac artery is patent. This patient suffered from severe claudication (100 m). **B,** The "up and over" technique for recanalization. Recanalization is performed from the contralateral side to ensure that the recanalized tract joins the true lumen at the proximal end of the occlusion. **C,** Endoluminal anastomosis. Following proximal stent deployment, the distal end of the endovascular graft emerges from the arteriotomy site, at which point it is cut to an appropriate

length. An endoluminal anastomosis (EA) is then carried out. CFA—common femoral artery. **D,** Completion angiogram. The external iliac artery is recanalized with the endovascular graft. The proximal stent (*arrows*) is placed at the orifice of the internal iliac artery (I), thus preserving this artery.

the iliac artery; 4) common and external iliac and femoral arteries that are either of sufficient caliber to allow passage of the introducer sheath or amenable to balloon dilatation to facilitate passage; 5) iliac vessels that are not excessively tortuous; 6) excluded segment of aorta is clear of aberrant vessels, such as an indispensable accessory renal artery; 7) patient not dependent on the inferior mesenteric artery for intestinal perfusion (because this vessel will be excluded from the circulation); and 8) no angle greater than 60° to 75° between the suprarenal aorta and the aneurysm's proximal neck, which is a requirement for some self-expanding devices [37•,38].

Choice of endovascular grafts based on anatomic classification and patient health status

Abdominal aortic aneurysms are classified into five distinct groups according to the morphology and the extent of the aneurysm (Fig. 13-6) [39•,40]. The appropriate endovascular graft for the treatment of a given aneurysm is chosen on the basis of this classification. In addition, because these procedures are still under investigation, each operation performed in the United States is done under a Food and Drug Administration Investigational Device Exemption, which allows the use of the device in either low-risk or high-risk patients. Therefore, the choice of device can be further specified according to the health status of the patient along with the anatomic classification, as mentioned previously. The Parodi, Montefiore, and Talent grafts are predominantly used for patients at high surgical risk (compassionate use). Conversely, the Chuter bifurcated graft, the Endovascular Technologies graft, the Vanguard graft, the White-Yu endovascular GAD graft [17,18•], and the Corvita graft are being evaluated in patients at good surgical risk.

Devices designed for type I abdominal aortic aneurysms

First-generation endovascular grafts were tube grafts that could treat only those aneurysms categorized as type 1 (Fig. 13-6) [14,15]. This type of stented graft was limited because patients with type I composed only 10% to 11% of all AAAs [16,40]. In

addition, the high incidence of incomplete aneurysm exclusion ("endoleaks") originating from the distal fixation site hampered the value of this type of graft. The Parodi tube graft, the Endovascular Technologies tube graft, the Vanguard tube graft, the Talent tube graft, the White-Yu Endovascular GAD graft [17,18•], and the Corvita tube graft are of this design.

Devices designed for type IIA and IIB abdominal aortic aneurysms

Recent developmental efforts in stent-graft design have focused on devices that can treat types IIA and IIB AAAs (Figs. 13-6 and 13-7A,B). These grafts are bifurcated and the distal fixation sites are in the common iliac arteries. The Chuter graft [19,20,21•] was the first graft that had a bifurcated design. In addition, the Endovascular Technologies bifurcated graft, the Vanguard graft [22••], the Talent graft, the White-Yu endovascular GAD bifurcated graft [18••], the Corvita bifurcated graft, and the AneuRx graft [23] fall into this category (Fig. 13-4).

Devices designed for type IIC abdominal aortic aneurysms

Abdominal aortic aneurysms with extensive iliac artery involvement can only be treated with an aortouni-iliac graft in combination with a standard femorofemoral bypass, placement of a contralateral iliac artery occluder device, and embolization of

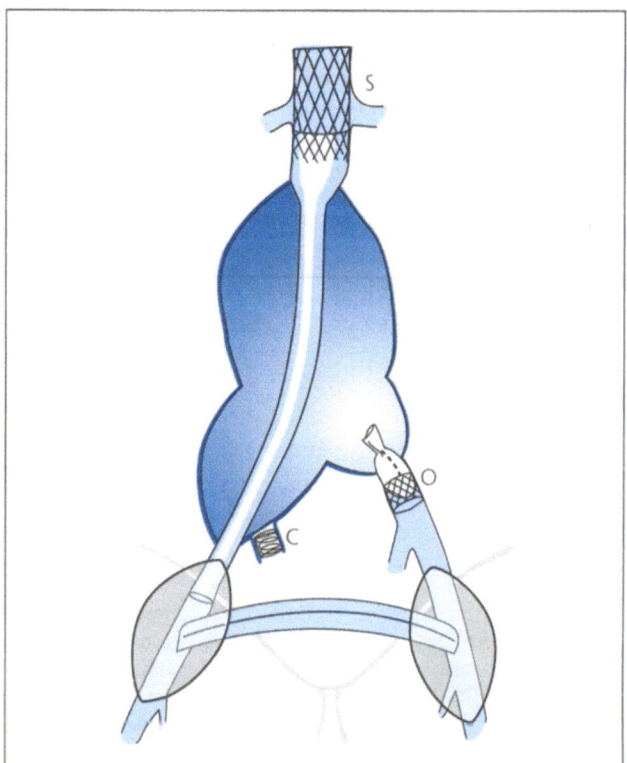

Figure 13-5 Completion of repair of an abdominal aortic aneurysm using the Montefiore graft. The bare portion of the proximal stent (S) is placed across the renal artery in order to maximize stent fixation. The distal end of the graft is hand-sewn to the femoral artery. Embolization coils (C) are placed in the internal iliac artery ipsilateral to graft insertion to prevent retrograde filling of the aneurysm. If possible, an occluder device (O) is placed in the common iliac artery so that at least one internal iliac artery is preserved.

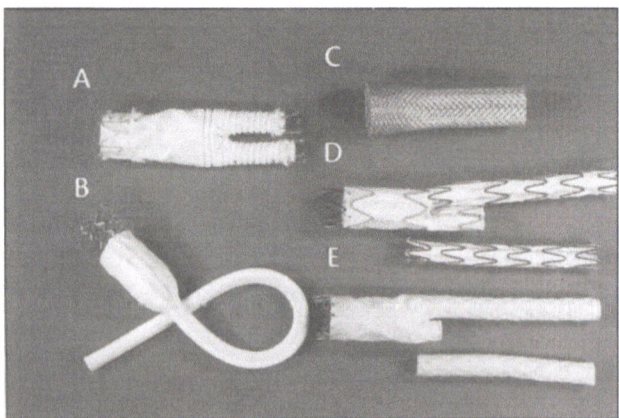

Figure 13-4 Various endovascular grafts used for abdominal aortic aneurysms. **A,** Endovascular Technologies (Menlo Park, CA) bifurcated graft. **B,** Montefiore graft. **C,** Corvita (Corvita Corp., Miami, FL) tube graft. **D,** Talent (World Medical Manufacturing Corp., Sunrise, FL) bifurcated graft. **E,** Vanguard (Meadox Medical, Oakland, NJ) bifurcated graft.

the ipsilateral hypogastric artery. The Parodi graft, the Montefiore graft, the Nottingham graft, the Leicester graft, and the Endovascular Technologies aortoiliac graft were designed to treat this type of AAA.

Devices designed for type III abdominal aortic aneurysms

Although type III AAAs are generally thought to be unsuitable for endovascular repair, certain endovascular grafts with bare proximal stents that have wide interstices permit the proximal fixation stent to be placed above the lowest renal artery. Such devices include the Montefiore graft (Fig. 13-5) [36] and the Talent graft.

Construction of the Montefiore device

The Montefiore device is constructed from 7- to 10-mm PTFE grafts. The proximal 4-cm portion of each graft is expanded to 30 mm to accommodate the diameter of the proximal aortic neck. Expansion is accomplished by means of a gradual dilatation using 5 atm of pressure with an esophageal dilatation balloon. The graft is then sutured to a Palmaz stent (P-5014) with four "U" stitches so as to overlap one half the length of the stent. A metallic marker is sutured to the proximal end of the graft material so that the end of the PTFE covering can be seen under the fluoroscope. The stent-graft is then crimped onto a 25- to 35-mm balloon and loaded into a 16- to 24-F sheath. The 35-mm balloon catheter has a second balloon at the tip of the catheter similar to the system previously described.

The occluder device, which is placed in the contralateral iliac artery to prevent retrograde filling of the aneurysm, is also made from PTFE and a Palmaz stent (Fig. 13-1*D*). PTFE suture material is used as two ligatures to occlude one end of the PTFE graft. A Palmaz stent (P-4014, P-308) is attached to the other end of the PTFE graft by means of four "U" stitches. The occluder device is loaded onto an angioplasty balloon and then inserted into a 14- to 18-F sheath.

Coil embolization of the hypogastric artery

Coil embolization of the hypogastric artery ipsilateral to the graft insertion site is carried out if the distal landing zone is distal to the internal iliac artery orifice. Coil embolization (Gianturco coils; Cook Inc., Bloomington, IN) is usually performed at the time of the preoperative angiogram, although it can be performed in the operating room at the time of graft insertion. Coil embolization is routinely performed for all Montefiore aortofemoral grafts.

Operative and adjunct techniques

Bilateral surgical exposure of the common femoral arteries is followed by insertion of a diagnostic catheter into the aorta through one of these vessels. The locations of the renal artery, aortoiliac bifurcation, and hypogastric arteries as well as the site for proximal graft implantation are identified. A 260-cm Amplatz Super Stiff wire (Medi-tech Inc.) is inserted up to the thoracic aorta. A delivery catheter containing the endovascular graft is then advanced over the wire. If difficulty is encountered advancing the device through a diseased, tortuous iliac artery, the following techniques may be used. If there is stenosis in the iliac system, balloon dilatation prior to insertion of the device may be undertaken. If the problem is caused by a tortuous iliac artery, one of the following techniques may be applied. First,

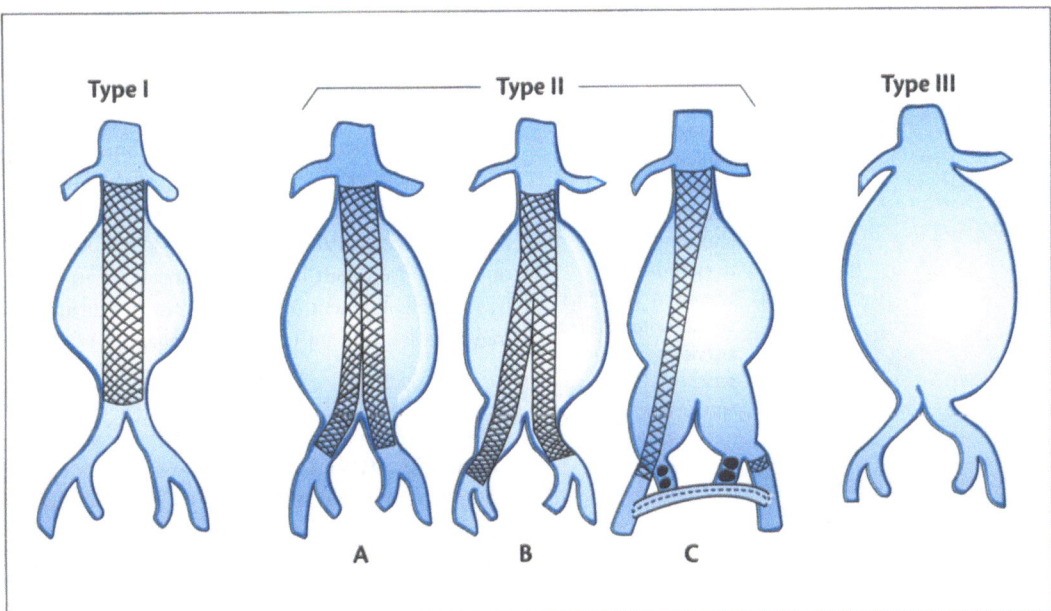

Figure 13-6 Morphometric classification of abdominal aortic aneurysms (AAAs) and possible endovascular graft configurations. Type I is an AAA with sufficient proximal (> 15 mm) and distal (> 10 mm) aortic necks (tube graft). Type IIA has a proximal neck greater than 15 mm and absence of distal iliac involvement (bifurcated graft). Type IIB has a proximal neck greater than 15 mm with proximal common iliac artery involvement (bifurcated graft). Type IIC has a proximal neck greater than 15 mm with iliac artery involvement to the iliac bifurcation (aortouni-iliac graft with contralateral iliac occlusion, femorofemoral bypass, and coil embolization of the hypogastric arteries). Type III has a proximal neck of less than 15 mm (grafts that permit suprarenal stent placement).

dissection of the external iliac artery from the surrounding tissue through a groin incision is carried out. This maneuver will usually straighten any tortuosity in the external iliac artery. If this maneuver fails, a snare wire is introduced from a left brachial artery puncture site to capture the guidewire introduced from the groin. By applying tension on both ends of the "through and through" guidewire, most of the tortuosity of the aortoiliac system can be significantly reduced and the introduction of the delivery system is usually successful.

Following confirmation of the location of the lowest renal artery, the proximal stent is deployed. If a self-expanding device is used, the usual technique of deployment is to retrieve the outer sheath while holding the inner pusher rod in place. With balloon-expandable devices, the stent is deployed by inflating the proximal balloon following outer sheath retrieval. During proximal stent deployment, it has been recommended that the patient's blood pressure be lowered to a mean of 60 to 70 mm Hg in order to minimize any force being applied to the stent that might result in misdeployment. However, we found that lowering the blood pressure had minimal effect on the stabilization of the proximal stent. Rather, controlling outflow had a major effect in reducing the force applied to the proximal stent, thereby facilitating accurate stent deployment [41]. Therefore,

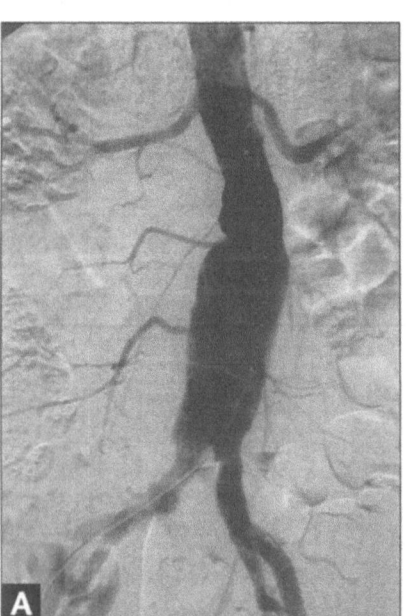

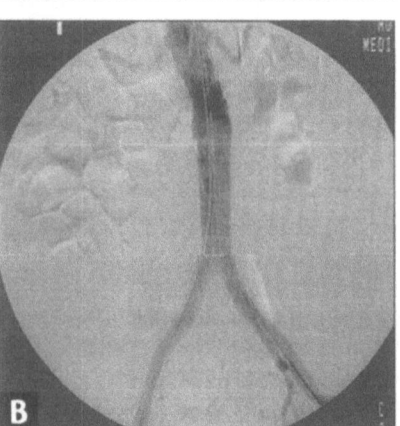

Figure 13-7
Endovascular repair of an abdominal aortic aneurysm. **A,** Preoperative angiogram revealed an aortic aneurysm with an ideal proximal neck. The aneurysm measured 6.5 cm on CT scan. **B,** Completion angiogram. A Vanguard (Meadox Medical, Oakland, NJ) bifurcated graft was implanted to exclude the aneurysm. The renal and the internal iliac arteries were preserved and the endoleak was not detected.

at present we occlude the outflow by applying a vascular clamp on the contralateral femoral artery or by placing an occlusion balloon in the contralateral common iliac artery (the ipsilateral iliac artery is usually completely occluded by the delivery device) and do not lower the blood pressure, which in some cases may be dangerous and time-consuming. In some instances we have also obtained temporal asystole by means of an intravenous bolus injection of adenosine (20 to 30 mg).

The cephalad end of the graft material in the Montefiore graft has a metallic marker for visualization under the fluoroscope. The graft is deployed so that this marker is placed just below the lowest renal artery. The bare stent above the marker covers the orifice of the renal artery.

If a bifurcated modular device is used, a guidewire must be placed into the short limb of the graft in order to facilitate deployment of the contralateral limb. This guidewire can be placed through the ipsilateral or contralateral femoral artery or through the brachial wire. Either an SOS Omni or a Cobra catheter (Medi-tech Inc.) is used for the contralateral approach. A Berenstein or a multipurpose catheter is used if working through the ipsilateral side. The amount of overlap between the main graft and the limb is determined by where the distal landing zone of the limb should be.

If a Montefiore graft is used, the main endovascular graft is deployed and an occluder device is placed in the contralateral common or external iliac artery, depending on the presence or absence of a common iliac artery aneurysm. Finally, a standard femorofemoral crossover graft is constructed.

Completion arteriograms and intravascular ultrasound (IVUS) are performed to assure technical satisfaction and the absence of an endoleak. IVUS can identify many lesions such as compression of the endovascular graft or dissection of the iliac artery caused by insertion of the graft, both of which are not always apparent on angiograms [42]. Graft compression and arterial dissection are treated by additional balloon dilatation or by the placement of either a Palmaz stent or a Wallstent (Schneider Inc., Minneapolis, MN). Endoleaks are treated by one of the following techniques. If an endoleak is caused by low deployment of the proximal stent, a PTFE-covered Palmaz stent is deployed proximal to the previously deployed graft to seal the leakage. If an endoleak is caused by underdeployment of the stent, further dilatation of the proximal stent is sufficient to seal the leakage.

ENDOVASCULAR REPAIR OF ILIAC ANEURYSMS

Endovascular repair of an isolated iliac aneurysm may be performed using the same concepts and similar devices as described for the repair of AAAs. However, there are only a few devices that are constructed for this purpose. These include the Passager, which is basically the same device as the extension limb of the Vanguard graft, and the Montefiore grafts. The Montefiore graft for the treatment of iliac aneurysms is mainly constructed from Palmaz stents (P-5014, P-308, P-294) and PTFE grafts (6 to 8 mm) in a manner similar to that previously described. The repairs are performed with one of the various techniques shown in Figure 13-8, depending on the anatomy of the aneurysm.

DISCUSSION

Endovascular graft repair has been investigated in clinical trials since 1991. During this period, a variety of devices were developed, and a guideline for their use [43] and reporting standards [44] were established. However, a number of questions regarding the use of endovascular grafts were raised, most of which still remain unanswered. These questions include the ethical and legal aspects of their use [45], who should perform these procedures, and, most importantly, their effectiveness.

Following the first successful report of endovascular grafting for the treatment of AAAs by Parodi and coworkers [14], the indications for endovascular grafting were expanded to include arterial occlusive disease [28•,29•,30,35,46], occluded grafts [47], peripheral aneurysms [48,49], and traumatic arterial lesions [34,50].

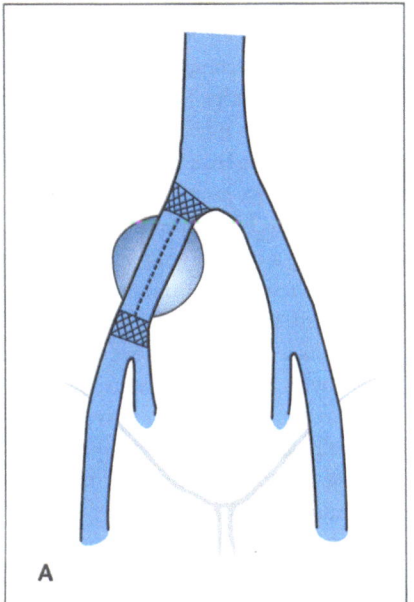
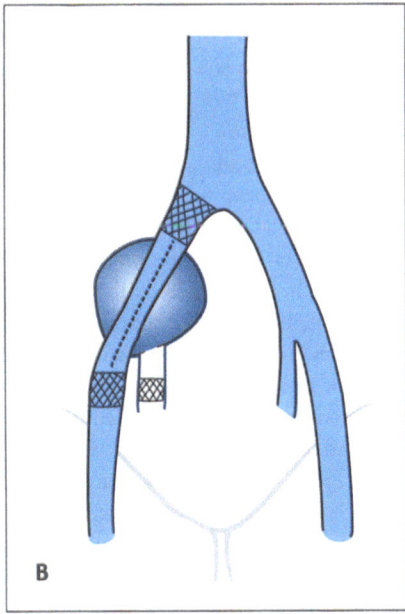
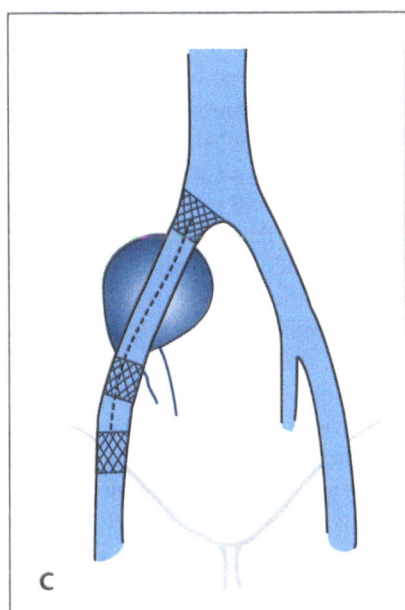
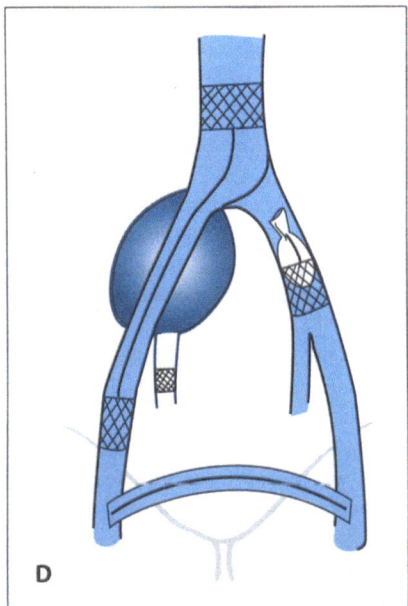
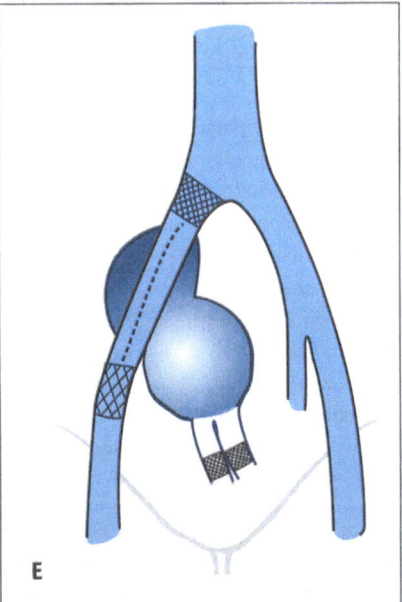
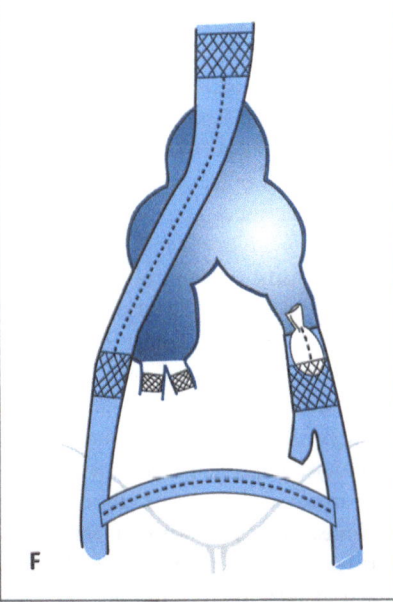

Figure 13-8 Techniques for the endoluminal repair of aortoiliac aneurysms. **A,** A localized common iliac artery aneurysm treated with stents anchoring the endovascular graft proximal and distal to the aneurysm. **B** and **C,** If the aneurysm of the common iliac artery extends to the hypogastric vessel, either placement of occlusion coils in the internal iliac artery or deployment of an additional stent within the endovascular graft is performed to prevent retrograde flow from the hypogastric artery into the common iliac artery aneurysm. **D** and **F,** In cases in which there is no proximal neck of the iliac aneurysm or in cases with common iliac artery aneurysms with aortic aneurysms, the treatment is carried out in a manner similar to that for abdominal aortic aneurysms. **E** and **F,** If a wide-mouth opening to an internal iliac artery aneurysm is present, the anterior and posterior divisions of the hypogastric artery are individually coil embolized and the endovascular graft is secured with a stent above and below the origin of the aneurysmal artery, functionally excluding it from the circulation. In any of these four reconstruction techniques, the second (distal) stent that is responsible for fixing the distal portion of the graft to the arterial wall may be eliminated by extending the endovascular graft to the common femoral artery and performing an endoluminal anastomosis. (*Adapted from Marin et al.* [48].)

Based on the currently available reported results, some of these indications, such as endovascular grafting for traumatic central arterial lesions, aortoiliac occlusive disease, and isolated iliac aneurysmal disease in patients at high surgical risk as described in this chapter, already appear to be justified. Although the treatment of AAAs with endovascular grafts appears to hold a major interest for both physicians and manufacturers, the safety and long-term efficacy of this treatment remain to be proven. Problems include the mortality rate and the significant rate of complications, including endoleaks and distal embolization; in addition, the standard aneurysm repair techniques are proven to be safe and durable. Further investigation is required before endovascular repair of AAAs is widely used.

Several additional issues are of concern regarding the endovascular repair of aortic aneurysms, including the use of embolization coils to occlude the hypogastric artery. It is generally believed that occlusion of the hypogastric artery may be harmful and even lethal. Iliopoulos and coworkers [51] described their experience with this occlusion, which led to lethal complications such as lower extremity paralysis, buttock necrosis, anal and bladder sphincteric dysfunction, and colorectal ischemia. However, we were unable to confirm this result [52]. We intentionally occluded 48 hypogastric arteries to facilitate the endovascular repair of abdominal aortic and iliac artery aneurysms, and only 9% resulted in consequences, all of which were nonlethal. These complications included three buttock claudications and one colonic mucosal ischemia. None required additional intervention and all resolved with conservative therapy. Therefore, we currently believe that unilateral coil embolization of the hypogastric artery can be safely performed. Bilateral hypogastric artery occlusion may be required in cases in which bilateral common iliac arteries are aneurysmal. The safety of this procedure has yet to be proven.

Another issue is the management of endoleaks. There seems to be uniform agreement that large endoleaks should be aggressively treated. In fact, rupture of AAAs with large endoleaks following endovascular repair has been reported [14,53]. However, the appropriate treatment of endoleaks that have spontaneously sealed remains a matter of considerable debate. To address this issue, experimental aneurysms were created in canines and repaired with endovascular grafts with small endoleaks [54]. These endoleaks were 4 mm in diameter, spontaneously sealed, and could not be detected on postoperative angiograms. The aneurysmal pressure was chronically measured with a pressure transducer implanted in the aneurysmal wall. This study revealed that aneurysmal pressure in the control groups that had complete endovascular repair without endoleaks decreased significantly, whereas the pressure in the animals with endoleaks remained elevated at 80% of systemic pressure. Based on these results, we believe that angiographic closure of an endoleak does not provide protection from rupture and, therefore, all endoleaks that are detected regardless of closure should be treated with either standard repair or placement of a covered stent.

Although there are several issues that have yet to be answered, the procedure provides a means of treating patients whose comorbid illnesses make conventional repair dangerous or impossible. In addition, shrinkage of the AAA has been observed when these grafts were successfully deployed [55,56••,57,58]. Long-term follow-up of patients treated with endovascular grafts is not yet available, but the initial early and midterm results are promising.

CONCLUSIONS

The field of minimally invasive vascular surgery is rapidly expanding. Existing techniques using a noninvasive approach are being refined on a monthly basis and new applications are being developed. Although some progress has been made, the field of endovascular surgery remains wide open for new innovations. The adaptation of previously existing techniques, such as stenting and percutaneous transluminal angioplasty, to form stented grafts has allowed significant progress in the minimally invasive treatment of vascular disease. The ability to treat such diverse entities as aneurysmal, occlusive, and traumatic arterial lesions with a common, technical approach is especially appealing. In addition, the current capability of inserting a stented graft at a site distant from the disease with less anesthesia, tissue trauma, blood loss, and perhaps a coincident decrease in hospital stay and cost likely foreshadows the future of vascular surgery. Although continued investigation and comparison with more conventional techniques are called for, the stented graft has, nonetheless, arrived and has defined the course of minimally invasive vascular surgery for the decade to come. It should be kept as an important tool in the armamentarium of vascular surgeons.

REFERENCES AND RECOMMENDED READING

Recently published papers of particular interest have been highlighted as:
•   Of interest
••   Of outstanding interest

1.   DeBakey ME, Crawford ES, Cooley DA, *et al.*: Aneurysm of abdominal aorta: analysis of results of graft replacement therapy one to eleven years after operation. *Ann Surg* 1964, 160:622–639.

2.   Crawford ES, Saleh SA, Babb JW III, *et al.*: Infrarenal abdominal aortic aneurysm: factors influencing survival after operation over a 25-year period. *Ann Surg* 1981, 193:699–709.

3.   Szilagyi DE, Smith RF, DeRusso FJ, *et al.*: Contribution of abdominal aortic aneurysmectomy to prolongation of life. *Ann Surg* 1966, 164:678–679.

4.   AbuRahma AF, Robinson PA, Boland JP, *et al.*: Elective resection of 332 abdominal aortic aneurysms in a southern West Virginia community during a recent five-year period. *Surgery* 1991, 109:244–251.

5.   Johnson KW, Scobie TK: Multicenter prospective study of non-ruptured abdominal aortic aneurysms: population and operative management. *J Vasc Surg* 1988, 7:69–81.

6.   Veith FJ, Gupta SK, Wengerter KR, *et al.*: Changing arteriosclerotic disease patterns and management strategies in lower-limb-threatening ischemia. *Ann Surg* 1990, 212:402–414.

7.   Snyder WH III, Thal ER, Perry MO: Peripheral and abdominal vascular injuries. In *Vascular Surgery*, edn 2. Edited by Rutherford RB. Philadelphia: WB Saunders; 1984:460–500.

8.   Lim RC Jr, Trunkey DD, Blaisdell FW: Acute abdominal aortic injury: an analysis of operative and postoperative management. *Arch Surg* 1974, 109:706–711.

9. Mattox KL, Feliciano DV, Birch J, *et al.*: Five thousand seven hundred sixty cardiovascular injuries in 4459 patients: epidemiologic evaluation 1958 to 1987. *Ann Surg* 1989, 209:698–707.

10. Thompson JE, Hollier LH, Patman RD, *et al.*: Surgical management of abdominal aortic aneurysms: factors influencing mortality and morbidity: a 20 year experience. *Ann Surg* 1975, 181:654–661.

11. McCombs PR, Roberts B: Acute renal failure following resection of abdominal aortic aneurysm. *Surg Gynecol Obstet* 1979, 148:175–178.

12. Hollier LH, Reigel MM, Kazmier FJ, *et al.*: Conventional repair of abdominal aortic aneurysm in the high-risk patient: a plea for abandonment of nonresective treatment. *J Vasc Surg* 1986, 3:712–717.

13. Gardner RJ, Gardner NL, Tarnay TJ, *et al.*: The surgical experience and a one to sixteen year follow-up of 277 abdominal aortic aneurysms. *Am J Surg* 1978, 135:226–230.

14. Parodi JC, Palmaz JC, Barone HD: Transfemoral intraluminal graft implantation for abdominal aortic aneurysms. *Ann Vasc Surg* 1991, 5:491–499.

15. Moore WS, Vescera CL: Repair of abdominal aortic aneurysm by transfemoral endovascular graft placement. *Ann Surg* 1994, 220:331–341.

16. Chuter TAM, Green RM, Ouriel K, *et al.*: Infrarenal aortic aneurysm morphology: implications for transfemoral repair. *J Vasc Surg* 1994, 20:44–50.

17. May J, White G, Waugh R, *et al.*: Treatment of complex abdominal aortic aneurysms by a combination of endoluminal and extraluminal aortofemoral grafts. *J Vasc Surg* 1994, 19:824–833.

18.•• White GH, Yu W, May J: Three year experience with the White-Yu endovascular GAD graft for transluminal repair of aortic and iliac aneurysms. *J Endovasc Surg* 1997, 4:124–136.

The authors report their results with the original stented graft (endovascular GAD graft) used to treat 76 abdominal aortic aneurysms. Although a 14% endoleak rate was encountered following tube graft repair, no endoleak was seen when an aortoiliac or a bifurcated graft was used.

19. Chuter TAM, Donayre C, Wendt G: Bifurcated stent-grafts for endovascular repair of abdominal aortic aneurysm: preliminary case reports. *Surg Endosc* 1994, 8:800–802.

20. Chuter TAM, Green RM, Ouriel K, *et al.*: Transfemoral endovascular aortic graft placement. *J Vasc Surg* 1993, 18:185–197.

21.• Chuter TAM, Wendt G, Hopkinson BR: European experience with a system for bifurcated stent-graft insertion. *J Endovasc Surg* 1997, 4:13–22.

The authors were the first to report the use of a bifurcated endovascular graft. This paper reports their follow-up results to 3 years using both their original graft and industry-made devices. The importance of selection criteria is mentioned.

22.•• Blum U, Voshage G, Lammer J, *et al.*: Endoluminal stent-grafts for infrarenal abdominal aortic aneurysms. *N Engl J Med* 1997, 336:13–20.

The largest series (154 patients) of endovascular graft repairs of AAAs published. The success rate, mortality rate, and complication rate (minor, 8%; major, 2%) were 86%, 0.7%, and 10%, respectively.

23. Allen RC, White RA, Zarins CK, *et al.*: What are the characteristics of the ideal endovascular graft for abdominal aortic aneurysm exclusion. *J Endovasc Surg* 1997, 4:195–202.

24. Yusef SW, Whitaker SC, Chuter TAM: Early results of endovascular aortic aneurysm surgery with aortouniiliac graft, contralateral iliac occlusion, and femorofemoral bypass. *J Vasc Surg* 1997, 25:165–172.

25. Thompson MM, Sayers RD, Nasim A: Aortomonoiliac endovascular grafting: difficult solutions to difficult aneurysms. *J Endovasc Surg* 1997, 4:174–181.

26. Nasim A, Thompson MM, Sayers RD, *et al.*: Investigation of the relationship between aortic stent position and renal function. *J Endovasc Surg* 1995, 2:90–91.

27. Ohki T, Veith FJ, Sanchez LA, *et al.*: Varying strategies and devices for endovascular repair of abdominal aortic aneurysms. *Semin Vasc Surg* 1997, 10:242–256.

28.• Marin ML, Veith FJ, Sanchez LA, *et al.*: Endovascular repair of aortoiliac occlusive disease. *World J Surg* 1996, 20:679–686.

This paper reports the midterm results of endovascular repair for aortoiliac occlusive disease resulting in critical ischemia.

29.• Ohki T, Marin ML, Veith FJ, *et al.*: Endovascular aortounifemoral grafts and femorofemoral bypass for bilateral limb-threatening ischemia. *J Vasc Surg* 1996, 24:984–997.

A novel endovascular procedure for bilateral aortoiliac occlusive disease in high-risk patients is described. The authors advocate the use of endovascular aortounifemoral grafts and femorofemoral bypass over simple stenting or axillobifemoral bypass in this group of patients.

30. Pernes JM, Auguste MA, Hovasse D, *et al.*: Long iliac stenosis: initial clinical experience with the Cragg Endoluminal Graft. *Radiology* 1995, 196:67–71.

31.• Diethrich EB, Papazogou K: Endoluminal grafting for aneurysmal and occlusive disease in the superficial femoral artery: early experience. *J Endovasc Surg* 1995, 2:225–239.

One of the few papers describing the use of endovascular grafts for infrainguinal arterial disease.

32. Spoelstra H, Casselman F, Lesceu O: Balloon expandable endobypass (B.E.E.B.) for femoral-popliteal atherosclerotic occlusive disease: a review of 55 patients. *J Vasc Surg* 1996, 24:647–654.

33. Marin ML, Veith FJ, Panetta TF, *et al.*: Transluminally placed endovascular stented graft repair for arterial trauma. *J Vasc Surg* 1994, 20:466–473.

34. Ohki T, Veith FJ, Marin ML, *et al.*: Endovascular approaches for traumatic arterial lesions. *Semin Vasc Surg* 1997, 10:272–285.

35. Ohki T, Marin ML, Veith FJ: Use of endovascular grafts to treat non-aneurysmal arterial disease. *Ann Vasc Surg* 1997, 11:200–205.

36.• Wain RA, Marin ML, Veith FJ, *et al.*: Endoleaks complicating endovascular graft treatment of aortic aneurysms: classification, risk factors, and outcome. *J Vasc Surg* 1998, 27:69–80.

This paper describes the authors' 4-year experience with stented grafts for the treatment of AAAs with special focus on endoleaks. A classification of endoleaks is proposed.

37.• Moore WS: The EVT tube and bifurcated endograft systems: technical considerations and clinical summary. *J Endovasc Surg* 1997, 4:182–194.

Update on the results of the oldest manufactured stented graft for AAA repair.

38. Chuter TAM, Risberg Bo, Hopkinson BR: Clinical experience with a bifurcated endovascular graft for abdominal aortic aneurysm repair. *J Vasc Surg* 1996, 24:655–666.

39.• Schumacher H, Allenberg JR, Eckstein HH: Morphological classification of abdominal aortic aneurysm in selection of patients for endovascular grafting. *Br J Surg* 1996, 83:949–950.

A prospective anatomical evaluation of 194 AAAs. An anatomic classification of AAAs that might be useful for patient selection for endovascular repair is advocated.

40. Schumacher H, Eckstein HH, Kallinowski F, *et al.*: Morphometry and classification in abdominal aortic aneurysms: patient selection for endovascular and open surgery. *J Endovasc Surg* 1997, 4:39–44.

41. Ohki T, Lu Z, Veith FJ, *et al.*: Effect of blood pressure and arterial outflow on the stabilization of proximal stent deployment during endovascular aortic aneurysm repair: does lowering pressure facilitate accurate deployment. *J Endovasc Surg* 1998, 5(suppl):1–24.

42. Lyon RT, Marin ML, Veith FJ, *et al.*: Intravascular ultrasound for intraoperative assessment of endovascular graft procedures. *Proceedings of the 11th Annual Meeting of the Eastern Vascular Society.* Atlantic City, NJ, May 2–4, 1997.

43   Veith FJ, Abbott WM, Yao JST, *et al.*: Guidelines for development and use of transluminally placed endovascular prosthetic grafts in the arterial system. *J Vasc Surg* 1995, 21:670–685.

44.   Ahn SS, Rutherford RB, Johnston KW, *et al.*: Ad Hoc Committee for Standardized Reporting Practices in Vascular Surgery for The Society For Vascular Surgery/International Society for Cardiovascular Surgery: Reporting standards for infrarenal endovascular abdominal aortic aneurysm repair. *J Vasc Surg* 1997, 25:405–410.

45.   Veith FJ, Marin ML: Ethical and legal issues related to endovascular graft investigation and early usage. *J Endovasc Surg* 1997, 4:66–71.

46.   Marin ML, Veith FJ, Cynamon J, *et al.*: Transfemoral endovascular stented graft treatment of aorto-iliac and femoropopliteal occlusive disease for limb salvage. *Am J Surg* 1994, 168:154–162.

47.   Sanchez LA, Marin ML, Veith FJ, *et al.*: Placement of endovascular stented grafts via remote access sites: a new approach to the treatment of failed aortoiliofemoral reconstructions. *Ann Vasc Surg* 1995, 9:1–8.

48.   Marin ML, Veith FJ, Lyon RT, *et al.*: Transfemoral endovascular repair of iliac artery aneurysms. *Am J Surg* 1995, 170:179–182.

49.   Tazavi MK, Dake MD, Semba CP, *et al.*: Percutaneous endoluminal placement of stent-graft for the treatment of isolated iliac artery aneurysms. *Radiology* 1995, 197:801–804.

50.   Marin ML, Veith FJ, Panetta TF, *et al.*: Percutaneous transfemoral stented graft repair of a traumatic femoral arteriovenous fistula. *J Vasc Surg* 1993, 18:299–302.

51.   Iliopoulos JI, Horanitz PE, Pierce GE, *et al.*: The critical hypogastric circulation. *Am J Surg* 1987, 154:671–675.

52.   Marin ML, Veith FJ, Ohki T, *et al.*: Intentional internal iliac artery occlusion to facilitate endovascular repair of aortoiliac aneurysms and occlusions. *Proceedings of the 21st Annual Meeting of the Southern Association for Vascular Surgery.* Coronado, CA, January 22–25, 1997.

53.   Lumsden AB, Allen RC, Chaikof EL, *et al.*: Delayed rupture of aortic aneurysms following endovascular stent grafting. *Am J Surg* 1995, 170:174–178.

54.   Marty B, Sanchez LA, Ohki T, *et al.*: Significance of endoleak on aneurysmal pressure. *J Vasc Surg* 1998, in press.

55.   May J, White GH, Yu W, *et al.*: A prospective study of changes in morphology and dimensions of abdominal aortic aneurysms following endoluminal repair: a preliminary report. *J Endovasc Surg* 1995, 2:343–347.

56.•• Matsumura JS, Pearce WH, McCarthy JW, *et al.*: Reduction in aortic aneurysm size: early results after endovascular graft placement. *J Vasc Surg* 1997, 25:113–123.
This paper reports 1-year follow-up following endovascular repair of AAAs, with special reference to the change in aneurysmal diameter. The diameter of AAAs without endoleaks or with endoleaks that sealed decreased in size. However, it increased in those with persistent endoleaks. This paper highlights the importance of endoleaks.

57.   Malina M, Ivancev K, Chuter TAM, *et al.*: Changing aneurysmal morphology after endovascular grafting: relation to leakage or persistent perfusion. *J Endovasc Surg* 1997; 4:23–30.

58.   Balm R, Katee R, Blankensteijn JD, *et al.*: CT-angiography of abdominal aortic aneurysms after transfemoral endovascular aneurysm management. *Eur J Endovasc Surg* 1996, 12:182–188.

Minimally Invasive Techniques in Pediatric Surgery

Steven J. Fishman

Minimally invasive techniques are now broadly applied in the surgery of infants and children. During the early 1990s, the widespread zealous enthusiasm to perform minimally invasive procedures in adults was somewhat muted among pediatric surgeons. The techniques and procedures that were found to be useful in adults have now been applied in children. Innovative modifications have been developed to account for the smaller working areas and volumes in the pediatric patient. In addition, a different spectrum of pathology has led to the development of several pediatric-specific procedures. These newer procedures are undergoing rapid evolution, and additional techniques are continually introduced. Each new technique should be evaluated carefully to ensure that it can be performed safely and that the risk-benefit ratio favors a minimally invasive approach over preexisting procedures through standard incisions.

GENERAL CONSIDERATIONS

In general, the principles of laparoscopy and thoracoscopy in children are similar to those applied in adults. The availability of smaller, finer, and shorter instruments, ports, and telescopes has facilitated the adaptation of minimally invasive techniques to the smallest patients, even premature newborns. However, the pediatric practitioner is often forced to use instruments intended for larger patients. Commercial instrument development is geared toward the larger adult marketplace, with miniaturization occurring later or often not at all.

PROCEDURES

Although port locations are often standardized for the various procedures performed in adults, an individualized approach is frequently required in infants and children. Use of "standard" port sites in a very small body cavity may result in very short working distances, inability to fully insert the necessary working length of an instrument, and a cluster of short parallel instruments in close approximation to one another, rather then the instruments approaching the working area from multiple angles. The smallest patients require the greatest relative separation of port sites. The most favorable locations can often be best chosen after insertion of the telescope. The umbilical site remains popular for initial port placement. It should be understood that the urinary bladder is intra-abdominal in infants. The urachal remnant extending from the umbilicus to the dome of the bladder is often very short. The urinary bladder should always be emptied prior to laparoscopy in infants and small children. Lower abdominal ports should be placed carefully with intra-abdominal visualization to avoid bladder injury.

General anesthesia is almost always used during laparoscopy or thoracoscopy in children. Brief procedures can occasionally be performed in teenagers under conscious sedation. The general physiologic effects of pneumoperitoneum in children are similar to those in adults. However, children have an increased metabolic rate and greater oxygen demand coupled with a lesser pulmonary functional residual capacity than adults. Pneumoperitoneum can generally be established and maintained with safety when the anesthesiologist is experienced in caring for pediatric patients [1•]. Thoracoscopic procedures are greatly assisted by continuous or intermittent single-lung ventilation, allowing collapse of the ipsilateral lung. Double-lumen endotracheal tubes can generally be inserted in children weighing 40 kg or greater. Bronchial blockers or selective bronchial intubation with an endotracheal tube can be useful in smaller children. Pulmonary collapse can be assisted by external compression of the lung. I prefer an inflatable balloon-type retractor for this purpose, rather than a metal fan–type device, to avoid injuring the pulmonary parenchyma or mediastinal structures that can be in close proximity in a small patient. Many minimally invasive procedures are performed in infants and children in a similar manner to that used in adults. Some of these are mentioned briefly, followed by a more extensive discussion of pediatric-specific procedures.

Biliary procedures

Cholelithiasis is far less prevalent in the pediatric population than in adulthood. Nevertheless, cholecystectomy is not uncommonly required in childhood. Although hematologic disorders underlie the formation of gallstones in many children, idiopathic cholelithiasis remains most common. Familial hypocholesterolemias and prolonged neonatal dependence on total parenteral nutrition occasionally lead to gallstone formation. With the exception of altered port placement, cholecystectomy is performed in an identical fashion to that in adults. Age presents no limitation to the laparoscopic approach. I have performed laparoscopic cholecystectomy in children as young as 8 months of age. One's approach to the performance of intraoperative cholangiography depends to a great extent on the availability of personnel experienced and capable of performing endoscopic retrograde cholangiopancreatography (ERCP) and sphincterotomy in pediatric patients. I generally do not perform cholangiograms without a specific indication, because I can generally clear the common bile duct preoperatively or postoperatively by ERCP.

However, in institutions in which such expertise is not available, intraoperative cholangiography is more frequently performed [2]. Experience in laparoscopic choledochoscopy and common bile duct exploration in children is limited, but developing.

Laparoscopic-guided percutaneous cholangiography can be performed through the gallbladder, if present, in infants who are jaundiced and in whom the diagnosis of biliary atresia is considered. A normal cholangiogram establishing patency of the biliary ducts can avoid an otherwise routinely performed laparotomy in this situation. A liver biopsy can be obtained simultaneously.

Appendectomy

Appendectomy is performed laparoscopically by many surgeons. I perform most appendectomies in small patients through a standard incision, because a thin patient generally requires an incision of only 2 to 3 cm. Postoperative pain, return to normal diet, and hospital discharge are not different between the two approaches. I reserve laparoscopy for obese patients, who would otherwise require a significantly larger incision, or patients with a diagnostic dilemma. In particular, laparoscopy

facilitates simultaneous evaluation for potential pelvic pathology in adolescent girls with a history and physical examination that deem exploration, but are not classic for acute appendicitis.

Splenectomy

Laparoscopic splenectomy can be performed at any age. Again, careful consideration must be given to appropriate port placement. This is particularly challenging in a very small child with a large spleen. In such a case, most of the ports must be placed as inferiorly as possible, often approaching the groins. I have found the harmonic scalpel to be of great utility in dividing the short gastric vessels and the splenic peritoneal attachments. It is narrower than a linear stapling device, facilitating division of the very small highest short gastric vessels. In addition, its working length is significantly shorter than a stapler, making it easier to place and observe in the small field of dissection in a younger child. However, I do prefer to use the stapler to divide the splenic artery and vein.

Gastric fundoplication

As in adults, gastric fundoplication is frequently performed laparoscopically in children without age limitation. A standard Nissen fundoplication with a single row of sutures securing the wrapped stomach anterior to the esophagus can be performed satisfactorily in this matter. However, I prefer to place three vertical rows of sutures, with the additional two rows securing the wrapped stomach to the esophagus in the left and right posterolateral positions. In addition, after completing a wrap, I place another row of sutures securing the right side of the wrapped fundus down to the right crus of the diaphragm. I believe this more extensive procedure provides significantly greater protection from long-term slippage or disruption of the wrap [3]. Current intracorporeal suturing techniques prohibit the timely performance of this procedure laparoscopically, which requires the placement of over 25 sutures. I currently believe that the long-term advantages of a fundoplication with multiple rows of sutures outweigh the benefits of a minimally invasive approach, and thus I continue to perform the operation through an open incision.

Esophagomyotomy

Esophageal achalasia uncommonly presents in childhood. However, esophagomyotomy has been performed in children both laparoscopically and thoracoscopically. I prefer the thoracic approach because it does not disrupt the gastric attachments near the angle of His, which may theoretically lead to less postoperative gastroesophageal reflux. I have performed this procedure on children as young as 8 years of age, with excellent results.

Pulmonary resection

Primary malignancies of the lung are exceedingly rare in childhood. However, thoracoscopic pulmonary wedge resection is frequently performed for diagnosis and resection of metastatic malignant nodules. Diagnostic biopsies are also performed for diffuse inflammatory and infectious processes. Complete resection of a congenital cystic adenomatoid malformation of the lung can be performed. In addition, pulmonary sequestrations have been resected thoracoscopically. It is important to specifically identify and secure systemic vessels supplying a sequestration. Thoracoscopic exploration in otherwise healthy teenagers with recurrent spontaneous pneumothoraces usually reveals pulmonary blebs. These are most frequently found in the uppermost portion of the superior segment of the lower lobes or the apex of the upper lobes. Chemical or mechanical pleurodesis or pleurectomy can be performed simultaneously.

Empyema débridement

Empyema resulting from infection of parapneumonic effusions is relatively common in children. Although antibiotic administration, thoracentesis, and chest tube drainage are often effective therapy, there has been a recent trend toward early thoracoscopic evaluation, evacuation, irrigation, débridement of loculations, and chest tube insertion [4]. Early cleansing of the pleural space has led to fewer recurrent or persistent infections and earlier discharge from hospitalization. The need for repetitive thoracenteces and multiple chest tube insertions into loculated cavities has also been alleviated.

Nephrectomy

Wilms' tumors, the most common solid organ tumors of childhood, generally present as very large renal masses and are removed through standard open surgical techniques. However, laparoscopic nephrectomy by either transperitoneal or retroperitoneal approaches is becoming more popular for the removal of multicystic dysplastic kidneys and nonfunctioning kidneys associated with hydronephrosis.

Diagnostic laparoscopic exploration

Diagnostic laparoscopic exploration is useful for indications similar to those in adulthood. These indications include abdominal trauma and chronic and acute abdominal pain.

SPECIFIC PEDIATRIC CONCERNS
Inguinal hernias

In contrast to adult herniorrhaphy, pediatric inguinal herniorrhaphy is almost always performed through a standard incision. Pediatric groin hernias are almost exclusively indirect, require a

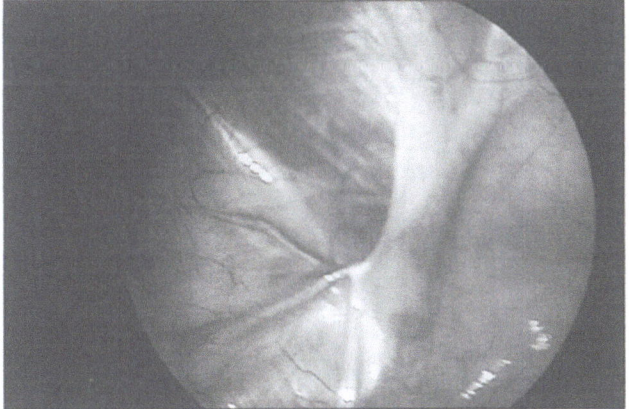

Figure 14-1 Left inguinal hernia viewed laparoscopically with telescope inserted through open right inguinal hernia sac. (*See* Color Plate.)

very small incision in the groin crease, are brief in duration, and cause minimal postoperative discomfort. There would be no significant benefit to performing standard pediatric inguinal herniorrhaphies laparoscopically. Conversely, manipulation or insertion of prosthetic material near the vas deferens and testicular vessels might risk future fertility. In addition, unnecessary incisions in the peritoneum may result in small bowel obstruction, which does not occur after standard inguinal herniorrhaphy. It is reasonable, however, to repair a hernia discovered incidentally in a female patient during laparoscopy performed for another reason. This can be performed by inverting and ligating or clipping the patent processus vaginalis.

Bilateral inguinal hernias are extremely common in infants and young children. It has long been common practice for many pediatric surgeons to perform a contralateral groin incision for exploration after repairing an inguinal hernia. If a contralateral hernia is found, it is then repaired. Although laparoscopy has been of little utility in repairing pediatric inguinal hernias, it has gained widespread popularity in the evaluation of the contralateral groin at the time of herniorrhaphy. This is generally performed through the open hernia sac during repair of the clinically apparent hernia. After separation of the clinically apparent hernia sac from the vital spermatic cord structures up to the level of the internal ring, the sac is opened. A moistened small flexible catheter is advanced through the sac into the peritoneal cavity. Carbon dioxide is insufflated through this catheter. I generally maintain an airtight seal by holding the sac between my thumb and forefinger. Others prefer to place a pursestring suture in the sac prior to passing the catheter. A moistened telescope without a sheath is advanced through the sac into the peritoneal cavity. The insufflation catheter can be removed prior to passing a telescope, but I find that leaving it in place often facilitates passage of the rigid telescope by holding the neck of the sac open. I use a 4-F 70°-angled telescope. In almost all cases, the internal structures of the contralateral groin can be seen well. In infants, it is helpful to empty the urinary bladder with manual suprapubic pressure after the induction of anesthesia, but prior to beginning the operation. Otherwise, the full bladder may make visualization of the contralateral groin difficult. The presence of a patent processus vaginalis is easily determined (Fig. 14-1), although there is generally a small flap of peritoneum that can overlie even a closed processus (Fig. 14-2A). An angled telescope makes visualization beyond this flap possible. In addition, gentle pressure on the groin externally will assist in visualizing this region in its entirety (Fig. 14-2B). Insufflation of the peritoneal cavity and palpation of the contralateral groin for air alone, without telescopic visualization, yields surprisingly inaccurate evaluation of the contralateral groin. Telescopic visualization should always be performed for certainty. In a series of 518 patients with a clinically apparent unilateral inguinal hernia and an unknown status of the contralateral groin, Holcomb and coworkers [5••] found a contralateral patent processus vaginalis in 47% of children under 1 year of age and 37% of children over 1 year of age. Identifying clinically inapparent contralateral hernias allows for the performance of bilateral herniorrhaphy, avoiding the need for future procedures. Excluding the presence of a contralateral hernia avoids unnecessary open groin exploration in those whose explorations would prove to be negative.

Identification and management of the undescended testicle

Approximately one in four boys with an incompletely descended testicle will have no palpable testicle in the scrotum or groin on physical examination in the office. In the prelaparoscopic era, imaging was often used to determine the existence or location of a nonpalpable testicle. In cases of bilateral nonpalpable testicles, hormonal studies are often used to determine whether testicles are present, although it is difficult to definitively establish the diagnosis of anorchia on this basis. Open groin and retroperitoneal exploration was generally used to definitively determine whether a testicle was present and to relocate it into the scrotum, if found. Management of the nonpalpable testicle has been simplified by diagnostic laparoscopy and laparoscopic orchiopexy. All children should be examined under anesthesia prior to performance of laparoscopy, because occasionally a testicle that is nonpalpable in the office can be identified in the inguinal canal under anesthesia. Palpable, but incompletely descended testicles, are best handle by standard orchiopexy using a groin incision.

A clear liquid diet for 24 hours and a single suppository are provided prior to laparoscopic exploration for an intra-abdominal testicle and potential orchiopexy. A urinary catheter and rectal tube are placed to decompress the bladder and bowel to maximize visualization of the pelvis and retroperitoneum. A 2- or 5-mm telescope is placed through an umbilical laparoscopic port. The structures in the region of the internal inguinal ring are carefully examined. Comparison to the normal side in cases of unilateral undescended testicle is often helpful. An intra-abdominal testis is usually easily identified (Fig. 14-3); however, nonvisualization on initial examination demands further investigation. If the testicle is not seen near the internal ring, it may be found higher in the pelvis, behind the colon, or anywhere in the retroperitoneum along the expected course of the testicular vessels. To definitively determine the existence and location of a testis, the vas deferens and spermatic vessels must be identified. A child can be concluded to have a "vanishing testis," probably resulting from *in utero* torsion, only if the spermatic vessels and vas deferens are seen to fade away as they converge on the internal inguinal ring (Fig. 14-4). If the vas

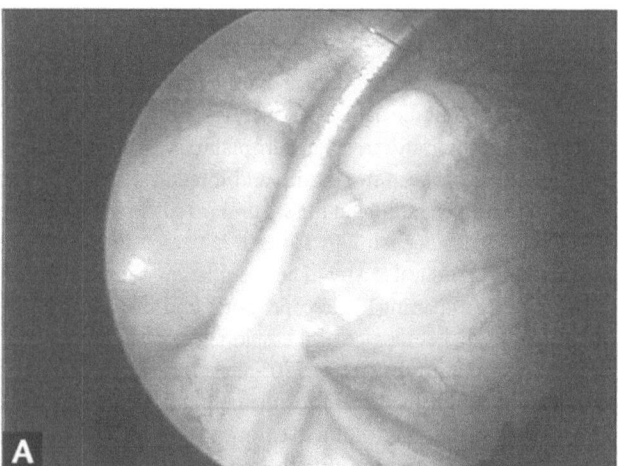

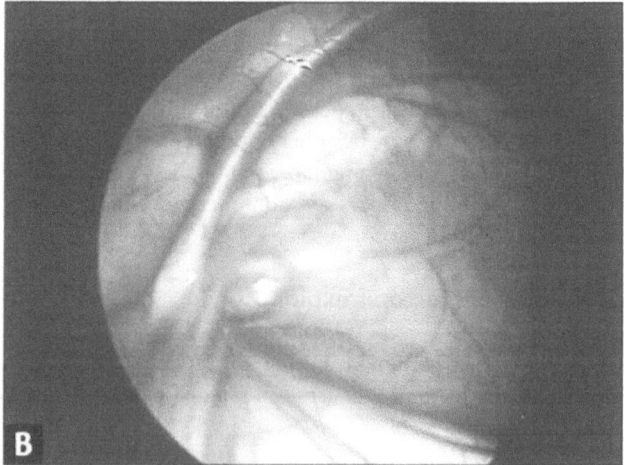

Figure 14-2 Laparoscopic examination for contralateral inguinal hernia. **A,** Laparoscopic view of right groin through left inguinal hernia sac. Peritoneal flap just lateral to inferior epigastric vessels giving the suggestion of an indirect hernia. **B,** External digital pressure over the deep inguinal ring deflects peritoneal flap, confirming the absence of a hernia. (*See* Color Plates.)

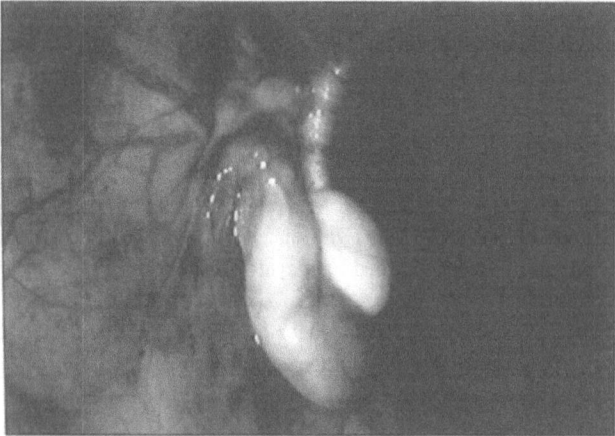

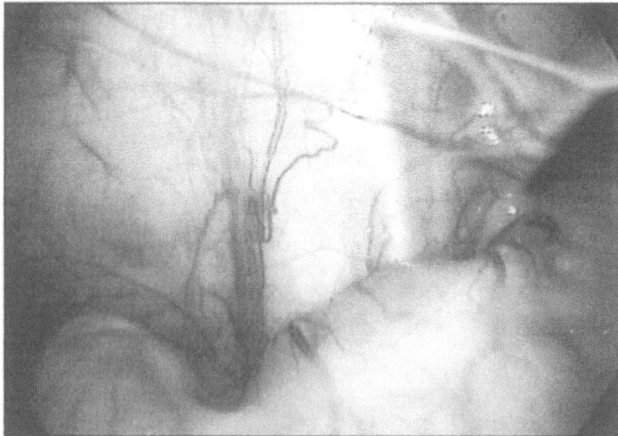

Figure 14-3 Intra-abdominal nonpalpable testicle. (Courtesy of Dr. Craig Peters. *From* Moore *et al.* [16]; with permission.)

Figure 14-4 Fading spermatic vessels and vas deferens converging on a "vanishing testicle." (Courtesy of Dr. Craig Peters. *From* Peters and Kavoussi [6••]; with permission.)

deferens and spermatic vessels exit the internal ring, inguinal exploration by incision should be performed to determine whether there is a viable testicle or small testicular remnant. A viable testicle should be relocated to the scrotum and a diminutive testicular nubbin removed.

Once an intra-abdominal testicle is identified, the decision must be made whether to perform a primary laparoscopic orchiopexy with intact spermatic vessels or to divide the spermatic vessels to mobilize the testicle in a Fowler-Stephens fashion. Peters and Kavoussi [6••] found that under the age of 3 years, testes located 2.5 cm or less cephalad to the peritoneal ring can be mobilized into the scrotum with the spermatic vessels intact. Higher testicles are more likely to require division of the testicular vessels and a Fowler-Stephens orchiopexy. Older children are also more likely to require a Fowler-Stephens procedure.

Once an intra-abdominal testicle is identified, operative ports are placed depending on the size of the patient and location of the testicle. For small children, an ipsilateral subcostal port in the midclavicular line is generally placed. Another is placed in the contralateral midclavicular line at the level of the anterior superior iliac spine. For a primary orchiopexy with intact spermatic vessels, the testicle is mobilized from its gubernacular attachments upward. The peritoneum lateral to the spermatic vessels is incised as high as possible. The peritoneum inferomedial to the vas deferens is then similarly incised, thus allowing mobilization of a triangular flap bounded by the vessels superiorly and vas deferens inferiorly from the lateral pelvic side wall. Additional length can be obtained on the vascular pedicle by then dividing the triangular peritoneum between the vas deferens and the vessels (Fig. 14-5). A tract through which the testicle will be passed into the scrotum is created by dissecting just over the pubic tubercle, medial to the obliterated umbilical artery, until the instrument advances into the scrotum. A standard dartos pouch is then created through a small dependent scrotal incision. Holding sutures, which will later be used to secure the testicle to the dartos, are placed. The instrument in the scrotum is then advanced through an incision in the dartos between the holding sutures. A 5-mm cannula is advanced over the tip of the instrument protruding out the

bottom of the scrotum and then further advanced up through the tunnel and into the peritoneal cavity. The mobilized testicle is then grasped through this port and the sheath and testicle withdrawn out through the new canal and the bottom of the scrotum. The testicle is then secured in the dartos pouch in a standard fashion.

A laparoscopic Fowler-Stephens orchiopexy is generally performed in two stages. It is preferable to avoid mobilization of the testicle during the first stage, in which the testicular vessels are clipped in continuity slightly above the testicle. An interval of approximately 6 months allows maturation of the collateral vasal circulation to the testicle. During the second stage of the procedure, the testicular vessels are transected and the testicle mobilized on a broad pedicle of peritoneum around the vas deferens. The testicle is then brought down into the scrotum in a similar fashion to that of a primary orchiopexy.

Meckel's diverticulectomy

A Meckel's diverticulum, whether diagnosed preoperatively or discovered incidentally at laparoscopy, can often be removed with ease. Any attachment to the umbilicus should be detached. The vitelline artery or its remnant running from the mesentery to the diverticulum should be divided to allow the Meckel's diverticulum to hang freely from the antimesenteric surface of the ileum. Gentle compression and palpation of the diverticulum with laparoscopic instruments can usually demonstrate a "step-off" between the thick gastric mucosa in the diverticulum, if present, and the thinner intestinal epithelium. If there is no gastric mucosa, or all gastric mucosa can be included with the specimen, a linear stapler can be applied across the base of the diverticulum (Fig. 14-6). The ileum should be carefully inspected to ensure that the staple line has not caused any narrowing. The excised specimen must be opened and carefully examined to ensure that all gastric mucosa has in fact been removed. If the configuration of the diverticulum or prominent gastric mucosa prevents excision with a stapler, open or laparoscopic-assisted techniques may be used to perform a wedge excision of the antimesenteric surface of the bowel or a segmental small bowel resection.

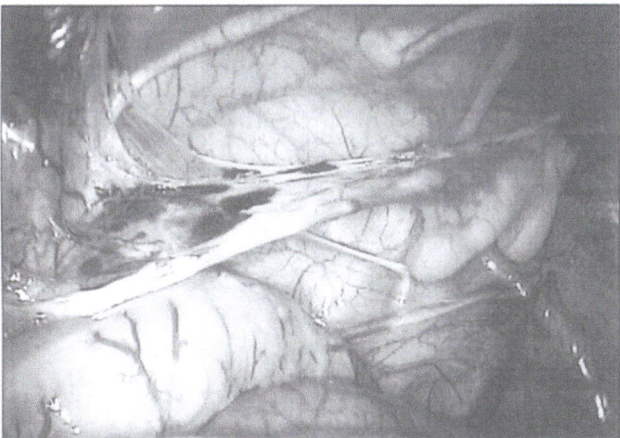

Figure 14-5 Intra-abdominal testicle mobilized on testicular vessels and vas deferens. (Courtesy of Dr. Craig Peters. *From* Peters [17]; with permission.)

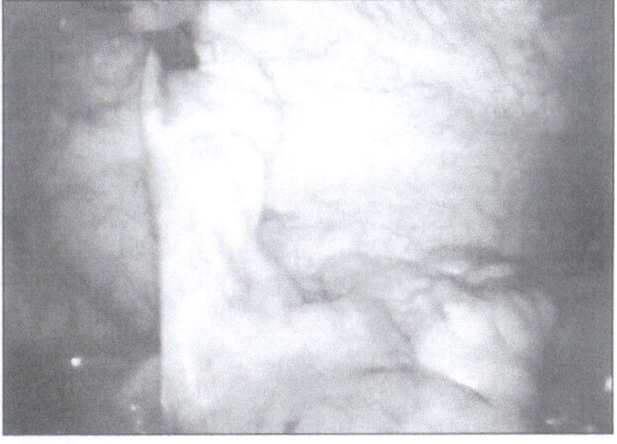

Figure 14-6 Positioning of a Meckel's diverticulum for amputation with a linear stapler. (*See* Color Plate.)

Coloanal pull-through for Hirschsprung's disease

The three most popular types of coloanal pull-through procedures for Hirschsprung's disease have all been modified for minimally invasive approaches. In the laparoscopic Swenson procedure, the colorectum is mobilized down to the anus laparoscopically and the full thickness of the bowel everted through the anus. The everted bowel is opened at the level of proposed anastomosis and the proximal ganglionic bowel pulled through from below for anastomosis [7]. In the laparoscopic Duhamel procedure, the colorectal mobilization is also performed laparoscopically and anastomosis performed in a transanal fashion to the posterior aspect of the residual native anorectal stump [8]. Georgeson and coworkers [9•] elegantly modified the Soave endorectal pull-through. In this procedure, the necessary length of colon is mobilized laparoscopically, dividing the blood supply as necessary. A transanal circumferential mucosal incision is performed 5 to 10 mm above the dentate line. A submucosal dissection is then performed proximally up the rectum while maintaining traction on the mucosal tube. The submucosal dissection is extended until the level of the laparoscopic rectal mobilization is met. The muscular sleeve is transected at this point, allowing the proximal colon to be pulled through the distal rectal muscular sleeve, which has been stripped of its mucosa. Importantly, the residual rectal sleeve is incised vertically posteriorly to allow the colon to be pulled through without constriction. A full-thickness frozen section rectal biopsy is performed to confirm the presence of ganglion cells at the level of proposed anastomosis. The colon is then transected above the biopsy site and a hand-sewn anastomosis of the colon performed to the anus at the level of the transected mucosa just above the dentate line. In experienced hands, this operation takes no longer than a standard Soave operation performed by laparotomy. It can be performed at any age, including in the newborn.

Ovarian procedures

Ovarian torsion can be suspected on history and physical examination, but is difficult to confirm or exclude radiographically or ultrasonographically. Laparoscopy allows for rapid definitive diagnosis. Detorsion and oophoropexy, as well as a contralateral oophoropexy, if desired, can be performed simply. Many surgeons are now choosing to detorse almost all ovaries, regardless of their appearance, however, an oophorectomy may be performed laparoscopically if desired. Although many ovarian masses in children are massive, the smaller benign lesions can be dissected from the ovary and excised laparoscopically.

Ventriculoperitoneal cerebrospinal fluid shunt placement

Although the distal end of most ventriculoperitoneal cerebrospinal fluid shunts can be placed through a small abdominal incision without intraperitoneal visualization, laparoscopy can be useful in patients who have had previous abdominal operations or multiple previous shunts, obliterating portions of the free peritoneal cavity. An appropriate portion of the peritoneal cavity can be identified or created and the shunt tubing passed through a percutaneously inserted peel-away sheath after the shunt tubing has been tunneled down from the head in the subcutaneous plane (Fig. 14-7). Disconnected shunt tubing can also be easily removed laparoscopically [10].

Pyloromyotomy

Rammstedt pyloromyotomy for hypertrophic pyloric stenosis in infants has been performed for decades through a very small incision in the upper abdomen or umbilicus. This operation can be performed laparoscopically [11]. Very few pediatric surgeons have chosen to adopt this technique because it provides little improvement in postoperative course or scarring, and the experience to date is too limited to be certain that the extremely high rates of safety and efficacy in the open technique are maintained with a minimally invasive approach.

Correction of intestinal malrotation

Ladd's procedure to reorient the bowel in children with intestinal rotation and fixation abnormalities is designed to minimize the incidence and recurrence of midgut volvulus. This procedure, which involves division of the retroperitoneal

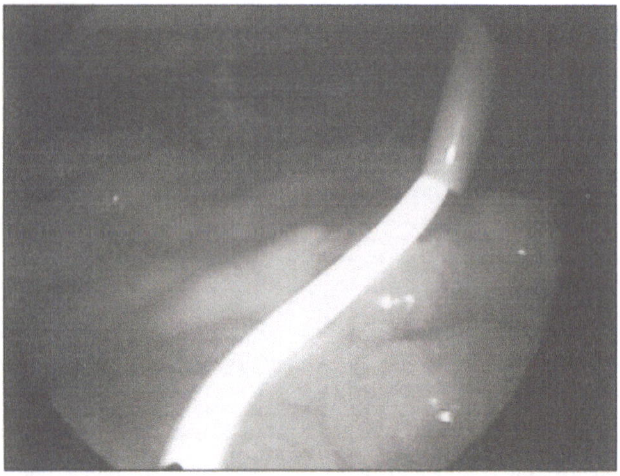

Figure 14-7 Distal end of ventriculoperitoneal shunt inserted through peel-away sheath. (*See* Color Plate.)

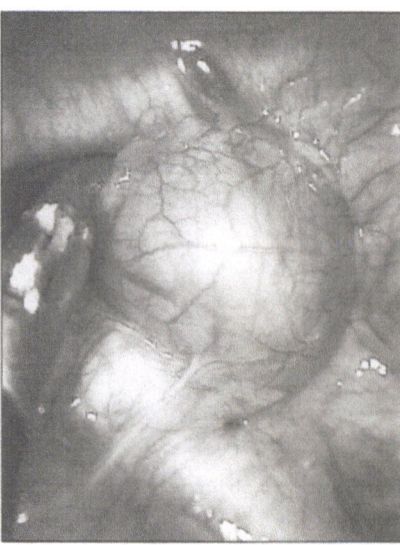

Figure 14-8 Apical mediastinal mass excised thoracoscopically. Histologic examination revealed benign ganglioneuroma. (*See* Color Plate.)

attachments of the duodenum and proximal colon and reorientation of the small bowel and colon, has been performed laparoscopically [12]. It is unlikely that the laparoscopic Ladd's procedure will gain widespread popularity. Many pediatric surgeons believe that the success of Ladd's procedure depends on the formation of intra-abdominal adhesions to prevent midgut volvulus.

Mediastinal masses

Many pediatric mediastinal masses can be approached for biopsy or excision thoracoscopically. Bronchogenic, esophageal duplication, thymic, and pericardial cysts have all been removed thoracoscopically. Mediastinal lymph nodes can be biopsied or excised for tissue diagnosis. Small teratomas and neurogenic tumors can also be approached thoracoscopically (Fig. 14-8).

Division of patent ductus arteriosis and vascular rings

Thoracoscopic techniques have now been used to divide a patent ductus arteriosis in children of all sizes, including small premature newborns [13]. Vascular rings causing extrinsic tracheoesophageal compression have also been divided thoracoscopically or by video-assisted thoracotomy in cases requiring division of patent vascular structures [14]. Caution must be exercised to identify and protect the recurrent laryngeal nerve in performing these procedures. In addition, enthusiasm to perform these procedures using minimally invasive techniques must not override the primary concern of patient safety. Divided patent vascular structures must be oversewn rather than clipped to avoid potentially fatal hemorrhage.

Correction of spinal deformities

Scoliosis requiring excision of intervertebral disks and posterior spinal fixation has traditionally been performed by open thoracotomy followed by posterior spinal exposure. The thoracotomy can be avoided by performing the disk excisions thoracoscopically [15].

Multiple segmental disks can be removed. In children with severe spinal curves, I find it helpful to spread the ports as much as possible to allow nearly perpendicular access to each disk space, regardless of its orientation to the curve. The upper- and lower-most ports should be placed under thoracoscopic vision to ensure safe access, avoiding injuries below the diaphragm or in the thoracic inlet. The diskectomies can be performed without dividing the segmental intercostal vessels. If division is desired, the use of a harmonic scalpel is preferable to clips, which are easily dislodged during disk manipulation. The mid- and upper-thoracic spine can be approached in a retropleural thoracoscopic fashion. The advantage of this technique is to prevent the dislodgment of bone allograft, which may be used for vertebral fusion, into the pleural space. It is difficult but not impossible to continue a retropleural dissection to the level of the diaphragm. Thoracoscopic exposure can be augmented by retroperitoneal exposure of the lumbar spine for extensive curves.

REFERENCES AND RECOMMENDED READING

Recently published papers of particular interest have been highlighted as:

- •   Of interest
- •• Of outstanding interest

1.• Holtzman RS: Special considerations of anesthesia for endo-urologic procedures and laparoscopy in children. In *Smith's Textbook of Endourology*. Edited by Smith AD. St. Louis: Quality Medical Publishing; 1996:1293–1306.
Reviews anesthetic considerations for pediatric laparoscopy.

2. Holcomb GW III, Sharp KW, Neblett WW III, *et al.*: Laparoscopic cholecystectomy in infants and children: modifications and cost analysis. *J Pediatr Surg* 1994, 29:1900–1904.

3. Price MR, Janik JS, Wayne ER, *et al.*: Modified Nissen fundoplication for reduction of fundoplication failure. *J Pediatr Surg* 1997, 32:324–326.

4. Stovroff M, Teague G, Heiss KF, *et al.*: Thoracoscopy in the management of pediatric empyema. *J Pediatr Surg* 1995, 30:1211–1215.

5.•• Holcomb GW III, Morgan WM III, Brock JW III: Laparoscopic evaluation for contralateral patent processus vaginalis: part two. *J Pediatr Surg* 1996, 31:1170–1173.
This large series of laparoscopic contralateral groin exploration during inguinal herniorrhaphy demonstrates the ease and utility of this technique. It also highlights the poor reliability of peritoneal insufflation alone. Forty-one percent of over 500 pediatric patients were demonstrated to have clinically inapparent contralateral inguinal hernias.

6.•• Peters CA, Kavoussi LR: Laparoscopy in children and adults. In *Campbell's Urology*, edn 7. Edited by Walsh PC, Retik AB, Vaughan ED Jr., Wein AJ. Philadelphia: WB Saunders Company; 1997:2875–2911.
A clear and thorough review of the history, indications, technique, and outcome of laparoscopic exploration and orchiopexy for nonpalpable testicles.

7. Curran TJ, Raffensperger JG: Laparoscopic Swenson pull-through: a comparison with the open procedure. *J Pediatr Surg* 1996, 31:1155–1156.

8. Smith BM, Steiner RB, Lobe TE: Laparoscopic Duhamel pullthrough procedure for Hirschsprung's disease in childhood. *J Laparoendosc Surg* 1994, 4:273–276.

9.• Georgeson KE, Fuenfer MM, Hardin WD: Primary laparoscopic pull-through for Hirschsprung's disease in infants and children. *J Pediatr Surg* 1995, 30:1017–1022.
Excellent description and illustration of a laparoscopic modified anorectal mucosectomy and endorectal coloanal pull-through.

10. Holcomb GW III, Smith AP: Laparoscopic and thoracoscopic assistance with CSF shunts in children. *J Pediatr Surg* 1995, 30:1642–1643.

11. Alain JL, Grousseaud D, Longis B, *et al.*: Extramucosal pylorotomy by laparotomy. *Eur J Pediatr Surg* 1996, 6:10–12.

12. Gross E, Chen MK, Lobe TE: Laparoscopic evaluation and treatment of intestinal malrotation in infants. *Surg Endosc* 1996, 10:936–937.

13. Burke RP: Video-assisted thoracoscopic surgery for patent ductus arteriosis. *Pediatrics* 1994, 93:823–825.

14. Burke RP, Rosenfeld HM, Wernovsky G, *et al.*: Video-assisted thoracoscopic vascular ring division in infants and children. *J Am Coll Cardiol* 1995, 25:943–947.

15. Holcomb GW III, Mencio GA, Green NE: Video-assisted thoracoscopic diskectomy and fusion. *J Pediatr Surg* 1997, 32:1120–1122.

16. Moore RG, Peters CA, Bauer SB, *et al.*: Laparoscopic evaluation of the nonpalpable testis: a prospective assessment of accuracy. *J Urol* 1994, 151:728–731.

17. Peters CA: Laparascopy in pediatric urology: challenge and opportunity. *Semin Pediatr Surg* 1996, 5:16–22.

Thoracoscopy and Video-assisted Thoracic Surgery

Michael T. Jaklitsch
Raja M. Flores
Malcolm M. DeCamp, Jr.

Thoracoscopy was first described by Jacobeus [1] in 1910, when he used an electrically illuminated cystoscope to lyse adhesions within the pleural space in the application of collapse therapy for tuberculosis. The mediastinoscope inserted into the pleural space was substituted for the cystoscope by several generations of thoracic surgeons prior to the current technologic revolution. These early instruments, however, were hampered by poor lighting and optics, which limited applications to pleural biopsies, drainage of effusions, and lysis of pleural adhesions [1–3].

The level of thoracoscopic sophistication achieved in the 1990s has been the result of several overlapping technologies: improved lighting with fiberoptic cables, video projection of the telescopic image to a television screen, improved stapling and dissection instruments, standardized use of single-lung ventilation anesthesia, and preoperative chest CT and magnetic resonance imaging (MRI) to guide the placement of incisions. With the advent of video cameras and projected images, all members of the surgical team can simultaneously see through the thoracoscope and participate in the operation [4]. Benign and malignant disease can now be diagnosed and treated within the lungs, pleural spaces, pericardium, mediastinum, and diaphragm with minimally invasive techniques [5•]. The goal of all thoracoscopic procedures is to obtain diagnostic tissue and treat intrathoracic disease while minimizing the amount of soft tissue destruction, and thus operative morbidity. The experience gained with these techniques has dramatically expanded their application to thoracic illness, and has led to common use of a more descriptive term: *video-assisted thoracic surgery* (VATS) [6].

This chapter highlights basic concepts in the application of minimally invasive surgery to specific thoracic diseases. We have found the indications for VATS techniques to be expanding, and thus have added lung volume reduction techniques and diaphragmatic repair techniques. Additionally, we have tried to add some of the refinements in previous techniques that have become standard within our operating room. Minimally invasive techniques have brought a modern revolution in surgical procedures to general thoracic surgery, and patients have reaped the rewards.

GENERAL PRINCIPLES

The bony thoracic cage consists of the vertebral bodies and pedicles, 12 thoracic ribs, and the sternum. For conceptual purposes, the cavity of each hemithorax can be thought of as a triangular-based pyramid. One vertex is at the apex, one vertex at the junction of the anterior rib cage with the anterior mediastinum, one vertex at the junction of the posterior rib cage and mediastinum, and one vertex at the lateral insertion of the diaphragm to the ribs in the midaxillary line. This structure creates the diaphragmatic, mediastinal, anterior, and posterior faces of the pyramid.

CHAPTER

15

Port access to the pyramid is generally limited to the anterior and posterior faces. Access through the thoracic inlet is prevented by the overlying clavicle, subclavian vessels, and brachial plexus. Access through the diaphragmatic base is possible through subcostal incisions or low thoracic interspace incisions, but there is a risk of injury to intraperitoneal structures, and perforation of the diaphragm may be required. Additionally, the overlying scapula limits port access through the posterolateral region of the first four interspaces.

Each rib is an arch of bone with a posterior joint on both the vertebral body and pedicle of each thoracic vertebrae. The first five ribs attach separately to the bony sternum with a separate costal cartilage. The costal cartilages of the sixth to 10th ribs fuse together to create the anterior costal margin. The 11th and 12th ribs do not have an anterior attachment and are referred to as "floating ribs." Each intercostal space is asymmetric, with a wider interspace at the anterior costocartilagenous junction and a tighter interspace at the posterior costovertebral junction. The widest space between ribs is typically the anterior fourth interspace, followed by the anterior fifth and third interspaces [7].

All VATS procedures should be performed in a setting that allows rapid conversion to standard open thoracotomy. This setting includes appropriate anesthesia and thoracic surgical personnel and instruments. Specifically, a full complement of open thoracotomy instruments as well as specialized thoracoscopic instruments need to be readily available. Limited incisions prevent quick control of the lung hilum and great vessels of the mediastinum, and the surgeon must always be prepared for an emergency thoracotomy.

There should be at least one video monitor that is positioned to allow a clear field of vision for all members of the operative team. We prefer the use of two monitors positioned to allow clear vision without body contortion of the surgeon or assistants.

The type of endotracheal intubation can be individualized. Pleuroscopic procedures such as drainage of large parapneumonic effusions, pleural biopsies, and lysis of pleural adhesions frequently can be accomplished with a single-lumen endotracheal tube. Resections of lung parenchyma and proper visualization of mediastinal structures generally require single-lung ventilation with either a double-lumen endotracheal tube or bronchial blocker. Our preference for a left-sided double-lumen endotracheal tube for both right and left procedures is based on the increased length and decreased diameter of the left main bronchus. The geometry of the left main bronchus facilitates tube placement and decreases the likelihood of tube displacement during positioning of the patient into the lateral decubitus position. Further, it decreases the chance of unintentional occlusion of the right upper lobe orifice, which is typically 2 cm from the carina. If intubation with a double-lumen endotracheal tube is difficult, a 5-mL vascular embolectomy catheter can serve as a bronchial blocker. Positioning of both the double-lumen tube and the bronchial blocker is confirmed by flexible bronchoscopy.

The majority of port positions are confined to either the anterior axillary, midaxillary, or posterior axillary lines. For this reason, the patient is generally placed in a full lateral decubitus position. Legs are padded with pillows and the hips secured to the table with 4-inch tape. A dependent axillary roll is placed to prevent undue stretch on the brachial plexus of the contralateral arm. We use two rolls pulled tight beneath the patient to produce a convex lateral border to the ipsilateral hemithorax. This enlarges each intercostal space. Alternatively, the operating table can be broken at the midthorax with the head and feet lower than the midportion of the chest. A concave thorax will narrow the intercostal spaces, hinder port placement, and increase the likelihood of an intercostal neuralgia postoperatively.

Access to all intercostal spaces is possible when the patient is properly prepped and draped. A single port in the anterior fifth intercostal space may be sufficient for pleural procedures. Two ports with a double-instrument port in the anterior fifth intercostal space and an accessory port in the mid or posterior axillary line can be successful in wedge resections of the lateral and apical portions of the lung. In general, three or more ports are required for other thoracic surgical procedures. Regional intercostal nerve blocks with 0.5% bupivacaine with epinephrine should include the interspace above and below each port placement.

Initial port placement is performed sharply, usually in the seventh or eighth intercostal space in the midaxillary line. This port placement gives an excellent view of the majority of the hemithorax and makes a convenient chest-tube site with dependent drainage at the conclusion of the operation. The dome of the diaphragm is an anterior structure, and ports anterior to the anterior axillary line and below the fifth intercostal space may prove to be beneath the diaphragm.

If using single-lung ventilation, the operative lung is deflated during the prepping and draping of the patient. Incision is with a scalpel. An O-ring forcep placed within the wound retracts the skin and subcutaneous fat and exposes the underlying muscle. Dissection is then carried straight down to the underlying rib at a 90° angle to the course of the bone. The pleural space is entered with a finger inserted over the top of the rib to avoid injury to the intercostal neurovascular bundle and potentially adhesed lung tissue. A reuseable port with trocar is placed through the chest wall and the trocar removed. Room air is allowed to enter the chest through the hollow port. Unlike laparoscopy, the bony thorax precludes the need for insufflation of air to distend the soft tissues of the chest wall. No gas is insufflated into the chest, because this has been associated with hemodynamic instability [8]. Deflation of the lung is almost always possible with suction through the airway. If the pleural space is adhesed, an alternative port placement is attempted, or the procedure is converted to an open thoracotomy. If a free pleural space is entered, the 30° scope is inserted and the hemithorax is carefully inspected. This inspection includes the lung parenchyma for nodules, the parietal pleura for implants or plaques, the diaphragm position, and mediastinal abnormalities.

Additional port placement is generally in a triangular pattern, with each port occupying first-, second-, and third-base positions and the target lesion occupying home plate [9]. The trocar sites should be placed at a sufficient distance to achieve a panoramic view of the chest and prevent instrument crowding. Additional incisions in the chest wall are viewed directly with the camera to check hemostasis. A small amount of seepage of blood into the thorax can dramatically absorb light and affect the quality of the optical image.

The best panoramic view within the thorax is obtained with a 30° scope. In general, the surgeons manipulate the viewing scope with the nondominant hand and the stapler or dissector simultaneously with the dominant hand. The assistant "delivers" the lesion to the surgeon with the retracting instruments. We do not hesitate to move the video camera from port to port to gain a new angle of perspective on the dissection. All of our ports are open, hollow, reusable tubes.

A chest tube is generally inserted through the most dependent port at the conclusion of the procedure. The tube is placed to the apex under direct vision, to prevent a trapped pneumothorax at the apex of the lung when the patient is vertical. Each port site is inspected from within the chest to check for hemostasis. The chest is irrigated and aspirated of blood and pleural fluid. The lung is reinflated while visualized with the camera to check for regional atelectasis. Then each port is closed in three layers of absorbable suture: muscle, Scarpa's fascia, and skin. The chest tube port is partially closed around the tube.

LUNG DISEASE
Benign lung disease
Spontaneous pneumothorax

Spontaneous pneumothorax (SP) is a common clinical problem accounting for one in 100 hospital admissions. SP is considered primary if patients have no history of underlying lung pathology. Nearly all of these are the result of ruptured, subpleural bullae. A secondary SP is a nontraumatic pneumothorax in a patient with significant underlying lung pathology. In tertiary North American hospitals, 50% to 64% of SPs requiring treatment are secondary [10]. At our institution, 289 patients have required admission for SP in the past 7 years, representing one admission every 9 days. Smoking increases the risk of spontaneous pneumothorax 10- to 20-fold.

Although most primary SPs and up to half of secondary SPs may be managed nonoperatively with tube drainage with or without sclerosis, a substantial number of patients require operative intervention. We advocate surgery for all patients with an air leak persisting longer than 3 days, recurrent pneumothorax, history of bilateral or contralateral pneumothorax, or patients with incomplete lung expansion after drainage. The optimal surgical approach is a three-port thoracoscopic technique under single-lung anesthesia focused on the upper lobe and superior segment of the lower lobe (Fig. 15-1A–C). We routinely resect all visible bullae and perform a mechanical pleural abrasion (Fig. 15-2A,B). For patients with secondary SP—especially those taking corticosteroids, with significant immunodeficiency or altered wound healing—a parietal pleurectomy is also advocated to prevent recurrence. With this algorithm, the median postoperative hospital stay is 3 to 4 days with a 2% risk of recurrence.

Giant bullae

Emphysema is a major public health problem, afflicting at least 2 million Americans [11]. Whereas most of these patients have diffuse parenchymal destruction, a small subset suffer from dyspnea related to large or dominant bullae. These giant bullae can rapidly expand over weeks to months and cause compression of more normal functioning lung tissue.

Bullectomy accomplished via a standard thoracotomy has been the accepted approach to therapy for giant bullae for the past four decades [12]. The disadvantages of such a major intervention center on the morbidity of the incision in these patients with limited pulmonary reserve. Splinting secondary to excessive pain leads to an increased risk of postoperative respiratory failure that necessitates ventilatory support, which in turn engenders a substantial risk of prolonged postoperative air leak.

Based on these historical observations, we continue to advocate giant bullectomy for patients with dyspnea and documented compressive atelectasis, but prefer a thoracoscopic approach. Using a minimally invasive technique, we can limit postoperative pain and improve respiratory mechanics, thereby decreasing respiratory complications and postoperative length of stay [13•].

The operative approach to giant bullae requires a three-port technique similar to that used for thoracoscopic management of SP. Most dominant bullae involve the upper lobes, which require a midaxillary seventh intercostal space camera port, a second axillary port, and a third parascapular, posterior operating port. Patients with alpha$_1$-antitrypsin deficiency often develop basilar bullae. In this case, the port strategy is inverted with an axillary camera port and anterior and posterior basilar operating ports. When approaching basilar lesions, we prefer to place the video monitors at the patient's foot to avoid surgeon or assistant disorientation. The bulla is grasped at its apex and once controlled may require puncture to manipulate. Rolling the thin bullous tissue allows the surgeon to identify the critical area of transition from bulla to more normal lung tissue. Stapled resection with or without exogenous buttressing material is then performed at the transition zone. The more normal lung parenchyma holds staples better than the thin bullous tissue, thereby decreasing risk of prolonged air leak. We minimize manipulation of other aspects of the lung to avoid further disruption of the pleura. Most patients are extubated in the operating room at the conclusion of the procedure. Limiting the time of positive pressure ventilation helps minimize any postoperative air leak.

Lung volume reduction surgery

Surgical intervention to palliate dyspnea in patients with diffuse emphysema is an ongoing controversy. Several prominent centers have reported good results in highly selected patient groups undergoing lung volume reduction surgery via sternotomy [14] or thoracoscopy [15]. Whether these early results will endure and whether such intervention prolongs survival or is cost effective is the focus of a multicenter, nationwide trial cosponsored by the National Institutes of Health and the Healthcare Financing Administration.

Successful lung volume reduction surgery requires a motivated patient who can complete a course of preoperative cardiopulmonary rehabilitation. We prefer a thoracoscopic approach modeled after the approach to giant bullous disease. Stapled resection of poorly perfused, hyperinflated areas of lung is performed via three or four ports. We have reported our initial experience using the defunctionalized, bullous lung stapled

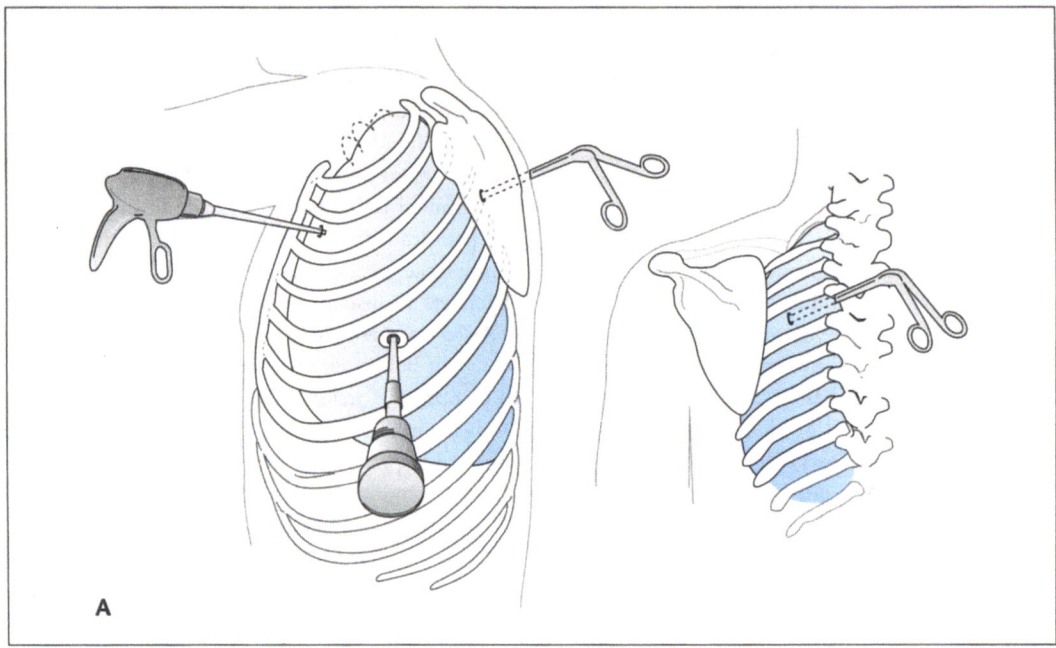

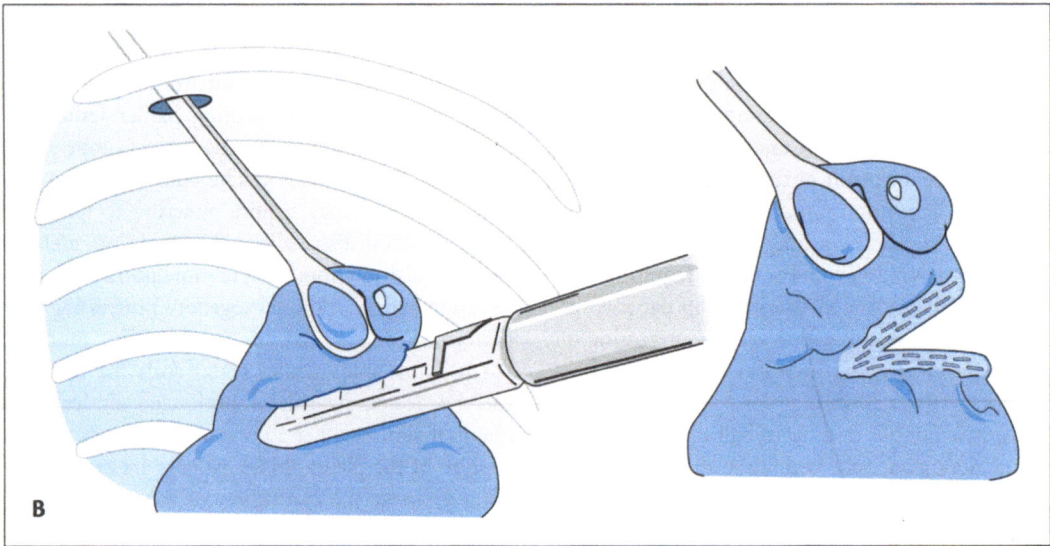

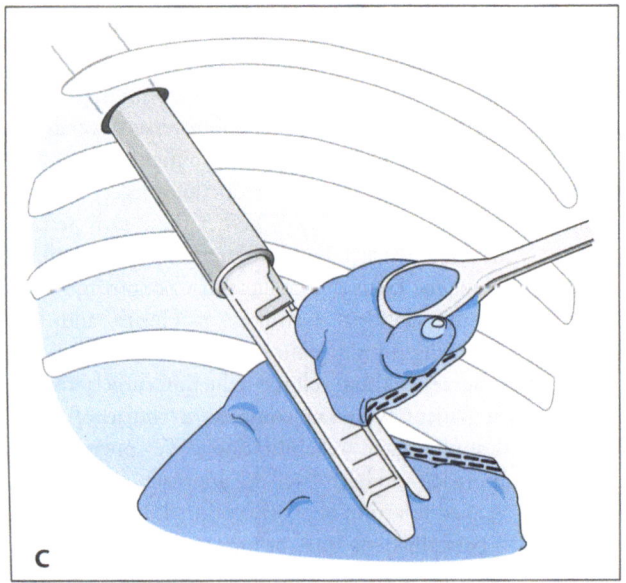

Figure 15-1 Operative approach to thoracoscopic bullectomy. **A,** The optimal surgical approach is a three-port technique under single-lung anesthesia focused on the upper lobe and superior segment of the lower lobe. **B,** Apical bullectomy is initiated using a ring forcep and an edoscopic stapler. **C,** The bullectomy is completed by exchanging the port positions of the forcep and stapler.

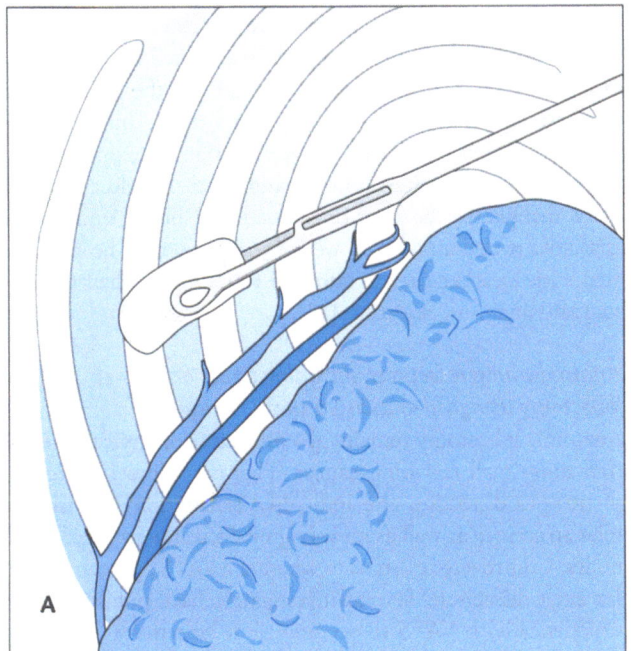
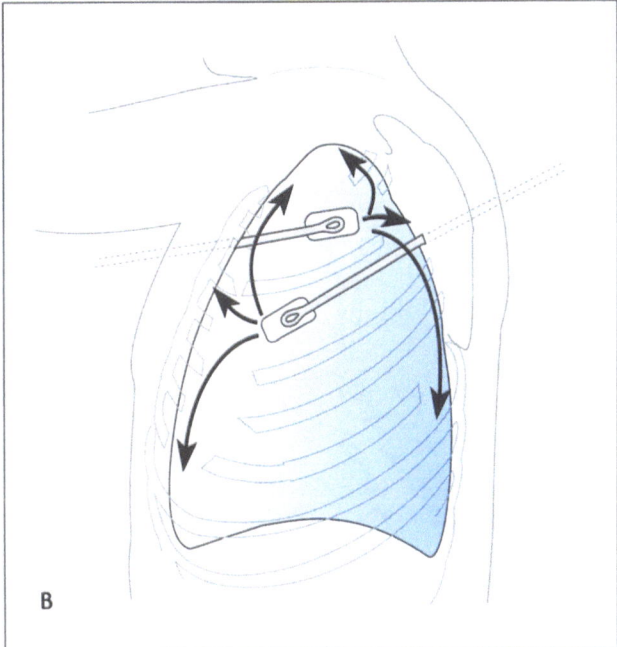

Figure 15-2 All visible bullae are rountinely resected, and a mechanical pleural abrasion is performed. **A** and **B**, Technique of mechanical pleurodesis.

to itself to form a plicated, autologous buttress. This plication allows us to avoid cutting the diseased bullous lung and appears to be an effective strategy to minimize postoperative air leak (Fig. 15-3)[16].

Interstitial lung disease

A wide variety of diseases may present as diffuse interstitial lung disease: infections, vasculopathies, allergic responses, pulmonary eosinophilia, disseminated neoplasm, radiation pneumonitis, and pulmonary fibrosis. Thoracoscopy and VATS are excellent methods of obtaining a diagnosis in many situations. However, prior to using these methods, lesser invasive means of establishing a diagnosis must be exhausted. Sputum induction, bronchoalveolar lavage (BAL), needle biopsy, and transbronchial biopsy in addition to a thorough clinical evaluation may lead to a definitive diagnosis, precluding the need for open or VATS biopsy. Once the differential diagnosis has been narrowed down to several possibilities, the necessity of histologic confirmation and the risk of the specific diagnostic procedure must be weighed against the risk of empiric treatment.

Vasculitic processes are quite difficult to assess bronchoscopically and are best diagnosed by thorascopic wedge biopsy. For other processes, a transbronchial biopsy should be considered before venturing to the operating room. If this is nondiagnostic or contraindicated (patients with coagulopathy or pulmonary hypertension), then an open or thoracoscopic biopsy is appropriate after a suppurative process is excluded by sputum analysis or BAL.

Sputum induction is a very simple and risk-free procedure that can be done at the bedside. It is useful in common bacterial infections, but is unrewarding on many occasions. BAL lavage is safe in patients who can withstand fiberoptic bronchoscopy. Pulmonary parenchymal diseases can be successfully diagnosed with this technique [17]. Transbronchial biopsy has a 59% diagnostic yield and is limited by small sample size and the patchy nature of many pulmonary diseases [18]. The risk of pneumothorax and hemorrhage is 5%. Cutting needle biopsy has a diagnostic yield varying from 52% to 89% [18]. The major complication is pneumothorax in up to 20% of cases.

Open lung biopsy has been the most reliable method of establishing a diagnosis, with a diagnostic yield as high as 92%. General anesthesia and single-lumen endotracheal intubation are used. Mortality ranges from 0.3% to 70%, with most patients succumbing to the intrinsic disease within 30 days [19].

Thoracoscopic lung biopsy provides the same diagnostic yield with less surgical morbidity. This technique gives the surgeon the ability to inspect the entire pleural surface and allows increased accessibility of different lung regions for biopsy, compared with an anterolateral thoracotomy. However, this procedure is limited to patients who can tolerate single-lung ventilation. Diagnostic yields are 92% to 100% [20]. Patients experience reduced postoperative pain and a statistically significant decrease in hospital stay and complication rate when compared with open lung biopsy [21].

Thoracoscopic lung biopsy for diffuse interstitial or multifocal nodular lung disease is usually performed with a two- or three-port access technique. A preoperative chest CT scan is useful to guide port placement. In the case of an infiltrative or fibrotic process, we advocate biopsy of the "transition zone" between normal and severely affected lung. The densely infiltrated or honeycombed areas reflect the end stage of a process and may not define a discreet cause. Dependent lung areas should be avoided in critically ill patients to prevent confusion of pathology with simple atelectasis or congestive failure.

The judicious use of the thoracoscopic biopsy as a means of diagnosing diffuse interstitial lung disease may allow patients

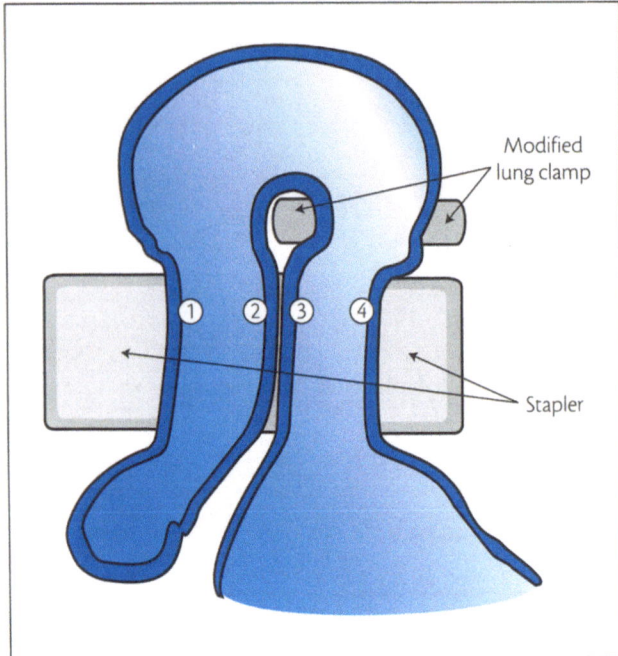

Figure 15-3 Diagram of the folded lung with the lung clamp and stapler in place. Note the four layers of visceral pleura that buttress the staple line.

with untreatable lung disease to be spared the side effects of steroid or antimetabolite therapy, and may guide specific therapy for patients with treatable abnormalities.

Lung nodules and cancers

Solitary pulmonary nodules

New solitary pulmonary nodules are a common clinical finding usually detected by plain chest radiographs obtained for unrelated indications. In addition, the common use of CT has resulted in the discovery of even more unsuspected lung nodules. These lesions most commonly present in the outer third of the lung and present a diagnostic conundrum to treating physicians. Conventional options for solitary pulmonary nodule management have been observation with serial radiographs versus endoscopic or image-guided fine-needle aspiration (FNA). In a patient with any significant smoking history, observation of a new solitary pulmonary nodule is not justified because more than 50% of these lesions will be malignant. The diagnostic yield of bronchoscopy for peripheral nodules is less than 20%. CT-guided FNA has an 85% diagnostic accuracy, but a 20% pneumothorax risk.

In contrast to endoscopic or image-guided biopsy, thoracoscopy allows for excisional biopsy. A precise histologic evaluation of the entire nodule eliminates the confusion that cytology alone often confers. Resecting the entire nodule also provides additional tissue for microbiologic studies or immunohistochemistry as indicated.

Nodules appropriate for thoracoscopic resection are generally restricted to the outer third of the lung parenchyma. Deeper lesions may be approached if they lie near a fissure. Resection is usually accomplished via a three-port technique as described by Landreneau and coworkers [9]. The target lesion should be

excised using endoscopic staplers with a rim of normal lung parenchyma. All specimens should be extracted from the chest in an impenetrable bag to prevent seeding of the pleural space or chest wall with tumor [22]. If a benign, infectious, or metastatic lesion is defined by frozen section histology, then no additional surgical intervention is indicated. Should a new primary malignancy be confirmed, patients should undergo an anatomic resection. Stapled wedge resections have been associated with local recurrence rates 2.5 times higher than those of standard anatomic resection [23].

Anatomic lung resections, including upper and lower lobectomy using video-assisted thoracic surgery

Anatomic lobectomy remains the procedure of choice for localized non–small cell lung cancer. This procedure requires the meticulous dissection and individual isolation and division of hilar structures as well as sampling or dissection of hilar lymph nodes. Controversy exists as to whether a VATS approach allows for such dissection. Several investigators have published their experience with VATS to accomplish a lobectomy. They have demonstrated a VATS lobectomy to be associated with less acute pain [24,25], less chronic pain [13•], better postoperative ventilatory function [26], and less shoulder dysfunction [13•] as compared with thoracotomy. Postoperative length of hospital stay is shorter for VATS lobectomy in one study [24], but in the only randomized trial there was no difference [27]. No long-term comparisons regarding cancer-related survival are published. We continue to advocate VATS lobectomy for patients with peripheral tumors, without hilar adenopathy. If initial thoracoscopic inspection reveals excessive pleural adhesions or poorly developed fissures, we have a low threshold to convert to a standard, muscle-sparing open thoracotomy.

Right-sided lobectomies commonly require a four-port technique. Upper and middle lobectomies are more difficult than resections of the lower lobe. Left-sided lobectomies are typically performed with a three-port technique. Once the decision to proceed with lobectomy is made, we place our auxillary VATS incision (< 8 cm) over the fissure centered on the anterior axillary line. This incision allows for use of both standard and thoracoscopic instruments during hilar dissection and provides an atraumatic egress for the specimen once it has been resected. The remaining incisions are for port access only, with the inferior-most port reserved for a chest drain following resection.

For a right upper lobectomy, we routinely dissect the anterior hilar pleura and divide the upper lobe veins first. This technique exposes the commonly large truncus branch of the right pulmonary artery supplying the apical and anterior segments, which is divided with a single application of the endovascular stapler. We then carry our pleural dissection over the apex of the hilum to the subcarinal space exposing the upper lobe bronchus as it arises laterally from the main stem bronchus. The bronchus is transected, allowing the lobe to be retracted caudally and exposing the posterior segmental pulmonary arterial branch, which can be stapled, clipped, or tied. Fissures are then developed with staplers, completing the lobectomy.

On the left side, a similar approach is used, although it is often useful to place the camera in the axilla looking "down" on the hilum. Our preferred sequence of division of hilar structures for a left upper lobectomy is the superior vein first followed by the segmental arteries to the upper lobe as the fissure is developed from superior to inferior, leaving the bronchus for last.

Lower lobectomy using VATS involves a more predictable dissection and is generally simpler to successfully complete. We place our auxiliary incision one interspace lower than for upper lobectomy and can usually visualize and dissect the pulmonary artery and bronchus directly. The pulmonary arterial branches to the superior segment are normally ligated separately on the left to spare the lingular blood supply, but can often be taken with the basilar arteries on the right side if there is adequate separation from the middle lobe arteries. The fissure is then completed, followed by mobilization of the inferior pulmonary ligament and transection of the inferior pulmonary vein. We routinely cover dependent bronchial stumps with vascularized pleura or pericardial fat.

PERICARDIAL AND PLEURAL EFFUSIONS

Malignant pleural effusions are a debilitating complication of metastatic cancer. Several liters of pleural fluid can fill the chest and completely compress the ipsilateral lung with subsequent ventilation-perfusion mismatching. The result is profound dyspnea and the constant feeling of smothering. Intermittent thoracentesis is ineffective due to the reaccumulation of fluid within days and the loss of protein in the effusate. Chest tube placement at the bedside with subsequent sclerosis is generally effective for patients with documented malignancy and a free pleural space. Thoracoscopy has the added benefits of allowing pleural biopsies to establish the diagnosis of a malignant effusion, the breakdown of loculations within the chest to produce a more uniform pleurodesis, and the application of the sclerotic agent in a uniform manner and with the patient under general anesthesia [28].

The patient is placed in supine position with a roll under the ipsilateral hip, or else in a full thoracotomy position. Split-lung anesthesia is not required, and the procedure can be performed satisfactorily with a single-lumen endotracheal tube. A mediastinoscope is used as a single thoracoscopic instrument access, generally in the fifth intercostal space anteriorly. Pleural adhesions are broken down bluntly or with cautery through the working lumen of the mediastinoscope. Up to 4 g of sterile talc is insufflated under direct vision once the pleural fluid is completely drained and biopsies obtained. Usually a single posterior chest tube is left in place.

Malignant pericardial effusions are frequently associated with malignant pleural effusions. The average life expectancy of patients with malignant pleuropericardial effusions is generally measured in weeks. Maximum palliation is the treatment goal. This includes maximum drainage of fluid, prevention of reaccumulation of fluid, and minimal morbidity. Minimally invasive thoracic surgical techniques offer the opportunity to simultaneously treat pericardial and pleural fluid collections with very low morbidity. Further, 10% to 20% of patients with a malignant pleural effusion have the neoplasm undiagnosed at the time of symptomatic presentation [29]. Thoracoscopic management of these effusions offers the advantage of providing pleural biopsies to diagnose the malignancy.

The standard open approach to a pericardial window is through a subxyphoid approach. A vertical paramedian incision is made just to the left side of the xyphoid cartilage and extended cephalad toward the sternum. The sixth costal cartilage is sometimes divided to provide additional exposure. A sturdy retraction system and headlight is frequently required to adequately visualize the pericardium, and exposure is frequently difficult. However, this technique can be used on the awake patient using only local anesthesia. We continue to use this technique in unstable patients who cannot tolerate anesthesia. The safety of both the subxyphoid and thoracoscopic drainage techniques can be improved in patients with impending cardiac tamponade by preoperative echo-guided catheter placement and partial drainage of the pericardial effusion.

The standard subxyphoid approach has been associated with a 20% to 30% failure rate within 3 months. Some authors advocate a larger window, stripping the entire anterior pericardium from phrenic nerve to phrenic nerve to prevent recurrence. However, recurrence has been documented to occur posteriorly in such patients.

Thoracoscopy offers superior visualization and potential for a larger window than the subxyphoid technique. Thoracoscopy does require general anesthesia with single-lung ventilation in most patients. The patient is placed in either a full lateral decubitus position or supine with a 30° elevation to the ipsilateral side. The thoracoscopic ports can be placed over either the right or left chest, and the choice is generally in favor of the same side as a unilateral pleural effusion. The distended pericardium can fill a surprisingly large intrathoracic space, so the camera port needs to be placed in the midaxillary line at a point maximally displaced from the pericardium. A right-sided approach may be superior to the left in this regard, because a distended pericardial sac can reach the left lateral chest wall. A VATS technique is frequently useful in these cases with a small parasternal utility incision allowing multiple-instrument access to the pericardium. Alternatively, a successful thoracoscopic technique has been used with a fifth intercostal space midaxillary line camera port and fourth and seventh anterior axillary line instrument ports.

A distended and pressurized pericardium is difficult to grasp with an instrument. We have had the most success with a small ratcheted clamp (Frazier clamp) or a nerve hook to tent up the pericardial edge. This allows a scissors to initiate the window. Alternatively, aspiration of the fluid with an 18-gauge needle may produce enough pericardial laxity to assist the initial incision. A bare area of pericardium anterior to the phrenic nerve is the usual initial site of the window. Loculated posterior fluid collections may require an additional window to be cut in the pericardium behind the phrenic nerve. This requires a left-sided thoracoscopic or VATS approach.

In patients with a simultaneous pericardial effusion and malignant pleural effusion, we have combined thoracoscopy with drainage of the pleural effusion, pericardial window, and talc poudrage of the hemithorax. We have not seen evidence of epicardial irritation from the talc in these patients. Further, the patient benefits from multiple therapeutic interventions while under a single general anesthetic.

MEDIASTINAL DISEASES

Anterior mediastinum

Minimally invasive thoracic surgery is useful in the diagnosis and excision of a variety of common diseases of the anterior mediastinum. Diagnostic biopsies of anterior mediastinal masses can identify lymphomas and germ cell tumors that are in turn definitively treated with nonsurgical therapies. Therapeutic excisions are possible for bronchogenic cysts, pericardial cysts, thymic cysts, and normal thymus in patients with myasthenia gravis [30]. Aspiration alone is insufficient therapy for cysts because the mucosal lining is not removed and recurrences are frequent. Thoracoscopic techniques allow surgical extirpation while avoiding the morbidity associated with open thoractomy.

Patients are routinely ventilated with a double-lumen endotracheal tube. This allows a clear view of the mediastinum. For minimally invasive access to the anterior mediastinum, we prefer the patient in a 45° off-center position. This is accomplished with a roll under the ipsilateral posterior ribcage and hip, with the ipsilateral arm suspended from an overhead brace. The patient is taped across the anterior superior iliac spine to secure this position during rotation of the operating room table.

The anterior mediastinum is a small space bordered by the sternum anteriorly, the pericardium posteriorly, the innominate vein superiorly, and the phrenic nerves laterally. Safe resection of anterior mediastinal structures depends on the clear delineation of the small veins draining into the innominate vein and superior vena cava.

We routinely approach the anterior mediastinum from the left side because the left ventricle provides excellent anatomic orientation. Others advocate a right-sided approach to clearly visualize the junction of the superior vena cava with the innominate vein.

Thymic cysts are approached with three ports. The camera port is placed in the fifth intercostal space, anterior axillary line. One instrument port is placed medial to the cyst, generally in the fifth or sixth intercostal space, midclavicular line. An additional instrument port is placed lateral to the lesion in the fifth intercostal space, midaxillary line. The camera port has to be placed more laterally in the left chest in patients with cardiomegaly on preoperative chest radiography.

Lateral traction is placed on the thymic cyst and, with the phrenic nerve visualized, dissection is begun along the pericardium through the medial working port. Dissection is started inferiorly and extended toward the innominate vein. Once feeding vessels are isolated along the medial surface, they are clipped and divided. Generally, several small veins drain toward the innominate vein from the posterosuperior aspect of the cyst.

Bronchogenic cysts are removed in a similar fashion. Abnormal budding of the embryologic tracheobronchial tree causes these cysts to form. These cysts are located in the mediastinum without direct communication to the airways. Bronchogenic cysts tend to be hypovascular, and the dissection is usually easier than with thymic cysts. These cysts are generally found in the subcarinal space, in the groove between the trachea, and the superior vena cava on the right, and between the left mainstem bronchus and the pulmonary artery on the left. The phrenic and vagus nerves should be clearly identified during the resection, as well as the back wall of the superior vena cava. The azygous vein can be divided by a vascular endoscopic stapler to facilitate this dissection. Generally, a narrow stem between the cyst and the bronchus can be delineated and clipped prior to resection. Subcarinal cysts are best approached from the right. The intact cyst can then be placed within an endoscopic bag for removal from the chest.

Patients with new onset of myasthenia gravis symptoms should undergo a chest CT scan. Myasthenic patients with thymoma are best treated by complete resection via a limited or complete sternotomy. Those patients without evidence of thymic hyperplasia or thymoma are potential candidates for thoracoscopic thymectomy. The patient is placed in a 45° off-center position with a roll beneath the left rib cage. Dissection begins with a small cervical incision similar to the one used for cervical mediastinoscopy. The left and right upper poles of the thymus are dissected from surrounding structures through the neck. Thoracoscopic port placement is then similar to that described previously for thymic cysts. The lateral port is used for retraction while dissection is begun along the left inferior pole through the medial port. In turn, the right lobe is grasped and pulled to the left and dissected from the underlying pericardium. The thymic veins drain into the innominate vein and lie deep to the upper poles of the gland. The lower poles frequently have to be flipped back onto the upper poles to expose these veins. The veins are divided using endoscopic clips. A partial pericardial resection can also be accomplished thoracoscopically if the gland is adhesed to the anterior pericardium.

Middle mediastinum

The role of thoracoscopy within the middle mediastinum is primarily the accurate assessment of the mediastinal lymph nodes. Patients with lung cancer confined to the lung itself have a 5-year life expectancy of approximately 60% with surgical resection alone, whereas patients with mediastinal nodal involvement have only a 23% chance of surviving 5 years [31].

Accurate assessment of the middle mediastinal nodes has become an important decision-making point in our care of lung cancer patients. Patients without mediastinal node involvement advance to surgical resection, whereas preresection irradiation and chemotherapy are most commonly chosen for patients with mediastinal nodal spread.

Compared with surgical biopsy specimens of mediastinal nodes, preoperative chest CT and MRI scans are only accurate 70% of the time [32]. Errors in accurate staging by CT scans include both false-positive enlarged nodes that are reactive and false-negative nodes with micrometastases.

The American Thoracic Society classifies the middle mediastinal nodes with a standardized lymph node map [33]. Important mediastinal nodes include stations 2 (high paratracheal), 4 (tracheobronchial angle), 5 (aortopulmonary window), 6 (preaortic), 7 (subcarinal), 8 (paraesophageal), and 9 (inferior pulmonary ligament). Further, the side of the node is designated in the shorthand notation of the station (ie, station 4R is the right tracheobronchial angle node). The issue of contralateral nodal involvement from the site of the primary tumor is quite important in distinguishing between stage IIIA (ipsilateral nodes) and stage IIIB (contralateral nodes).

Cervical mediastinoscopy is the conventional way of surgically staging the middle mediastinal nodes. The patient is positioned supine. A 4-cm transverse incision is made one fingerbreadth above the sternal notch, and dissection carried down sharply to the pretracheal fascia. The surgeon then passes a finger bluntly anterior to the trachea as far as the carina. A mediastinoscope is inserted and biopsies are taken of nodal stations 4R, 7, 4L, and possibly 2R and 2L. The advantage of this surgical approach is the ability to sample the contralateral and ipsilateral nodes through a single incision.

Stations 5 and 6 cannot be reached by standard cervical mediastinoscopy and generally require a separate parasternal incision over the left second costal cartilage. This procedure is called anterior mediastinotomy or the Chamberlain procedure. Stations 5 and 6 are the initial mediastinal drainage of the left upper lobe, and should be sampled to adequately stage cancers of this part of the lung.

Neither cervical mediastinoscopy nor anterior mediastinotomy allows access to the paraesophageal (station 8) or inferior pulmonary ligament (station 9) nodes. These nodes drain portions of the lower lobes. Further, the subcarinal nodal packet (station 7) is a pyramid lying in the crotch of the right and left mainstem bronchi when the patient is lying supine. Only the apex of that pyramid can be biopsied with cervical mediastinoscopy [34]. The larger base of the pyramid of nodes lies below the plane of the scope and is inaccessible. Stations 8, 9, and posterior station 7 are all accessible to a thoracoscope.

Thoracoscopic lymph node biopsy of the middle mediastinum is straightforward. The patient is placed in a lateral thoracotomy position. Stations 2 and 4 are accessible on the right, and station 2 on the left. The increased access to stations 7, 8, and 9 on the right and stations 5 through 9 on the left is an advantage of the thoracoscopic technique. Transpleural thoracoscopic approach to the aortopulmonary window gives better visualization than an anterior mediastinotomy. Further, thoracoscopic inspection of the hemithorax can identify diffuse pleural seeding or the relationship of a hilar tumor to important mediastinal structures. Finally, a thoracoscopic approach can be used to avoid reoperating in a scarred field to restage those patients who have undergone previous cervical mediastinoscopy followed by preresection chemotherapy or radiation therapy. The disadvantages are that the contralateral nodes are not accessible and palpation of the nodes is not possible.

Although thoracoscopic staging of the mediastinal nodes has not replaced cervical mediastinoscopy as our standard approach to patients with suspected lung cancer, the addition of this technique to our surgical armamentarium has allowed us to successfully apply the technique to correctly stage selected patients.

Posterior mediastinum

Posterior mediastinal masses include benign duplication foregut cysts, neurogenic tumors, and malignant tumors of the pleura and lung. Esophageal duplication cysts result from abnormal budding of the embryologic foregut. An esophageal duplication cyst lies next to or within the esophagus, is covered with two muscle layers, and is lined with a foregut epithelium [35]. Approximately 60% of these cysts occur around the distal third of the esophagus, 20% at the mid-third, and 20% around the upper third. These cysts are generally asymptomatic and discovered through unrelated diagnostic studies. Therapy is complete surgical excision of the cyst and its contents to prevent enlargement, secondary infection, or rupture.

Esophageal cysts are satisfactorily removed with a thoracoscopic technique. The patient is placed in the semiprone position for all posterior mediastinal thoracoscopy procedures. Port placement is similar to that described later for other esophageal procedures. Briefly, the camera port is generally in the fifth interspace anterior axillary line, and the two instrument ports are over the seventh rib in the posterior axillary line and within the third interspace between the posterior and midaxillary lines. The pleura overlying the esophagus is divided, and the azygous vein is divided during approaches from the right hemithorax. The goal is the complete removal of the cyst while avoiding mucosal injury to the esophagus. Doubt regarding the integrity of the esophageal mucosa can be dispelled by the simultaneous placement of a flexible esophagoscope with air insufflation within the esophagus, while visualizing the external dissection area.

Neurogenic tumors are approached with the same constellation of thoracoscopic ports. These tumors are smooth walled and tend to be in intimate association with either the sympathetic chain or the vertebral bodies. Preoperative MRI is required to rule out the involvement of the neural canal. The posterior parietal pleura overlying the tumor is incised and the inferior border dissected free of surrounding tissue. If the tumor arises from the sympathetic chain, the chain is divided above an endoscopic clip to minimize cautery damage to the remaining nerves. As the tumor is dissected upward, the upper pedicle is identified, which is the superior remnant of the sympathetic chain. This in turn is divided below an endoscopic clip and the specimen removed.

Malignant tumors of the pleura and lung within the posterior mediastinum can be accurately staged with thoracoscopic techniques. By definition, these tumors are of an advanced stage. Preoperative chest imaging has limited ability to judge invasion of vascular or bony structures. The mediastinal pleura is incised over the tumor, and its relationship to vascular, neural, and bony structures is established. These relationships are important in accurately staging and assessing the resectability of advanced cancers. Further, this staging can be combined with mediastinal nodal biopsies. This approach has proven to be an invaluable asset in accurately staging selected patients.

ESOPHAGEAL DISEASE
Achalasia

An inappropriate increased resting pressure of the lower esophageal sphincter, incomplete relaxation of the lower sphincter during swallowing, and aperistalsis of the body of the esophagus are the three primary components of achalasia [36]. Patients typically develop progressive dysphagia for both liquids and solids and regurgitate undigested food. Endoscopically guided pneumatic dilatation of the lower esophageal sphincter is effective in relieving symptoms in 75% of patients [37]. The remaining 25% who are not sufficiently relieved of their symptoms are referred for surgical intervention.

The goal of surgical therapy is the destruction of the spasmodic lower esophageal sphincter. Destruction of too much of this sphincter mechanism, however, can lead to disabling gastroesophageal reflux. This surgical morbidity has been avoided by making a small myotomy and limiting the mobilization of the distal esophagus and thus the paraesophageal soft tissues. This prevents the migration of the lower esophageal sphincter from the positive-pressure abdominal cavity to the negative-pressure thoracic cavity with consequent reflux.

Video-assisted esophageal myotomy allows standard surgical treatment of achalasia without a thoracotomy. The patient is placed in the right lateral decubitus position and the left chest is prepped and draped as for a routine thoracotomy. Single-lung anesthesia is required. A four-port approach is required; including a fifth intercostal interspace anterior axillary camera port, a sixth or seventh interspace anterior axillary port to depress the diaphragm, a third port in the axilla to retract the left lower lobe anteriorly and cephalad, and a seventh interspace, posterior axillary port to dissect the esophagus and perform the myotomy. The mediastinal pleura over the distal third of the esophagus is incised, but the esophagus is not dissected free of the surrounding structures. The myotomy is initiated with an endoscopic scissors to prevent damage to the underlying mucosa. Dissection is facilitated by either a gastroscope in the lumen of the esophagus with insufflation of air or an illuminated bougie. A right-angle hook is used to retract the circular muscle fibers away from the underlying mucosa prior to their division. The myotomy is extended onto the first part of the stomach, but care is taken not to disrupt the phrenoesophageal attachments for 270° around the distal esophagus. An endoscopic Kittner instrument is then used to bluntly dissect the circular muscle fibers laterally away from the myotomy line for approximately 1.5 cm. This separation of the divided circular muscle from the mucosa prevents recurrence of dysphagia, which is usually the result of rehealing of the myotomized lower sphincter. A single right-angle pleural drain is left in the chest.

Benign esophageal masses

Benign esophageal masses typically appear as a smooth-contoured filling defect on barium swallow. This is very different from the shaggy and shelf-like appearance of a typical esophageal carcinoma on barium swallow. These symptoms are generally caused by obstruction. Such benign lesions should be removed when diagnosed to prevent further enlargement and exacerbation of symptoms. The most common benign esophageal mass is a leiomyoma of the muscular wall.

Thoracoscopic enucleation of benign masses has been a convenient surgical approach that avoids the morbidity of thoracotomy. The left chest approach is used for tumors of the lower third of the intrathoracic esophagus (30 to 40 cm from the incisors). The right chest approach is used for tumors of the mid and upper third of the intrathoracic esophagus. This approach avoids the obstructed view that can be created by the arch of the aorta within the left chest.

The goal of surgical resection is the complete enucleation of the tumor while preserving the integrity of the esophageal mucosa. An endoscope can be used to distend the esophagus with air insufflation during thoracoscopic resection of the mass, facilitating the plane of dissection between the mass and the mucosa. Also, this technique is useful in identifying when a small mucosal defect has been created, which is a relative indication to convert to open thoracotomy and primary repair of the mucosa.

The camera port is generally placed in the fifth intercostal space posterior axillary line. Two instrument ports are generally in the fourth and sixth intercostal spaces in the anterior axillary line. A fan retractor to hold back the lung or diaphragm can be inserted through an additional port. The mediastinal pleura is incised over the esophagus, and the azygous vein may be divided if directly overlying the tumor. The longitudinal muscle layer is split and one end of the tumor is lifted away from the underlying mucosa. The tumors tend to be round and difficult to grasp. Once the tumor is enucleated, an endoscopic bag is used to facilitate extraction of the tumor from the chest. With this technique, the chest tube can be discontinued on the same day and the patient discharged after an overnight stay.

Esophageal cancer

There is currently no standardized treatment of esophageal cancer in the United States. Improved long-term survival has been reported with preresection chemoradiation therapy [38], which has led enthusiasts to advocate preresection chemoradiation for all patients with esophageal cancer. Such therapy, however, carries considerable morbidity. Depth of esophageal wall invasion by tumor or the involvement of regional lymph nodes have proven to be the most important predictors of long-term outcome in esophageal cancer [39]. Preresection assessment of depth of wall invasion and regional lymph nodes may allow better allocation of neoadjuvant therapy. Thoracoscopy has allowed us to evaluate the mediastinal nodes and local invasion of surrounding mediastinal structures [40]. This technique has complemented our use of chest and abdominal staging CT scans as well as endoesophageal ultrasounds.

To stage a newly diagnosed esophageal cancer, the patient is placed in the full, left lateral decubitus position, and split-lung anesthesia is achieved. A camera port is placed in the fifth intercostal space, posterior axillary line. Three additional instrument ports are placed in the third and fourth intercostal spaces of the midclavicular line and the seventh intercostal space anterior axillary line. An atraumatic fan retractor is used to retract the lung or diaphragm to expose the paraesophageal region and inferior pulmonary ligament.

The pleura overlying the esophagus is opened for the entire length and the azygous vein is divided. Important nodal stations include the paraesophageal nodes, subcarinal node, paratracheal nodes, and inferior pulmonary ligament nodes. These are sampled with a grasper and an endoscopic clip is placed at the base of the nodes (Fig. 15-4). Further, the esophagus can be mobilized and full-thickness invasion of the wall can be determined along the ipsilateral side. We have used endoesophageal ultrasound to evaluate the contralateral side.

In a prospective, multi-institutional trial, this surgical staging technique was technically successful in 95% of patients. Of

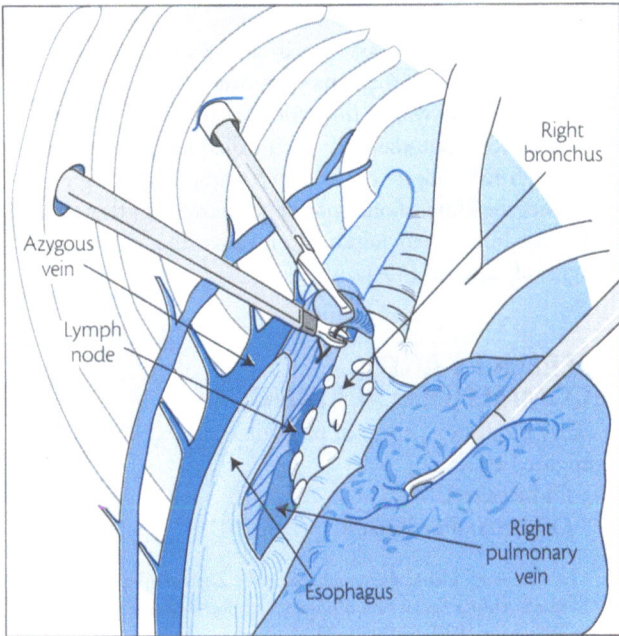

Figure 15-4 View through the camera of the sampling of the azygous node. The mediastinal pleura overlying the esophagus has been opened, and the deflated lung retracted anteriorly. The entire node is removed by gentle traction with an endoscopic forceps while a hemostatic clip is placed at the pedicle.

those patients undergoing immediate surgical resection because preresection staging suggested no nodal involvement or full-thickness wall invasion, 88% were correctly staged in comparison with the final pathologic specimen [40]. Further, the routine addition of laparoscopic staging of the celiac nodes may improve the diagnostic accuracy of surgical staging.

There is also no standardized way to perform an esophagectomy in this country. Some surgeons advocate the blunt dissection of the mediastinal esophagus through a laparotomy and cervical incision (transhiatal esophagectomy). Other groups recommend direct dissection of the mediastinal esophagus through a right thoracotomy combined with a laparotomy, finishing with a midthoracic gastroesophageal anastomosis (Ivor-Lewis esophagectomy). We have advocated direct surgical dissection through three incisions, including a right thoracotomy, laparotomy, and cervical incision with a cervical gastroesophageal anastomosis [41].

One of the proposed advantages of direct surgical dissection of the intrathoracic esophagus is improved intrathoracic lymph node toilet. Additionally, there is a poorly visualized portion of the intrathoracic dissection around the azygous vein and carina with the transhiatal technique, and surgical misadventures have been reported.

We have used a video-assisted dissection of the intrathoracic esophagus in selected patients during the first portion of a modified transhiatal esophagectomy. This has successfully replaced the thoracotomy incision in these patients. The azygous vein is directly ligated, and esophageal perforators that branch directly from the aorta are controlled with hemoclips. Adhesions to the back of the membranous trachea can be sharply dissected. Further, we believe there is enhanced visualization of the subcarinal and

paraesophageal nodes as compared with that seen during a transhiatal dissection. Extensive mediastinal invasion is a relative indication to convert to open thoracotomy.

Patient position and port placement is the same as described previously for preresectional surgical staging of the esophagus. Split-lung ventilation is necessary to obtain adequate visualization of the paraesophageal area. The esophagus is initially mobilized at the level of the pericardium, and a Penrose drain (Sherwood Medical, St Louis, MO) is placed around the organ for retraction. The vagus nerves are kept separate from the specimen to avoid traction injury on the recurrent laryngeal nerves. After the entire esophagus has been mobilized, one Penrose drain is tied with a suture and placed at the apex of the chest to be retrieved through the cervical incision. A second Penrose drain is likewise tied and placed at the diaphragmatic hiatus to be retrieved through the laparotomy incision to facilitate the additional dissection. A chest tube is placed to the apex under direct vision. The ports are closed and the patient is repositioned supine for a completion transhiatal esophagectomy.

DIAPHRAGM

Disease of the diaphragm presents as an apparent elevation on plain chest radiography. Differential diagnosis usually consists of a diaphragmatic-based mass, diaphragmatic hernia, or phrenic nerve palsy. Thoracoscopy is an effective method of diagnosing and treating diaphragmatic disease. It can be used to biopsy diaphragmatic masses, and for both diaphragmatic plication [42] and hernia repair.

Paralysis of a hemidiaphragm can be quite well tolerated in the adult, because the diaphragmatic muscle only contributes between 10% and 25% of respiratory function [43]. In patients with underlying respiratory disease, however, the unilateral compression of the ipsilateral lower lobe can significantly contribute to dyspnea. In these cases, diaphragmatic plication offers therapeutic benefit.

It is important to remember that the dome of the paralyzed diaphragm can be quite high in the anterior thorax, even though the costal insertion is unchanged. We have successfully used a two-port technique for diaphragmatic plication. The double-instrument port is in the wide anterior fifth intercostal space. This port will allow access of both the video camera and the endoscopic needle driver. The camera is placed and the thorax inspected. Specifically, the entire course of the phrenic nerve as it runs along the anterior border of the superior vena cava and then onto the pericardium anterior to the hilum is visualized to rule out an organic cause of phrenic nerve palsy. An accessory port is then placed in the fifth or sixth intercostal space, posterior axillary line. An O-ring forcep passed through the accessory port can help "tent-up" the muscle of the diaphragm. This facilitates the safe passage of the nonabsorbable suture through a muscle pleat without injury to underlying abdominal structures. Three to five pleats are made in the diaphragm with a nonabsorbable heavy suture. These interrupted sutures are placed from the posterolateral to the anteromedial borders of the diaphragm (ie, furthest away from the camera back toward the camera). Approximately eight to 10 sutures are placed. We tie each suture as placed to facilitate the next suture placement and to prevent suture entanglement. Tying of the sutures gathers the lateral borders of the muscle together within the pleats and displaces the diaphragm downward toward the thoracic base. The ultimate tightness of the plication depends on the width of the first and last pleat.

Diphragmatic hernia repair is similar, although generally requires an additional port. A retraction device such as the endoscopic Kittner instrument is used to reduce the abdominal contents through the diaphragmatic defect, whereas an additional instrument such as an O-ring forcep is used to lift up the muscle margin. The endoscopic needle driver is then passed through first one muscle edge and then the opposite muscle edge. Generally, an additional pleating of the diaphragmatic muscle on each side of the defect gives additional strength to the sutured repair.

There may be a role for nonabsorbable mesh repair of very large defects, which would require undue tension on the muscle edges if repaired primarily. A sheet of marlex is cut outside of the chest in an estimate of the size of the defect, then passed through a port. An endoscopic needle driver could then be used to tack down the mesh into position in an interrupted suture technique.

EXPANDING INDICATIONS

Minimally invasive thoracic surgery techniques have offered new diagnostic and therapeutic options for patients with intrathoracic disease. Previous clinical algorithms have been predicated on the considerable morbidity associated with open thoracotomy. For instance, most patients with a new intrapulmonary nodule or infiltrate were frequently followed up with serial radiographs or transthoracic needle biopsies. These same patients are now frequently referred for excisional biopsy, which improves diagnostic accuracy with minimal morbidity.

Prior to 1991, thoracoscopy at Brigham and Women's Hospital consisted of visualization and biopsy of pleural-based disease through a rigid mediastinoscope. Beginning in July 1991, we have applied video thoracoscopy to our practice and accumulated prospective outcome data. Currently, 50% to 60% of our operative case load is managed with video-assisted techniques.

Between July 1991 and June 1994, 895 patients underwent VATS procedures at the Brigham and Women's Hospital, Boston. The cumulative operative mortality for this series was 1%. New morbidity occurred in 14% of cases, and conversion to a limited open thoracotomy was required in 1.4%. Average length of hospital stay was 3 days for closed thoracoscopy and 5 days after a video-assisted technique, compared with an average length of stay after open thoracotomy of 7.2 days [5•].

Although our initial clinical experience with these techniques was gained in low-risk patients, we soon discovered that the decrease in associated surgical trauma decreased the operative risk in certain patient subgroups. Age has previously been found to be an independent risk factor for death after thoracotomy, with a 7% to 8% expected operative mortality for pulmonary resection among patients aged 70 or older [44]. Between July 1991 and June 1994, we performed 307 separate minimally invasive thoracic surgery procedures on 296 patients between the ages of 65 and 89 years. Specifically, 88 patients were over 75 years of age and 33 patients were over 80 years of age. The operative mortality within this series was less than 1%, and the major morbidity rate was 7%. The median length of stay within this high-risk subgroup was 4 to 5 days, depending on age. Age alone, therefore, should not be a deterrent to thoracic surgical procedures when minimally invasive thoracic surgery is thoughtfully applied [45•].

REFERENCES AND RECOMMENDED READING

Recently published papers of particular interest have been highlighted as:

• Of interest
•• Of outstanding interest

1. Jacobaeus H: Ueber die Moglichkeit die Zsytoskopie bei Untersuchung Seroser Hohlungen Anzuwenden. *Munch Med Wochenschr* 1910, 57:2090–2092.
2. Jacobaeus HC: The practical importance of thoracoscopy in surgery of the chest. *Surg Gynecol Obstet* 1922, 34:289–296.
3. Jacobaeus HC: The cauterization of adhesions in pneumothorax treatment of tuberculosis.*Surg Gynecol Obstet* 1921, 33:493–500.
4. Lewis RJ, Caccavale RJ, Sisler G: Special report: video-endoscopic thoracic surgery. *NJ Med* 1991, 88:473–475.
5.• DeCamp MM, Jaklitsch MT, Mentzer SJ, *et al.*: The safety and versatility of video-thoracoscopy: a prospective analysis of 895 consecutive cases. *J Am Coll Surg* 1995, 181:113–120.
The largest single institution experience of thoracoscopic applications and objective outcomes. Eight hundred ninety-five cases are reviewed from the Thoracic Surgery Division of the Brigham and Women's Hospital. Data includes rates of conversion, major and minor morbidities, operative mortality, and lenght of stay with nonrandomized comparisons to open thoracotomy patients from the same institution.
6. McKneally MF, Lewis RJ, Anderson RP, *et al.*: Statement of the AATS/STS Joint Committee on Thoracoscopy and Video Assisted Thoracic Surgery. *J Thorac Cardiovasc Surg* 1992, 104:1.
7. Gray H: *Anatomy, Descriptive and Surgical*, edn 15. Edited by Pick TP, Howden R. New York: Bounty Books; 1997:1257.
8. Kaiser LR: Video-assisted thoracic surgery: current state of the art. *Ann Surg* 1994, 220:720–734.
9. Landreneau RJ, Mack MJ, Hazelrigg SR, *et al.*: Video-assisted thoracic surgery: basic technical concepts and intercostal approach strategies. *Ann Thorac Surg* 1992, 54:800–807.
10. Wait M, Estrara A: Changing clinical spectrum of spontaneous pneumothorax. *Am J Surg* 1992, 164:528–531.
11. American Lung Association: *Facts about emphysema*. New York: American Lung Association; 1990.
12. Brantigan OC, Kress MB, Mueller EA: The surgical approach to pulmonary emphysema. *Dis Chest* 1961, 39:485–499.
13.• Landreneau RJ, Mack MJ, Hazelrigg SR, *et al.*: Prevalence of chronic pain after pulmonary resection by thoracotomy or video-assisted thoracoscopy. *J Thorac Cardiovasc Surg* 1994, 107:1079–1086.
Report of a comparative trial between VATS and lateral thoracotomy patients in regard to chronic pain using a visual analog scale. Within 1 year of operation, the video-assisted patients had subjective improvement compared with open thoracotomy patients, yet their pain medication requirements were similar. After 1 year, there was no difference in pain-related morbidities.

14. Cooper JD, *et al.*: Bilateral pneumectomy (volume reduction) for chronic obstructive pulmonary disease. *J Thorac Cardiovasc Surg* 1995, 109:106–116.

15. Keenan RJ, Landreneau RJ, Sciurba FC, *et al.*: Unilateral thoracoscopic surgical approach for diffuse emphysema. *J Thorac Cardiovasc Surg* 1996, 111:308–315.

16. Swanson SJ: No-cut thoracoscopic lung plication: a new technique for lung volume reduction surgery. *J Am Coll Surg* 1997, 185:25–32.

17. Ferguson MK: Thoracoscopy for diagnosis of diffuse lung disease. *Ann Thorac Surg* 1993, 56:694–696.

18. Burt ME, Flye MW, Webber BL, *et al.*: Prospective evaluation of aspiration needle, cutting needle, transbronchial, and open lung biopsy in patients with pulmonary infiltrates. *Ann Thorac Surg* 1981, 32:146–151.

19. Gaensler EA, Carrington CB: Open biopsy for chronic diffuse infiltrative lung disease: clinical, roentgenographic, and physiological correlations in 502 patients. *Ann Thorac Surg* 1980, 30:411–426.

20. Miller D, Allen M, Trastek V, *et al.*: Video thoracoscopic wedge excision for diffuse interstitial lung disease. *Chest* 1992, 102(suppl):169S.

21. Feron PF, Landreneau RJ, *et al.*: Comparison of open versus thoracoscopic lung biopsy for diffuse infiltrative pulmonary disease. *J Thorac Cardiovasc Surg* 1993, 106:194–199.

22. Fry WA, Siddiqui A, Pensler JM, Mostafavi H: Thoracoscopic implantation of cancer with a fatal outcome. *Ann Thorac Surg* 1995, 59:42–45.

23. Ginsberg RJ, Rubinstein LV: Randomized trial of lobectomy versus limited resection for T1N0 non-small cell lung cancer: Lung Cancer Study Group. *Ann Thorac Surg* 1995, 60:615–622.

24. Giudicella R, *et al.*: Video-assisted minithoracotomy versus muscle sparing thoracotomy for performing lobectomy. *Ann Thorac Surg* 1994, 58:712–718.

25. Yim APC, Ko K, Chan W, *et al.*: Video-assisted thoracoscopic anatomic lung resections: the initial Hong Kong experience. *Chest* 1996, 109:13–17.

26. Landreneau RJ, Hazelrigg SR, Mack MJ, *et al.*: Postoperative pain-related morbidity: video-assisted thoracic surgery versus thoracotomy. *Ann Thorac Surg* 1993, 56:1285–1289.

27. Kirby TJ, Mack MJ, Landreneau RJ, *et al.*: Lobectomy: VATS vs muscle-sparing thoracotomy. A randomized study. *J Thorac Cardiovasc Surg* 1995, 109:997–1002.

28. DeCamp M, Mentzer S, Swanson SJ, Sugarbaker DJ: Malignant effusive disease of the pleura and pericardium. *Chest* 1997, 112:291S–295S.

29. Rusch VW, Mountain C: Thoracoscopy under regional anesthesia for the diagnosis and management of pleural disease. *Am J Surg* 1987, 154:274–278.

30. Sugarbaker DJ: Thoracoscopy in the management of anterior mediastinal masses. *Ann Thorac Surg* 1993, 56:653–656.

31. Mountain CF: Revisions in the international system for staging lung cancer. *Chest* 1997, 111:1710–1717.

32. Sugarbaker DJ, Strauss GM: Advances in surgical staging and therapy of non-small-cell lung cancer. *Semin Oncol* 1993, 20:163–172.

33. Tisi GM, Friedman PJ, Peters RM, *et al.*: American Thoracic Society, Medical Section of the American Lung Association: clinical staging of primary lung cancer. *Am Rev Respir Dis* 1983, 127:659–664.

34. Pearson FG, *et al.*: Significance of positive superior mediastinal nodes identified at mediastinoscopy in patients with resectable cancer of the lung. *J Thorac Cardiovasc Surg* 1982, 83:1–11.

35. Jones DR, Graeber GM: Cysts and duplications in adults. In *Thoracic Surgery*. Edited by Pearson EG, Deslauriers J, Ginsberg RJ, *et al.* New York: Churchill Livingstone; 1995:1399–1410.

36. Sugarbaker DJ, Kearney DJ, Richards WG: Esophageal physiology and pathophysiology. *Surg Clin North Am* 1993, 73:1101–1118.

37. Vantrappen G, Janssens J: To dilate or to operate? That is the question. *Gut* 1983, 24:1013–1019.

38. Orringer MB, Forastiere AA, Perez-Tamayo C, *et al.*: Chemotherapy and radiation therapy before transhiatal esophagectomy for esophageal carcinoma. *Ann Thorac Surg* 1990, 119:348–355.

39. Jaklitsch MT, Harpole DH, Healey EA, Sugarbaker DJ: Current issues in the staging of esophageal cancer. *Semin Radiat Oncol* 1994, 4:135–145.

40. Krasna MJ, *et al.*: Thoracoscopic staging of esophageal cancer: a prospective, multi-institutional trial. *Ann Thorac Surg* 1995, 60:1337–1340.

41. Sugarbaker DJ, DeCamp MM, Liptay MJ: Surgical procedures to resect and replace the esophagus. *Maingot's Abdominal Operations*, edn 10 (vol 1). Edited by Zinner MJ, Schwartz SI, Ellis H. Stamford, CT: Appleton & Lange; 1997:885–910.

42. Mouroux J, Padovani B, Poirier NC, *et al.*: Technique for the repair of diaphragmatic eventration. *Ann Thorac Surg* 1996, 62:905–907.

43. Wade OL: Movements of the thoracic cage and diaphragm in respiration. *J Physiol* 1954, 124:193–212.

44. Ginsberg RJ, Hill LD, Eagan RT, *et al.*: Modern thirty-day operative mortality for surgical resections in lung cancer. *J Thorac Cardiovasc Surg* 1983, 86:654–658.

45.• Jaklitsch MT, DeCamp MM, Liptay MJ, *et al.*: Video-assisted thoracic surgery in the elderly: a review of 307 cases. *Chest* 1996, 110:751–758.

Objective single institution outcome data from the application of a variety of thoracoscopic techniques to the high-risk elderly population.

Laparoscopy for Urologic Conditions

Kevin R. Loughlin
Michael P. O'Leary

CHAPTER

16

Laparoscopic surgery can be divided into three areas: diagnostic, extirpative, and reconstructive. Because much of urologic surgery is reconstructive, and because radiologic imaging techniques continue to refine the accuracy of urologic diagnoses, the role of laparoscopy in urologic practice has contracted somewhat in the past few years.

However, there are specific areas of urologic surgery in which laparoscopic applications have expanded. Laparoscopy is used extensively in pediatric urology for the diagnosis and operative correction of undescended testicles as well as the laparoscopic removal of obstructed or poorly functioning kidneys. Another major new application of laparoscopy in urology has been laparoscopic adrenalectomy for both benign and malignant conditions of the adrenal gland. In this chapter we review laparoscopic varicocelectomy, pelvic lymphadenectomy, and nephrectomy. In addition we discuss the expanding role of laparoscopy in pediatric urology. Finally, we review the experience with laparoscopic retroperitoneal lymph node dissection, lymphocele drainage, ureterolysis, ureteral reimplantation, bladder diverticulectomy, cystectomy, ileal conduit, urinary incontinence surgery, and adrenalectomy.

LAPAROSCOPIC VARICOCELECTOMY

Laparoscopic varicocele ligation has been performed by many urologists, and reports from several medical centers have been published. The data suggest that laparoscopic varicocele ligation is therapeutically equivalent to open surgical (inguinal and retroperitoneal) and radiographic (embolization) techniques. Laparoscopic varicocelectomy appears to reduce postoperative morbidity [1–3]. Experimental work in a canine model by Klee and coworkers [4] verified that successful ligation of the gonadal veins can be achieved laparoscopically. Whether it is necessary to identify and preserve the testicular artery during laparoscopic varicocelectomy remains controversial. Loughlin and Brooks [5] reported on the use of a laparoscopic Doppler probe that they believe facilitates the identification and preservation of the testicular artery (Fig. 16-1). Matsuda and coworkers [6] claim that the testicular artery does not have to be preserved; they clip the testicular artery and veins en bloc. Further multicenter experience is needed to resolve whether the testicular artery should be preserved during laparoscopic varicocele ligation. Because the testicular artery is preserved during open surgical repair or radiographic embolization procedures, intuition would suggest that the laparoscopic surgeon do the same.

Technique

The technique of laparoscopic varicocele ligation is straightforward. The procedure is usually performed using general anesthesia, although Matsuda and coworkers [6] recently reported using local anesthesia alone for laparoscopic varicocelectomy. A urethral catheter is placed to empty the bladder, and a Veress needle is placed at the umbilicus to inflate the peritoneal cavity with approximately 5 L of carbon dioxide. Alternatively, a mini-laparotomy can be performed at the inferior margin of the umbilicus, and the trocar can be placed into the peritoneum under direct vision. Three

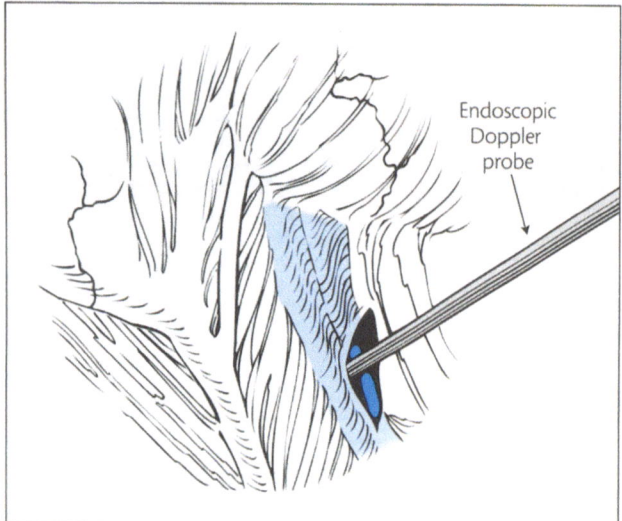

Figure 16-1 Endoscopic Doppler probe is used to identify spermatic artery. (*From* Loughlin and Brooks [5]; with permission.)

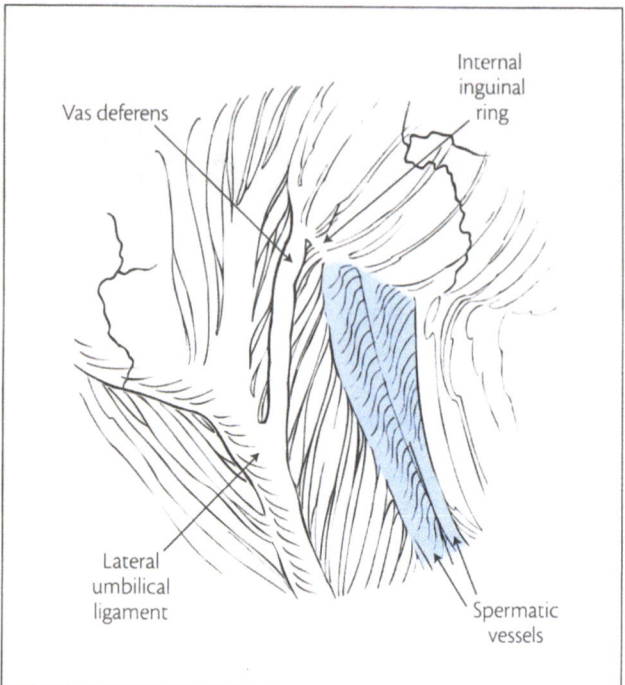

Figure 16-2 Anatomy of spermatic cord above the internal inguinal ring. (*From* Loughlin and Brooks [5]; with permission.)

laparoscopic trocars are placed for unilateral varicoceles. Four laparoscopic trocars are placed for bilateral varicocele repair. Ten-millimeter trocars are positioned at the umbilicus and at two finger breadths above the symphysis pubis. A 5-mm trocar is placed lateral to McBurney's point on the side of the varicocele. A laparoscopic videoendoscope is placed through the umbilical trocar port, and the procedure is performed using a video monitor.

The next step is to identify the pertinent anatomy. The intraabdominal vas deferens can be seen joining the spermatic cord above the internal inguinal ring (Fig. 16-2). The gonadal vessels are visualized easily in the retroperitoneum. The posterior peritoneum is excised with cautery, laser, or endoscopic scissors. The gonadal vessels are then mobilized; however, reliably identifying the spermatic artery and its branches is sometimes difficult through the laparoscope. Therefore, we prefer to use the laparoscopic Doppler probe mentioned previously to facilitate identification of the spermatic artery during laparoscopic varicocele ligation. The Doppler probe is 28.58 cm long and fits through a 5-mm laparoscopic trocar port. It is connected to a speaker that can be placed on or off the surgical field at the discretion of the surgeon. After identifying the gonadal artery, the surgeon isolates the gonadal vein or veins using blunt dissection with atraumatic graspers. A disposable endoscopic clip applier is used to ligate the gonadal vein or veins while sparing the artery. The pneumoperitoneum is vented and the trocars are removed. Subcuticular stitches are used to close the puncture sites on the abdominal wall.

LAPAROSCOPIC PELVIC LYMPHADENECTOMY

Laparoscopic pelvic lymphadenectomy has the potential to aid in the staging of prostate cancer. Most urologists embrace the philosophy that if the pelvic lymph nodes are involved in prostate cancer, cure cannot be achieved with radical prostatectomy or radiation therapy, and hormonal therapy is indicated in these patients for palliation.

Two crucial questions need to be answered before laparoscopic pelvic lymphadenectomy can be accepted. First, can a laparoscopic node dissection be performed safely? Second, can a laparoscopic node dissection be performed as completely as an open node dissection? Kavoussi and coworkers [7] reported a retrospective multicenter review of 372 patients who underwent laparoscopic pelvic lymph node dissections. The complication rate was 15%. A total of 55 complications occurred (14 intraoperatively and 41 postoperatively). Complications included vascular injury ($n = 11$), viscus injury ($n = 8$), genitourinary problems ($n = 1$), functional or mechanical bowel obstruction ($n = 7$), lower extremity deep venous thrombosis ($n = 5$), infection or wound problems ($n = 5$), lymphedema ($n = 5$), anesthetic complications ($n = 2$), and obturator nerve palsy ($n = 2$).

Vascular injuries occurred during both trocar placement and dissection. Trocar injuries were most commonly associated with the epigastric vessels. Green and coworkers [8] described a useful method to manage trocar injuries. Bowel injury occurred in three patients. It was recognized intraoperatively in one, and postoperatively in two. Ureteral injuries were noted in two patients; one was recognized intraoperatively, and an open repair was performed in the other patient in conjunction with a radical retropubic prostatectomy. The second case was not recognized until 3 days postoperatively, when the patient became febrile and a CT scan revealed a fluid collection in the pelvis consistent with a urinoma. The patient underwent an open repair of the ureter.

Many of the complications occurred early in the experience of the respective institutions. Urologists performing laparoscopic pelvic node dissections, however, must be aware that significant complications occurred throughout the collective experience of the eight institutions. Adherence to good laparoscopic technique and familiarity with the anatomy are the most reliable ways to avoid complications.

The second question—whether laparoscopic pelvic node dissection is as complete as open pelvic lymph node dissection—was addressed by Parra and coworkers [9]. The authors compared 12 open and 12 laparoscopic pelvic node dissections and found no statistical difference in the number of nodes removed by either technique. Experience in our institution also showed that laparoscopic and open node dissections were comparable in efficacy [10].

However, recent work by Steiner and Marshall [11], which describes an open "mini-laparotomy," pelvic lymphadenectomy through a 6-cm intraumbilical incision, has weakened the argument for laparoscopic node dissection. Their technique combines the advantages of open surgery with the decreased morbidity of a small incision.

Technique

The technique of mini-laparotomy is described as follows. The pneumoperitoneum is established in the standard manner. Trocar placement is then performed. The size and location of trocar sites for the procedure vary with the surgeon's preference. Most use the diamond configuration (Fig. 16-3). An alternative used by some surgeons is the so-called fan configuration for trocar placement (Fig. 16-3). This configuration allows the surgeon and the surgical assistant to manipulate instruments with both hands during the dissection. It is also helpful in obese patients or in those with a prominent urachus. The size of the trocars used at each site may vary. A 10-mm trocar is usually placed in the umbilicus for the videoendoscope. An additional 10- or 11-mm trocar is placed in at least one other site for tissue removal. Another 10- or 11-mm port is used for the endoscopic clip applier. Usually, 5-mm trocars are used for the remaining trocar sites. After completion of trocar placement, the laparoscopic landmarks for pelvic node dissection are identified. These landmarks include the medial umbilical ligament (remnant of the obliterated umbilical artery), urachus, bladder, vas deferens, iliac vessels, spermatic vessels, and internal ring (Fig. 16-4). The next maneuver is to incise the posterior peritoneum parallel and lateral to the medial umbilical ligament (Fig. 16-5). Early identification of the ureter is important to avoid ureteral injury. The vas deferens is then divided to facilitate operative access to the obturator space. Using primarily blunt dissection, the iliac vein and artery are identified. The nodal tissue overlying the external iliac vein is then teased medially to expose the internal obturator muscle. A laparoscopic vein retractor can be used to retract the external iliac vein laterally and permit easier, more complete dissection of the nodal tissue beneath the vein. The dissection proceeds with removing tissue off the vein distally until Cooper's ligament and the pubic bone are identified.

Blunt dissection is continued and the medial border of the packet is identified by clearing off the pubic bone just lateral to the medial umbilical ligament. Electrocautery is used to fulgurate small vessels and lymphatics, and the distal extent of the packet is freed from the pubic bone. The packet is pulled proximally and freed from the underside of the pubic bone. At this point, the obturator nerve is identified (Fig. 16-6).

Because nodal tissue can be quite bulky and difficult to grasp, adequate forceps (eg, the endoscopic Russian forceps), can ensure a more reliable grasp of the specimen. With blunt dissection, the obturator nerve is cleaned off proximally, and endoscopic clips are used to divide the distal portion of the dissection. At the completion of the laparoscopic pelvic lymphadenectomy, the iliac artery, vein, pubic bone, and obturator nerve can be seen clearly. The field is checked for hemostasis, and the dissection is performed in an identical manner on the opposite side. The trocars are removed, and the puncture sites are closed in the usual manner.

LAPAROSCOPIC NEPHRECTOMY

Clayman and coworkers [12] pioneered the development of laparoscopic nephrectomy. They reported their cumulative experience of 16 cases of laparoscopic nephrectomy. Thirteen patients had benign disease, one had a solid renal mass that ultimately

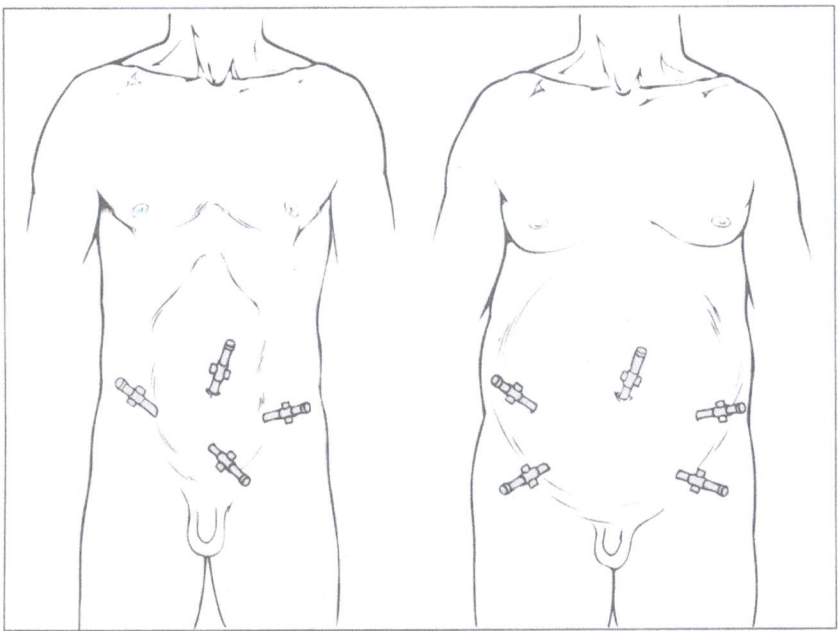

Figure 16-3 Two alternatives for trocar placement for pelvic lymphadenectomy. The diamond configuration is shown on the *left*, and the fan configuration on the *right*. (*From* Loughlin and Kavoussi [10]; by permission of J. Foerster, Fort Collins, CO.)

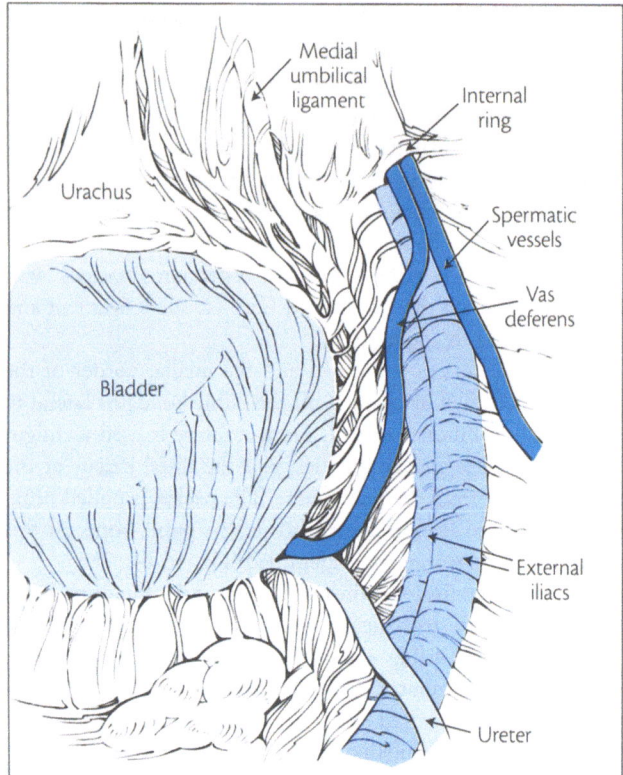

Figure 16-4 Pelvic anatomy viewed laparoscopically. (*From* Loughlin and Kavoussi [10]; by permission of J. Foerster, Fort Collins, CO.)

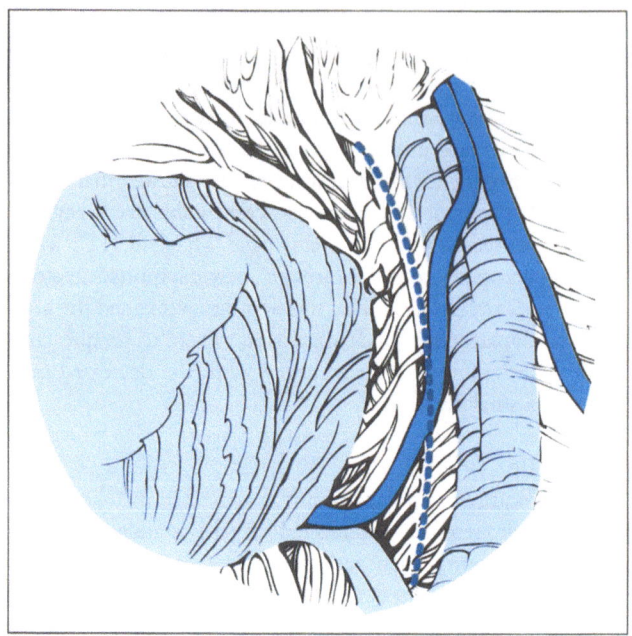

Figure 16-5 Posterior peritoneum is incised parallel and lateral to medial umbilical ligament to start dissection. (*From* Loughlin and Kavoussi [10]; by permission of J. Foerster, Fort Collins, CO.)

proved to be an oncocytoma, and two patients had transitional cell carcinoma of the upper tract. Several obstacles are preventing this technique from being more widely embraced. The first is the time factor. The average operating time was 5.6 hours, which is considerably longer than for an open nephrectomy. The second is the handling of the renal pedicle. Clayman and coworkers [12] have used endoscopic clips (Endoclip, US Surgical Corporation, Norwalk, CT) to control the renal artery and vein. Ehrlich and coworkers [13] used an endoscopic stapler to control the pedicle. Despite the fact that Clayman and coworker's group did not report any significant intraoperative or postoperative bleeding because of inadequate pedicle control, many urologists are uneasy with this aspect of the operation. The third and perhaps most serious concern is the applicability of this technique to cases of renal malignancy. Currently, the adrenal gland is not included in the laparoscopic radical nephrectomy; although this exclusion is probably more a theoretical concern in lower pole and midpole tumors, it would be a limiting factor in upper pole tumors.

Tumor spillage during laparoscopy is a practical, not a theoretical, concern. Several reports [14–18] documented tumor implantation during laparoscopy. Clayman and coworkers tried to solve this problem by developing an entrapment system for the kidney [12] and the lymph nodes [19]. These systems consist of impermeable bags inserted through the laparoscopic trocar. The surgical specimen is placed within the bag or pouch and a drawstring around the opening of the bag allows for closure and acts as a handle to remove the pouch from the abdominal cavity through the laparoscopic trocar. In nephrectomy, the renal specimen is fragmented and aspirated using a specially

designed electrical tissue morcellator placed through the neck of the kidney sack. The development of this type of technology decreases but does not eliminate the potential for tumor spillage. Undoubtedly, more work is needed to address the concern of tumor implantation, if this technique is to be applied to malignant renal tumors.

Technique

The patients early in the series all underwent preoperative renal artery embolization [12]; however, this procedure is no longer done. After induction of general anesthesia, a 7-F occlusion balloon catheter is passed up the ureter of the kidney to be removed. A bladder drainage catheter is also used as well as a nasogastric tube. The patient is placed in a supine position. A Veress needle is placed at the umbilicus, and a carbon dioxide pneumoperitoneum is created in the usual manner. Then two 11-mm laparoscopy ports are placed, one at the umbilicus and one immediately subcostal along the midclavicular line. A 5-mm port is also placed in the midclavicular line, 2 to 3 cm below the level of the umbilicus. The patient is then placed in the lateral decubitus position and secured to the operating table. Two 5-mm ports are placed in the anterior axillary line, one on a level with the umbilicus and one off the tip of the eleventh or twelfth rib.

Dissection commences by incising the line of Toldt and resecting the colon medially. The ureter is then identified and secured with a 5-mm locking forceps. The lower pole lateral surfaces, upper pole lateral surfaces, and upper pole of the kidney are dissected free. The adrenal gland is left in place.

The kidney is then lifted upward, which places the renal hilum on traction. The renal artery and vein are then dissected. Three endosurgical clips are placed on the distal portion of each vessel, and two clips are placed on the proximal portion of each vessel; an endoscopic scissors is then used to divide the vessels.

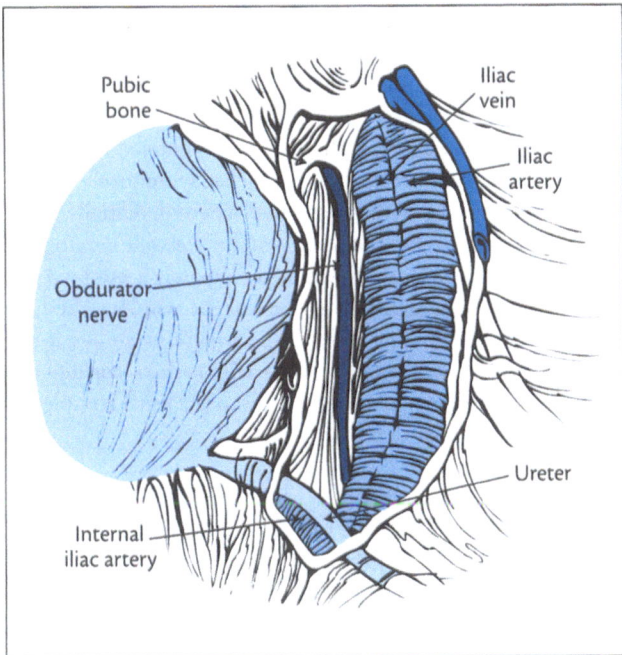

Figure 16-6 Completion of node dissection. (*From* Loughlin and Kavoussi [10]; by permission of J. Foerster, Fort Collins, CO.)

The ureter is divided between two metal clips and the kidney is free. An impermeable nylon surgical sack (Cook Urological, Spencer, IN) is introduced through an 11-mm port. Three 5-mm graspers are used to open the mouth of the sack, and the kidney is pushed into the open sack. The drawstrings on the sack are grasped by a 5-mm forceps and pulled through the 11-mm umbilical port, thereby closing the neck of the sack on the kidney. The mouth of the sack is then brought out through the skin, and the metal shaft of the electrical tissue morcellator is introduced into the sack. The morcellator is activated, and the renal tissue is fragmented and aspirated [19]. When all the renal tissue is removed, the empty sack is removed from the abdomen. The port sites are closed in the standard fashion.

In the two cases of transitional cell carcinoma [12], the ureter was dissected down to the bladder, and a laparoscopic GIA stapler (Endo-GIA, US Surgical Corporation, Norwalk, CT) was used to include the distal ureter and a cuff of bladder. Clayman and coworkers [12] and Gaur and coworkers [20] also described a retroperitoneal approach to laparoscopic nephrectomy. A key advance to this approach has been the use of a retroperitoneal balloon dissector that facilitates the development of working space within the retroperitoneal space.

LAPAROSCOPIC PEDIATRIC UROLOGY

In some respects, children may be better suited for laparoscopic procedures than adults because of their decreased intra-abdominal and retroperitoneal fat. The major application of laparoscopy in pediatric urology thus far, however, has been in the management of undescended testicles [21–23]. Diamond and Caldamone [21] demonstrated the value of laparoscopy in three situations. For unilateral impalpable testes, laparoscopy identified testicular absence in 27%; intra-abdominal testes were found in

16%. For bilateral undescended testes (one or both impalpable), laparoscopy was diagnostic in 75% of cases (17% had blind-ending spermatic vessels above the internal ring, 58% had intra-abdominal testes). Finally, in patients with previous negative inguinal exploration, laparoscopic diagnosis was made in 100% of cases. Laparoscopy also enables the pediatric urologist to plan a surgical approach and incision if an orchiopexy is to be done. In a young child, if an intra-abdominal testis is confirmed, a Fowler-Stephens procedure can be considered, whereas if laparoscopy demonstrates the testis is just above or at the internal inguinal ring, then the traditional transinguinal incision and approach can be used. In the older child or adolescent in whom the surgeon believes orchiectomy is preferable to orchiopexy, the orchiectomy can be accomplished laparoscopically [23].

In a recent survey by Peters [24•], 75% of pediatric urologists questioned responded that they were using laparoscopy in their practice. However, even in this group, the average number of laparoscopic procedures performed per year was 19. Nonetheless, it appears that laparoscopy is firmly established in pediatric urology, and its applications will likely expand in the future.

LAPAROSCOPIC RETROPERITONEAL NODE DISSECTION

The proper role for laparoscopic retroperitoneal node dissection in the management of testicular cancer is still unclear. Several case reports [25,26] demonstrate the feasibility of the procedure; however, increased operating time is a consideration in applying laparoscopic techniques to a procedure. Although Hulbert and Fraley [25] reported a laparoscopic retroperitoneal node dissection that took 4 hours, Rukstalis and Chodak [26] reported a case that required 8.5 hours to complete. As with pelvic node dissection, the question has also been raised as to the completeness of the laparoscopic retroperitoneal node dissection. Although Rukstalis and Chodak [26] harvested 28 nodes and Hulbert and Fraley [25] report 29 and 17 nodes in their two cases, laparoscopic retroperitoneal node dissection does not now include suprahilar nodes, and dissecting out the nodal tissue behind the aorta and vena cava is difficult laparoscopically.

Therefore, laparoscopic retroperitoneal node dissection appears, at least for now, best applied to patients without evidence of bulky disease in the retroperitoneum who would otherwise be candidates for observation rather than surgical exploration. Although the laparoscopic procedure does not currently appear to be as thorough a dissection as the open node dissection, it offers the opportunity to have some pathologic documentation of nodal status in patients considered for observation. The technique for laparoscopic retroperitoneal node dissection has not been standardized and is still evolving; therefore, the reader is referred to the case reports [25,26] for the authors' individual techniques.

LAPAROSCOPIC MANAGEMENT OF LYMPHOCELES

Lymphoceles are not uncommon after renal transplantation; an incidence of 0.6% to 18% has been reported [27–29].

Lymphoceles can also occur after pelvic lymphadenectomy, and an incidence of 5.6% has been reported in this circumstance [30]. Most of these patients are asymptomatic and do not require treatment. When the lymphocele becomes symptomatic or is associated with fever and potential infection, however, drainage of the lymphocele is indicated. Several investigators have reported successful laparoscopic drainage of lymphoceles [31–33]. Khauli and coworkers [33] report a cogent analysis of the indications for laparoscopic management of lymphoceles. An adaptation of their proposed algorithm for management appears in Figure 16-7.

Technique

The technique of lymphocele drainage is described as follows. After the induction of general endotracheal anesthesia, the surgeon places a urethral catheter to drain the bladder, and a nasogastric tube is then inserted. A Veress needle is inserted into the peritoneal cavity in the left upper quadrant to avoid the transplant allograft. A pneumoperitoneum is achieved in the usual manner. The Veress needle is removed, and an 11-mm trocar sheath is inserted through the same site into the peritoneal cavity. The videoendoscope is placed through this port, and two additional 5-mm ports are inserted under direct vision in the periumbilical area in the right upper quadrant at the level of the midclavicular line. The abdomen is carefully inspected, and the renal transplant and associated lymphocele are visualized. They appear as two extrinsic bulges in the retroperitoneum. The lymphocele is distinguishable by its superolateral location to the graft and the soft consistency on probing. In addition,

the lymphocele transmits light readily when the light source is placed at its wall.

The patient is then placed in Trendelenburg position to allow the small bowel to fall cephalad and to accentuate the visibility of the lymphocele. The lymphocele is then entered using electrocautery. The peritoneum and its attached lymphocele wall are grasped, and the incision is extended circumferentially using endoscopic scissors. An ellipse of lymphocele wall is removed, thereby creating a window that is approximately 7 cm by 3 cm. After careful coagulation of the edges of the window, the lymphocele is inspected, and all internal loculations are lysed and excised to create a single cavity. The cavity is then irrigated and inspected for adequate hemostasis prior to the usual completion of the laparoscopic procedure.

LAPAROSCOPIC URETEROLYSIS

Kavoussi and coworkers [34] published a case report of laparoscopic ureterolysis. This procedure was performed in a 15-year-old girl with right flank pain. Her intravenous pyelogram demonstrated moderate right hydronephrosis and medial deviation of the right midureter, which suggested the diagnosis of retroperitoneal fibrosis. A CT scan confirmed a retroperitoneal mass. The patient underwent laparoscopic ureterolysis via a transperitoneal approach. An external ureteral stent was placed to help identify the ureter as is done with laparoscopic nephrectomy.

The ureter was successfully mobilized laparoscopically, and laparoscopic biopsy forceps were used to obtain multiple biopsy specimens of the periurethral tissue. The pathology revealed

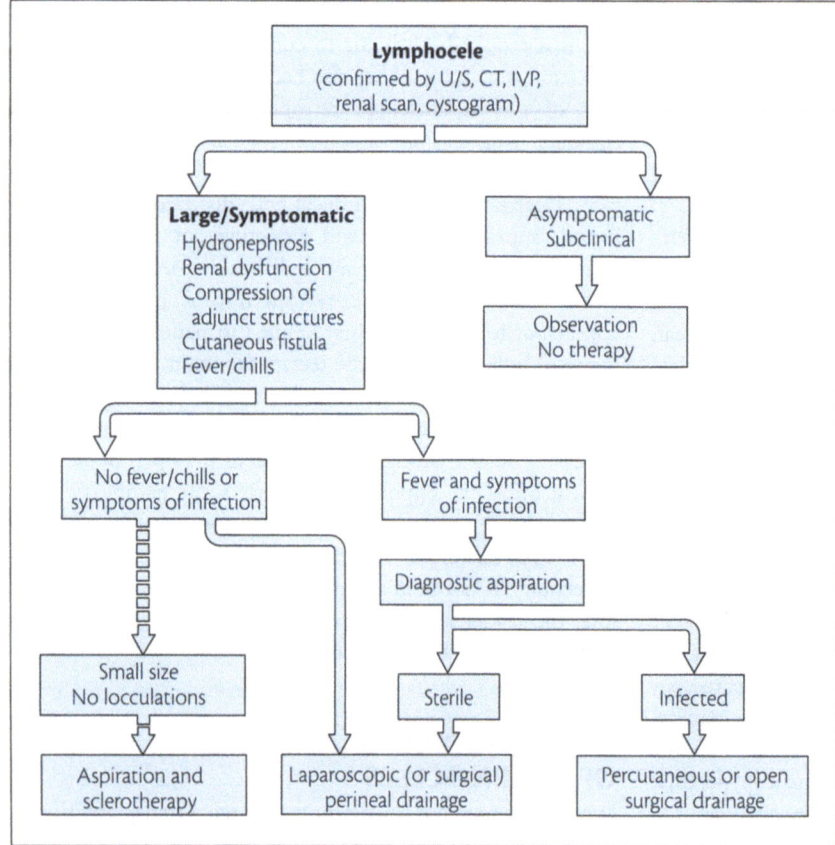

Figure 16-7 Management algorithm suggested for posttransplant lymphoceles. U/S—ultrasound; IVP—excretory urography. (*Adapted from* Khauli *et al.* [33].)

chronic inflammation and fibrosis. The procedure was successful, but the patient remained hospitalized for 6 days. Again, the total operative time of 5.5 hours was considerably longer than a comparable open procedure would require. Only additional experience will help determine how applicable laparoscopic ureterolysis will become in the future.

LAPAROSCOPIC URETERAL REIMPLANT

Nezhat and coworkers [35] published a case report of a laparoscopic ureteral reimplant for ureteral obstruction secondary to endometriosis. Given the current status of laparoscopic instrumentation, this technique seems extremely arduous and is unlikely to achieve widespread acceptance. Another limitation of the technique reported by the authors is that a nonrefluxing reimplant could not be performed laparoscopically. Clearly in children and young women, a nonrefluxing reimplant is required. Major advances in instrumentation are needed before this procedure can be done routinely laparoscopically.

LAPAROSCOPIC DIVERTICULECTOMY

Parra and coworkers [36] reported a case in which a large bladder diverticulum was excised laparoscopically in an 87-year-old man. The indication for removal was chronic infection. An endoscopic stapler was used to divide the diverticulum at the base. The outcome was successful, but again there was a prolonged operative time of 4.8 hours, which in an 87-year-old person seems imprudent. This procedure appears to be another laparoscopic technique with limited applications.

LAPAROSCOPIC CYSTECTOMY

Parra and coworkers [37] also reported a case in which a laparoscopic cystectomy was performed in a retained bladder of a 27-year-old paraplegic woman with recurrent pyocystis. Again, although this case was successful, few patients present with pyocystis in a retained bladder. In selected cases, this approach may be a useful alternative to open surgery, but many of these patients can be drained transvaginally with much less potential morbidity than with the laparoscopic procedure.

LAPAROSCOPIC ILEAL CONDUIT

Kozminski and Partamian [38] reported the first laparoscopic ileal loop conduit. The procedure was performed for palliation of obstruction in an 83-year-old man with fibrosarcoma of the prostate. The ileal loop itself was fashioned laparoscopically using endoscopic stapling devices. To perform the ureteral anastomosis, however, the distal ureters and a portion of the conduit had to be brought in through a trocar site, and an extracorporeal, hand-sewn, ureteroileal anastomosis was performed on each side.

The report emphasizes the limitation of laparoscopic instrumentation at this time. Laparoscopic suturing is cumbersome, and the ureteroileal anastomoses could not have been completed easily laparoscopically. Until either tissue-welding techniques or better suturing techniques are available, only limited applications

are available for laparoscopic reconstructive surgery such as that outlined in this case report.

LAPAROSCOPIC BLADDER NECK SUSPENSION

Albala and coworkers [39] reported their technique of laparoscopic bladder neck suspension to treat female urinary stress incontinence. They performed the procedure successfully in 22 patients. Using standard laparoscopic technique, they placed Ethibond 2-0 sutures (Ethicon, Somerville, NJ) between the periurethral tissue and pubic bones and tied the sutures endoscopically. Although they reported a successful series with few complications, laparoscopic bladder neck suspension appears to offer no advantage over several widely used transvaginal needle suspension techniques [40–42].

The role of laparoscopy in urologic surgery continues to evolve. Laparoscopic instrumentation remains a major factor in limiting further applications of laparoscopic techniques in urology. Many urologists are committed to laparoscopic surgery, and undoubtedly new techniques will be developed in the near future.

RETROPERITONEAL APPROACH TO UROLOGIC DISEASE

The majority of laparoscopic urologic procedures are done transperitoneally. However, in an attempt to decrease morbidity, many urologists are now using a retroperitoneal approach for some laparoscopic urologic procedures. The retroperitoneal approach affords the potential advantage of decreased visceral and vascular injuries as well as a lower incidence of postoperative ileus. Several techniques have been used to develop an extraperitoneal space: blunt dissection, balloon distention, and gasless techniques.

Blunt dissection

Blunt dissection with an operating laparoscope was the earliest technique used. However, this technique did not gain wide acceptance because visualization was impaired due to blood and tissue fluid on the laparoscope lens.

Balloon distention

There are several commercially available balloon systems that can be inserted through trocar ports to create an extraperitoneal space (PDB System, Origin Medsystems, Menlo Park, California) [43]. These balloons can hold up to 1000 mL of air or fluid and can facilitate the dissection of the extraperitoneal space.

GASLESS TECHNIQUE

Gasless laparoscopy avoids the creation of a pneumoperitoneum. Instead, an infraumbilical incision is made and the extraperitoneal space is entered [44•]. New commercially available instruments that are placed through the incision can maintain mechanical retraction (Laparolift and Laparofan: Origin Medsystems). In this system, the Laparofan is inserted through the lower abdominal incision and then it is opened as a fan parallel to the abdominal wall. The Laparofan is then connected to the Laparolift, which is attached to the side of the operating table. The Laparolift is motorized and can raise the abdominal wall upward, thus facilitating dissection in the extraperitoneal space. As technology continues to improve, gasless laparoscopy will become easier and its applications will expand.

LAPAROSCOPIC ADRENALECTOMY

Laparoscopic adrenalectomy is gaining increasing acceptance among urologic surgeons. Although large adrenal lesions, prior abdominal surgery, and patient obesity are considered relative contraindications for laparoscopy, the indications for laparoscopic adrenalectomy appear to be expanding. Staren and Prinz [45•] reported a favorable experience with laparoscopic adrenalectomy. Their series included three patients with adrenal adenomas, six with pheochromocytomas, five with aldosteronomas, and one patient with a hemorrhagic adrenal cyst. Other authors [46] have reported similar encouraging results with laparoscopic adrenalectomy. Although operative time seems to be longer with the laparoscopic versus open approach, laparoscopy does seem to reduce patient morbidity as measured by hospital stay and decreased analgesia requirement.

The technique for laparoscopic adrenalectomy varies somewhat from institution to institution. Most urologists place the patient in full flank position and a pneumoperitoneum is achieved by entry into either upper quadrant with a Veress needle. Usually four 10-mm trocar ports are placed approximately 2 finger-breadths subcostally and are lateral to the rectus abdominis muscle. An important technical point is to make certain the short right adrenal vein is securely clipped when a laparoscopic right adrenalectomy is performed.

REFERENCES AND RECOMMENDED READING

Recently published papers of particular interest have been highlighted as:
-    Of interest
- ••   Of outstanding interest

1. Aaberg RA, Vancaillie TG, Schuessler WW: Laparoscopic varicocele ligation: a new technique. *Fertil Steril* 1991, 56:776–777.

2. Hagood PG, Mehan DJ, Worischeck JH, *et al.*: Laparoscopic varicocelectomy: preliminary report of a new technique. *J Urol* 1992, 147:73–76.

3. Donovan JF, Winfield HN: Laparoscopic varicocele ligation. *J Urol* 1992, 127:77–81.

4. Klee LW, Brito CG, Bihrle F, *et al.*: Laparoscopic spermatic vein ligation in dogs. *J Endourol* 1991, 5:341–344.

5. Loughlin KR, Brooks DC: The use of a Doppler probe to facilitate laparoscopic varicocele ligation. *Surg Gynecol Obstet* 1992, 174:326–328.

6. Matsuda T, Horii Y, Higashi S, *et al.*: Laparoscopic varicocelectomy: a simple technique for clip ligation of the spermatic vessels. *J Urol* 1992, 147:636–638.

7. Kavoussi LR, Sosa E, Chandhoke P, *et al.*: Complications of laparoscopic pelvic lymph node dissection. *J Urol* 1993, 149:322–325.

8. Green L, Loughlin KR, Kavoussi LR: Management of epigastric vessel injury during laparoscopy. *J Endourol* 1992, 6:99–101.

9. Parra RO, Andrus C, Boullier J: Staging laparoscopic pelvic bode dissection: comparison of results with open pelvic lymphadenectomy. *J Urol* 1992, 127:875–878.

10. Loughlin KR, Kavoussi LR: Laparoscopic lymphadenectomy in the staging of prostate cancer. *Contemp Urol* 1992, 4:69–82.

11. Steiner MS, Marshall FF: Mini-laparotomy pelvic lymphadenectomy (minilap): alternative to standard and laparoscopic pelvic lymphadenectomy. *Urology* 1993, 41:201–206.

12. Clayman RV, Kavoussi LR, McDougal EM, *et al.*: Laparoscopic nephrectomy: a review of 16 cases. *Surg Laparosc Endosc* 1992, 2:29–34.

13. Ehrlich RM, Gershman A, Mee S, *et al.*: Laparoscopic nephrectomy in a child: expanding horizons for laparoscopy in pediatric urology. *J Endourol* 1992, 6:463–465.

14. Cava A, Roman J, Gonzalez O, *et al.*: Subcutaneous metastasis following laparoscopy in gastric adenocarcinoma. *Eur J Surg Oncol* 1990, 16:63–67.

15. Dubrante Z, Wittman T, Karascony G: Rapid development of malignant metastases in the abdominal wall after laparoscopy. *Endoscopy* 1978, 10:127–130.

16. Stockdale AD, Pocock TJ: Abdominal wall metastases following laparoscopy: a case report. *Eur J Surg Oncol* 1985, 11:373–375.

17. Pezet D, Fondriner E, Rotman N, *et al.*: Parietal seeding of carcinoma of the gallbladder after laparoscopic cholecystectomy. *Br J Surg* 1992, 79:845–847.

18. Keate RF, Shaffer R: Seeding of hepatocellular carcinoma to the peritoneoscopy insertion site. *Gastrointest Endosc* 1992, 38:203–205.

19. Kavoussi LR, Clayman RV: Organ entrapment system for removing nodal tissue during laparoscopic pelvic lymphadenectomy. *J Urol* 1992, 147:879–880.

20. Gaur DD, Agarwal DK, Purohit KC: Retroperitoneal laparoscopic nephrectomy: initial case report. *J Urol* 1993, 149:103–105.

21. Diamond DA, Caldamone AA: The value of laparoscopy for 106 impalpable testes relative to clinical presentation. *J Urol* 1992, 148:632–638.

22. Plotzker ED, Rushton HG, Belman AB, *et al.*: Laparoscopy for nonpalpable testes in childhood: is inguinal exploration also necessary when vas and vessels exit the inguinal ring? *J Urol* 1992, 148:635–638.

23. Thomas MD, Mercer LC, Saltzstein EC: Laparoscopic orchiectomy for unilateral intra-abdominal testis. *J Urol* 1992, 148:1251–1253.

24.• Peters CA: Complications in pediatric urological laparoscopy: results of a survey. *J Urol* 1996, 155:1070–1073.
A good overview of how to avoid and manage common complications encountered in pediatric urologic laparoscopic surgery.

25. Hulbert JC, Fraley EE: Laparoscopic retroperitoneal lymphadenectomy: new approach to pathologic staging of clinical stage 1 germ call tumors of the testis. *J Endourol* 1992, 6:123–125.

26. Rukstalis DB, Chodak GW: Laparoscopic retroperitoneal lymph dissection in a patient with stage 1 testicular carcinoma. *J Urol* 1992, 148:1907–1910.

27. Howard RJ, Simmons RL, Najarian JS: Prevention of lymphoceles following renal transplantation. *Ann Surg* 1976, 18:166–169.

28. Schweizer RT, Sho SI, Koutz SL, *et al.*: Lymphoceles following renal transplantation. *Arch Surg* 1972, 104:42–44.

29. Braun WE, Banowsky LH, Stratton RA, *et al.*: Lymphocytes associated with renal transplantation: report of 15 cases and review of the literature. *Am J Med* 1974, 57:714–718.

30. McDowell GC, Babain RJ, Johnson DE: Management of symptomatic lymphocele via percutaneous drainage and sclerotherapy with tetracycline. *Urology* 1991, 37:237–239.

31. Waples MJ, Wegenke JD, Vega RJ: Laparoscopic management of lymphocele after pelvic lymphadenectomy and radical retropubic prostatectomy. *Urology* 1992, 39:82–84.

32. Bardor SF, Montie JE, Jackson CL, *et al.*: Laparoscopic surgical technique for internal drainage of pelvic lymphocele. *J Urol* 1992, 147:908–909.

33. Khauli RB, Mosenthal AC, Caushaj PF: Treatment of lymphocele and lymphatic fistula following renal transplantation by laparoscopic peritoneal window. *J Urol* 1992, 147:1353–1355.

34. Kavoussi LR, Clayman RV, Brunt LM, *et al.*: Laparoscopic ureterolysis. *J Urol* 1992, 127:426–492.

35. Nezhat C, Nezhat F, Green B: Laparoscopic treatment of obstructed ureter due to endometriosis by resection and ureteroureterostomy: a case report. *J Urol* 1992, 148:865–868.

36. Parr RG, Jones JP, Andrus CH, *et al.*: Laparoscopic diverticulectomy: preliminary report of a new approach for the treatment of bladder diverticulum. *J Urol* 1992, 128:869–871.

37. Parra RO, Andrus CH, Jones FP, *et al.*: Laparoscopic cystectomy: initial report of a new treatment for the retained bladder. *J Urol* 1992, 148:1140–1144.

38. Kozminski M, Partamian KO: Case report of laparoscopic ileal loop conduit. *J Endourol* 1992, 6:137–141.

39. Albala DM, Schuessler WW, Vancaillie TG: Laparoscopic bladder neck suspension. *J Endourol* 1992, 6:137–141.

40. Stamey TA: Endoscopic suspension of the vesical neck for urinary incontinence. *Surg Gynecol Obstet* 1973, 135:547–559.

41. Raz S: Modified bladder neck suspension for female stress incontinence. *Urology* 1981, 17:82–85.

42. Gittes RF, Loughlin KR: No-incision pubovaginal suspension for stress incontinence. *J Urol* 1987, 138:568–570.

43. Gomella LG: Laparoscopy: retroperitoneal approach to urologic disease. *Mediguide to Urology* 1997, 91:1–7.

44.• O'Leary MP, Rubenstein SC: Gasless laparoscopy. In *Principles of Endosurgery.* Edited by Loughlin KR, Brooks DC. Boston: Blackwell Science; 1996: 72–80.
A good step-by-step description of the technique of gasless laparoscopy.

45.• Staren ED, Prinz RA: Adrenalectomy in the era of laparoscopy. *Surgery* 1996, 120:705–709.
A review of the current experience with laparoscopic adrenalectomy.

46. Linus DA, Stylopoulos N, Boukis M, *et al.*: Anterior, posterior, or laparoscopic approach for the management of adrenal diseases? *Am J Surg* 1997, 173:120–125.

Physiologic Changes Occurring During Laparoscopy, Including Port Site Implantation

Mark A. Talamini
Michael F. Kutka

CHAPTER

17

Laparoscopic surgery continues to provide new modalities to the repertoire of the general surgeon. Unfortunately, we do not yet have full knowledge regarding the physiology associated with the application of the laparoscope in general surgery. This chapter outlines the current state of knowledge regarding the physiology of laparoscopy.

HISTORY

Laparoscopy has been used since the early part of this century. It was first performed by Kelling [1] in 1901, but has developed rapidly since the 1950s in Europe and since the 1960s in the United States. This development coincided with technologic advances in optics, which allowed for improved visualization. Prior to these advances, many problems existed. The use of a light source within the abdomen was fraught with difficulty. Burns and the risk of electrocution presented a serious problem in the early development of laparoscopy. As a result, for most of this century laparoscopy remained within the realm of experimental surgery, where it was initially embraced by gynecologists. Beginning in the 1960s, research into the physiology of laparoscopic surgery was limited to the study of short procedures performed by gynecologists. Their cohort was primarily young healthy women who were undergoing tubal ligations. The first laparoscopic cholecystectomy was performed in 1985 in Europe by Mühe, who by 1987 had a series of 94 cases [2]. Following this advance, general surgeons embraced laparoscopic surgery here in the United States. In the late 1990s, new applications of laparoscopic surgery continue to evolve, sometimes rendering early physiology research obsolete. Patient demographics now vary, encompassing a broader age range and longer operative times for increasingly complex procedures. Therefore, a reexamination of the physiology encountered in laparoscopy is necessary.

OBSERVED PHYSIOLOGIC CHANGES

At the initiation of pneumoperitoneum for laparoscopy there is a change in the abdominal environment owing to the use of an insufflation gas. Several studies have compared a variety of gases for this purpose. The consensus at present is that CO_2 is the least noxious gas available. Attempts at using an inert gas such as helium have not become widespread because of the small but dangerous risk of gas embolism. Carbon dioxide is well known to be absorbed rapidly by blood components and does not present as much a risk for embolism as do gases that are not readily absorbed. Unfortunately, CO_2 absorption does increase systemic PCO_2, potentially causing acidosis. Arterial sampling during pneumoperitoneum will reflect these changes as an increased PCO_2 and a decreased pH. The anesthesiologist must therefore counteract the effects of absorbed CO_2 by increasing the ventilation rate. Some patients, particularly older individuals or those with preexisting pulmonary disease or increased lung dead space, may have difficulty eliminating such a CO_2 load, regardless of increased minute ventilation.

Cardiovascular changes

The mechanical effects of pneumoperitoneum, hemodynamic stimulation by absorbed CO_2, and volume shifts caused by positioning are the primary forces imposed by laparoscopy on the cardiovascular system [3]. Most investigators agree that CO_2 pneumoperitoneum causes an increase in heart rate, mean arterial pressure, systemic vascular resistance, and a decrease in cardiac output (Table 17-1).

There is a biphasic effect on venous return to the heart at the time of insufflation. Initially a transient increase due to compression of the abdominal capacitance vessels occurs, which is followed by impedance of venous return from the abdomen and lower limbs due to mechanical pressure. This impedance combines with an increase in cardiac filling pressures due to transmitted compression from the elevated diaphragm [4•]. In human and animal models, it has been shown that insufflation pressures below 20 mm Hg result in few changes of significance in cardiac physiology [5–7].

Moderate hypercapnia is considered a stimulus to the cardiovascular system through central effects from adrenaline and noradrenaline release. However, this effect is opposed by the peripheral depression in target organs caused directly by CO_2 and indirectly through a lowered pH environment. If the PCO_2 increases above 60 mm Hg, direct cardiodepressive effects predominate. This can quickly lead to cardiovascular pathology including dysrhythmias and collapse. To minimize hypercapnia it is important to increase minute ventilation, avoid the formation of subcutaneous emphysema, and use insufflation pressures

Table 17-1

Cardiovascular function during CO_2 pneumoperitoneum

Function studied	Study method	Sample details	Results and observations
CI and MABP	Thermodilution	15 Healthy	Induction and head-up tilt: 25% reduction; further reduction of 50% of awake values at start of insufflation, followed by gradual restoration but no compensatory tachycardia; MABP increased
CI and MABP	Doppler pulse from esophageal probe	21 Healthy, 4 CAD	Variable reduced (average ~25%) with head-up position and insufflation, and partial restoration with time; MABP and HR increased
CI and MABP	Bioimpedance	10 ASA 1–3, no CAD	Initially decreased ventricular preload and CI then gradual improvement by tachycardia; MABP increased
CI and MABP	Ejection fraction by TEE	13 Healthy	Insufflation in the supine position: no change in EF, HR, or LVEDV; subsequent tilt: LVEDA decreased, thus SV and CI must have decreased
CI and MABP	Bioimpedance	15 Healthy and 1 CABG	-30% With positioning and insufflation; MABP increased
CI and MABP	TEE pulse Doppler	18 Healthy	-24% With positioning and insufflation; MABP increased
CI and MABP	TEE pulse Doppler	16 Healthy	No change at peak; $PaCO_2$ (43.7 mm Hg); MABP increased
CI and MABP	Thermodilution	5 Cardiac patients	50% Reduction with positioning and insufflation; partial restoration with time; no change in BP
CI and MABP	Thermodilution	9 ASA 3–4: no details	Initial reduction with positioning and insufflation, then normalization; BP increased
CI and MABP	Thermodilution	15 Cardiac patients (ASA 3–4)	Marked reduction during insufflation phase; BP increased
PAOP and CVP	Pulmonary artery catheterization	Healthy	Initial 60% increased; initial doubling and elevated throughout; increase related to insufflation pressure
PAOP and CVP	Pulmonary artery catheterization	Cardiac history or ASA 1–4	Initial increase during insufflation in both reports
SVR	Calculated		Markedly increased at start of insufflation, then gradual, partial restoration

ASA—American Society of Anesthesiologists; BP—blood pressure; CABG—coronary artery bypass graft; CAD—coronary artery disease; CI—cardiac index; CVP—central venous pressure; EF—ejection fraction; HR—heart rate; LVEDA—left ventricular end diastolic area; LVEDV—left ventricular end diastolic volume; MABP—mean arterial blood pressure; PAOP—pulmonary artery occluded pressure; SV—stroke volume; SVR—systemic vascular resistance; TEE—transesophageal echocardiography.

Adapted from Wahba et al. [4•]; with permission.

that are minimal but adequate for visualization. During prolonged laparoscopic procedures, the surgeon should introduce brief periods of desufflation, perhaps every 30 minutes or so. Patients with potentially inadequate respiratory and cardiovascular reserve must be carefully selected. Westerband and coworkers [8] showed a 30% decrease in the cardiac index of patients undergoing laparoscopic cholecystectomy. They did not observe any clinical sequelae, and the cardiac index returned to normal following surgery, suggesting that most patients can tolerate such a transient effect.

Our group has demonstrated that a 30% drop in the cardiac output occurs during mediastinal dissection for laparoscopic Nissen fundoplication in a pig model (Table 17-2) (Paper presented at the Society of University Surgeons Meeting, Milwaukee, 1998). We observed this effect using CO_2 or helium as the insufflation agent. Cardiac output depression was originally believed to be a result of the metabolic effects of absorbed CO_2; however, our findings indicate that there may be a role played by the mechanics of intramediastinal gas, which is unique to laparoscopic Nissen fundoplication. Other rare and unusual system effects have also been observed. For example, Mitchell and Jamieson coworkers [9] described a case of celiac and mesenteric artery thrombosis after laparoscopic Nissen fundoplication. They conjectured that a CO_2 pneumoperitoneum along with a congenitally narrowed celiac axis contributed to the development of thrombosis in the celiac axis. The authors also mentioned two cases of mesenteric infarction after laparoscopic cholecystectomy that resulted in death.

Respiratory changes

Pneumoperitoneum directly affects respiratory compliance through increased intra-abdominal pressure, which leads to elevation of the diaphragms. The head-down tilt exaggerates this effect, thus the head-up tilt may alleviate it somewhat. Overall, there is a resultant increase in intrathoracic pressure and airway pressure. Basilar atelectasis causes a right to left shunt and ventilation perfusion mismatch [10]. During laparoscopic surgery, a 30% decrease in respiratory compliance was demonstrated in otherwise healthy individuals [11•]. In a study of laparoscopy patients using N_2O as the insufflation gas, Haydon and coworkers [12] suggested that the main cause of decreased arterial oxygen saturation in the setting of local anesthesia and intravenous sedation was hypoventilation. This effect has been shown to be fully reversible following human laparoscopic cholecystectomies. In fact, laparoscopy patients regain their lung function more quickly than laparotomy patients following surgery [13,14].

Carbon dioxide is stored in visceral and muscle tissue as well as being carried in the blood stream. This accumulation may take several hours to dissipate after a prolonged laparoscopic procedure [15–17]. Postoperative laparoscopic cholecystectomy patients can have an increased respiratory rate compared with open cholecystectomy patients for up to 3 hours after the procedure. Only after 3 hours does expired CO_2 reach preoperative levels [17].

Other effects

Approximately 30% of laparoscopic complications are related to physiologic or cardiovascular changes induced by a CO_2 pneumoperitoneum [18]. Gas embolism, as detected by transesophageal echocardiography, is surprisingly common during laparoscopic cholecystectomy, but does not usually cause cardiorespiratory instability [19•]. In their study reporting this finding, Derouin and coworkers [19•] speculate that embolism occurs during two distinct periods: first during peritoneal insufflation, and second during gallbladder dissection. Life-threatening gas embolism, however, is exceedingly rare and occurs in fewer than one in 10,000 procedures [20]. It can be recognized by the sudden appearance of hypotension, cyanosis, hypoxia, dysrhythmias, pulmonary edema, or a rapid change in end-tidal

Table 17-2

Physiologic parameters observed in laparoscopic Nissen fundoplication (pig model)

Parameter	CO_2 (n = 6)*		He (n = 6)*	
	Baseline[†]	LNF[‡]	Baseline[†]	LNF[‡]
Cardiac output	2.93 ± 0.38	1.72 ± 0.26[§]	2.47 ± 0.25	1.35 ± 0.08[§]
Mediastinal pressure	0.73 ± 1.16	14.47 ± 3.39[§]	0.87 ± 0.26	8.23 ± 2.35[§]
Pulmonary capillary wedge pressure	12.00 ± 1.27	16.10 ± 1.11[§]	10.67 ± 0.76	17.93 ± 1.67[§]
Central venous pressure	5.73 ± 1.17	11.70 ± 1.11[§]	7.00 ± 1.43	13.2 ± 1.69[§]
Systemic vascular resistance	2906 ± 469	4958 ± 594	2765 ± 421	5057 ± 506[§]
Minute ventilation	5.80 ± 4.48	8.33 ± 5.73[§]	5.38 ± 7.06	5.30 ± 8.90

*Pneumoperitoneum at 13 mm Hg.

[†]Steady-state anesthesia reading.

[‡]Mean value of surgical readings.

[§]$P<0.05$ versus baseline (one-way analysis of variance plus Dunnett's method); data are mean ± SEM.

LNF—laparoscopic Nissen fundoplication.

CO_2 concentration. Characteristically this occurs at the onset of pneumoperitoneum. Treatment involves immediate dessuflation, 100% oxygen administration, head-down and right-side-up positioning, and possible attempts at aspiration of gas from the right ventricle. In some rare instances, insufflation of a pneumoperitoneum has triggered vasovagal activity in otherwise healthy individuals. Severe depression of heart rate and blood pressure develop, but immediate administration of atropine usually returns the hemodynamic parameters to normal.

Pneumoperitoneum in experimental animals causes intracranial pressure to increase [21]. An intraperitoneal pressure of 15 mm Hg caused a 28% increase in the intracranial pressure over baseline. This effect is worsened in the head-down position. Increases in intracranial pressure secondary to laparoscopic surgery generally do not pose a problem for healthy individuals. In healthy human laparoscopic cholecystectomy patients, blood flow velocity through the middle cerebral artery (an index of cerebral blood flow) can increase as much as 50%, probably because of the increase in $PaCO_2$ [22]. However, in an individual with severe preexisting cranial trauma, the rise in intracranial pressure can result in significant pathology. In the aforementioned experiment, Josephs and coworkers [21] also used a head-injured animal model to demonstrate that a 16% increase in the intracranial pressure occurred with a 15 mm Hg pneumoperitoneum. This could cause a catastrophic drop in cerebral perfusion pressure, thus negating any potential benefit of a laparoscopic approach in the head-injured patient.

The kidney is also affected by pneumoperitoneum. Oliguria is common during laparoscopic procedures. Studies show that superficial renal cortical blood flow decreases on average 60% in kidneys compressed by pneumoperitoneum. Blood flow returns to its preinsufflation level 2 hours following pressure release [23•]. The fact that urine output does not visibly return immediately after dessuflation implies that humoral factors play a role. In 50% of women undergoing diagnostic laparoscopy, the antidiuretic hormone level increases markedly. Some speculate that stretch receptors in the abdomen cause the increase in antidiuretic hormone [24]. In a porcine model, the two significant contributors to both hepatic and renal blood flow reduction were the reverse Trendelenburg positioning of the patient and insufflation pressures that exceeded 12 mm Hg [25•].

Hypothermia is a risk during prolonged laparoscopic procedures. Large volumes of gas are expended through the peritoneal cavity of the patient [26], and it is estimated that core body temperature drops by 0.3°C for every 50 L of CO_2 used. Warming the gas and applying heating pads and blankets can prevent this problem [27].

EXTRAPERITONEAL INSUFFLATION

Extraperitoneal laparoscopy is used as a surgical approach for some pelvic and flank organs. Potential side effects include increased CO_2 absorption secondary to the potentially large extraperitoneal area exposed to gas [28] and the increased risk of gas dissection into the mediastinum or pleural cavity. The latter can occur because there is no peritoneal membrane to limit the gas. An advantageous characteristic to extraperitoneal insufflation

is the finding that lower insufflation pressures can be used. Further investigation is required into this newest application of laparoscopic surgery.

SELECTION OF INSUFFLATION GAS

The search for a gas superior to CO_2 has led to investigations into the effects of N_2O and helium for the formation of a pneumoperitoneum. At present the gas of choice remains CO_2 because of its rapid rate of absorption, its high solubility, and because it does not support combustion.

Research into the consequences of a pneumoperitoneum on the cardiac output and systemic vascular resistance suggest the effects are independent of the type of gas used. When insufflation pressure reaches 20 mm Hg, portal flow decreases to 65% and hepatic flow decreases to 45% of preinsufflation rates [29,30]. These decreases are believed to be caused by a vasoconstriction of the vascular bed in combination with an increase in resistance to blood flow across the liver. In the case of hypervolemic or euvolemic patients, this change probably would not represent a life-threatening situation, but in the hypovolemic or hypotensive patient, the reduction in portal and hepatic blood flow could produce bowel ischemia and liver necrosis. One study compared argon, CO_2, and helium and showed that insufflation pressure and tilting of the patient had a more profound effect on human cardiovascular physiology than did choice of gas [25•]. Another early investigation compared oxygen with N_2O as an insufflation gas and found no differences in their effect on cardiac function in healthy individuals undergoing laparoscopy [31]. N_2O shares many absorption characteristics with CO_2, but it is less irritating to the peritoneum. Presently, N_2O and air are considered undesirable for interventional laparoscopic surgery because of their potential for combustion or explosion in the presence of cautery [32]. Therefore, N_2O use is reserved for diagnostic laparoscopy with the patient under local anesthesia. Monoatomic gases, *eg*, xenon and krypton, are unsuitable because of their anesthetic effect [33]. In the future, helium may be used as an insufflation gas in those individuals with a compromised respiratory system. Helium does not affect $PaCO_2$ nor pH to the extent that CO_2 does. Additionally, helium emboli may behave similarly to CO_2 emboli because of rapid diffusibility and minimal effect on pulmonary mechanics [34,35]. Research into gasless laparoscopy continues and may prove the most benign form of intervention. Unfortunately, lifting devices still are unable to afford the degree of visualization provided by gas.

PORT SITE IMPLANTATION

Port site metastases have been reported to occur in patients anywhere from 7 days to up to 10 months after laparoscopy, depending on the type of primary (Table 17-3). Unfortunately, experimental work investigating laparoscopy in the setting of malignancy to date has supported the theory that CO_2 insufflation is associated with the intra-abdominal dissemination of free cells, coating of trocar shafts with tumor cells [36], and increased rates of metastases arising in trocar wounds [37•,38].

Table 17-3

Reports of port site recurrences after laparoscopic procedures in various malignancies

Reason for laparoscopic procedure	Organ involved	Original stage*	Peritoneal seeding at diagnosis	Interval to recurrence
Diagnosis	Stomach	IV	No	1 wk
Biopsy	Liver	Not stated	No	37 mo
Biopsy	Liver	Not stated	No	5 mo
Cholecystectomy	Pancreas	Unknown	No	4 mo
Biopsy	Burkitt's lymphoma	Not applicable	Yes	Days

*American Joint Committee on Cancer staging system.
Adapted from Johnstone et al. [44••]; with permission.

There appears to be no link between specific ports and the risk of metastases. In laparoscopic surgery, any healing wound site represents an area of high proliferation that is ideal for tumor growth. The catalyst causing this dispersal of tumor at the microscopic level has yet to be clearly identified. Open surgery differs in this respect because the reported incidence of incisional metastases is extremely low. Unfortunately, this implies that use of a specimen bag to remove tumor pathology will not eliminate the risks of implantation. Most of the common intra-abdominal tumors, such as colorectal, gastric, pancreatic, gallbladder, urinary, and ovarian have been described in port-site metastases [39–43]. Tumors have ranged in grade from low malignant potential to poorly differentiated carcinoma. Ascites was not necessary for implantation to occur nor was macroscopic disease (Table 17-4). Reported incidence of laparoscopic seeding varies from 0% to 21% in the literature [44••].

Comparison studies may provide some clues regarding the cause of this disturbing phenomenon. When compared with open laparotomy wounds, there appears to be a fivefold increase in seeding in laparoscopy trocar wounds [45•]. Using gasless laparoscopy in a rat model reduces the incidence of wound site metastases to that seen in open surgery [46•]. This may encourage the development of gasless techniques for laparoscopic staging of tumors in humans. This finding also supports the theory that there is a beneficial immunologic role in laparoscopic surgery. This may be related to the degree of physiologic insult to the patient. Also advocating for a laparoscopic approach and reinforcing this immunologic advantage is the fact that in animal models, researchers have shown a decreased growth rate in the primary tumor of those undergoing gasless or CO_2 laparoscopy versus that of laparotomy animals [45•,47]. The immunologic advantage may be related to the size of the wounds, but this has yet to be confirmed. Studies have demonstrated that a period of relative immunosuppression follows major surgery performed through a laparotomy incision [48–52], and in one experiment this relative immunosuppression lasted from 6 to 9 days postoperatively [53]. Experimental data support the use of laparoscopy for staging purposes because the tumor is not directly manipulated. In one study, nonlaceration of the primary tumor resulted in no evidence of port site metastases in animal models [54]. This finding is probably of little clinical relevance, however, because of the technical difficulties of laparoscopic dissection, which may unexpectedly lead to tumor laceration.

DETRIMENTAL EFFECTS OF LAPAROSCOPY
Cosmetic

Port-site hernias are rare and really only occur following use of larger 10- to 12-mm trocars as opposed to 5-mm cannulas. Rates of occurrence vary in the literature from 0.02% to 5% [55,56]. Herniation has been known to occur both shortly after surgery and following a prolonged postoperative period [57]. Prevention through the use of a periumbilical fascial defect repair is recommended, although this can be difficult in the obese patient. It is worth extending the skin incision to maximize the fascial repair if necessary. A variety of creative laparoscopic tools are now available to aid this difficult task.

Other effects

A variety of other events can occur during laparoscopic procedures that have profound physiologic implications. Bowel injuries caused by needle entry or trocars occur during laparoscopic cholecystectomy with a 0.14% incidence [58]. Retroperitoneal great vessel injury occurs during laparoscopic cholecystectomy with an incidence of 0.05% [58], and usually can be attributed to trocar insertion. Intra-abdominal vessel injury during laparoscopic cholecystectomy also occurs with a 0.25% incidence [58], and is more likely to be caused by Veress needle insertion. Mortality from these injuries depends on early diagnosis and intervention. One literature review reported a 37% mortality rate among those patients with delayed recognition of a vascular injury [59•].

Traumatic organ injury from instrumentation has also been described. This includes insult to the liver and other organs. Laceration of the liver can occasionally cause life-threatening bleeding, but more often obscures the view of the operative field and may more often cause conversion to an open procedure.

Table 17-4

Reported abdominal wall tumor implantation in women with ovarian cancer

Adenocarcinoma grade	Postsurgical time, d	Ascites	Gross disease	Instrument
Not reported	14	Yes	Yes	Veress needle
Not reported	8	Yes	Yes	Trocar
Low malignant potential	21	Yes	Yes	Veress needle
Low malignant potential	21	Yes	Yes	Trocar
Low malignant potential	14	No	Yes	Trocar
Poorly differentiated	14	Yes	Yes	Trocar
Not reported	14	Yes	Yes	Trocar
Poorly differentiated	56	No	No	Trocar

Adapted from Childers et al. [39]; with permission.

Trauma to the heart during a laparoscopic Nissen fundoplication has resulted in dysrhythmias [60].

During diagnostic laparoscopy, deep venous thrombosis or pulmonary embolus occur in 0.2 per 1000 procedures [61]. These events are probably caused by altered physiology during laparoscopy; animal studies have shown a progressive and significant decrease in lower limb blood flow during laparoscopy, which seems to confirm this explanation. The introduction of reverse Trendelenburg positioning accentuates this effect; only after desufflation and return to a neutral supine position does lower limb blood flow return to normal [62].

Pneumomediastinum, pneumothorax, and subcutaneous emphysema are also reported complications of laparoscopic surgery [63]. Massive subcutaneous emphysema as a cause for iatrogenic respiratory acidosis has been described in both laparoscopic cholecystectomy [64] and laparoscopic hernia repair [65]. In one large laparoscopic survey, pneumomediastinum and pneumothorax occurred in 0.08% and 0.03% of cases, respectively [66]. The question is, then, how does the CO_2 escape the abdomen to enter these contiguous body cavities? Some have suggested that this escape occurs either through persistent fetal structures, barotrauma, directly through existing anatomy (eg, the esophageal hiatus or the pleural hilum), or along the perivascular sheath of blood vessels. Others have suggested that gas can escape around ports and therefore into extraperitoneal tissues. In one case report, the development of delayed surgical emphysema, pneumomediastinum, and bilateral pneumothoraces was believed to be the result of prolonged postoperative vomiting [67].

Bronchospasm has been described in the setting of CO_2 pneumoperitonuem. The authors believe that pneumoperitoneum may induce vagally mediated bronchoconstriction through mechanical stimulation of intra-abdominal visceral afferent nerves. In both described cases, the wheezing began at the initiation of a CO_2 pneumoperitoneum and resolved shortly after desufflation [68].

A less dramatic but no less important physiologic shift can occur in the eye. Ocular pressure in glaucoma sufferers can reach dangerously high levels when the patient is placed in the head-down position [69]. Appropriate intraoperative treatment can avoid this problem if it is anticipated.

LAPAROSCOPIC SURGERY IN PREGNANCY

Until fairly recently, pregnancy was considered a relative contraindication to laparoscopic surgery. This belief is gradually changing. New research in animals has failed to show any long-term sequelae from CO_2 pneumoperitoneum at 15 mm Hg pressure in gravid ewes. There was no appreciable drop in cardiac output or mean blood pressure. Mild fetal hypertension and acidosis in the fetuses developed, but no hypoxia [70•]. The acidosis reached a steady state within 30 minutes, and the pH of both the mother and fetus returned to normal ranges by increasing ventilatory rate. When N_2O was used as the insufflation agent, there were no effects on fetal blood–gas values, heart rate, or blood pressure. Based on this finding, the authors proposed that hypercarbia from CO_2 causes the observed fetal tachycardia and hypertension. In animal studies and human case reports, however, there is no significant risk to a healthy fetus as long as the pneumoperitoneum pressure remains below 15 mm Hg. Laparoscopic cholecystectomy is described in 27 case reports in the literature [71•,72,73] in pregnant women. The procedures were carried out between 6 and 31 weeks estimated gestational age and there were no complications. Additionally, there are 13 case reports of laparoscopic appendectomy in pregnant patients at between 4 and 32 weeks estimated gestational age [44••,74]. None of these interventions resulted in abortion or premature delivery. When surgery on the gallbladder or appendix is indicated during pregnancy, a laparoscopic approach offers important advantages to the mother. There is decreased need for analgesia, less exposure of the fetus to potentially toxic agents, and the mother mobilizes rapidly, decreasing the incidence of deep venous thrombosis.

BENEFITS OF LAPAROSCOPY

The benefits of laparoscopy versus open surgery include cosmetic, physiologic, and societal advantages. Talamini and coworkers [75] have shown that laparoscopic staging of adeno-carcinoma of the esophagus complements the data gathered from esophageal ultrasound and noninvasive imaging studies. Laparoscopic bowel resection in patients with Crohn's disease may prove advantageous because these patients often require further surgery later in the course of their disease and they may have less abdominal adhesions from their laparoscopic surgery than from open surgery.

CONCLUSIONS

At this point in the evolution of minimally invasive surgery, it is pertinent to reflect on the impact that new techniques may have on the compromised patient, particularly as it relates to cardiac output and respiratory function. This can then be compared with the benefits of shorter recovery time and decreased opera-tive morbidity and mortality. Additionally, most patients prefer the minimal visible scarring that is a hallmark of laparoscopic surgery. There are many opportunities for the application of minimal access surgery in the future. As technology improves and new interventions develop, it will be important to fully evaluate this approach to surgery. Research provides an objective judge of the new technology and should be encouraged.

REFERENCES AND RECOMMENDED READING

Recently published papers of particular interest have been highlighted as:
•   Of interest
••   Of outstanding interest

1. Kelling G: Über Oesophagoskopie, Gastroskopie and Zolioskopie. *Munchene Medizinische Wochenschrift* 1902, 49:21–24.

2. Mühe E: Laparoskopische Cholezystekomie-Spatergebnisse. *Langenbecks Arch Chir Suppl Kongressbd* 1991, 416–423.

3. Wolf JS, Stoller ML: The physiology of laparoscopy: basic princi-ples, complications and other considerations. *J Urol* 1994, 152:294–302.

4.• Wahba RWM, Béïque F, Kleiman SJ: Cardiopulmonary function and laparoscopic cholecystectomy. *Can J Anaesth* 1995, 42:51–63.
In-depth retrospective review of cardiopulmonary physiology in laparo-scopic cholecystectomy. Compares the effects of CO_2 and N_2O when used as the insufflation gas.

5. Kelman GR, Swapp GH, Smith I, *et al.*: Cardiac output and arter-ial blood-gas tension during laparoscopy. *Br J Anaesth* 1972, 44:1155–1161.

6. Motew M, Ivankovich AD, Bieniarz J, *et al.*: Cardiovascular effects and acid-base and blood gas changes during laparoscopy. *Am J Obstet Gynecol* 1973, 115:1002–1012.

7. Lee CM: Acute hypotension during laparoscopy: a case report. *Anesth Analg* 1975, 54:142–143.

8. Westerband A, Van De Water JM, Amzallag M, *et al.*: Cardiovascular changes during laparoscopic cholecystectomy. *Surg Obstet Gynecol* 1992, 175:535–538.

9. Mitchell PC, Jamieson GG: Coeliac axis and mesenteric arterial thrombosis following laparoscopic Nissen fundoplication. *Aust N Z J Surg* 1994, 64:728–730.

10. Brady CE, Harkleroad LE, Pierson WP: Alterations in oxygen sat-uration and ventilation after intravenous sedation for perito-neoscopy. *Arch Intern Med* 1989, 149:1029–1032.

11.• Mäkinen MT, Yli-Hankala A: The effect of laparoscopic cholecys-tectomy on respiratory compliance as determined by continuous spirometry. *J Clin Anesthesia* 1996, 8:119–122.
Prospective analysis of lung physiology in the setting of laparoscopic cholecystectomy. Study limited to use of CO_2 and showed the effects of a CO_2 pneumoperitoneum to be completely reversible.

12. Haydon GH, Dillon J, Simpson KJ, *et al.*: Hypoxemia during diagnostic laparoscopy: a prospective study. *Gastrointest Endosc* 1996, 44:124–128.

13. Putensen-Himmer G, Putensen C, Lammer H, *et al.*: Comparison of postoperative respiratory function after laparoscopy or open laparotomy for cholecystectomy. *Anethesiology* 1992, 77:675–680.

14. Rademaker BM, Ringer J, Odoom JA, *et al.*: Pulmonary function and stress response after laparoscopic cholecystectomy: comparison with subcostal incision and influence of thoracic epidural analge-sia. *Anesth Analg* 1992, 75:381–385.

15. Lewis DG, Ryder W, Burn N, *et al.*: Laparoscopy: an investigation during spontaneous ventilation with halothane. *Br J Anaesth* 1972, 44:685–691.

16. Puri GD, Singh H: Ventilatory effects of laparoscopy under gener-al anesthesia. *Br J Anaesth* 1992, 68:211–213.

17. Tolksdorf W, Strang CM, Schippers E, *et al.*: The effects of the carbon dioxide pneumoperitoneum in laparoscopic cholecystecto-my on postoperative spontaneous respiration. *Anaesthetist* 1992, 41:199–203.

18. Loffer FD, Pent D: Indications, contraindications and complica-tions of laparoscopy. *Obstet Gynecol Surg* 1975, 30:407–411.

19.• Derouin M, Couture P, Boudreault D, *et al.*: Detection of gas embolism by transesophageal echocardiography during laparosco-pic cholecystectomy. *Anesth Analg* 1996, 82:119–124.
Noninvasive technique used to prospectively analyze cardiac output during laparoscopic cholecystectomy. Also reported an unexpectedly high incidence of subclinical emboli being showered into the lung circulation.

20. Chamberlain G, Carron-Brown J: Gynecological laparoscopy. In *Report of the Working Party of the Confidential Inquiry Into Gynecological Laparoscopy*. London: Royal College Of Obstetricians and Gynaecologists; 1978:116–117.

21. Josephs LG, Este-McDonald JR, Birkett DH, *et al.*: Diagnostic laparoscopy increases intracranial pressure. *J Trauma* 1994, 36:815–819.

22. Litwin DEM, Girotti MJ, Poulin EC, *et al.*: Laparoscopic chole-cystectomy: trans-Canada experience with 2201 cases. *Can J Surg* 1992, 35:291–296.

23.• Chiu AW, Chang LS, Birkett DH, Babayan RK: The impact of pneumoperitoneum, pneumoretroperitoneum, and gasless laparoscopy on the systemic and renal hemodynamics. *J Am Coll Surg* 1995, 181:397–406.
Prospective animal study that showed the effects of insufflation on renal and systemic hemodynamics.

24. Punnonen R, Viinamaki O: Vasopressin release during laparoscopy: role of increased intra-abdominal pressure. *Lancet* 1982, i:175–176.

25.• Junghans T, Böhm B, Gründel K, Schwenk W, Möller J: Does pneumoperitoneum with different gases, body positions, and intraperitoneal pressures influence renal and hepatic blood flow? *Surgery* 1997, 121:206–211.
Comprehensive animal study looking at the effects of different insuffla-tion gases and body positions on liver and renal blood flow.

26. Ott DE: Laparoscopic hypothermia. *J Laparoendosc Surg* 1991, 1:127–131.

27. Ott DE: Correction of laparoscopic insufflation hypothermia. *J Laparoendosc Surg* 1991, 1:183–186.

28. Kent RB: Subcutaneous emphysema and hypercarbia following laparoscopic cholecystectomy. *Arch Surg* 1991, 126:1154–1156.

29. Diebel LN, Wilson RF, Dulchavsky SA, Saxe J: Effect of increased intraabdominal pressure on hepatic arterial, portal venous, and hepatic microcirculatory blood flow. *J Trauma* 1992, 33:279–282.

30. Shuto K, Kitano S, Yoshida T, *et al.*: Hemodynamic and arterial blood gas changes during carbon dioxide and helium pneumoperitoneum in pigs. *Surg Endosc* 1995, 9:1173–1178.

31. McKenzie R, Wadhwa RK, Bedger RC: Noninvasive measurement of cardiac output during laparoscopy. *J Reprod Med* 1980, 24:247–250.

32. Robinson JS, Thompson JM, Wood AW: Laparoscopy explosion hazards with nitrous oxide. *Br Med J* 1975, 3:764–765.

33. Cullen SC, Gross EG: The anesthetic properties of xenon in animals and human beings with additional observations on krypton. *Science* 1951, 113:580–582.

34. Khan MA, Alkalay I, Suetsugu S, Stein M: Acute changes in lung mechanics following pulmonary emboli of various gases in dogs. *J Appl Physiol* 1972, 33:774–777.

35. Leighton TA, Liu S-Y, Bongard FS: Comparative cardiopulmonary effects of carbon dioxide versus helium pneumoperitoneum. *Surgery* 1993, 113:527–531.

36. Thomas WM, Eaton MC, Hewett PJ: A proposed model for the movement of cells within the abdominal cavity during CO_2 insufflation and laparoscopy. *Aust N Z J Surg* 1996, 66:105–106.

37.• Mathew G, Watson DI, Rofe AM, *et al.*: Wound metastases following laparoscopic and open surgery for abdominal cancer in a rat model. *Br J Surg* 1996, 83:1087–1090.
Animal study on the effects of open laparoscopy on tumor growth and spread.

38. Jones DB, Guo L-W, Reinhard MK, *et al.*: Impact of pneumoperitoneum on trocar implantation of colon cancer in hamster model. *Dis Colon Rectum* 1995, 38:1182–1188.

39. Childers JM, Aqua KA, Surwit EA, *et al.*: Abdominal wall tumor implantation after laparoscopy for malignant conditions. *Obstet Gynecol* 1994, 84:765–769.

40. Gleeson NC, Nicosia SV, Mark JE: Abdominal wall metastases from ovarian cancer after laparoscopy. *Am J Obstet Gynecol* 1993, 169:522–523.

41. Pezet D, Fondrinier E, Rotman N, *et al.*: Parietal seeding of carcinoma of the gallbladder after laparoscopic cholecystectomy. *Br J Surg* 1992, 79:230.

42. Andersen JR, Steven K: Implantation metastases after laparoscopic biopsy of bladder cancer. *J Urol* 1995, 153:1047–1048.

43. Wexner SD, Cohen SM: Port site metastases after laparoscopic colorectal surgery for cure of malignancy: a plea for caution. *Br J Surg* 1995, 82:295–298.

44.•• Johnstone PAS, Rohde DC, Swartz SE, *et al.*: Port site recurrences after laparoscopic and thoracoscopic procedures in malignancy. *J Clin Oncol* 1996, 14:1950–1956.
Retrospective analysis of port site recurrences after laparoscopic and thoracoscopic procedures for malignancy.

45.• Allendorf JDF, Bessler M, Kayton ML, *et al.*: Increased tumour establishment and growth after laparotomy vs laparoscopy in a murine model. *Arch Surg* 1995, 130:651–653.
Excellent animal study showing a beneficial immune advantage to laparoscopic surgery over open surgery.

46.• Watson DI, Mathew G, Ellis T, *et al.*: Gasless laparoscopy may reduce the risk of port-site metastases following laparoscopic tumour surgery. *Arch Surg* 1997, 132:166–168.
Animal study that showed that CO_2 insufflation increased the likelihood of wound metastases versus open surgery.

47. Allendorf JDF, Bessler M, Kayton ML, *et al.*: Tumour growth after laparotomy or laparoscopy: a preliminary study. *Surg Endosc* 1995, 9:49–52.

48. Akiyoshi T, Koba F, Arinaga S, *et al.*: Impaired production of interleukin-2 after surgery. *Clin Exp Immunol* 1985, 59:45–49.

49. Christou NV, Mannick JA, West MA, *et al.*: Lymphocyte-macrophage interactions in the response to surgical infections. *Arch Surg* 1987, 122:239–251.

50. Cole WH, Humphrey L: Need for immunologic stimulators during immunosuppression produced by major cancer surgery. *Ann Surg* 1985, 202:9–20.

51. Hjortsø NC, Kehlet H: Influence of surgery, age and serum albumin on delayed hypersensitivity. *Acta Chir Scand* 1986, 152:175–179.

52. Lennard TWJ, Shenton BK, Borzotta A, *et al.*: The influence of surgical operations on components of the human immune system. *Br J Surg* 1985, 72:771–776.

53. Hammer JH, Nielsen HJ, Moesgaard F, Kehlet H: Duration of postoperative immunosuppression assessed by repeated delayed type hypersensitivity skin tests. *Eur Surg Res* 1992, 24:133–137.

54. Watson DI, Mathew G, Ellis T, *et al.*: Gasless laparoscopy may reduce the risk of port-site metastases following laparoscopic tumor surgery. *Arch Surg* 1997, 132:166–168.

55. Howard F, Sweeney TR: Omental herniation after laparoscopy: a case report. *J Reprod Med* 1994, 39:415–416.

56. McMurrick PJ, Polglase AL: Early incisional hernia after use of the 12mm port for laparoscopic surgery. *Aust N Z J Surg* 1992, 63:574–575.

57. Horgan PG, O'Connell PR: Subumbilical hernia following laparoscopic cholecystectomy. *Br J Surg* 1993, 80:1595.

58. Deziel DJ, Millikan KW, Economou SG, *et al.*: Complications of laparoscopic cholecystectomy: a national survey of 4292 hospitals and an analysis of 77,604 cases. *Am J Surg* 1993, 165:9–14.

59.• Nordestgaard AG, Bodily KC, Osborne RW, Buttorff JD: Major vascular injuries during laparoscopic procedures. *Am J Surg* 1995, 169:543–545.
Good review of reported major vascular injuries seen in laparoscopic surgery.

60. Swide CE, Nyberg PF: Cardiac trauma: an unusual cause of dysrhythmias and electrocardiographic changes during laparoscopic Nissen fundoplication. *Anesthesiology* 1996, 85:209–211.

61. Chamberlain G, Carron-Brown J: Gynaecological laparoscopy. In *Report of the Working Party of the Confidential Enquiry Into Gynaecological Laparoscopy*. London: Royal College Of Obstetricians And Gynaecologists; 1978:116–117.

62. Jorgensen J, Gillies RB, Lalak NJ, Hunt DR: Lower limb venous hemodynamics during laparoscopy: an animal study. *Surg Laparosc Endosc* 1994, 4:32–35.

63. Hasel R, Arora SK, Hickey DR: Intraoperative complications of laparoscopic cholecystectomy. *Can J Anaesth* 1993, 40:459–464.

64. Kent RB: Subcutaneous emphysema and hypercarbia following laparoscopic cholecystectomy. *Arch Surg* 1991, 126:1154–1156.

65. Waisbren SJ, Herz BL, Ducheine Y, *et al.*: Iatrogenic respiratory acidosis during laparoscopic preperitoneal hernia repair. *J Laparoendosc Surg* 1996, 6:181–183.

66. Brühl W: Complications of laparoscopy and liver biopsy under vision: the results of a survey. *German Medical Monthly* 1967, 12:31–32.

67. Bremner WGM, Kumar CM: Delayed surgical emphysema, pneumomediastinum and bilateral pneumothoraces after postoperative vomiting. *Br J Anaesth* 1993, 71:296–297.

68. Kersten JR, Kane K, Koon R: Bronchospasm during pneumoperitoneum. *Anesth Analg* 1995, 81:1099–1101.

69. Gartner S, Beck W: Ocular tension in the Trendelenburg position. *Am J Ophthalmol* 1965, 59:1040–1043.

70.• Curet MJ, Vogt DA, Schob O, *et al.*: Effects of pneumoperitoneum in pregnant ewes. *J Surg Res* 1996, 63:339–344.
Animal study that demonstrated some intraoperative changes in fetal and placental blood flow, pH, uterine blood flow, and end-tidal CO_2. No long-term sequelae was noted and the fetuses were carried to term with a normal delivery.

71.• Lemaire BMD, Van Erp WFM: Laparoscopic surgery during pregnancy. *Surg Endosc* 1997, 11:15–18.
Seven case reports of laparoscopic surgery in pregnant patients are presented and a review of the current literature is included.

72. Comitalo JB, Lynch D: Laparoscopic cholecystectomy in the pregnant patient. *Surg Laparosc Endosc* 1994, 4:268–271.

73. Edelman DS: Alternative laparoscopic technique for cholecystectomy during pregnancy. *Surg Endosc* 1994, 8:794–796.

74. Schreiber JH: Laparoscopic appendectomy in pregnancy. *Surg Endosc* 1990, 4:100–102.

75. Talamini MA, Kutka MF, Heitmiller R, *et al.*: Laparoscopic staging of esophageal cancer alters neoadjuvant therapy. *J Gastrointest Surg* 1998, in press.

Suturing and Tissue Approximation

Shawn M. Garber
Jonathan M. Sackier

During the early stages of a surgeon's education, the techniques of tying knots and suturing and anastomosing tissue occupy a great deal of time and effort. Indeed, progress from assistant to surgeon is predicated upon one's ability to smoothly and reliably perform these tasks.

The initial enthusiasm for minimally invasive surgery was engendered by the development of laparoscopic cholecystectomy, an operation that could be performed without a single intracorporeal tie or suture.

If one wishes to tackle anything other than cholecystectomy, then it is imperative that the methods of securing knots, placing sutures, and approximating tissue be learned. Indeed, it is also true that such skills may be germane to gallbladder surgery—how else might one seal a rent in the gallbladder or close a dilated cystic duct?

There are many differences between laparoscopic and open suturing. The appreciation of these differences allows surgeons to learn to adapt to the laparoscopic operating environment. The first difference is the lack of depth perception in laparoscopy, as the procedure is viewed on a two-dimensional video screen. Secondly, there is a lack of direct manual contact with the tissue. The remote technique of handling needle and thread with two instruments is considerably hampered by the length and rigidity of the instruments. It is difficult to achieve the correct needle position in the jaws of the needle holder or to drive it through the tissue in any desired direction, and it is challenging to maintain adequate suture tension. Restricted instrument mobility in laparoscopic surgery is another obstacle; for example, when passing a needle through tissue, the surgeon is confined by the cannula placement to a single arc of rotation perpendicular to the axis of the instrument. Finally, the laparoscopic view is limited to a portion of the body cavity and it is critical that instruments and needle always be followed to prevent iatrogenic injury.

The best method of tissue approximation is determined by the type of procedure being performed and the technical skills of the surgeon. These methods include intracorporeal suturing, extracorporeal knotting, endoscopic staplers, endoscopic clips, automatic suturing devices, fibrin glue, and the biofragmentable anastomosis ring.

TRAINING

For the new generation of surgeons, suturing and knot-tying skills will be incorporated into residency programs. For practicing surgeons, a dedicated course of study will be the first step and should be followed by regular practice.

After suitable didactic presentations, much can be accomplished with inanimate models. Initially the surgeon should become familiar with the instruments and sutures. Placing pretied Roeder loops on foam models and then practicing extracorporeal Roeder ties is a good first step. One may then place individual sutures in a surgical glove with ink dots to mark the exact spot where the needle should penetrate.

Animal models are suitable for practicing ties on vessels, such as those that supply the porcine spleen, or for closing induced gastric perforations. Obviously, one can finely hone the techniques to fashion sutured or stapled anastomoses in animals, although some of the newer inanimate models are also well suited for this training.

PREREQUISITES OF ENDOSCOPIC HAND SUTURING

The cannulae used for needle holder and suture forceps must not be positioned too close to each other or the laparoscope, nor too distant from the operative field of view. The distance between the two operating cannulae should be equal to half the length of the instruments. The appropriate angle between the suture holder and the needle driver is 60° [1•]. The performance of laparoscopic hand suturing is hampered by the friction between the cannula sealing cap, valve, and the instrument's shaft. A 10-mm reducer sleeve for placing the needle and needle holder into the abdomen is recommended (Fig. 18-1). Because visibility and the space of the operative field are limited, correct selection of suture material is important: for instance, certain color sutures are difficult to see; others with "memory" are taxing to use. Knot substitutes potentially may improve the ability for intracorporeal knot tying; however, only some of the available devices have sufficient tensile strength to ensure a reliable knot.

INSTRUMENTATION

Suture material

All varieties of suture material are available for laparoscopic use. The length of the suture is important. For intracorporeal knots, 9 inches of suture—long enough to allow knotting yet not so long as to be cumbersome—seems to be ideal. When performing extracorporeal knots, there must be adequate suture length to extend through the cannula to reach the operative field and then return again through the cannula with enough remaining suture to create a knot. For intracorporeal interrupted or running sutures and specifically for intracorporeal knotting, a polyfilament suture should be used. Extracorporeal slipknots tied with silk and polyamide have been found to be less secure than the equivalent knots tied with dacron, lactomer, and polydioxanone [2]. There are many different types of laparoscopic designed sutures, including prethreaded needles composed of a "ski needle" with a pretied Roeder knot and a knot pusher attached (Fig. 18-2*A*), prethreaded needles composed of a straight needle on the proximal tip that has been prethreaded with suture and is

attached distally to a knot pusher (Fig. 18-2*B*), and pretied loops with an attached knot pusher (Fig. 18-2*C*). These special needles are easier to grasp because they have a three-sided straight shaft and a slightly curved cylindrical tip. A short straight needle or standard curved needles may also be used (Fig. 18-3).

Needle holders

Two needle holders should be used for laparoscopic suturing. The devices designed by Szabo and Berci (Karl Storz, Culver City, CA) allow precise and relatively easy performance of suturing and tying of internal knots. The handle is designed like a Castro-Viejo needle holder and can be opened from any rotational position. The axial shape enables rotation of the instrument 360°, which allows the precise maneuvers necessary for laparoscopic suturing. There are many patterns of needle holder available, and the aspiring laparoscopic surgeon should try those that are available and find which suits his or her preferences.

Suturing

At least two operating cannulae are necessary for laparoscopic suturing. These must be appropriately placed in relation to one another and to the third port for the laparoscope. Two needle holders are generally used. The suture is introduced into the

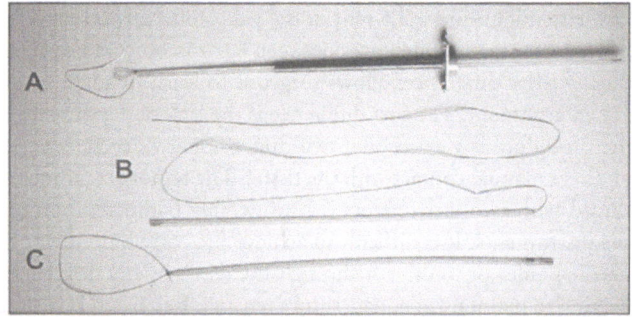

Figure 18-2 Laparoscopic designed sutures. **A,** Prethreaded needle composed of a "ski needle" with a pretied Roeder knot and a knot pusher attached. **B,** Prethreaded needle composed of a straight needle on the proximal tip that has been prethreaded with suture and is attached distally to a knot pusher. **C,** Pretied loop with an attached knot pusher.

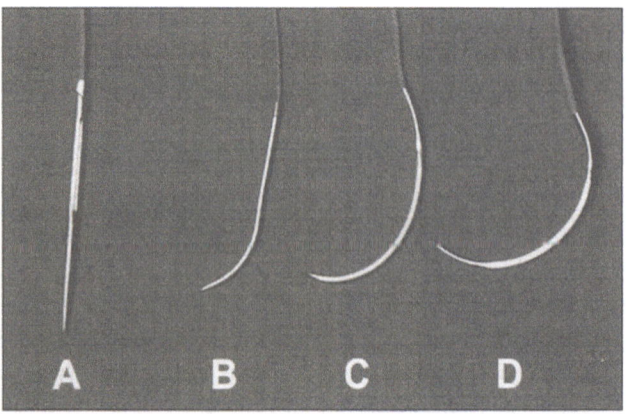

Figure 18-3 The most popular needles are a straight needle (**A**) and ski needle (**B**). The curved needles (**C, D**) are useful, but are more difficult to load in the needle holder and require more skill on the part of the surgeon.

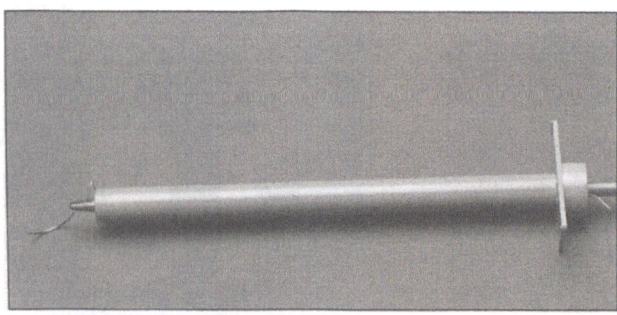

Figure 18-1 The needle holder is placed through 10-mm reducer sleeve, grasps the needle, and is backloaded into the reducer sleeve.

abdomen by grasping it with either holder adjacent to the needle and backloading it into a 10-mm sleeve. Several important principles are mandated for trouble-free suturing:

1. Any grasp is better than none—do not let go of the needle.
2. Always keep the needle in view.
3. Protect adjacent tissue.
4. Close camera work aids depth of field perception.
5. Minimize handling of the suture material.

If the surgeon is right-handed, the needle is grasped with the right-hand needle holder (active) and driven through the tissue from right to left. The left-hand needle holder (receptive) recovers the needle from the tissue following its passage. The needle should be mounted perpendicular to the needle holder with its tip oriented vertically. Supination of the right (active) wrist will pass the needle cleanly through without tearing the tissue to be secured.

Knot tying

Externally created slip knots

The Roeder knot was initially developed for tonsillectomy, but was modified by Semm [3] for use during pelviscopic surgery. In the modified form, it is the most widely used extracorporeal knot used in laparoscopic surgery (Fig. 18-4A–D). To form an externally created slip knot, the suture is passed around the structure to be ligated and brought back out through the same sheath while the other needle holder acts as a pulley to prevent scissoring (Fig. 18-5). After creation of the knot, some of the excess suture tail is cut off, and the knot is pushed into the field using a hollow pushrod.

Preformed slip knots are also available commercially and packaged as the Endo-loop (Ethicon Endosurgery Inc., Cincinnati, OH) or the Surgitie (US Surgical Corporation, Norwalk, CT). These sutures are packaged with the long tail of the loop threaded through a plastic pushrod, the end of which is snapped off to release the tail of the suture. This slip knot is useful for ligating structures that have already been divided or for closing holes in structures in which the two opposing edges of the defect can be grasped and drawn together. To use the preformed slip knot, forceps are placed through the loop to grasp the structure to be ligated. The pushrod is then broken and inserted to tighten the loop down around the base of the structure while the tissue itself is picked up and placed on tension inside the loop. The tip of the pushrod should be placed at the

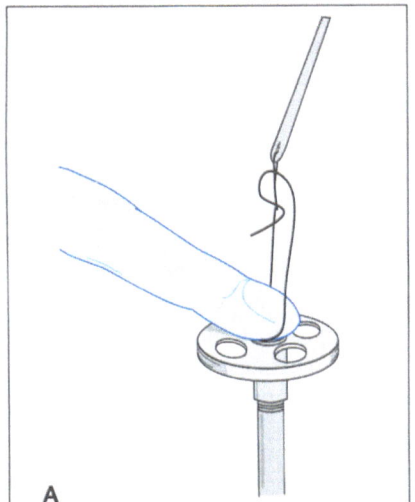

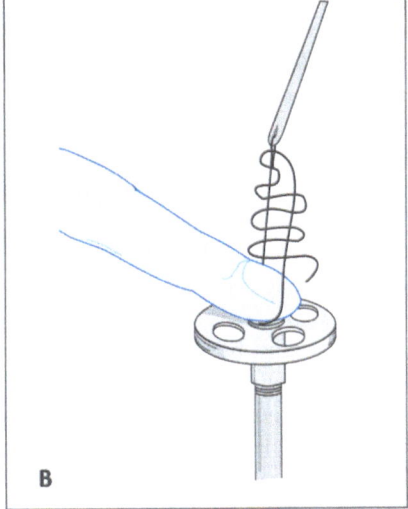

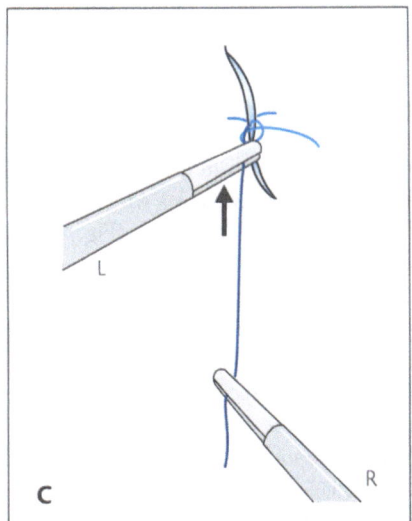

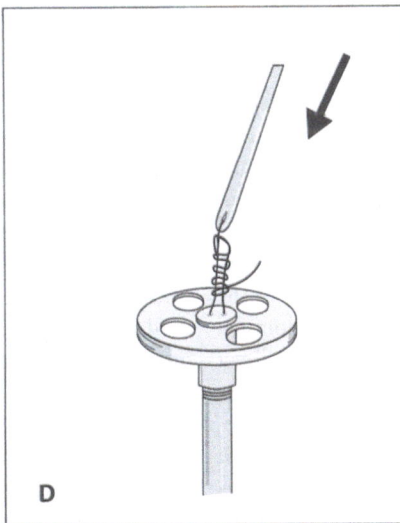

Figure 18-4 When tying a Roeder knot, the orifice of the reducer sleeve should be occluded by the assistant. A single throw is taken and held between the thumb and index finger (**A**). The short thread is wound around the loop three times (**B**), and then passed between the two threads exiting the cannula and under itself (**C**). The knot is then pushed into the abdomen using a knot pusher (**D**). (L—left hand; R—right hand.)

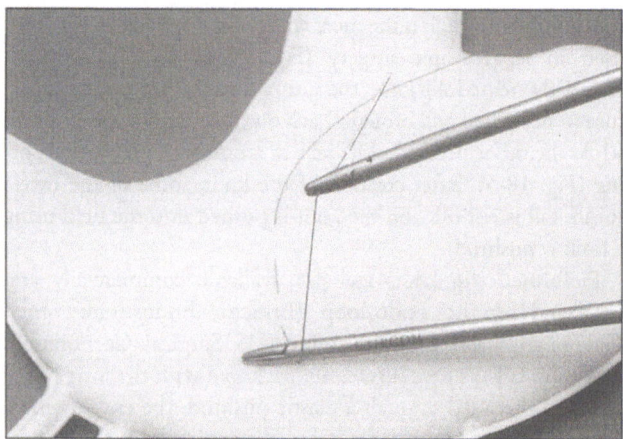

Figure 18-5 When placing extracorporeal knots, one needle holder should act as a pulley to prevent scissoring of the tissues when pulling the needle out of the abdomen.

point where the knot is to lay. Because it is not a classic square knot, Semm [4] recommended placement of a minimum of three preformed slip knots in which vasculature is involved. This technique works well for closing perforations of the gallbladder wall, for closure of a large cystic duct, and for ligating the base of the appendix. Nathanson and coworkers [5] suggested that use of preformed slip knots on the cystic duct stump decreases the incidence of postoperative bile leakage. An alternative to decrease postoperative bile leakage is clip placement and cystic duct division followed by preformed slip knot placement over the medial end of the cystic duct [6]. Additionally, it has been suggested [7] that metal clips to occlude the cystic duct could be replaced by chromic catgut pretied Roeder loops to avoid the complication of a clip migrating into the common duct. Such errant clips may become the nidus for a stone [7], although even absorbable clips have been known to cause ductal obstruction [8]. As a general rule, sutures that must be placed under tension or whose integrity is vital may be tied externally as more force can be applied. For extracorporeal Roeder knots, additional intracorporeal knots should be placed to prevent the Roeder knot from slipping.

Intracorporeal square knot

Internal knotting requires a great deal of training and patience for efficiency. After passage of the suture from right to left, the short tail of the suture remains to the right of the tissue defect. Either a simple overhand knot or a surgeon's knot may be used for the first throw, depending on the ease with which the suture slips. The suture tail must be kept short and placed in a position where it can be grasped easily. When the suture has been passed through the tissue from right to left, the right needle holder regrasps the suture adjacent to the needle and the suture is cut. The needle is then removed from the abdominal cavity by withdrawing the needle into the sleeve under direct visualization, and then removing the sleeve along with the needle and needle holder. Some surgeons prefer to leave the needle attached during tying to help form the loop necessary for knot tying. Care must be taken to avoid puncturing or lacerating abdominopelvic structures and to ensure that either the

needle or the suture attached to the needle are always grasped by a needle holder.

The long suture end is then grasped at right angles to the right needle holder. Next, the suture is wrapped over and around the left needle holder. While wrapping, the right hand should be rotated clockwise to assist in forming a loop. The left hand then grasps the short end of the suture and pulls down the knot. For the next throw, the left needle holder grasps the long end of the suture at right angles, and the suture is wrapped around the right needle holder. The left hand should rotate counter clockwise to help form the loop (Fig. 18-6A–E). If the knot becomes loose it can be converted into a slip knot (Fig. 18-7A–D). The suture is grasped above and below the knot and pulled to convert to a slip knot. The knot is then cinched down by sliding it with a needle holder directly above the knot and reconverting it to a locking square knot by pulling on the two ends. When performing laparoscopic procedures that result in significant tension on suture lines, consideration should be given to using the stronger laparoscopic knots, such as the intracorporeal two-turn flat square knot, instead of the weaker Roeder knot [9]. Four half stitches are the most secure configuration for laparoscopically tied knots and are stronger than three half stitches and a surgical knot. The extracorporeal tied slip knot (Roeder loop) is significantly less secure than four half stitches [10].

Knot substitutes

It is possible to replace external knots with knot clips. The Lapraty knot clip (Ethicon Endosurgery Inc.) is made of bioabsorbable polydioxanone suture and can therefore be used in various situations, but it does involve additional costs. The friction of the Lapraty is only suitable when pressed on size 3-0 polyfilament thread; it is useful to start and end a running suture. These knot clips are useful for placing the first suture to take the tension off the tissues for the subsequent knots. Some surgeons use these for placing the first suture during a laparoscopic Nissen fundoplication.

Clips and clip appliers

Most surgeons are familiar with using the endoscopic clip appliers during laparoscopic cholecystectomy. The traditional titanium clip appliers in general use a 10-mm cannula. Recently, a 5-mm clip applier became available (Ligaclip Allport, Ethicon Endosurgery Inc.) that allows the placement of three 5-mm and one 10-mm port during laparoscopic cholecystectomy, replacing the traditional approach of two 5-mm and two 10-mm ports. Right-angle clip appliers are available, which enhance visualization of the clip applier's back jaw (Fig. 18-8). Traditional titanium clips do have some disadvantages, mainly their poor lateral grip after application to the pedicle, which can lead to displacement when they are brushed accidentally during manipulations. However, ligature clips are acceptable for small pedicles, provided they are applied precisely. Two or three clips should be placed next to one another to secure the pedicle.

Clips for tissue approximation include the 10-mm endohernia multiple staplers, whose U-shaped clip is deformed to a closed square. Although their efficacy in endoscopic hernia repair with

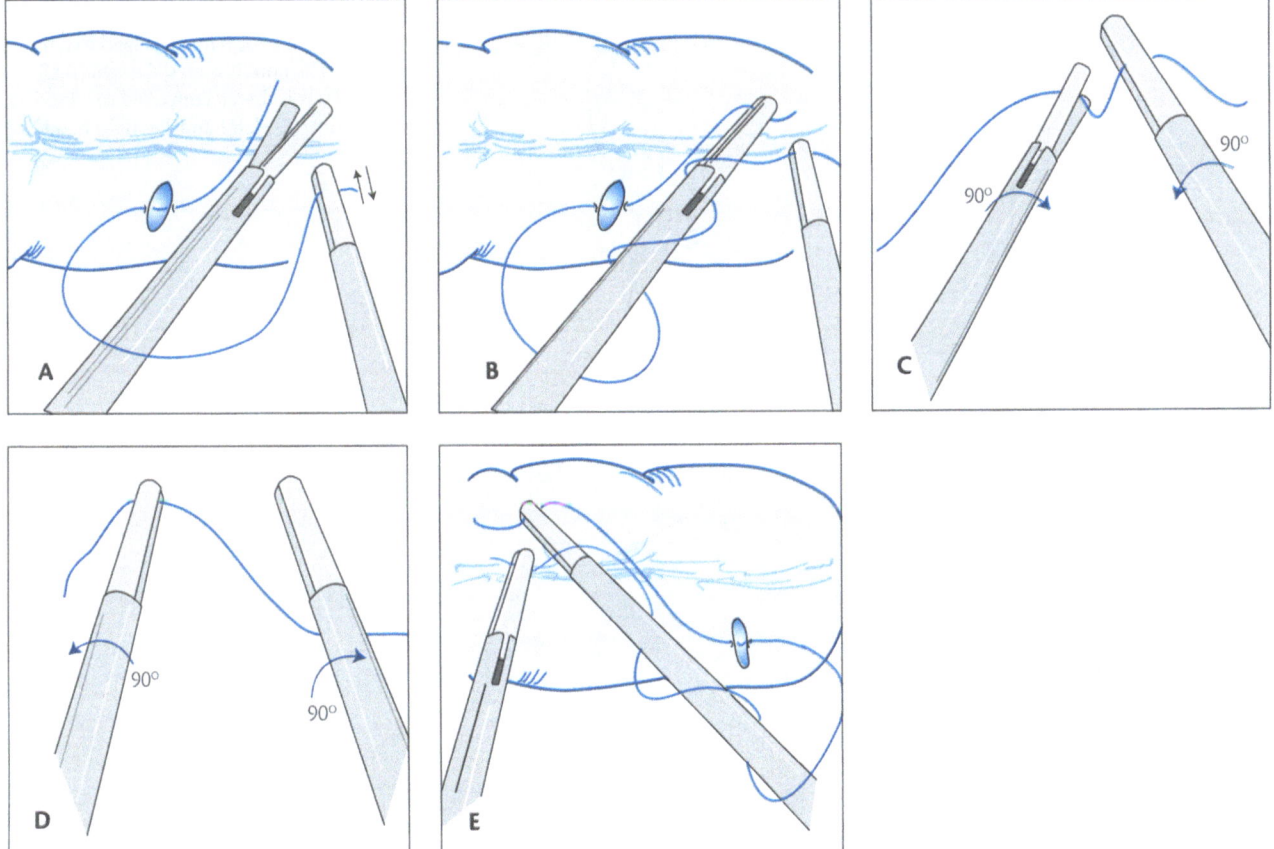

Figure 18-6 When tying an intracorporeal knot, the needle point or end of the stitch is grasped at right angles to the right needle holder and brought back to the right, adjacent to the short end of the needle (**A**). Next, the suture is wrapped over and around the left needle holder. While wrapping, the right hand should be rotated clockwise to assist in forming the loop. The left hand then grasps the short end of the suture and pulls down the knot (**B**). The needle or the long end of the suture is then transferred to the left-hand needle holder with both needle holders in the vertical position (**C**). The same maneuvers are repeated on the left (**D,E**). The left needler holder should rotate counterclockwise to help form the loop.

mesh has been proven, the long-term effects caused by these clips to the surrounding tissue are still unclear. Another alternative is the tack applier (Origin Medical, Menlo Park, CA), which consists of corkscrew tacks for securing a mesh during laparoscopic hernia repair and has the advantage of insertion through a 5-mm cannula.

Sewing devices

The requirements for an endoscopic sewing device are that it is reliable, fast, and safe, and provides easy tissue approximation with atraumatic needle and thread design. The needle should be easily held and one should be able to stitch in various directions (axial and radial), with various knotting techniques at reasonable cost per procedure. The device should be easily maintained and cleaned if it has reusable parts.

A needle with two pointed trocars and a central cross-bore as thread housing was introduced many years ago to surgery. However, this shuttle needle requires transfer between two needle drivers. A breakthrough for the management of needle and thread is achieved by shuttling the needle between the jaws of the same instrument. One such disposable product (Endostitch, US Surgical Corporation) has been available since 1994 (Fig. 18-9).

This 10-mm instrument is equipped with double-action jaws, each of which has a gripping system for the needle that is oper-

ated by an attached lever at the axial handle. These gripping elements are simple stainless steel bands that fit into cross-sectional grooves pressed into the needle proximal to the trocar point. This instrument has been shown to reduce the time needed for placement of stitches and knot tying [11].

Endosurgical stapling

Surgical stapling systems were developed and used for decades in Eastern Europe and the Soviet Union, but have been late in coming to the United States. The ancients used ants to close wounds, which was probably the inspiration for the Von Petz and later surgical staplers. The history of stapler development began in the early 1900s and continues today [12–14]. The laparoscopic 30-mm linear stapling and cutting device was first introduced in the United States in 1990.

The development of this endoscopic instrument had to overcome many obstacles, including the need to decrease the size of the instrumentation to fit available cannulae, operation of the stapler remote from the handle, availability of interchangeable cartridges with varying staple size, ability to operate the instrument with one hand, ability to be able to ligate small and large vessels, and the need for rotary articulation of the stapler to apply staples at the appropriate angles. Successful cooperation

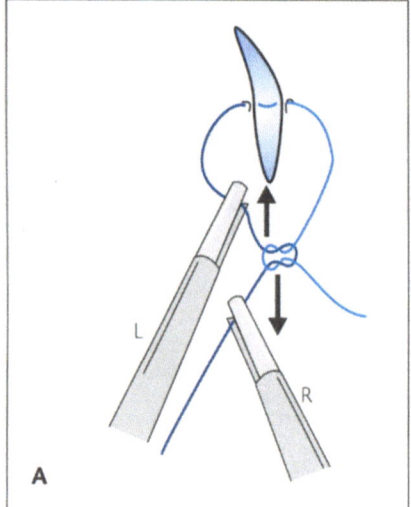

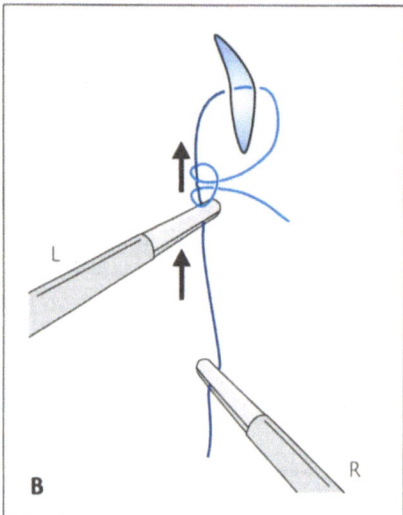

Figure 18-7 The slip knot conversion. The locking square knot is first changed to a slip knot (**A**). The knot is then slid down (**B,C**). The slip knot is then reconverted to a locking square knot. (L—left hand; R—right hand.)

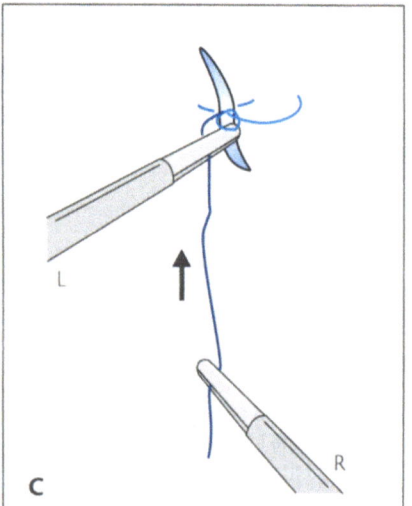

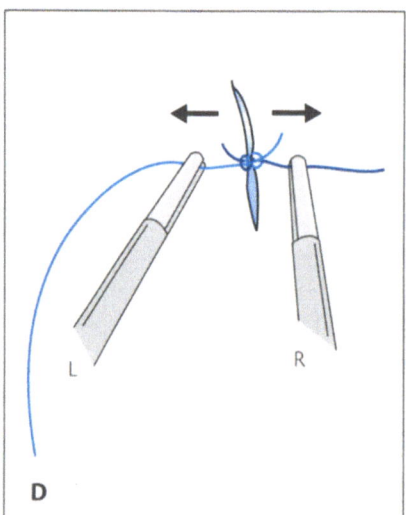

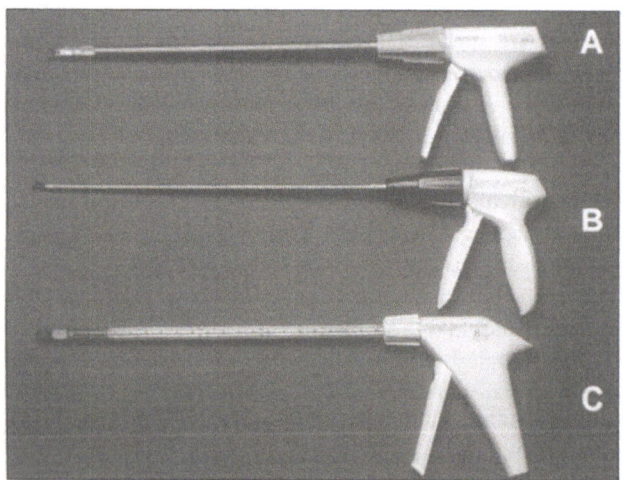

Figure 18-8 Clip appliers. **A**, Traditional 10-mm clip applier (Endopath Endoscopic Multifeed Stapler [Ethicon Endosurgery Inc., Cincinnati, OH]). **B**, The 5-mm clip applier (Ligaclip Allport, Ethicon Endosurgery Inc.). **C**, A right-angle clip applier (Ligaclip Rightangle 8 mm, Ethicon Endosurgery Inc.).

between clinicians and biomedical engineers produced the linear stapler and cutting devices. The staples vary in size, depending on whether vascular or nonvascular tissue is being transected. Vascular staples compress to 1 mm and nonvascular staples compress to 1.5 mm on firing. The 30-mm linear stapler and cutting device needs to be placed through a 12-mm cannula.

There are 45-mm and 60-mm staplers on the market that are placed through a 12-mm and 18-mm cannulae, respectively (Figure 18-10*A,B*).

The nature of most laparoscopic instruments requires a length adequate to reach through the cannula to within the abdomen. Once the jaw of a linear stapler and cutting device is closed, the instrument may be used as a lever to manipulate the tissues. Unnecessary tissue trauma can be caused by injudicious use of such force. It is at times difficult to visualize the most distal portion because of the length of the stapler, but this is vital to ensure that it is free of underlying vital structures; an angled laparoscope is valuable in this regard. A 30-mm linear stapler and cutting device can be used during laparoscopic appendectomy to staple across the base of the appendix and the mesoappendix (Fig. 18-11), or to fashion a side-to-side anastomosis (Fig. 18-12).

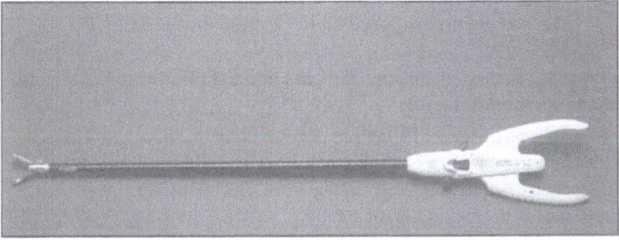

Figure 18-9 An Endostitch (US Surgical Corporation, Norwalk, CT) shuttle needle device.

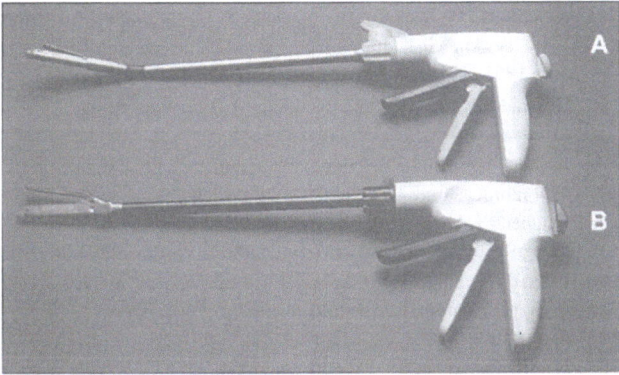

Figure 18-10 Linear stapler and cutting devices. **A,** A 35-mm linear stapler and cutting device with a tip that articulates (ETS-Flex-35 mm, Ethicon Endosurgery Inc., Cincinnati, OH). **B,** A 45-mm linear stapler and cutting device (Endopath EZ-45 mm, Ethicon Endosurgery Inc.).

Since the advent of surgical stapling there have been many skeptics, initially because of the shift from sutures, but more recently because of the cost of such devices. Some data suggest that the use of staplers, whether at laparotomy or laparoscopy, shorten operative procedure times and thus results in cost savings, although this may not be true for all surgical applications [15,16••]. In a study involving 65 patients comparing the use of automatic stapling devices, bipolar coagulation, and ligature placement in performing laparoscopic oophorectomy, there were found to be no differences in operative time, hospital admission rates, or complications among the three groups [17]. A new linear stapler and cutting device has been developed with the ability to articulate the angle of the stapler. Such a modification may improve the ability to reach difficult areas without placing an additional cannula (Fig. 18-10A).

Fibrin glue

The use of fibrin tissue adhesives has been proposed in many surgical disciplines. Hemostasis has been achieved using fibrin glue in hepatic and splenic lacerations, in partial nephrectomy, and for sealing vascular anastomoses [18,19]. Laparoscopic surgical techniques have recently been developed as alternatives to traditional open surgical approaches. Fibrin glue has been used for laparoscopic ureteral resection and anastomosis [20], to control hemorrhage via diagnostic laparoscopy for splenic trauma [21], laparoscopic repair of perforated peptic ulcer [22], and laparoscopic choledochojejunostomy [23]. Fibrin glue might offer promise in the future to assist with anastomoses, tissue approximation, and hemostasis.

Biofragmentable anastomosis ring

The biofragmentable anastomosis ring (BAR) was introduced in 1985 [24]. This device is similar to the original metal Murphy's button, which was first described in 1892. The BAR is a double-segmented ring originally designed for colonic anastomoses and is constructed of polyglycolic acid impregnated with barium sulfate. The bowel segments to be anastomosed are anchored with purse-string sutures, after which the halves are compressed digitally. A circumferential serosa-to-serosa contact is formed with even compression without any tissue piercing material at the anastomotic

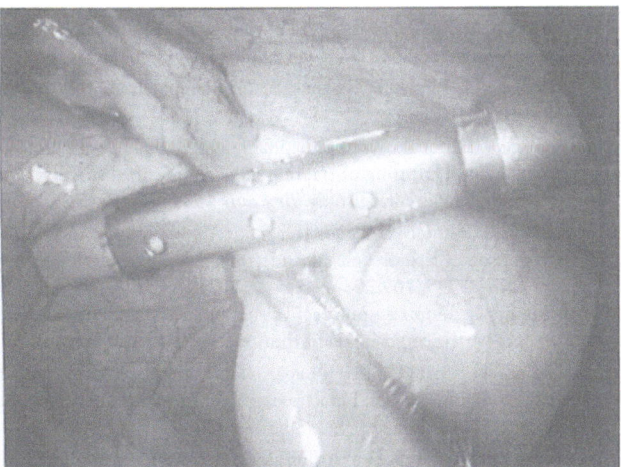

Figure 18-11 Demonstration of transecting the base of the appendix using a 30-mm linear stapler and cutting device during a laparoscopic appendectomy. (*See* Color Plate.)

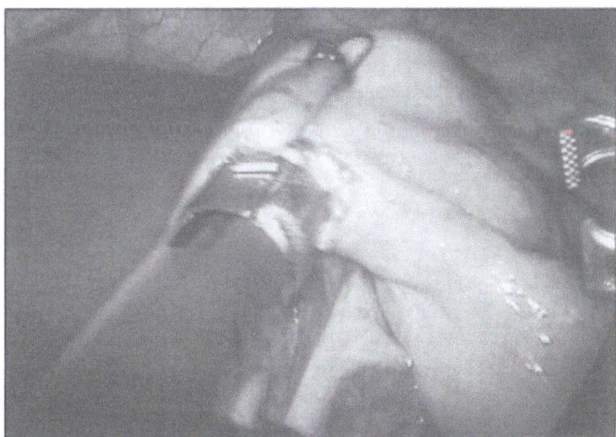

Figure 18-12 Demonstration of a side-to-side gastrojejunostomy anastomosis using a 30-mm linear stapling and cutting device in a patient with pyloric stenosis secondary to Crohn's disease. (*See* Color Plate.)

line. The ring fragments in about 3 weeks, and the pieces are expelled with the feces. This method has proven its value in several trials of colonic surgery as well as for small bowel anastomosis [25–27]. In addition, this device has been used to perform laparoscopic intestinal surgery in an animal model [28], and has also been reported for laparoscopic-assisted left hemicolectomy [29]. This technology might be useful in helping to perform anastomoses if the device can be altered for laparoscopic use.

THE FUTURE OF LAPAROSCOPIC SUTURING AND TISSUE APPROXIMATION

Much research has been done on the value of three-dimensional vision systems, which may improve laparoscopic suturing by less-experienced surgeons. Telemanipulation and telepresence is a field that is being applied to perform complex human tasks either within remote areas, such as outer space or deep beneath the ocean, or inaccessible and inhospitable fields, such as radioactive or biologically contaminated areas. Work is in progress in the development of robots that can perform the fine suturing required during endoscopic coronary artery bypass surgery. The "Zeus" robot (Computer Motion Inc., Goleta, CA), a robotic enhancement device designed to perform and fine-tune the movements made by human hands, might be useful for minimally invasive cardiac surgery and possibly other roles in laparoscopic surgery in the near future (Fig. 18-13).

CONCLUSIONS

Laparoscopic surgery is evolving, and its applications are growing to include most abdominal operations. Tissue approximation by means other than mechanical clips or staples is becoming increasingly important. Today's surgeon is driven by the desire to perform a given procedure under laparoscopic guidance as well as, if not better than, under laparotomy. The ability to suture laparoscopically and to use all the stapling techniques available greatly adds to the level of comfort and confidence of the endoscopic surgeon. If surgeons do not feel comfortable with laparoscopic suturing and stapling, they should question whether or not the procedure should be performed endoscopically.

REFERENCES AND RECOMMENDED READING

Recently published papers of particular interest have been highlighted as:

- •   Of interest
- ••   Of outstanding interest

1.• Hanna GB, Shimi S, Cuschieri A: Optimal port locations for endoscopic intracorporeal knotting. *Surg Endosc* 1997, 11: 397–401.
This study accurately demonstrates the optimal placement of ports for intracorporeal knot tying.

2. Shimi SM, Lirici M, Velpen V, *et al.*: Comparative study of the holding strength of slipknots using absorbable and nonabsorbable ligature materials. *Surg Endosc* 1994, 8:1285–1291.

3. Semm K: *Operationslehre fur Endoskopische Abdominal-chirurgie Operative Pelviskopie, Operative Laparoskopie.* Stuttgart: FK Schattauer Verlag; 1984.

4. Semm K: *Operative Manual for Endoscopic Abdominal Surgery.* Chicago: Year Book Medical Publishers; 1987.

5. Nathanson LK, Easter DW, Cuschieri A: Ligation of the structures of the cystic pedicle during laparoscopic cholecystectomy. *Am J Surg* 1991, 161:350–354.

6. Cuschieri A: Laparoscopic treatment of gallbladder disease. *Minimally Invas Ther* 1992, 1:115–123.

7. Janson JA, Cotton PB: Endoscopic treatment of bile duct stone containing a surgical staple. *HPB Surg* 1990, 3:67–71.

8. Onghena T, Vereecken L, Vanden Dweyk, *et al.*: Common bile duct foreign body: an unusual case. *Surg Laparosc Endosc* 1992, 2:8–10.

9. Dorsey JH, Sharp HT, Chovan JD, *et al.*: Laparoscopic knot strength: a comparison with conventional knots. *Obstet Gynecol* 1995, 86:536–540.

10. Kadirkamanathan SS, Shelton JC, Hepworth CC, *et al.*: A comparison of the strength of knots tied by hand and at laparoscopy. *J Am Coll Surg* 1996, 182:46–54.

11. Adams JB, Schulam PG, Moore RG, *et al.*: New laparoscopic suturing device: initial clinical experience. *Urology* 1995, 46:242–245.

12. Hultl H: II Kongress der Ungarischen Gesellschaft fur Chirugie, Budapest, May 1908. *Pester Med Chir Presse* 1909, 45:108–122.

13. Von Petz A: Zur Technik der Magenresektion: Ein neuer Magen-Darmnahapparat. *Zentralbl Chir* 1924, 51:179.

14. Friedrich H: Ein neuer Magen-Darm-Nahapparat. *Zentralbl Chir* 1934, 61: 504.

15. George WD, for the West of Scotland and Highland Anastomosis Study Group: Suturing or stapling in gastrointestinal surgery: a prospective randomized study. *Br J Surg* 1991, 78:337–341.

16.•• Ortega A, Hunter JG, Peters JH, *et al.*: A prospective, randomized comparison of laparoscopic appendectomy with open appendectomy. *Am J Surg* 1995, 169:208–213.
This is the first randomized prospective study that revealed a clear advantage for laparoscopic appendectomy over open appendectomy.

17. Daniell JF, Kurtz BR, Lee J: Laparoscopic oophorectomy: comparative study of ligatures, bipolar coagulation and automatic stapling devices. *Obstet Gynecol* 1992, 80:325–328.

18. Levinson AK, Swanson DA, Johnson DE, *et al.*: Fibrin glue for partial nephrectomy. *Urology* 1991, 38:314–316.

19. Kram HB, Hermenegildo PO, Yamaguchi MP, *et al.*: Fibrin glue in renal and ureteral trauma. *Urology* 1989, 33:215–218.

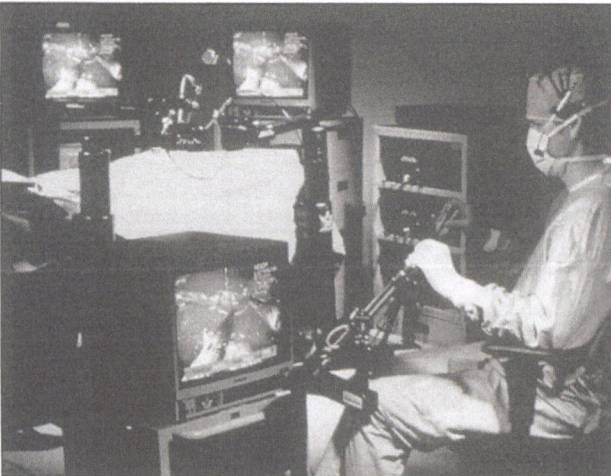

Figure 18-13 The "Zeus" robot (Computer Motion Inc., Goleta, CA) performs and fine tunes the movements made by human hands.

20. McKay TC, Albala DM, Gehrin BE, *et al*.: Laparoscopic ureteral reanastomosis using fibrin glue. *J Urol* 1994, 152:1637–1640.

21. Tricarico A, Tartaglia A, Taddeo F, *et al*.: Videolaparoscopic treatment of spleen injuries. *Surg Endosc* 1994, 8:910–912.

22. Lau WY, Leung KL, Zhu XL, *et al*.: Laparoscopic repair of perforated peptic ulcer. *Br J Surg* 1995, 82:814–816.

23. Jones DB, Brewer JD, Meininger TA, *et al*.: Sutured or fibringlued laparoscopic choledochojejunostomy. *Surg Endosc* 1995, 9:1020–1027.

24. Cahill CJ, Betzler M, Gruwez JA, *et al*.: Sutureless large bowel anastomosis: European experience with the biofragmentable anastomosis ring. *Br J Surg* 1989, 76:344–347.

25. Zederfeldt B, Jiborn H, Ekelund G: Sutureless colonic anastomoses. *Langenbecks Arch Chir* 1990, 375:181–185.

26. Gullichsen R, Ovaska J, Rantala A, *et al*.: Small bowel anastomosis with the biofragmentable anastomosis ring and manual suture: a prospective, randomized study. *World J Surg* 1992, 16:1006–1008.

27. Gullichen R, Havia T, Ovaska J, *et al*.: Colonic anastomosis using the biofragmentable anastomotic ring and manual suture: a prospective randomized study. *Br J Surg* 1992, 79:578–580.

28. Sackier JM, Jessup G, Krenz H, *et al*.: Biofragmentable anastomosis ring for laparoscopic bowel surgery. *Surg Endosc* 1994, 8:1190–1194.

29. Sackier JM, Slutzki S, Wood C, *et al*.: Laparoscopic endocorporeal mobilization followed by extracorporeal sutureless anastomosis for the treatment of carcinoma of the left colon. *Dis Colon Rectum* 1993, 36:610–612.

Gasless Laparoscopy

Albert K. Chin
Edmund K.M. Tsoi
Claude H. Organ, Jr.

The term *gasless laparoscopy* describes the technique of performing laparoscopic procedures without the use of pressurized gas for abdominal distention. In gasless laparoscopy, initial or concurrent gas insufflation is not used; instead, mechanical lifting of the abdominal wall maintains an endoscopic operating cavity. Substitution of mechanical support for pneumoperitoneum allows laparoscopic tools to revert to open surgical instrumentation, as gas sealing is no longer a requirement. This technical difference has significant impact on surgical control and coordination. The potential for performing more complicated endoscopic procedures is increased. The learning curve for new techniques may be decreased. Lastly, removal of the requirement to maintain full gas insufflation for adequate visualization may increase the safety and reliability of laparoscopic surgery. In gasless laparoscopy, a constant level of visualization is achieved throughout the procedure, independent of gas leakage and application of suction aspiration. We believe that the investment of effort required to learn the technique of gasless laparoscopy is well compensated by the multiple benefits bestowed by this approach.

THE DEVELOPMENT OF GASLESS LAPAROSCOPY

Mechanical abdominal support systems have gone through various stages of development. The earliest systems used simple devices as adjuncts to gas insufflation in obese patients or in those with other factors requiring additional abdominal lifting. The hinged T retractor was first described by Gazayerli [1] in 1991. Inserted through a trocar port in a straight configuration, the retractor contained a distal cross-member that unfolded to brace the abdominal wall and permit point retraction in conjunction with gas insufflation. Semm and Lehmann-Willenbrock [2] use a similar device to provide assisted abdominal displacement during laparoscopic procedures.

The next stage of development in mechanical abdominal wall lifting involved systems inserted into the insufflated belly. Once positioned, the pneumoperitoneum was evacuated, leaving only the mechanical means to support the laparoscopic cavity. Kitano and coworkers [3] described a U-shaped retractor that entered the abdomen in the subxiphoid region, passed through the falciform ligament, and exited below the right costal margin. A long 5-mm diameter stainless steel trocar is passed through the abdominal wall and falciform ligament under laparoscopic guidance. The trocar pulls a guide tube into place, and the U-shaped retractor is inserted into the guide tube, following the path of the stainless steel trocar. The U-shaped retractor has openings along its length to allow smoke evacuation via a connected suction line. It is elevated by a winch supported on a framework over the patient's chest.

Other devices used prior to the establishment of a pneumoperitoneum include the Tri-X system, described by Francois and Mouret [4], and the coat-hanger system, developed by Maher [5]. Both systems use rigid wire forms that are threaded into the abdomen via single incisions. The Tri-X system has a vertical post that bends into a horizontal loop; the loop is inserted intra-abdominally to lift a planar section of abdominal wall. The coat-hanger device contains a curved cross-member that enters the abdominal cavity in the suprapubic region lateral to the epigastric vessels on one side, and exits lateral to the epigastric vessels on the contralateral side. The system is hoisted by a connecting chain to suspend the abdominal wall.

The final stage of development in gasless laparoscopy consisted of systems that do not require gas insufflation during any portion of the procedure. As early as 1991, Nagai and coworkers [6] described insertion of multiple Kirschner wires through the subcutaneous tissue below the right costal margin and the supraumbilical area to lift the abdominal wall for laparoscopic cholecystectomy. The wires were connected to chains that were hoisted by a winch placed on the side rail of the operating table. Another Japanese researcher, Hashimoto [7], devised a technique that used two wires to define a plane in the subcutaneous space of the right upper quadrant. Both wires entered the body via an incision in the right side of the abdomen, midway between the costal margin and the iliac crest. One wire proceeded transversely to the midline, then angled superiorly toward the subxiphoid region. The other wire ran below the costal margin and intersected the angled wire in two places. Both wires remained subcutaneous; no exit incision was made. Suture strands were passed through the skin, underneath the wire, and back out the skin in four places. Suspension of the suture strands from the curved framework of a Kent retractor (Shinko Optical Ltd., and Takasago Medical Ltd., Japan), which formed a cross-structure above the patient, elevated the plane of abdominal wall delineated by the two wires.

Chin and coworkers [8] developed a planar elevation system whose lifting surface was formed by two legs of a device that fanned out into a V-shaped retractor (Laparofan, Origin Medsystems Inc., Menlo Park, CA). The fan retractor was connected to a motor-driven arm, which provided vertical displacement for abdominal wall lifting (Fig. 19-1). Tsoi and Organ [9••] performed the first gasless laparoscopic cholecystectomy with this device in 1993. This system is the only externally powered gasless lifting device in use today.

INSTRUMENTS USED IN GASLESS LAPAROSCOPY

Instruments applied in gasless laparoscopic procedures include 1) retractors, which provide contact with the abdominal wall; 2) suspension mechanisms, which supply the lift; 3) internal bowel and organ retractors; 4) dissection balloons for preparation of extraperitoneal cavities; and 5) surgical instruments, both generic and specific to gasless laparoscopic surgery.

Abdominal wall retractors

These retractors range from wires and metal rods to plastic fans and inflatable rings. Systems that use subcutaneous wire or cable (Nagai) use placement of abdominal wall retractors at multiple sites. This is necessary because a combination of lift at several different points is needed to yield a planar surface of elevation. Conversely, rigid metal rod forms that are shaped to define a planar lifting surface (Tri-X system) enter the abdomen or subcutaneous space via a single incision.

The deployable fan retractor (Laparofan) is constructed of a composite of stainless steel rod and high-strength plastic. The plastic blade deforms under loading to contact the abdominal wall in a physiologically conforming curvature. This curvature prevents the tips of the fan from protruding into and traumatizing the abdominal wall. The inflatable balloon retractor provides a symmetrical area of lift extending circumferentially around the insertion point. Inflation of the lifting ring with air yields both rigidity and cushioning for abdominal wall retraction. The inflatable retractor is compressed in a sheath in its deflated state to allow insertion through a 15-mm incision. A pull cord attaches to its outer circumference to facilitate removal at the end of the procedure.

Suspension mechanisms

Suspension devices are of two types. The first type is a rigid framework positioned over the patient's chest or abdomen. The frames attach to side rails on the operating table and provide a structure for attachment of retraction wires or chains connected to retracted devices. The frame may also support winches that wind up retracting wires to lift the belly wall.

The second type of suspension device is the powered mechanical lift (Laparolift, Origin Medsystems Inc.), which elevates the fan retractor or balloon retractor via push-button control. The mechanical lift produces simple vertical displacement by means of a motor-driven screw actuator. A built-in gauge halts lifting when the force reaches 18 kg, which is the force equivalent to gas insufflation at 15 mm Hg pressure in an average-sized abdominal cavity.

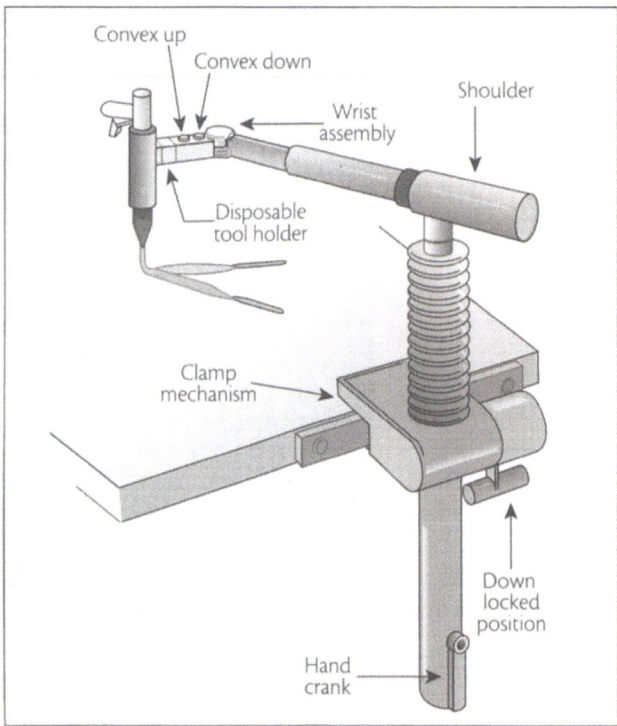

Figure 19-1 Abdominal wall retractor (Laparolift; Origin Medsystems Inc., Menlo Park, CA) and Laparofan (Origin Medsystems Inc.). (*Courtesy of* Origin Medsystems, Inc.)

Bowel retractors

In gasless laparoscopy, absence of positive gas pressure in the peritoneal cavity results in a greater degree of bowel distention than with a pneumoperitoneum. Bowel retraction becomes important to the procedure, because its absence may result in inadequate endoscopic visualization. Two types of laparoscopic bowel retractors are available. The first type is a device with multiple flat metal blades that spread apart to form a retractor surface (EndoRetract, US Surgical Corporation, Norwalk, CT). Care must be exercised while closing this retractor to avoid pinching bowel between the blades. The retractor must also be used gently when retracting organs such as the liver, because the rigid retractor tips may injure soft tissue.

The second type of bowel retractor uses an inflatable balloon to form the retracting surface (ExtraHand, Origin Medsystems Inc.). Inflation of the outer border of the balloon generates a flat continuous surface for bowel and organ retraction. The balloon is initially sheathed to allow insertion through a 10-mm entry site. Air inflation of the retraction device forms a structure that is moderately flexible, to provide atraumatic contact with body tissue.

Dissection balloons

Dissection balloons are used to create cavities in the extraperitoneal space for gasless endoscopic retroperitoneal and preperitoneal procedures (Fig. 19-2) [10••]. A balloon-mounted cannula is advanced into the extraperitoneal plane through a 15-mm incision. The balloon is inflated to dissect an operating cavity approximately 1 L in size or greater; a laparoscope residing inside the balloon monitors the dissection process (Fig. 19-3). Following dissection, a lifting fan or balloon retractor is placed through the incision and elevated by the mechanical arm to support the ceiling of the cavity. A balloon bowel retractor is inserted to displace the side or the floor of the cavity. In the retroperitoneum, the side of the cavity is retracted medially; in the preperitoneum, the floor of the cavity is retracted dorsally.

Two types of dissection balloons are available. The first type is a round elastomeric balloon used to form a spherical cavity. It is used to dissect a central preperitoneal cavity for bladder neck suspension procedures, a paramedian preperitoneal cavity for unilateral hernia repair procedures, and a retroperitoneal cavity for nephrectomy procedures. The second type of dissection balloon is a relatively inelastic balloon of spherical or elliptical

shape. It holds a constant shape on inflation, and in the case of the elliptical balloon, it is useful for forming an elongated cavity. The elliptical dissection balloon may be used to dissect a laterally extending preperitoneal cavity for bilateral inguinal hernia repair, or an elongated retroperitoneal cavity for aortobifemoral bypass graft placement or diskectomy and spinal fusion. The inelastic balloons are gathered in a perforated sheath in their deflated state to provide a small profile for balloon insertion, whereas the elastomeric balloon contracts around the shaft of the cannula without the need for an outer sheath. Inflation of the balloons is performed using a squeeze bulb.

Surgical instruments

Gasless laparoscopy allows the laparoscopic surgeon to use conventional styles of open surgical instruments in an endoscopic setting. Both curved and straight instruments may be introduced through small skin incisions, because gas leakage is no longer an issue. Simple, valveless sleeves may be inserted through the incision to maintain a path through the abdominal wall for multiple instrument exchanges. If these flexible sleeves are cut lengthwise along one axis, instruments can be opened to their maximal extent within the incision without restriction by the sleeves.

Conventional instruments that have proved to be most useful in gasless laparoscopy include long straight and right-angled clamps, Babcock clamps, sponge sticks, long-handled scalpels, and long needle holders. Tissue retraction, dissection, and clamping may be performed in a manner similar to open surgery. Suturing may be performed with the use of familiar needle holders, and needle exchange is less cumbersome compared with laparoscopic needle holders.

Specialized open surgical instruments may be applied in gasless laparoscopy, facilitating complex endoscopic procedures. Vascular cross-clamps may be introduced via a 2-cm abdominal incision during endoscopic retroperitoneal aortobifemoral bypass. In a retroperitoneal approach to endoscopic diskectomy and spinal fusion, orthopedic rongeurs, curettes, and periosteal elevators may be inserted, making an otherwise difficult or impossible procedure applicable to routine usage.

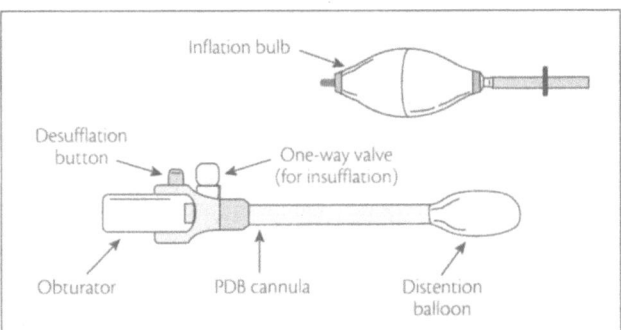

Figure 19-2 A dissecting balloon. (*Courtesy of* Origin Medsystems Inc., Menlo Park, CA.)

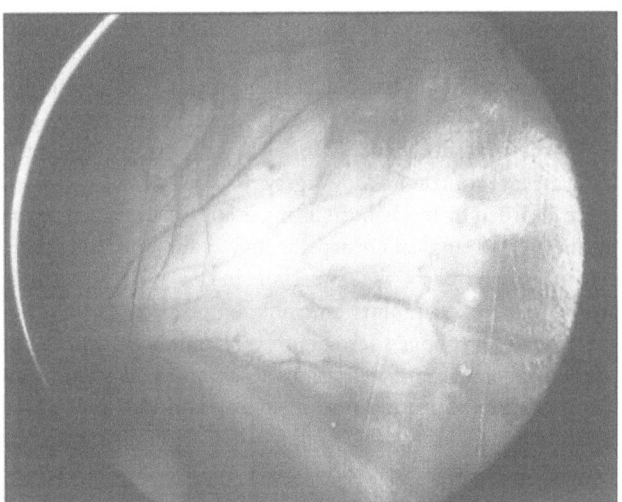

Figure 19-3 Laparoscopic view of the retroperitoneal space during balloon dissection. (*See* Color Plate.)

A full complement of specialized instruments directed toward gasless laparoscopy have yet to be developed. Gasless laparoscopic instruments require a length equivalent to long open surgical instruments, however, they need not encompass the length used in present laparoscopic instruments. Planar lifting allows surgeons to be closer to the operative site, whereas gas insufflation bulges the abdominal wall to a greater extent, necessitating extreme instrument working lengths.

The feature that has yet to be incorporated into a specialized gasless laparoscopic instrument is a ring-handled instrument with a pivot point operable through a 15- to 20-mm incision. Conventional ringed instrument handles open too widely to be used through a small instrument. A novel type of instrument with an axial actuator may need to be developed for the gasless application.

RATIONALE FOR GASLESS LAPAROSCOPY

Improved operative ergonomics was the primary impetus for development of gasless laparoscopic systems. The requirement for gas-tight seals and specialized instruments imposed by pneumoperitoneum restricts the mobility and coordination of the surgeon. Increased lever arms resulting from excess instrument lengths compromise surgical control. As discussed in the preceding section, returning to conventional instrument configurations allows the surgeon to manipulate tissue in a more familiar and predictable fashion. The ability to apply curved and angled instruments broadens the capability of the laparoscopic surgeon to retract and dissect tissue. With gasless laparoscopy, a single entry site may accommodate the insertion of two or more instruments; for example, an endoscope plus suction cannula plus grasper. This further decreases the invasiveness of laparoscopic surgery. Difficult endoscopic maneuvers such as suturing are aided by the ability to apply conventional needle holders. A surgical knot may be placed with an index finger instead of a knot pusher in some instances, allowing the surgeon to appreciate suture tension directly.

Gasless laparoscopy is advantageous in preserving endoscopic visualization throughout the laparoscopic procedure. With a pneumoperitoneum, visualization is dependent on the adequacy of gas insufflation. Significant gas leakage or high flow suction aspiration leads to collapse of the operating cavity with conventional insufflated laparoscopy. In contrast, gasless laparoscopy establishes a mechanical structure at the outset of the procedure, and abdominal wall retraction remains unchanged throughout the surgery. Control of the operating space afforded by mechanical lifting is appreciated in the event of unexpected surgical mishaps, as it gives surgeons the opportunity to approach the situation in an orderly fashion. Inadvertent vascular injury does not require immediate laparotomy; instead, sponge stick compression, saline irrigation, and suction aspiration may be applied to control and identify the source of bleeding for subsequent isolation and repair in a laparoscopic manner. The ability to insert multiple instruments via single abdominal incisions means that compression may be maintained on bleeding sites while dissection instruments are inserted through existing incisions to expose transected vessels for hemostasis.

Gasless laparoscopy offers surgeons the ability to insert a finger into the peritoneal cavity for endoscopic palpation. This ability, unavailable with pneumoperitoneum, allows tactile appreciation of abdominal pathology, and assists the surgeon with endoscopic suturing and soft tissue dissection. Localization of organs, masses, and vascular structures may be performed with the aid of digital palpation, rather than relying on visual discrimination alone, or elucidation by diagnostic modalities such as ultrasonography. The mechanical lift may be lowered partially to allow the palpating finger to reach tissues of interest, while laparoscopic visualization continues via a cavity with a dropped ceiling.

A gasless approach may also assist with the task of tissue resection and tissue removal. To preserve the benefits of limited incisional size in laparoscopic surgery, organ removal must be performed through a small opening. Laparoscopic morcellators grind up tissue for removal through trocar ports. Tissue removal through the tubular structure of a morcellator expends significant time. With gasless laparoscopy, an internal organ may be grasped by multiple surgical clamps and sectioned into narrow strips using a long-handled scalpel for extraction through a limited incision. Bulk tissue removal is performed in nephrectomy, splenectomy, and uterine myomectomy. Ligation of the vascular supply, followed by internal sectioning of tissue and piecemeal removal of cut segments, permits efficient laparoscopic organ excision.

Gasless laparoscopy addresses adverse physiologic effects inherent in pneumoperitoneum. Carbon dioxide instillation may result in reactive bradycardia or even cardiac arrest [11,12]; fortunately, the incidence of this complication is extremely low. Positive intra-abdominal pressure may result in pneumothorax [13] or pneumomediastinum, subcutaneous emphysema [14,15], gas embolism [16,17], and venous stasis [18]. With prolonged laparoscopic procedures, there is increased potential for hypercapnia and acidosis. The effects of pneumoperitoneum on the fetus in utero are uncertain; thus surgeons are reluctant to apply gas insufflation to the pregnant patient.

Laparoscopic procedures performed with a pneumoperitoneum carry a requirement for general anesthesia. Diaphragmatic pressure exerted by gas insufflation must be counteracted by positive pressure ventilation. With the advent of gasless laparoscopy, lower abdominal and pelvic procedures become amenable to regional or even local anesthetic use. This extends the application of laparoscopy to higher risk patients in whom surgical intervention may be contraindicated.

GENERAL TECHNIQUE

The technique for placement of the Laparolift is discussed because of our familiarity with this system. Application of alternate gasless systems may vary significantly, as outlined earlier in the section on devices.

Using an "opened" laparoscopy technique, entry into the abdomen for laparoscopic procedures is performed via a 2-cm skin incision located at the umbilicus or periumbilical area. Following peritoneal incision, a gloved finger is inserted into the abdomen and swept circumferentially to rule out the presence of adhesions. If a lifting fan retractor is used, it is inserted into the incision in a closed configuration with the blades maintained parallel to the abdominal wall. The fan is inserted in a cranial direction for upper abdominal procedures, and in a caudal direction for lower abdominal and pelvic procedures. Prior to deployment of the fan retractor, the closed blades are swept from side to side to detect the presence of bowel or omentum lodged on the retractor. If no resistance is detected, the retractor is opened and the wedge lock secured into position. The wrist portion of the draped mechanical arm is attached to the dovetail connector on the fan retractor, and the arm partially elevated, using the push-button control. A valveless sleeve is inserted behind the fan blades into the abdominal cavity, and the laparoscope advanced through the sleeve to view the position of the lifting blades and to verify that no bowel has been trapped by the fan retractor. Additional ports are placed under direct vision for instrument access. A bowel retractor may be introduced for bowel or organ retraction as needed. The inflatable balloon retractor contains a 5-mm diameter shaft that may fit behind the blades of the lifting fan, adjacent to the endoscope.

If the balloon lift is used in lieu of the fan retractor, it is advanced into the abdomen via the periumbilical incision. The rolled-up balloon is completely inserted, and the connector attached by the lifting strap to the balloon is pulled to center the balloon around the incision. Inflation of the balloon by means of the squeeze bulb releases the balloon from the surrounding perforated sleeve, and deploys the balloon about the incision. The abdominal wall is lifted as before by attaching the mechanical arm to the connector on the balloon lift.

Clinical and surgical applications of gasless laparoscopy

Gasless laparoscopy was first applied to transabdominal procedures, for general surgical and gynecologic indications. Subsequently, it was found useful for extraperitoneal endoscopic applications, particularly for retroperitoneal surgery. In both instances, the mechanical lift is used to elevate the abdominal wall to gain endoscopic exposure. In gasless extraperitoneal surgery, secondary retraction is also acquired to displace the peritoneum, which walls off bowel and peritoneal contents from the dissected extraperitoneal space.

Gasless laparoscopic cholecystectomy

The first gasless laparoscopic procedures were performed on patients undergoing cholecystectomy. Early reports by Nagai and coworkers [6] and Hashimoto and coworkers [7] describe wire-lifting techniques for maintaining right upper quadrant retraction in laparoscopic cholecystectomy. Although multiple reports detail the Japanese experience with wire suspension in laparoscopic cholecystectomy, the experience was not duplicated in other parts of the world. An increased thickness of the abdominal wall in European and North and South American patient populations precludes use of these systems as a general approach.

Gasless laparoscopic cholecystectomy has been performed with the use of the lifting fan retractor and mechanical arm (Laparolift) in a series of 450 patients between January 1994

and July 1997 in Lisbon, Portugal. Queiroz-Medeiros and coworkers (Abstract presented at the European IHPBA Congress, Hamburg, 1997) used this modality in consecutive patients, with preoperative diagnosis of carcinoma being the only exclusion criteria. The rate of conversion to open laparotomy was 3.3% (15 patients) in this series.

The cholecystectomy procedure begins with the placement of a lifting fan retractor via an umbilical incision, with the 15-cm long blades directed toward the right upper quadrant. The patient is placed in a significant degree of reverse Trendelenburg. On elevation of the abdominal wall, two additional ports are placed; both ports are valveless, flexible, and sleeves. A 10-mm port is placed 2 cm below the left costal margin in the midclavicular line. This port may accommodate conventional surgical clamps used to grasp the gallbladder, scissors, or needle holders. A 5-mm port is placed 2 cm below the right costal margin. Insertion of electrocautery dissection hooks or probes may proceed through either port. In a minority of cases, a 5-mm port may be added in the right anterior axillary line at the level of the umbilicus. In obese patients with a deeply placed hilum obscured by bowel, an extra retractor may provide downward retraction of the colon.

Dissection proceeds with elevation of the gallbladder and isolation of the cystic duct and artery in the usual fashion. Long right-angled clamps may be inserted to dissect these structures prior to ligation and transection. Gasless laparoscopic techniques are useful in cases that involve shrunken, sclerotic gallbladders, which are difficult to manipulate using the delicate jaws of laparoscopic graspers. Good control of such organs may be achieved using the aggressive grasp of a standard Kelly or Crafoord clamp.

The gallbladder is dissected from the liver bed as traction is maintained by the clamp. If desired, the gallbladder may be placed in a specimen bag and opened to allow bile to be aspirated and stones to be crushed prior to its removal. A pair of gallstone forceps or heavy clamps may be used to crush large stones. The gasless environment also aids in the placement of a cholangiography catheter if an intraoperative cholangiogram is performed. Multiple clamps may stabilize the common bile duct for catheter insertion, and the catheter may be clamped in place during the study.

Gasless laparoscopic bowel resection

A gasless approach addresses several concerns regarding laparoscopic bowel surgery. The foremost of these concerns may be the reported incidence of port site metastatic seeding following laparoscopic resection of malignant bowel. It is hoped that *in vivo* experiments demonstrating decreased occurrence of metastases at remote abdominal sites with the use of gasless laparoscopic techniques will apply to human patients as well. The lack of active gas flow in gasless laparoscopy may prevent malignant cell dislodgment and movement within the peritoneal cavity.

Gasless laparoscopic colectomy allows limited digital palpation to be used for localization of the primary lesion and evaluation of surrounding lymph nodes. It presents surgeons with the opportunity to apply standard open LDS stapling devices (US

Surgical Corporation) to divide omentum and mesentery, decreasing the cost of the procedure by limiting the use of expensive laparoscopic GIA devices (US Surgical Corporation).

An initial incision at the umbilicus allows placement of the lifting fan retractor or the lifting balloon retractor. The patient is tilted away from the site of planned resection. For a right hemicolectomy, the table is rolled to the left. For access to the cecum, the patient is placed in Trendelenburg position; for manipulation of the hepatic and splenic flexures, in reverse Trendelenburg.

Right hemicolectomy

The mechanical lifting arm is placed on the right side of the operating table, and the surgeon and assistant stand on the left side of the table. Following insertion of the 30° endoscope behind the umbilical lifting retractor, a specimen removal incision is made in the right lower quadrant. This incision is a muscle-splitting incision, approximately 3 cm in length. A third incision is made in the midline suprapubic region for placement of a 10-mm flexible port. This port accommodates a pair of curved endoscopic shears plus an inflatable bowel retractor for displacement of small bowel from the resection site. An endoscopic bowel grasper is introduced adjacent to the laparoscope at the umbilical incision, to grasp the cecum and pull it toward the midline. The right colon is mobilized using electrocautery shears to cut the peritoneal reflection, and sponge sticks to dissect the colon from the abdominal wall. A standard Babcock clamp may be inserted via the specimen removal incision, used to grasp the ascending colon, and retract it as dissection proceeds to the hepatic flexure. At this point in the procedure it is helpful to insert the endoscope through the suprapubic port for better visualization of the hepatic flexure and transverse colon. A sponge stick is used to tilt up the liver, and mobilization is continued past the point of transection on the transverse colon.

An LDS stapler is introduced through the specimen removal site and used to divide the omentum at the transection site. Two Babcock clamps are then introduced through the specimen removal incision, clamped on either side of the transection site, and elevated to suspend the transverse colon. The mesentery is divided using an LDS stapler; alternatively, laparoscopic clips may be applied to mesenteric vessels, and division performed with laparoscopic shears. The mobilized colon is externalized via the specimen removal incision, resected, and reanastomosed. Hand sewing, stapling devices, or biofragmentable anastomotic devices may be applied. The bowel is returned to the abdominal cavity. The mesenteric defect is repaired with a running stitch of absorbable suture, and the incisions are closed to complete the procedure.

Left hemicolectomy and sigmoid colectomy

For these procedures, the lifting arm is placed on the left side of the operating table, and the surgeons stand on the right side of the table. The lifting fan retractor is directed cephalad for procedures involving the splenic flexure, and caudad for sigmoid resections. The 3-cm long specimen removal incision is placed in the left lower quadrant if an extracorporeal anastomosis is performed. If a transanal stapler is used, the specimen removal incision is placed in the right lower quadrant and used as the main operating port. Mobilization of the left colon is

done in a similar manner to the technique described for right colectomy. If a standard EEA device (US Surgical Corporation) is used with a low anterior resection, the anvil is sewn into the proximal end of the transected bowel outside the specimen removal site, and dropped back into the abdomen. The transanal stapler is inserted, and the mating ends connected to achieve the anastomosis. The mesenteric defects are closed as before, followed by the abdominal incisions.

Abdominoperineal resection and Hartmann's procedure

The patient is placed in Trendelenburg position for these procedures, and the bony pelvis aids in providing a cavity for good visualization of the rectum. Mobilization of the rectum is performed to the level of the levator ani muscle with the aid of a standard GIA stapler. The specimen removal incision in the left lower quadrant doubles as a colostomy site. Closure of the distal rectum may be accomplished using an open TA stapler (US Surgical Corporation) inserted through the specimen removal port. The perineal resection proceeds in the standard open fashion. With abdominal lifting, visualization from an abdominal perspective is preserved throughout performance of the perineal dissection.

Transverse colectomy

In transverse colectomy, the lifting fan retractor is placed in the subxiphoid region with the legs extending inferiorly. Midabdominal ports are placed bilaterally, and the specimen removal incision located at the umbilicus. The first step in this procedure is removal of omentum attached to the segment of transverse colon to be resected, using an LDS stapler. Babcock clamps are inserted through the lateral incisions on each side and clamped to the transverse colon at the proximal and distal points of transection. The two clamps are lifted to suspend the colon and allow division of the mesentery, using the LDS stapler. An open surgical GIA stapler is inserted into the specimen removal incision and the colon is transected at the distal resection site. The cut end of the colon is brought out through the incision, and the bowel is transected at the proximal resection site. The anastomosis is performed extracorporeally, and the colon is returned to the abdominal cavity. The mesentery is reapposed with a reabsorbable running suture, and the belly incisions closed as the last step of the procedure.

Gasless laparoscopic Nissen fundoplication

The largest series of gasless laparoscopic Nissen fundoplication procedures has been performed by Benchetrit (Personal communication) in Lyon, France. His experience totals 86 cases between January 1996 and June 1997.

The patient is placed in a partial lithotomy position on the operating table, supine with the hip flexed and the thigh abducted. The surgeon is positioned between the patient's legs and the mechanical lift is clamped to the operating table above the patient's right shoulder. The surgical assistant stands on the left side of the patient. If the French laparoscopic position is not used, the primary surgeon may stand on the right side of the patient.

A 2-cm incision is made, 3 cm below the xiphoid process, and a 15-cm long lifting fan retractor is deployed with its blades directed inferiorly. Five additional ports are placed.

The endoscope is inserted through a port below the left costal margin, at the midclavicular line. A 10-mm port placed below the right lateral costal margin accepts a balloon retractor for the liver. Instrument ports, 10 mm in diameter, are placed below the left lateral costal margin, and 4 cm above the umbilicus in the midline. The single 5-mm port is placed in the right upper quadrant at the midclavicular line.

The initial step involves retraction of the left lobe of the liver to expose the proximal portion of the stomach. The lesser omentum attached to this area is dissected free using laparoscopic clips and shears or an LDS stapler. Dissection is continued to isolate the right crus of the diaphragm, and to separate it from the right wall of the esophagus. A long pair of right-angled clamps may be useful for this process, as well as laparoscopic dissectors. Dissection is continued along the anterior aspect of the esophagus, the left, and finally the posterior wall. A 6- to 7-mm length of esophagus should be isolated at the completion of dissection. A Penrose drain is used to loop the esophagus and assist with its manipulation during the remainder of the procedure.

Reduction of the enlarged hiatus is performed next, using several sutures to reappose the left and right diaphragmatic crus. When this has been completed, a gastric wrap is created around the esophagus. Long conventional needle holders may be used to place suture ties through both sides of the gastric wrap. The needle is prepositioned outside the body and introduced through the midline or left lateral port. A 5-mm probe should be inserted between the esophagus and the gastric wrap to verify that the repair has not been made excessively tight. A nasogastric tube is placed under endoscopic guidance, and removed at the end of the operative day or the first postoperative morning.

Gasless laparoscopic trauma surgery

A gasless approach allows evaluation of trauma patients who may have predisposing conditions contraindicating use of pneumoperitoneum. Unsuspected diaphragmatic and abdominal venous injuries that may lead to tension pneumothorax and gas embolism, respectively, upon gas insufflation, do not present a difficulty with gasless laparoscopy.

Incomplete evaluation of occult bowel injuries is another fear of laparoscopic trauma surgeons. Smith [19•] circumvents this problem by using an abdominal lifting fan via a periumbilical incision to conduct generalized abdominal inspection. This is followed by extension of the incision to 5 cm, allowing 1-m lengths of bowel to be exteriorized, examined, and returned to the abdomen in turn, until the full length of viscera has been scrutinized.

Examination of the abdominal cavity in both blunt and penetrating trauma is performed by inserting the endoscope in the periumbilical incision, behind the lifting fan blades. Evaluation proceeds in sequence, with the fan blades rotated to each of the four quadrants to provide sufficient distention for adequate manipulation of involved organs. Additional ports are inserted as needed to introduce graspers or needle holders; the latter may allow direct repair of lacerations to the diaphragm or bowel injuries. Laparoscopic repair of complex bowel injuries remain inadvisable, due to the potential of widespread peritoneal contamination complicating a simple puncture or perforation.

GYNECOLOGIC APPLICATIONS

Gasless laparoscopic vaginal hysterectomy

Gasless laparoscopic-assisted vaginal hysterectomy (LAVH) has significant benefits over LAVH performed under a pneumoperitoneum. With gas insufflation, incision of the vaginal cuff results in immediate total-loss incision of endoscopic visualization due to the magnitude of gas leakage. With mechanical abdominal lifting, intra-abdominal visualization is maintained at its initial level throughout the procedure, enabling controlled surgical dissection to occur as tissue incision proceeds from an external approach.

The gasless laparoscopic hysterectomy procedure is performed with the patient in a lithotomy position and in 30° of Trendelenburg. The lifting arm is placed at the patient's right shoulder, and the primary surgeon stands on the left side of the patient. A 15-mm umbilical incision is made to introduce the lifting fan retractor; a 10-cm long fan retractor will generally be the correct size, as the length of the pelvis is shorter than the length of the upper abdomen. Two 12-mm ports are inserted in the suprapubic region, in the midclavicular line bilaterally. If needed, an additional 10-mm port may be placed in the suprapubic midline. A uterine manipulator is inserted to allow external angulation of the uterus.

The round ligaments are transected, by the use of bipolar electrocautery forceps followed by scissor transection, or by the use of a GIA stapler. If the adnexa are to be removed, the infundibulopelvic ligaments are transected in a similar manner. The superior portion of the broad ligaments are then transected, followed by severing of the vesicouterine fold, and all uterine attachments to the bladder down to the level of the vaginal cuff. The uterine vessels are double clamped with curved clamps, transected, and suture ligated with extracorporeal ties.

The vaginal portion of the procedure is initiated with an anterior semicircular colpotomy, opening of the vesicovaginal space, and takedown of bladder attachments using clamps and suture ligation. The uterine manipulator is used to displace the uterus into the abdominal cavity and provide traction during dissection of the broad ligament, the cardinal ligament, and the uterosacral ligaments. These structures are clamped, transected, and ligated. Absorbable sutures are used to attach the posterior aspect of the vagina to the sectioned stumps of the uterosacral ligaments, to provide support of the vaginal vault. Following removal of the uterus, the vaginal cuff is closed vaginally. The lifting fan retractor is removed and the abdominal incisions closed.

Gasless laparoscopic myomectomy

A gasless approach is useful for laparoscopic resection of uterine leiomyomas when preservation of the uterus is desired and the patient is not subjected to formal hysterectomy. Gasless laparoscopy allows conventional surgical instruments to be introduced for manipulation of the uterus, enucleation of the myoma, removal of large fibroids from the abdominal cavity, and suture closure of the uterus following myoma resection. Many of the limitations of gas-insufflated laparoscopic myomectomy are removed, making the laparoscopic procedure an attractive alternative to laparotomy.

Laparoscopic myomectomy patients are placed in Trendelenburg and in a lithotomy position on the operating table. An indwelling bladder catheter and a uterine manipulator are placed. An inflatable balloon lift or a lifting fan retractor is inserted through a 2-cm periumbilical incision and elevated by the mechanical arm. Bilateral suprapubic ports are inserted, similar to the placement used for gasless hysterectomy. Enucleation of the myoma proceeds with scalpel incision of the serosa overlying the mass, down to the pseudocapsular plane. An Allis clamp or a Schroeder tenaculum is used to grasp the myoma while curved Mayo scissors dissect it from the uterine bed. An electrocautery probe with a long extension tip may be used for hemostasis and dissection. Large vessels are controlled with the use of bipolar electrocautery forceps. The resected fibroid is grasped with two single-toothed tenaculums and suspended within the abdominal cavity. A number 10 scalpel on a long handle is inserted into the belly and used to section the specimen into strips for removal through the trocar port. The uterine bed is closed with interrupted absorbable deep and superficial sutures.

EXTRAPERITONEAL GASLESS ENDOSCOPY

During the past few years there has been an increase in minimally invasive endoscopic approaches conducted in an extraperitoneal locale. Extraperitoneal endoscopic surgery offers advantages over transabdominal endoscopic approaches in a number of different procedures. Structures in the preperitoneal region may be accessed without entering the abdominal cavity, decreasing anesthesia requirements during the procedure and limiting the occurrence of postoperative adhesions. Retroperitoneal organs and tissue may be operated on without the need for substantial bowel retraction. The peritoneal sac provides bowel containment, facilitating access to anatomic structures outside the dorsal aspect of the abdominal cavity. Whereas an anterior laparoscopic approach requires multiple layers of bowel to be retracted in order to reach structures such as the aorta, a retroperitoneal approach permits a more direct access over a shorter distance.

The surgical approach to extraperitoneal endoscopic procedures involves a 2-cm skin incision, dissection of a small tract to the preperitoneal or retroperitoneal space, introduction and inflation of a balloon cannula to dissect a 1-L cavity in the desired extraperitoneal area, and insertion of the mechanical lift and ancillary retraction to maintain the operating cavity. The dissection balloon cannula (PDB, Origin Medsystems Inc.) contains a transparent balloon that accommodates an endoscope within its lumen. Balloon inflation dissects a cavity under direct endoscopic visualization, allowing verification of proper anatomic landmarks and correct dissection balloon cannula placement. The dissected cavity is clean and devoid of fatty connective tissue strands, enhancing the surgeon's ability to gain orientation in the extraperitoneal space.

The benefits of gasless laparoscopic surgery extend to endoscopic extraperitoneal surgery as well. The ability to apply conventional open surgical instrumentation in an endoscopic setting becomes more important during performance of complex endoscopic procedures on the aorta and the spine. The ability to achieve adequate bowel retraction and vascular control is critical to the performance of these procedures.

PREPERITONEAL PROCEDURES

Gasless laparoscopic inguinal hernia repair

A 2-cm paramedian infraumbilical incision is performed, and blunt dissection of the subcutaneous fat is conducted to expose the fascia of the anterior rectus sheath. A 2-cm incision is made in the anterior rectus sheath, and fibers of the rectus muscle are spread apart using straight or curved clamps to reveal the posterior rectus sheath. A dissection balloon cannula is inserted into the incision placed on top of the posterior rectus sheath, and advanced to the level of the pubic symphysis. If a unilateral inguinal hernia is to be repaired, a spherical balloon (PDB1) may be advanced to the involved side; for bilateral hernia repair, an elliptical balloon (PDB2) is placed in the midline and inflated to dissect an elongated cavity incorporating both inguinal regions. Landmarks appreciated by the intraluminal endoscope during the dissection process include the arched border of Cooper's ligament and, in some cases, the epigastric vessels. Following balloon dissection, a 10-cm long lifting fan retractor is introduced through the incision, opened, and elevated with the mechanical arm to support the ceiling of the preperitoneal cavity. An inflatable balloon retractor is inserted via the same incision and used to push down the peritoneum on the floor of the cavity, yielding an adequate operating space for hernia reduction and mesh placement. The patient is placed in 30° of Trendelenburg to allow bowel to fall away from the floor of the pelvic cavity. Two 5-mm ports are placed. They may both reside in the midline, with one port entering 2 cm above the pubic symphysis and the other one 4 cm above the first. Alternatively, the second 5-mm port may be placed laterally, in the midclavicular line.

Laparoscopic Kittner probes and graspers are used to clear fatty tissue from Cooper's ligament and delineate the iliac vessels at the lateral margins of the cavity. The internal inguinal ring is identified lateral to the epigastric vessels, and the hernia sac is dissected away from the cord structures and reduced, using one or more pairs of graspers. Prosthetic mesh is inserted into the cavity via the infraumbilical incision, unrolled into position covering the defect, and tacked in place. Spiral tacks are placed through the lateral border of the mesh into Cooper's ligament, up to the lateral corner of the mesh, and medially along the top edge of the mesh into the arching fibers of the aponeurosis of the transversus abdominis muscle. No tacks are placed below the iliopubic tract, to avoid nerve or vascular injury. Following mesh placement, the ports and retractors are removed, and the incisions closed to complete the procedure.

Gasless laparoscopic bladder neck suspension

The patient is placed in a modified lithotomy position on the operating table, with the legs abducted, and the thighs minimally flexed. An indwelling catheter is inserted into the bladder. Balloon dissection is used to form a preperitoneal cavity, as in inguinal hernia repair. The spherical balloon (PDB1) is advanced through an infraumbilical incision as described in the preceding section, and inflated in the midline. The cavity created by balloon dissection is maintained by insertion of the inflatable balloon lift (Airlift, Origin Medsystems Inc.), which is partially inflated to allow the balloon to provide a lifting surface while incorporating a fold along its transverse axis. Two 10-mm flexible ports are inserted after they have been split longitudinally to allow multiple instrument insertions through each port. The ports are placed bilaterally in the midclavicular line, 3 cm above the pubic symphysis.

A laparoscopic Kittner probe is inserted to isolate the periurethral area. The bladder is reflected medially from each side, and the fascia of the obturator internus muscle observed, as well as the arcus tendineus fascia (white line). The obturator vessels are identified, and the paravaginal tissue exposed. Dissection is also performed to delineate Cooper's ligament. The assistant surgeon places two fingers into the vagina, and elevates the lateral sidewalls. A suture is placed through the paravaginal tissue above the intravaginal finger, into the obturator internus or arcus tendineus fascia, and looped through the paravaginal tissue a second time. The suture is then placed through Cooper's ligament, and tied extracorporeally. Three or four sutures are placed on each side to accomplish the suspension.

An alternative to suture colpourethral suspension for urinary stress incontinence is mesh suspension, using 1-cm wide strips of prosthetic hernia mesh, which is attached to paravaginal tissue and Cooper's ligament using spiral hernia tacks (Origin Tacker, Origin Medsystems Inc.). The mesh-tacker technique shortens the procedure time by removing the need for intracorporeal suture placement. Experience to date suggests that the durability of the repair is comparable with suture suspension.

RETROPERITONEAL PROCEDURES
Gasless laparoscopic spine surgery
Lumbar diskectomy and spinal fusion is generally performed as a collaborative effort between an endoscopic general or vascular surgeon and a spine surgeon. The technique of balloon-assisted, endoscopic, retroperitoneal, gasless spine surgery has been termed *BERG* diskectomy and spinal fusion. Direct access to multiple levels of the lumbosacral spine, reliable bowel retraction, vascular control, and application of conventional spine instrumentation make this technique preferable to a transabdominal laparoscopic approach.

The patient is placed in a supine position on the operating table, and a sandbag is placed under the left hip. A 2-cm incision is made in the left flank at the anterior axillary line, midway between the costal margin and the iliac crest. Blunt dissection is performed with curved Metzenbaum scissors to access the retroperitoneal space. The external oblique, internal oblique, and transversus muscle fibers are spread apart, and the scissor tips are used to form and expand an opening through the lumbodorsal fascia into the retroperitoneal space. The inferior pole of the kidney may be palpable. The elliptical-shaped dissection balloon (PDB2) is advanced into the retroperitoneal space and inflated with the hand pump under endoscopic visualization (Fig. 19-4). Following dissection of a 1-L retroperitoneal cavity, the balloon is left in place and partially deflated. A 10-cm long lifting fan retractor is advanced through the flank incision on top of the dissection balloon, deployed, and lifted by the mechanical arm. The dissection balloon is deflated and removed from the body. An inflatable balloon retractor and an endoscope are inserted into the flank

incision, behind the legs of the lifting fan. The inflatable balloon retractor's malleable shaft is bent into a right angled configuration and used to retract the peritoneum medially, thus maintaining the side of the retroperitoneal cavity. A 15-mm paramedian incision is made, lateral to the dissected peritoneal edge. This incision is the primary operating port, used for insertion of various spinal instrumentation. If necessary, a second instrument port may be inserted in the left flank, 4 to 5 cm below the original flank incision.

Vascular structures in the proximity of the involved disk space are isolated and retracted medially. The left iliac artery lies anterolateral to the fourth and fifth lumbar interspaces, and sufficient length is mobilized to allow retraction. Lumbar segmental vessels may be isolated, ligated using a right angle clip applier, and transected. The median sacral artery may be clipped and transected during lumbosacral repair. The left ureter generally courses along the dissected peritoneal surface, and it is retracted medially along with the peritoneum. The sympathetic plexus and the presacral parasympathetic plexus lie on the anterior spine and may be retracted. Electrocoagulation near these structures is avoided to prevent erectile dysfunction and retrograde ejaculation.

Longitudinal fibers of the iliopsoas muscle are spread apart using a probe or dissectors to expose the disk space. Insertion of a Steinmann pin into the involved disk space and fluorographic visualization of the space verifies isolation of the correct level for repair. A long-handled scalpel is used to incise the annulus (Fig. 19-5), and the disk removed in a manner similar to open diskectomy, using a combination of pituitary rongeurs, Cobb elevators, and curettes. Endplate cutters are used to prepare the disk space for implant placement.

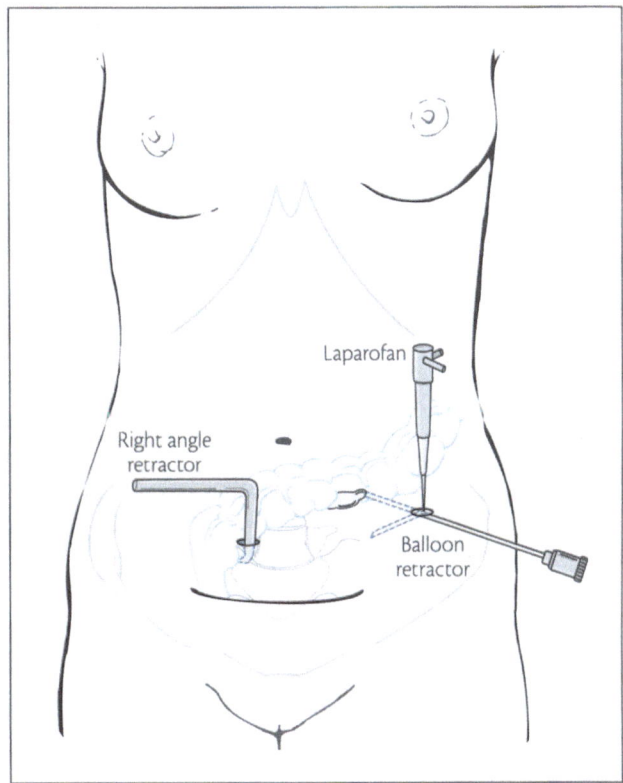

Figure 19-4 Placement of various retractors to expose the L$_5$ S$_1$ disk.

Once the disk has been resected, any choice of available implant may be placed. Femoral cortical allograft or titanium cages packed with harvested cancellous autograft may be tapped into position to achieve anterior fusion. If desired, a buttress plate may be placed by screw fixation into a pilot hole drilled in the superior vertebral body adjacent the implant. The flank and abdominal incisions are closed in two layers at the end of the procedure.

Gasless laparoscopic aortobifemoral bypass

Balloon-assisted, endoscopic, retroperitoneal, gasless aortobifemoral bypass uses an approach identical to that described for spinal reconstruction for dissection and support of the retroperitoneal operating cavity. Intermittent port locations are modified to allow introduction of an aortic cross-clamp and needle holders to execute the proximal anastomosis. The port for the aortic cross-clamp is placed 3 to 4 cm superior to the initial flank incision, while the two ports for anastomotic suture placement are placed lateral to the lifting fan retractor incision. One port is placed several centimeters superior to the level of the initial flank incision, whereas the other one is placed several centimeters inferior to the original incision; both ports are situated in the midaxillary line. A fifth port may be placed inferior to the lifting fan retractor port if an extra entry site is needed for kidney or peritoneal retraction.

Isolation of the aorta is performed with the aid of laparoscopic dissectors as well as conventional instruments such as right-angle clamps. The infrarenal aorta is mobilized a length sufficient to apply a double set of clamps, or approximately 5 cm. Lumbar branches originating from the aorta are carefully isolated, and titanium clips are applied with a right-angle clip applier (Accuclip, Origin Medsystems Inc.). The right-angled opening on the distal end of the clip applier allows the lumbar vessels to be hooked and controlled as clips are being placed on the vessel. This maneuver is useful for endoscopic ligation of deeply placed vessels. Transection of the lumbar branches allows mobilization of the infrarenal aorta, which is then cross-clamped. The distal stump may be ligated and transected using a laparoscopic stapler (Endo-GIA, US Surgical

Corporation), or a second cross-clamp may be applied, followed by aortic transection and oversewing of the cut distal end. A standard bifurcated graft is inserted into the retroperitoneal cavity, and an end-to-end anastomosis is performed using either an interrupted or running suture. For a running suture, two strands are used. The first one is applied to the far wall of the aorta, whereas a separate strand is used for the near wall. The two strands are tied together where they meet to complete the proximal anastomosis.

Bilateral groin incisions are performed next, in preparation for the distal anastomoses. Isolation of the common, deep, and superficial femoral arteries proceed in the standard fashion. Long, curved clamps are used to create a tunnel along the common iliac artery, into the retroperitoneal space, under endoscopic visualization from inside the cavity. A grasper transfers the distal end of the femoral limb to the long clamp, which pulls the graft limb out into the groin incision. The distal anastomoses are completed with an open surgical technique.

FUTURE DEVELOPMENTS IN GASLESS LAPAROSCOPY

Improved instrumentation that facilitates endoscopic tissue retraction and suturing will enable a greater segment of surgeons to accomplish advanced techniques in minimally invasive surgery. As procedures become increasingly complex, technologic developments may reduce that complexity.

Adequate tissue retraction is essential to the surgical process. In critical procedures such as aortic reconstruction, initial establishment of a proper endoscopic operating cavity allows the remainder of the surgery to be conducted smoothly. The design of superior gasless laparoscopic systems has placed an emphasis on reliable tissue retraction. Balloons or inflatable structures are being developed for sophisticated tissue dissection and tissue retraction. High-strength materials of minimal thickness allow low-profile balloons to be inserted into laparoscopic spaces, whereupon they may deploy into expanded forms for atraumatic tissue contact. With increased material tensile strength, resultant higher inflation pressures allow balloons to assume a smaller inflated profile, making these structures useful in an operative setting with limited working space.

Suture placement devices, or clip applicators that replace suture ligation, are other areas of active interest. Limitations in working space make conventional suture placement difficult and awkward. Low-profile instruments, which permit control of distal angulation and rotation, assist with the process of suturing. Clip applicators may speed up the process of tissue closure and tissue approximation. In critical situations, such as vascular anastomoses, the benefit of speed is well appreciated.

Mechanical lifting may be applied to yet further areas of the anatomy. Transabdominal lifting for abdominal procedures was followed by abdominal wall lifting for extraperitoneal procedures. We have applied mechanical lifting to elevate the sternum, creating a working space over the anterior surface of the heart. With the advent of minimally invasive direct coronary artery bypass and endoscopic coronary revascularization, sternal lifting may enlarge the mediastinal ceiling and allow increased

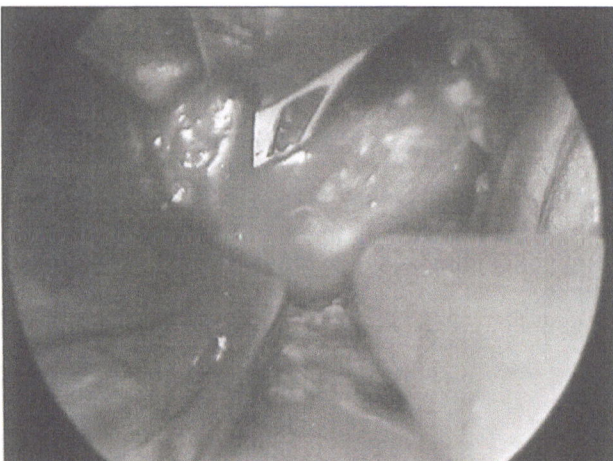

Figure 19-5 The annulus is incised with a long-handle scalpel. (*See* Color Plate.)

manipulation of the heart for various cardiac procedures previously performed through a median sternotomy. Cardiac defibrillator patch placement, epicardial mapping and ablation, transmyocardial revascularization, and coronary bypass are some of the procedures that may be assisted by mechanical lifting.

CONCLUSIONS

Gasless laparoscopy has expanded significantly from its initial use in laparoscopic cholecystectomy to applications in bowel resection, reflux surgery, gynecologic surgery, spine surgery, and vascular surgery. The features that make it beneficial to endoscopic abdominal surgery also apply to endoscopic retroperitoneal procedures. It is useful for the surgeon to become familiar with gasless laparoscopic techniques, as application of the same techniques will allow performance of more complex procedures. As developments in surgical technology continue, the boundaries of minimally invasive gasless endoscopy will likewise expand to include the most difficult and morbid procedures performed in an open setting today. Improved postoperative convalescence and reduced postoperative pain are the goals of this body of surgical research.

REFERENCES AND RECOMMENDED READING

Recently published papers of particular interest have been highlighted as:

- •   Of interest
- ••   Of outstanding interest

1. Gazayerli MM: The Gazayerli endoscopic retractor model 1. *Surg Laparosc Endosc* 1991, 1:98–100.

2. Semm K, Lehmann-Willenbrock E: Pelvioscopy and laparoscopy without overpressure: the aspiration pneumoperitoneum. In *Gasless Laparoscopy in General Surgery and Gynecology.* Edited by Paolucci V, Schaeff B. Stuttgart: Thieme; 1996.

3. Kitano S, Tomikawa M, Iso Y, *et al.*: A safe and simple method to maintain a clear field of vision during laparoscopic cholecystectomy. *Surg Endosc* 1992, 6:197–198.

4. Francois Y, Mouret P: Suspenseur de paroi et coelio-chirugie. *J Chir (Paris)* 1992, 129:492–493.

5. Wood C, Maher P, Hill D: Gasless synchronized laparovaginal hysterectomy. *Gynecol Endosc* 1995, 4:169–172.

6. Nagai H, Inabo T, Kamiya S, *et al.*: A new method of laparoscopic cholecystectomy: an abdominal wall lifting technique without pneumoperitoneum [abstract]. *Surg Laparosc Endosc* 1991, 1:26.

7. Hashimoto D, Nayeem SA, Kajiwara S, *et al.*: Laparoscopic cholecystectomy: a new approach without pneumoperitoneum. *Surg Endosc* 1993, 7:54–56.

8. Chin AK, Moll FH, McColl MB, *et al.*: Mechanical peritoneal retraction as a replacement for carbon dioxide pneumoperitoneum. *J Am Assoc Gynecol Laparosc* 1993, 1:62–66.

9.•• Tsoi EKM, Organ CH Jr: Abdominal wall lifting devices as alternatives to pneumoperitoneum. *Semin Laparosc Surg* 1995, 2:205–208.
This is a review article on the initial clinical application of abdominal lifting devices. The authors were members of the investigating team at the University of California, Davis-East Bay department of surgery using the planar lifting technique. This paper provides readers with the perspective of the investigators on this gasless technique.

10.•• Chin AK, Moll FH: Balloon-assisted extraperitoneal surgery. In *Retroperioneoscopy.* Edited by Darzi A. Oxford: Isis Medical Media; 1996.
The uses of an inflatable balloon in a retroperitoneal dissection enables surgeons to obtain rapid exposure for retroperitoneoscopy. This article describes the development and application of the balloon-assisted technique in a number of extraperitoneal procedures.

11. Myles PS: Bradyarrhythmias and laparoscopy: a prospective study of heart rate changes with laparoscopy. *Aust N Z Obstet Gynaecol* 1991, 31:171–173.

12. Doyle DJ, Mark PW: Laparoscopy and vagal arrest. *Anesthesiology* 1989, 44:448–453.

13. Pascual JB, Baranda MM, Tarrero MT, *et al.*: Subcutaneous emphysema, pseudomediastinum, bilateral pneumothorax and pneumopericardium after laparoscopy [letter]. *Endoscopy* 1990, 22:59.

14. Kent RB: Subcutaneous emphysema and hypercarbia following laparoscopic cholecystectomy. *Arch Surg* 1991, 126:1154–1156.

15. Pearce DJ: Respiratory acidosis and subcutaneous emphysema during laparoscopic cholecystectomy. *Can J Anaesth* 1994, 41:314–316.

16. Clark CC, Weeks DB, Gusdon JP: Venous carbon dioxide embolism during laparoscopy. *Anesth Analg* 1977, 56:650–652.

17. Yacoub OF, Cardona I, Coveler LA, *et al.*: Carbon dioxide embolism during laparoscopy. *Anesthesiology* 1982, 57:533–535.

18. Beebe DS, McNevin MP, Crain JM, *et al.*: Evidence of venous stasis after abdominal insufflation for laparoscopic cholecystectomy. *Surg Gynecol Obstet* 1993, 176;443–447.

19.• Smith RS: Evaluation and treatment of abdominal trauma. In *Gasless Laparoscopy in General Surgery and Gynecology.* Edited by Paolucci V, Schaeff B. Stuttgart: Thieme; 1996:68–75.
Laparoscopy has been shown to be a cost-effective technique to treat trauma patients. This article describes the author's experience in using the planar lifting technique in treating both blunt and penetrating abdominal trauma patients.

Virtual Reality for Image-guided Surgery

Ferenc A. Jolesz
Ron Kikinis
William M. Wells III
William E. Lorensen
Joachim Kettenbach

Recent advances in medical imaging techniques have led to an escalation in the use of image-based information by radiologists, clinicians, and surgeons. The increased availability of imaging modalities is of considerable use to the physician; however, these methods are still inherently limited because they provide images with information limited by the physical characteristics of the imaging device. Although the direct interpretation of images is sufficient, some situations require postprocessing for the extraction and use of the anatomic and physiologic information inherent in the three-dimensional medical images. This chapter reviews some applications that would benefit from improved use of effectively processed medical images.

DISEASE DIAGNOSIS

Early detection is often the key to effective treatment. Images of internal organs provide evidence of particular diseases that are manifested through structural or functional changes. The high resolution and high contrast available with ultrasound, CT, and magnetic resonance imaging (MRI) aid the diagnosis of a wide range of problems. Diagnosis can be improved not only with computerized tools that can highlight such diseases in single images, but also with methods that allow accurate comparison among images.

TREATMENT MONITORING

By taking multiple images of a subject over time, the physician can effectively track progress or regress of a medical condition and quickly determine the impact of treatment regimens. By using initial images as a baseline, such follow-up examination results in interpretations that are more specific to the disease process.

MULTIMODALITY INFORMATION INTEGRATION

Because different imaging modalities highlight different tissue types and different physiologic functions, it is often useful to fuse information from different imaging devices, such as blood vessels from angiograms, soft-tissue structures from MRI, bones from CT, or metabolic activity from single-photon emission CT (SPECT) or positron emission tomography. Differing resolutions, aspect ratios, possible distortions, and differences in coordinate frames pose difficult problems in interpreting these combined images.

AUGMENTED INTRAOPERATIVE VISUALIZATION

Visualization during surgery is incomplete because the surgeon cannot see the anatomy beyond the exposed surfaces. For example, conventional craniotomy is markedly constrained by the relatively small area of exposed brain surface, which lacks spatial clues that surgeons would need to comprehend all of the relevant anatomy. Such limitations of direct surgical visualization have several consequences. First, localization is not accurate and is even more compromised within the parenchyma. Second, the definition of exact trajectories for targeting is impossible without image guidance. Third, if the anatomic and pathologic boundaries are not clear (and thus accurate tumor localization is not possible), normal tissue has to be removed to ensure complete resection.

In many procedures, the surgeon has a limited view of the operating field and cannot visualize structures beyond the exposed surfaces. In minimally invasive surgeries, particularly during endoscopic procedures, the surgeon is also confronted with difficult hand-eye coordination problems because he or she is looking at a camera's view of the surgical field with a totally different reference frame than his or her own. In other cases, procedures are complicated by the similarity in visual appearance of different tissues (*eg*, tumor and healthy tissue), although such tissues have high contrast in some medical images. The best examples are breast cancer and brain glioma, which can be difficult to distinguish from normal tissue. Better use of the three-dimensional imaging can improve surgical visualization and help the surgeons overcome the limitations of existing procedures. In particular, enhanced reality visualization, in which the surgeon's field of view is augmented with additional structural information, can provide useful guidance in planning and executing the surgery.

INSTRUMENT TRACKING

Another application for bringing the imaging into the surgical process is to track the positions of surgical instruments and relate their location relative to images acquired preoperatively. For example, the correct placement of biopsy needles and minimally invasive surgical tools such as laparoscopes and remote cutting tools is problematic if they are out of the visual field. By tracking the three-dimensional position of these instruments, the position of the instrument can be shown on scans of the patient, such as MRI or CT.

INTRAOPERATIVE GUIDANCE

Because of the unavoidable changes of anatomy and tissue position during surgery, preoperatively acquired images have substantial limitation in guiding procedures intraoperatively. Real-time imaging or frequent image updates can provide the necessary corrections for these displacements. Intraoperatively acquired images can also be used for warping and fusing preoperative images to the shape of organs as they change during the surgical procedure. With the development of intraoperative MRI we can now combine the advantages of diagnostic imaging (definition of tumor margins, delineation of anatomy), real-time treatment monitoring (frequent image updates during open surgeries or real-time temperature-sensitive imaging of thermal ablations), multimodality image registration (with the possibility of elastic warping to the actual anatomic boundaries), visualization of the surgical field (in combination with enhanced reality

display from three-dimensional images), and instrument guidance (intraoperative tracking and interactive scanning).

To fully use the information available from medical images, and to optimally provide those to the diagnostic radiologist, surgeon, or clinician, we need to 1) extract the structural and functional information of particular relevance, and 2) provide that information in an effective manner. To achieve this desired goal, several key issues must be resolved, including image segmentation, image registration, and visualization.

Image segmentation

Segmentation converts the medical images into anatomically, functionally, or surgically identifiable structures that are more readily useful to the operator. This procedure involves the classification of particular tissue types, such as bone, fat, vessel, white matter, gray matter, or tumor. Such classification is based on the ability to discriminate among tissue types as well as anatomic knowledge of tissue structures and relationships. By providing automated tools for segmentation, we gain the ability to transform the raw image data into three-dimensional structures that more directly relate to the patient's anatomy.

Image registration

Registration involves the alignment of various image data sets (*eg*, MRI and CT scans) such that correspondences among them can be more easily identified. In this process, raw image data or the segmented images are transformed into new reference frames in which the geometric relationship between these structures is appropriate for the task. Such transformations are required for fusing information from multiple imaging modalities or mapping functionally, anatomically, or pathologically defined three-dimensional structures to the anatomy of the patient. The key problem in registration is to transform the segmented structures to new reference frames that best use the extracted information. This may mean registering multimodal inputs to a common coordinate frame, such as merging magnetic resonance angiographic data, MRI soft tissue reconstructions, and functional MRI inputs into a common coherent whole. Additionally, it may mean registering such a fused model of the patient's anatomy to the actual position of the patient, for use in image-guided surgery.

Visualization

Visualization is the display of transformed information to the observer in a useful manner. This term refers to the three-dimensional rendering and display of structures using interfaces through which the medical personnel can readily view and interpret the processed data. Image analysis tools must work synergistically with the clinician, providing sufficient interactivity, response, and feedback capabilities. The process of visualization and display are part of almost every use of computers in medicine, from inspection of an MRI series on an interactive console to the measurement of a patient's temperature or blood pressure. Visualization uses image processing, computer graphics, and interactive tools to separate relevant from extraneous information. The results of the visualization process can be computer-generated images, animated movies, or dynamic models with which the viewer can interact. No matter what form the processed data is in, the purpose of its presentation is to help the researcher, scientist, or physician better understand his or her data.

Although considerable progress has been made in these areas, all suffer from several drawbacks. In general, all of these methods are computationally expensive, and generally all still require some level of user interaction or guidance. The former problem will be alleviated to some extent by improvements in computational hardware, as well as by algorithm refinement. At the same time, however, better, more automated methods will also address this shortcoming. The ultimate goal is to provide fully automated methods for extracting important structural and functional information from the images, and to do this one must provide means for incorporating anatomic and other global knowledge into the process.

Although considerable progress has been made in combining computer vision techniques with medical image analysis methods, we are still not at the stage of providing fully automatic, rapid, accurate, and easily used tools for clinical applications.

The goal of image processing and virtual reality displays is to make the presentation of images easier by taking the raw imaging data, segmenting out relevant structures, and then generating three-dimensional computer-based reconstructions. This work has several potential applications:

- Making the work of radiologists more efficient by condensing information from several slices into one image rendering
- Facilitating the communication with referring physicians and enhancing their ability to translate imaging information into a surgical scenario
- Assisting surgeons in planning for surgical intervention
- Assisting in the follow-up
- Assisting in the investigation of pathology by revealing the subtle differences present in magnetic resonance or CT examinations that may not be apparent without processing

Although tissue specificity mostly depends on tissue characterization with a given physical system (ie, CT or MRI), anatomic specificity is primarily determined by postprocessing techniques. The development of methodology is primarily driven by specific medical questions. Nevertheless, all tools can be used for multiple purposes and build an integrated environment for medical image analysis.

COMPUTER-BASED IMAGE GUIDANCE

Image guidance, in general, can reduce the inherent invasiveness of surgery and improve localization and targeting by intraoperative imaging via ultrasound or, more recently, MRI. Alternatively, intraoperative image guidance can be based on previously acquired images using reference frames attached to the patient (frame-based stereotaxy), or images that have been registered to the patient (frameless stereotaxy). In the latter case, computers can navigate the operator through three-dimensional coordinates and thus fulfill the need for enhanced visibility during interventional radiologic and minimally invasive surgical procedures.

Image-derived information for treatment can be applied to every stage of the therapeutic process. The increasing demand for refinement of imaging and image representation for surgery requires unique methods for data acquisition, processing, and display, and the full understanding of the process of imaging and its applications to therapy. Image-based modeling requires computerized image-processing methods (segmentation, registration, and display) and image integration techniques, replacing the mental process of generating three-dimensional representations of the patient's anatomy. Although advanced imaging modalities and information processing or display methods are widely used in planning, monitoring, and guiding various therapies, these imaging techniques could be integrated into interventional and surgical procedures.

SURGICAL PLANNING AND SIMULATION

For full comprehension of image-based information, surgeons prefer appropriately rendered and interactively displayed three-dimensional data that resemble the visual information seen during surgical exploration. Automation of image processing, however, makes these novel approaches more and more feasible and practical. Depending on the particular application, preoperative planning implies not only image reconstruction, but also integration of various displays, image manipulation, and visualization tools that help simulate and plan an intervention.

The role of surgical planning in tumor surgery is to define the safest possible approach with the least possible damage to normal tissue. In this trajectory-optimization process, alternative navigational paths and movements through the physical space are tested and analyzed using a preoperative model. In craniofacial and orthopedic surgical applications, the role of surgical planning is the optimal execution of preoperative plans [1–6]. Further expansion of surgical planning and simulation techniques into other surgical fields requires more complex methods (eg, elastic warping) and more information about shape, position, and orientation that may correct or account for unavoidable tissue deformations and organ shifts during surgery [7]. Establishing a simulated procedural environment is also a critical step for creating an image-based virtual reality environment that allows the user to actively enter the three-dimensional environment and perform simulated procedures within it.

INTRAOPERATIVE IMAGE GUIDANCE USING PREOPERATIVE IMAGES

Surgery today relies conceptually on the same principles that it did 3000 years ago: the surgeons use their hands to directly control instruments and their eyes to observe feedback on the effect of their manipulations. Accordingly, surgeons need access to the site of an operation for both visualization and manipulation. The evolving modern trend in surgery is the development of minimally invasive approaches, in which the damage caused by accessing the surgical site is reduced. Rigid or flexible long-necked instruments are introduced into the target areas through natural openings or small incisions. These instruments typically carry some form of visualization equipment and provide some way to introduce instruments for procedures.

A skillfully prepared, geometrically correct preoperative plan and a well-developed simulation of the procedure are, in fact, components of an executional operational model that can be implemented in the operating room. Intraoperative image guidance is based on functional integration of the previously acquired and processed three-dimensional information and the corresponding anatomy of the patient within the same frame of reference. During the actual surgery, an interactive real-time display can demonstrate the otherwise hidden anatomic information that has been generated by a single modality or composed from multimodal volumetric images [7–10,11••,12]. Trajectories from the preoperatively prepared executional plans and models can also be exhibited (Fig. 20-1).

Intraoperative guidance requires matching of the two frames of reference. The actual coordinates within which the models exist must be mapped or registered into the physical space of the patient. Links between these two components are realized by combining image-to-patient registration and by tracking instruments within the operational field. These are the key ingredients of frameless stereotactic targeting methods, which capitalize on the interactive control of image planes and exploit the full information content of perceived three-dimensional space.

Patient-to-model registration is substantially different from multimodality coregistration. Image fusion requires matching all image-based geometric data in a single, unique coordinate system. The matched data coexist within a single virtual database, but for image-guided procedures they have to be registered into the physical space of the patient, too. In addition, these data should be overlaid or projected to the patient's exposed surface if surgical guidance is necessary. Various methods exist for patient-to-model registration. In the original, frame-based

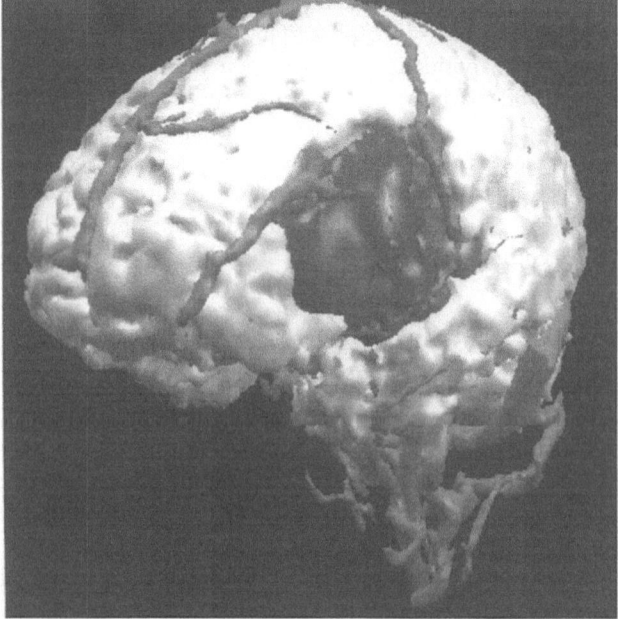

Figure 20-1 A three-dimensional reconstruction of a 37-year-old woman with an astrocytoma of the left frontal-temporal cortex. The tumor is in *green* and the blood vessels in *red*. (*See* Color Plate.)

stereotactic method, three-dimensional points (of the physical frame) are matched with two-dimensional points (seen on the images). Alternatively, surface points are matched with selected anatomic landmarks or external fiducial markers visible on both the images and on the patient. In these methods, the registration process requires pointers attached to position-sensing devices that establish the relationship between the reference frame of the patient and the images.

Other registration techniques match visible anatomic objects, features, or shapes represented on both the patient and the reconstructed images. Video camera–based methods detect visible features on the patient (ear, nose, eyes) appearing on both the reconstructed surfaces and on the video images [13]. Readjusting them to inner surfaces of the organs as they become exposed during surgery can refine skin surface–based registrations. For example, video registration can be improved by matching cortical vessels, visible on the surface of the exposed brain and on three-dimensional reconstructions based on magnetic resonance angiograms [14•]. Currently, we use laser scanning to obtain digitized surfaces and subsequently match three-dimensional curves with three-dimensional curves obtained with automated methods [15••].

To improve accuracy, the various registration methods can be combined. Multimodality data from MRIs, magnetic resonance angiography, SPECT, or positron emission tomography scans and spatially recorded functional physiologic and preoperative surgical planes can be registered to the patient in order to integrate all the available information intraoperatively [9,10].

Reliable and completely automated registration methods can integrate the image-based information with the patient's anatomy. Nevertheless, intraoperative three-dimensional position sensing and tracking is essential to account for the inevitable movements of the patients and the actual path of the surgical instruments. Without establishing the correspondence between the actual position of surgical instruments, anatomic landmarks, and image-derived three-dimensional anatomy, geometric accuracy is impossible and precise plans cannot be executed consistently. After initial registration, patient motion can be tracked by reregistration of the updated images if real-time imaging is available. In computer-assisted surgery, in which only previously acquired images are used, so-called navigational systems establish the relationship between the surgeon's movements and the image-based information within the physical space of the patient [16–22]. Using intraoperative two- and three-dimensional displays or virtual or enhanced (augmented) reality representations, navigation within the patient's body can be guided by both direct visibility and by the images themselves.

To follow the movements of the surgeon's hand or instruments, the position and orientation of passive mechanical arms can be continuously detected at the articulations by encoders [23]. Alternatively, various three-dimensional position sensors can be mounted on the patient or standard surgical tools [24,25••]. These noncontact devices can be used for tracking patient or physician movements or the path of rigid surgical instruments. Optical and ultrasound digitizers cannot transmit through the tissues; therefore, for detecting positions deep inside the body, they have to be placed on the proximal end of rigid instruments. Conventional electromagnetic sensors can be detected through the body, but cannot fit within needles or endoscopes unless they are miniaturized. Currently, a small-scale version of electromagnetic sensors has become available that can be attached to the tip of flexible catheters and inserted into the working channel of endoscopes (Acker and Jimenez, Paper presented at the Fourth Congress of Neurosurgical Surgeons, Montreal, 1996). The tracking technology, using single or multiple sensors, permits the use of instruments such as pointers or tracing tools and enables the physician to outline regions or define trajectories.

The most important aspect of the sensor technology and tracking is interactivity. Conventional stereotactic frames impede freedom of motion and use calculations instead of displays to define positions. In interactive frameless stereotaxy, the computer displays the position and the motion of the instruments accurately and immediately in correct orientation with respect to image-defined anatomic boundaries. Repetitive display of target, trajectory, and volume information allows interaction with the surgical plan and monitoring of the progress of the procedure.

Most of the navigational systems developed in the past decade are relevant only for interactive image-guided neurosurgery and endoscopic sinus surgery. The use of preoperative images for intraoperative image guidance is limited by the potential intraoperative changes in the anatomy. If the navigation is solely based on preoperative images, intraoperative tissue distortions, shifts and displacements (due to retraction of tissues, removal of tumor masses, loss of cerebrospinal fluid, hemorrhage, or edema) cause substantial errors. Modeling of elastic deformations and correction of the images is possible, but only within a limited range; beyond that, intraoperative imaging becomes necessary.

INTRAOPERATIVE IMAGE GUIDANCE USING MAGNETIC RESONANCE IMAGING

Magnetic resonance imaging, because of its high tissue contrast and spatial resolution as well as multiplanar and functional imaging capabilities, has the most appeal for monitoring and controlling therapy. Open configuration magnets, which permit full access to the patient and are equipped with instrument tracking systems, provide an interactive environment in which biopsies, percutaneous or endoscopic procedures, and minimally invasive interventions or open surgeries can be performed. In addition, various thermal ablations with image-based control of energy deposition can be performed to exploit the intrinsic sensitivity of MRI to both temperature and tissue integrity.

Magnetic resonance imaging provides images that are reflective of regional differences in proton concentrations and the physico-chemical environment of protons (eg, water protons show different magnetic resonance behavior from protons in larger molecules such as lipids, proteins, and so on; protons in hydration water show different magnetic resonance behavior than protons in unbound water). Pathologic changes in tissue composition often alter the proton distribution and can therefore be highlighted by MRI. Therefore, tumoral infiltration, edema, and bleeding can be distinguished from the surrounding healthy tissues.

More specific tissue characterization is being achieved by exogenous administration of MRI contrast agents. Gadopentate dimeglumine (Gd-DTPA) is a compound containing a paramagnetic ion (gadolinium) and a macromolecular chelating moiety (DTPA). The gadolinium ion modulates the magnetic resonance signal whereas the macromolecule moiety limits the molecule distribution in brain tissue to areas of disrupted blood-brain barrier. Postprocessing techniques enable the integration of this information into quantitative tissue characterization maps.

As the computer becomes a more integral part of the surgical process, the need to provide information to the surgeon in a convenient and intuitive way becomes greater. Nowhere is this relationship more obvious than in the interventional MRI system, in which image information acquired by MRI and augmented and annotated by computer data is a powerful tool for intraoperative planning and guidance.

In 1989, the magnetic resonance division of the Department of Radiology of Brigham and Women's Hospital and Harvard Medical School initiated a project to develop magnetic resonance–guided interventional procedures [26,27••,28,29,30••]. The components of this project included 1) the development of a new kind of MRI scanner, providing access to the patient during imaging; and 2) development of the computerized processing methods necessary for efficient presentation and analysis of data generated in such an environment.

General Electric Medical Systems (Milwaukee, WI) participated in the project by building an open magnet, called the SIGNA SP, for surgical applications. The SIGNA SP is a complete environment, including magnetic resonance–compatible instruments, magnetic resonance–compatible anesthesia, monitoring equipment, and so on. The first machine was installed at Brigham and Women's Hospital in March 1994. Since then, several surgical applications have been tested on it, including biopsies, ear, nose, and throat endoscopic procedures [25••,31,32], and open brain surgeries [33,34••].

Near real-time MRI imaging or frequent image updates during interventional and surgical procedures provide updates about patient anatomy or the changing position of movable organs, depicts the position of instruments, and without registration establishes the necessary relationship between the patient and the images. Advances in MRI with high-performance computing now permits the combination and integration of near-real time, high contrast and spatial resolution volumetric images with frameless stereotactic, interactive localization methods while performing image-guided therapy.

During the development of interventional MRI, several obstacles hindered the evolution of MRI-guided interventions. Its value for guiding biopsies of tumors best detectable by MRI was apparent, but the closed magnets—conventional at the time—made it a cumbersome procedure to perform. The incompatibility of the electromagnetic environment, the inaccessibility of patients within the magnets, and the expense of MRI impeded the widespread acceptance of MRI for percutaneous procedures. Advances in low-field open-configuration magnet design and recognition of the potential of MRI for monitoring and controlling thermal ablations and other percutaneous therapies initiated this new direction in interventional radiology. Because of the lack of direct visualization of thermal ablations, a three-dimensional imaging technique must be used to monitor these processes. Using temperature-sensitive MRI sequences during therapy, the progress of heat deposition and the resulting tissue alterations can be observed [35].

This unique potential of MRI provided the impetus for a mid-field open-configuration magnetic resonance system. The goal was to develop a new generation of imaging systems providing relatively unlimited access to the patient, near real-time monitoring, localization, targeting, interactive scanning, magnetic resonance–compatible instruments, and equipment necessary for an magnetic resonance–based interventional suite or operating room. An underlying promise of this project has been that MRI coupled with direct visualization can realize many interventional and surgical procedures better than either could do alone. A further premise is that such a combination of MRI and invasive procedures meets the present trend toward safe and accurate, image-guided minimally invasive therapies [36].

The configuration of magnet determines the scope and the ease with which interventional or intraoperative imaging can be performed. Most of the percutaneous procedures and open surgeries, however, require freehand techniques based on hand-eye coordination and need close and direct contact with the patient's exposed anatomy. The horizontal gap configuration

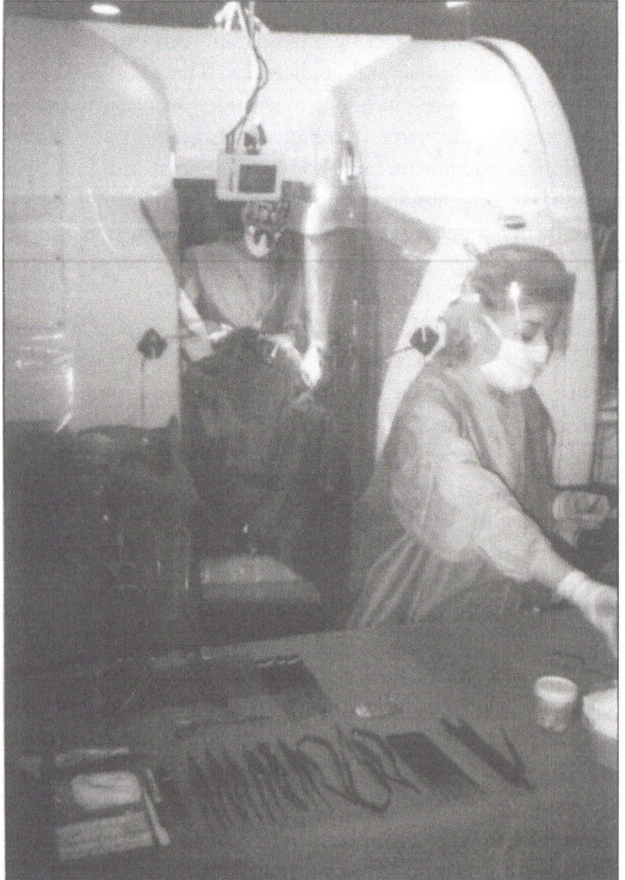

Figure 20-2 Performance in the open-magnet system. For surgery or interventional procedures, the open-magnet design permits direct clinical access to the patient and simultaneous interactive control of the magnetic resonance imaging process.

does not permit open procedures and makes more complicated percutaneous procedures difficult to perform. Only the vertical gap allows the physician to enter between the two components of the magnet and directly manipulate the patient's anatomy. This configuration allows the use of endoscopes, laparoscopes, and operating microscopes (Fig. 20-2).

The SIGNA SP interventional MRI system and the interventional-surgical suite in which it resides combines these key enabling technologies: superconductive magnetic resonance system, flexible transmit and receive coils, computer workstations, position sensors, intraoperative display, and audiovisual equipment [26,27••]. The facility is equipped with magnetic resonance–compatible anesthesia delivery and monitoring devices and instruments for biopsies, thermal ablations, endoscopies, and open surgical procedures. It incorporates and integrates functions related to imaging, image guidance, and therapy. The high-technology environment and its components represent a cross-fertilization between interventional radiology, minimally invasive therapy, and image-guided, computer-assisted surgery. Although the initial application domain included primarily percutaneous biopsy, the capability ultimately evolved into a broad range of interventional and surgical applications in which the combination of direct imaging and real-time image guidance was consolidated.

The most important characteristic of the interventional MRI system is the ability to interactively use imaging to localize, target, and monitor the procedure. The operator can define scan planes and their location as needed. This capability is similar to what can be done using sonography. The interactive image plane selection and definition implemented in the General Electric interventional MRI system (Flashpoint Scan Plane Pointer) uses an optical tracking system (light-emitting diodes localized by infrared-sensitive video equipment). This method has some aspects in common with frameless stereotactic or navigational systems. In particular, it provides direct control of scan plane location, orientation, and angulation with enough flexibility and convenience to perform freehand procedures and enough accuracy for stereotactic biopsies [26,27••]. The system is capable of capturing images along interactively defined coordinates to obtain geometrically correct information about the patient's anatomy and the location of instruments. This system has provided localization and targeting of brain biopsies even in extremely high-risk areas. Application of interactive MRI scan plane selection for performing biopsies of abdominal organs and other body parts also introduced the concept of frameless stereotaxy into the field of cross-sectional interventional radiology [29,37,38].

Interactive image-guidance within the interventional MRI system using optical or other tracking systems can be applied to a wide variety of interventional and surgical procedures. In all imaging modes, the information is acquired according to the position and orientation of the sensors and three orthogonal planes generated within a moving frame of reference. The most straightforward mode is interactive scanning, in which the operator intuitively moves the device in order to obtain a comprehensive view of the scanned three-dimensional volume. This mode resembles sonography except that the three orthogonal planes can be displayed without changing the actual position of the probe. In the localizing mode, the probe is used as a virtual pointer with a computer-displayed icon that can point to or outline an anatomic object within the body. This mode can also be used to trace contours of organs or margins of lesions or to obtain points or surfaces from inside the body for registration.

Using the targeting mode for biopsy, the tip or the shaft of a virtual needle is displayed on three orthogonal planes showing the expected path of the needle as an annotation. If the predicted position of the tip and the planned trajectory is acceptable by the physician, the real needle or probe can be advanced into the target. Using the tracking mode, the trail of instruments or the motion of body parts can be followed and displayed on the image [33].

For interactive image guidance, the images must be generated and displayed quickly enough to be used without disrupting or slowing down the procedure and before considerable changes occur within the operational field. The definition of real-time imaging or dynamic image update is relative and contingent on the time constants of the procedures or processes being imaged. Imaging needle placement may require update of multiple slices or planes. Monitoring thermal ablation of a tumor should incorporate a volume (several slices). Most localization, targeting, tracking, and monitoring requirements can be satisfied by the commonly available fast imaging techniques (fast spin echo, gradient echo). Several novel imaging techniques offer improved temporal resolution achieved by less redundant spatial encoding and without considerably affecting spatial resolution and signal-to-noise ratio. Magnetic resonance fluoroscopy and other dynamic imaging approaches are also available to use preexisting information for adaptive encoding of changing image data [39–42,43••,44].

MONITORING AND CONTROL OF MAGNETIC RESONANCE–GUIDED ABLATION THERAPY WITH INTERVENTIONAL MAGNETIC RESONANCE IMAGING

The greatest potential of MRI is in monitoring and delivering thermal energies using various thermal probes (*eg*, laser, radiofrequency, microwave, focused ultrasound, cryoprobe). This is a particularly important application of MRI guidance because achieving the full potential of these techniques requires not only good localization and targeting but also quantitative spatiotemporal control of energy deposition, which in turn requires monitoring of the thermal changes and the resulting tissue alterations.

Based on our extensive experience in thermal imaging and magnetic resonance–guided thermal ablations [41,42,43••,45,46], we have developed a computer-assisted monitoring technique based on temperature-sensitive MRI for interstitial laser therapy. Clinical applications involving tumor ablation in the brain and liver have already been initiated. The interventional MRI system was used to guide and monitor the accurate placement of the laser source (needle with optical fiber) at the targeted lesion. Newly developed software in the imaging system and the research workstation enabled rapid (27 to 221 ms) and on-line temperature image reconstruction. In the highlighted brain tumor case, subtraction images from T_1-weighted scans and proton chemical shift images clearly showed the

signal intensity peak at the tip of the laser guide. The preliminary study indicated that the presented system design is feasible for real-time and on-line monitoring of interstitial laser therapy.

INTRAOPERATIVE MAGNETIC RESONANCE IMAGING FOR OPEN SURGERIES

The simultaneous combination of direct vision and beyond the surface imaging is possible within a unique environment incorporating both the operating room and a MRI scanner. This integrated system allows more accurate localization and targeting during surgery. Definition of histopathologically correct tumor margins, comprehension of the full extent of disease processes, and accurate definition of anatomic landmarks may improve surgical efficiency and diminish the invasiveness. Complete resection of tumors, decreased vulnerability of surrounding tissues, and avoidance of critical structures should improve clinical outcome and reduce complication rates. By merging MRI with frameless stereotaxy, navigational tools, and multimodality image fusion, the combination of all available spatial information with real-time image update became possible. Use of this composite information during open procedures may revolutionize minimally invasive therapy and will lead to the development of new surgical strategies and approaches.

Our early neurosurgical experience based on close to 100 cases illustrates most of the anticipated benefits of intraoperative MRI [34••,38]. Interactive localization and targeting have not only provided on-line planning of optimal trajectories for biopsies, but also real-time image feedback during the needle advancement and tissue sampling (Fig. 20-2). Using this method, lesions within deep and high-risk regions (*eg*, hypothalamus, pineal region, or brainstem) have been biopsied [38]. Unavoidable hemorrhagic complication was immediately recognized, localized, and treated surgically by open craniotomy within the magnet. Intraventricular, relatively mobile and unstable targets have been reached safely, and cystic structures in various locations have been drained under continuous image control. The potential advantages of precise localization and optimized access route have also been demonstrated by combining an operative microscope with MRI-guided resection of deep-seated small tumors and cavernous hemangiomas. Surgical removal of extra-axial tumors may benefit from the delineation of surrounding, directly invisible anatomy.

When viewing the exposed brain surface without imaging, the neurosurgeon cannot define the spatial extent of the tumor, and even after surgically entering the brain tissue, the tumor is indistinguishable from normal cerebral tissue in most patients. Preoperative image data may help to demonstrate the extent of the tumor in some instances. During resection of large, deep tumors, however, brain structures may move and become deformed, negating the value of preoperative images. Using intraoperative optical tracking and refreshing the volumetric images, surgeons are able not only to locate the tumor margins, but completely resect the tumor while preserving the integrity of surrounding normal brain. Similar methods can be applied to resection of other intraparenchymal tumors such as breast cancer or soft tissue sarcoma, in which the margins are difficult to define with the naked eye.

Multimodality representation of morphology can be integrated from previous CT or MRI along with functional physiologic data (transcranial magnetic stimulation, magnetic resonance angiography, and functional MRI) and metabolic information (SPECT). These combined data can then be coregistered with intraoperative real-time MRI data. The resulting composite provides the surgeon the most comprehensive view of the operative field and helps not only to plan but also to execute the procedure. Coregistration of CT, magnetic resonance angiography, and MRI is especially helpful in skull-base surgery. The combination of functional MRI with cortical physiology is invaluable for executing surgical resection without sacrificing critical brain functions. SPECT registration to intraoperative MRI distinguishes metabolically active tumor parts from necrotic areas.

VIRTUAL ENDOSCOPY

Conventional endoscopic procedures demonstrate inner surfaces of hollow organs using direct visualization or video-assisted technology. The operator interactively explores the organs by navigating within them. Endoscopy is useful for the diagnosis of mucosal or epithelial lesions but provides minimal or no information about the extent of disease within or beyond the wall of the viewed organ. Another shortcoming of endoscopy is the lack of sufficient information in localizing lesions relative to surrounding anatomy.

Cross-sectional imaging has a lower resolution than endoscopy, but it is noninvasive and shows the anatomy beyond the wall. Nevertheless, cross-sectional CT or MRI does not allow contiguous viewing of the inside of the organs. Computerized image processing can render cross-sectional images into three-dimensional displays showing not only the outside configuration of organs, but also their inner surfaces. CT or MRI images can demonstrate the mucosal surfaces and can provide information on pathologic processes that go through and beyond organ walls. These images can also correct localization in relationship to surrounding anatomy.

Virtual endoscopy [47–50,51••] (Geiger and Kikinis, Paper presented at the Computer Vision, Virtual Reality and Robotics in Medicine, Nice, France, 1995) yields endoscopy-like visualization using cross-sectional imaging. Virtual endoscopy allows the contiguous exploration of surfaces and therefore improves diagnosis; it is also a navigational tool that can help the endoscopist during diagnostic or therapeutic procedures. Interactive virtual endoscopy displayed during endoscopic procedures can assist in the localization of the lesion, in determining its extent, and ultimately complement visualization during the invasive biopsy or surgical procedure performed with endoscopy (Figs. 20-3 and 20-4).

Virtual-reality techniques and visualization method may improve this new method. Endoscopic viewing is not restricted to the inner surfaces. The viewer may visualize through the walls and see the extent of lesions beyond it. The operator can also see the adjacent anatomic structures, which can assist in tumor staging and developing minimally invasive surgical strategies.

Correct localization and orientation relative to surrounding anatomy is also an important feature of virtual endoscopy. Complementing real endoscopy with virtual images, however, requires knowledge of the endoscope's location within the patient. Various tracking devices or sensors (mechanical, optical, or electromagnetic) can be attached to the endoscopes, or smaller sensors can be introduced into the working channels of endoscopes. Alternatively, endoscopic procedures can be performed within

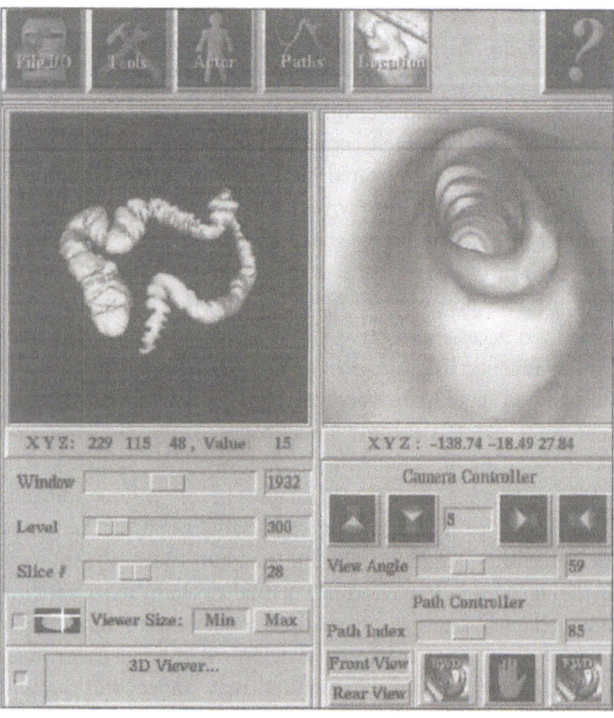

Figure 20-3 A virtual colonoscopy. **Left,** Global view. The program indicates the corresponding virtual camera position with the green line and also has the ability to display the corresponding computed tomographic slice. **Right,** The camera view is displayed. The control panel, on the lower portion of the screen, allows for adjustment of the view (lens) angle, camera direction, zoom, and more. (*See* Color Plate.)

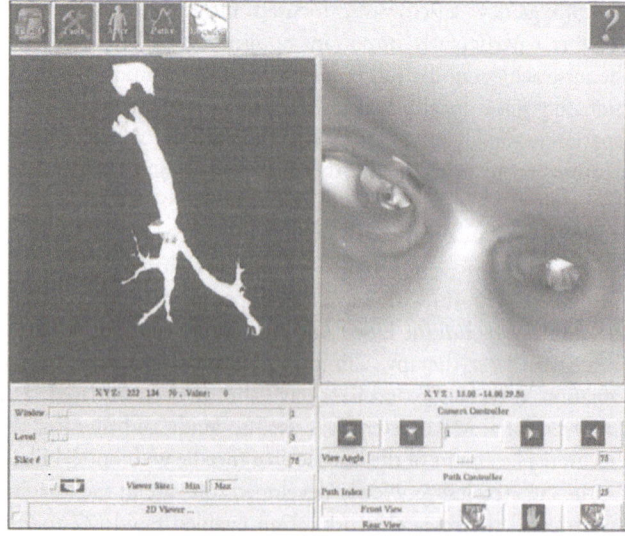

Figure 20-4 A virtual endoscopy of the trachea. **Left,** Global view with a virtual camera displaying the view direction. **Right,** Camera view looking at the carina and the right and left main stem bronchus. (*See* Color Plate.)

open interventional MRI systems. With this setting, the position of the endoscope defines the location of three orthogonal image planes. The magnetic resonance images are displayed simultaneously on two adjacent monitors or in a multiwindow-format display. This combination of endoscopy and cross-sectional imaging can also be achieved with virtual endoscopic presentation, which is based on previously acquired images. These images can be updated with real-time MRI obtained intraoperatively.

Virtual endoscopy is applicable for education and training. Because the endoscopic views are very different from the typical anatomic presentation seen in cross-sectional images or in an anatomy atlas, the virtual models are very useful for training endoscopists. Inexperienced users can learn the endoscopic anatomy and the correlated surrounding volumetric anatomy.

CONCLUSIONS

Full integration of advanced imaging in surgery will result in fundamental changes in therapeutic strategies and approaches. Advances in technology have already resulted in sweeping changes in diagnostic radiology, and more widespread use of modern therapeutic devices, computers, and advanced imaging technologies will have a far-reaching effect on surgery as well. Medical imaging can supplement the surgeon's visual field by providing intraoperative views of otherwise hidden structures.

The concept of image guidance demands a strategic shift in the focus of medical imaging from diagnosis to treatment. Continuous commitment from imaging experts, interventionists, and surgeons is necessary to expedite technologic development in our rapidly changing health care environment. Image-guided therapy offers the possibility of improving safety, efficacy, and cost-effectiveness of existing procedures, and it may result in new procedures that cannot be established outside of this environment.

REFERENCES AND RECOMMENDED READING

Recently published papers of particular interest have been highlighted as:

- • Of interest
- •• Of outstanding interest

1. Vannier MW, Marsh JL, Warren JO: Three dimensional CT reconstruction images for craniofacial surgical planning and evaluation. *Radiology* 1984, 1:179–184.

2. Cutting C, Bookstein EL, Grayson B, *et al.*: Three-dimensional computer assisted design of craniofacial surgical procedures: optimization and interaction with cephalometric and CT-based models. *Plast Reconstr Surg* 1986, 77:877–887.

3. Altobelli DE, Kikinis R, Mulliken JB, *et al.*: Computer-assisted three-dimensional planning in craniofacial surgery. *Plast Reconstr Surg* 1993, 92:576–585.

4. Jolesz FA, Kikinis R, Cline HE, Lorensen WE: The use of computerized imaging and image processing for neurosurgical planning. In *Astrocytomas*. Edited by Black PMcL, Lampson LA. Cambridge: Blackwell Scientific Publications; 1993:50–56.

5. Vogl TJ, Assal J, Bergman C: Three-dimensional MR reconstruction images of skull base tumors. *J Magn Reson Imag* 1993, 3:357–364.

6. Hu XP, Tan KK, Levin DN, *et al.*: Three-dimensional magnetic resonance images of the brain: application to neurosurgical planning. *J Neurosurg* 1993, 72:433–440.

7. Chernoff DM, Silverman SG, Kikinis R, *et al.*: Three-dimensional imaging and display of renal tumors using spiral CT: a potential aid to partial nephrectomy. *Urology* 1994, 43:125–129.

8. Zhang J, Levesque MF, Wilson CL, *et al.*: Multimodality imaging of brain structures for stereotactic surgery. *Radiology* 1990, 175:435–441.

9. Holman BL, Zimmerman RE, Johnson KA, *et al.*: Computer-assisted superimposition of magnetic resonance and high-resolution technetium-99m HMPAO and thallium-201 SPECT images of the brain. *J Nucl Med* 1991, 32:1478–1484.

10. Levin DN, Hu XP, *et al.*: The brain: integrated three-dimensional display of MR and PET images. *Radiology* 1989, 172:783–789.

11.•• Wells MW, Viola P, Atsumi H, *et al.*: Multimodal volume registration by maximation of mutual information. *Medical Image Analysis* 1996, 1:35–51.
A new technique is presented to register volumetric medical images such as MRI, CT, or positron emission tomography. This is achieved by adjustment of the relative position and orientation until the mutual information between the images is maximized. No reprocessing or segmentation is required because the algorithms are quite general and can foreseeably be used with a wide variety of imaging devices.

12. Kelly PJ, Kall B, Goerss S: Functional stereotactic surgery utilizing CT data and computer generated stereotactic atlas. *Acta Neurochir Suppl (Wien)* 1984, 33:577–583.

13. Gleason PL, Kikinis R, Altobelli D, *et al.*: Video registration virtual reality for nonlinkage stereotactic surgery. *Stereotact Funct Neurosurg* 1994, 63:139–143.

14.• Nakajima S, Atsumi H, Moriarty TM, Kikinis R, Jolesz, Black PML, *et al.*: Use of cortical surface vessel registration for image-guided neurosurgery. *Neurosurgery* 1997, 41:403–409.
Three-dimensional modeling and video registration using cortical surface vessels is practical and improves two-dimensional projection accuracy significantly over skin registration in neurosurgery.

15.•• Grimson WEL, Ettinger GJ, White SJ, *et al.*: An automatic registration method for frameless stereotaxy, image-guided surgery, and enhanced reality visualization. *IEEE Trans Med Imag* 1996, 2:129–140.
An automatic technique for registering segmented MRI or CT reconstructions (with any view of the patient on the operating table) was developed to help surgeons plan the exact location of incisions, to define the margins of tumors, and to precisely identify locations of neighboring critical structures. The method enables a visual mix of live video of the patient with the segmented three-dimensional MRI or CT model, supporting enhanced reality techniques for planning and guiding neurosurgical procedures, and interactive viewing of extracranial or intracranial structures nonintrusively. Extensions of the method include image-guided biopsies, focused therapeutic procedures, and clinical studies involving change detection over time sequences of images.

16. Kosugi Y, Watanabe E, Goto J, *et al.* An articulated neurosurgical navigation system using MRI and CT images. *IEEE Trans Biomed Eng* 1988, 35:147–152.

17. Kato A, Yoshimine T, Hayakawa T, *et al.*: A frameless, armless navigational system for computer assisted neurosurgery. *J Neurosurg* 1991, 74:845–849.

18. Roberts DW, Strohbehn JW, Hatch JF, *et al.*: A frameless stereotactic integration of computerized tomographic imaging and the operating microscope. *J Neurosurg* 1986, 65:545–549.

19. Koivukangas J, Louhisalmi Y, Alakuijala J, Oikarinen J: Ultrasound-controlled neuronavigator-guided brain surgery. *J Neurosurg* 1993, 79:36–42.

20. Kall BA, Kelly PJ, Goerss SJ: The computer as a stereotactic surgical instrument. *Neurol Res* 1986, 8:201–208.

21. Apuzzo ML, Sabshin JK: Computed tomographic guidance stereo-taxis in the management of intracranial mass lesions. *Neurosurgery* 1983, 12:277–285.

22. Zamorano L, Jiang Z, Kadi AM: Computer-assisted neurosurgery system: Wayne State University hardware and software configuration. *Comput Med Imaging Graph* 1994, 18:257–271.

23. Zinreich SJ, Tebo SA, Long DM, *et al.*: Frameless sterotactic inte-gration of CT imaging data: accuracy and initial applications. *Radiology* 1993, 188:35–42.

24. Mosges R, Klimek L: Computer-assisted surgery of the paranasal sinuses. *J Otolaryngol* 1993, 22:69–71.

25.•• Fried MP, Kleefield J, Gopal H, *et al.*: Image-guided endoscopic surgery: results of accuracy and performance in a multicenter clini-cal study using an electromagnetic tracking system. *Laryngoscope* 1997, 107:594–601.
The InstrTrak System, an electromagnetic tracking system, includes an automated registration technique for endoscopic sinus surgery. Advantages of this are elimination of the redundant CT scan, com-pensation for head movement, and the ability to use interchangeable instruments.

26. Schenck JF, Jolesz FA, Roemer PB, *et al.*: Superconducting open configuration MRI system for image-guided therapy. *Radiology* 1995, 195:805–814.

27.•• Silverman SG, Collick BD, Figueira MR, *et al.* Interactive MR-guided biopsy in an open-configuration MR imaging system. *Radiology* 1995, 197:175–181.
Magnetic-resonance–guided biopsy with a frameless stereotactic tech-nique is safe and accurate. Image feedback is near real time, and the procedure is interactive.

28. Jolesz FA: Interventional magnetic resonance imaging computed tomography and ultrasound. *Acad Radiol* 1995, 2:S124-S125.

29. Jolesz FA, Kahn T: Interventional MRI: state-of-the-art. *Appl Radiol* 1997, 26:8–13.

30.•• Jolesz FA: Image-guided procedures and the operating room of the future. *Radiology* 1997, 204:601–612.
This paper highlights the concept of image-guided therapy and the genuinely interdisciplinary approach of radiology in this emerging field.

31. Fried MP, Hsu L, Topulos GP, Jolesz FA: Image-guided surgery in a new magnetic resonance suite: preclinical considerations. *Laryncoscope* 1996, 106:411–417.

32. Fried MP, Kleefield J, Jolesz FA, *et al.*: Intraoperative image guidance during endoscopic sinus surgery. *Am J Rhin* 1996, 10:337–342.

33. Moriarty TM, Kikinis R, Jolesz FA, *et al.*: Magnetic resonance imaging therapy: intraoperative MRI. *Neurosurg Clin North Am* 1996, 44:323–331.

34.•• Black PM, Moriarty T, Alexander E III, *et al.*: Development and implementation of intraoperative magnetic resonance imaging and it neurosurgical applications. *Neurosurgery* 1997, 41:831–845.
Intraoperative MRI allows lesions to be precisely localized and targeted, hence the progress of a procedure can be immediately evaluated. This eliminates errors that can arise during frame-based and frameless stereo-tactic surgery when anatomic structures alter their position because of shifting or displacement of brain parenchyma but are correlated with images obtained preoperatively.

35. Jolesz FA, Shtern F: The operating room of the future: report of the National Cancer Institute workshop. Imaging-guided stereotactic tumor diagnosis and treatment. *Invest Radiol* 1992, 27:326–328.

36. Silverman G, Jolesz FA, Newman RW, *et al.*: Design and implementation of an interventional MR imaging suite. *AJR Am J Roentgenol* 1997, 168:1465–1471.

37. Alexander E, Kikinis R, Jolesz F: Intraoperative magnetic resonance imaging therapy. In *Image-Guided Neurosurgery: Clinical Applications of Interactive Surgical Navigation*. Edited by Barnett GH, Roberts D. St. Louis: Quality Medical Publishers; 1998: in press.

38. Alexander E, Moriarty TM, Kikinis R, Jolesz FA: Innovations in minimalism: intraoperative MR. *Clin Neurosurg* 1996, 43:338–352.

39. Matsumoto R, Oshio K, Jolesz FA: Monitoring of laser and freez-ing-induced ablation in the liver with T1-weighted MR imaging. *J Magn Reson Imag* 1992, 2:555–562.

40. Matsumoto R, Mulkern V, Hushek SG, Jolesz FA: Tissue tem-perature monitoring for thermal interventional therapy: com-parison of T1-weighted MR sequences. *J Magn Reson Imag* 1994, 4:65–70.

41. Bleier AR, Jolesz FA, Coheu MS, *et al.*: Real-time magnetic resonance imaging of laser heat deposition in tissue. *Magn Reson Med* 1991, 21:132–137.

42. Matsumoto R, Selig AM, Colucci VM, Jolesz FA: Interstitial Nd:YAG laser ablation in normal rabbit liver: trial to maximize the size of laser-induced lesions. *Lasers Surg Med* 1992, 12:650–658.

43.•• Cline HE, Hynynen K, Watkins RD, *et al.*: Focused US system for MR imaging-guided tumor ablation. *Radiology* 1995, 194:731–737.
A focused ultrasound system, implemented into an MR-scanner, has been used for image-guided tumor ablation in real time.

44. Duckwiler G, Lufkin RB, Teresi L, *et al.*: Head and neck lesions: MR-guided aspiration biopsy. *Radiology* 1989, 170:519–522.

45. Cline HE, Hynynen K, Hardy CJ, *et al.*: MR temperature map-ping of focused ultrasound surgery. *Magn Reson Med* 1994, 31:628–636.

46. Kettenbach J, Silverman SG, Hata N, *et al.*: Monitoring and visu-alization techniques for MR-guided laser ablations in open MR-system. *J Magn Reson Imag* 1998, in press.

47. Vining DJ, Shifrin RY, Grishaw EK, *et al.*: Virtual colonoscopy [abstract]. *Radiology* 1994, 193:446.

48. Davis CP, Ladd ME, Romanowski BJ, *et al.*: Human aorta: prelimi-nary results with virtual endoscopy based on three-dimensional MR imaging. *Radiology* 1996, 199:37-40.

49. Lorensen WE, Jolesz FA, Kikinis R: The exploration of cross-sec-tional data with a virtual endoscope. In *Interactive Technology and the New Health Paradigm*. IOS Press; 1995:221–230.

50. Virtual bronchoscopy: Relationships of virtual reality endo-bronchial simulation to actual brochoscopic findings. *Chest* 1996, 109:549-553.

51.•• Jolesz FA, Lorensen WE, Shinmoto H, *et al.*: Interactive virtual endoscopy. *AJR Am J Roentgenol* 1997, 169:1229–1235.
Merging of real and virtual endoscopy data may provide a more effective diagnostic workup. Knowledge of the location can be accomplished with sensors attached to the endoscope.

Medicolegal Perspectives on Laparoscopic Surgery

Kenneth A. Kern

Although the frequency of medical negligence litigation in general surgery remains stable, the development of minimally invasive surgical techniques has led to an explosive growth in litigation related to laparoscopic surgery. For example, since the widespread adoption of laparoscopic cholecystectomy by surgeons in 1990, litigation surrounding bile duct injury alone has surpassed similar litigation for open cholecystectomy by over 20-fold [1,2•3,4,5••]. In this regard, the Physician Insurers Association of America (PIAA), a trade association of malpractice insurance carriers, recently tabulated claims for laparoscopic cholecystectomy from 31 member companies who insure approximately 65,000 surgeons. Between 1990 and 1993, the PIAA recorded almost 331 claims for laparoscopic cholecystectomy, with 189 cases of bile duct injury (57%); of these, the mortality rate was 11% (21 deaths) [1,2•3,4,5••]. By comparison, in the 5 years between 1985 and 1990, only 35 cases of bile duct injury from open cholecystectomy were reported by member companies of the PIAA.

Given the increasing frequency of negligence litigation in laparoscopic surgery, we believe it is appropriate for surgeons to directly research and analyze the medicolegal outcomes of laparoscopic injuries. Of particular interest to surgeons is research focused on the medical aspects of litigated cases, their verdict outcomes, and their economic awards. Although the civil justice system proscribes the legal methods by which cases of negligence are decided, it does not dictate the clinical standards used to define medical malpractice. Indeed, only clinicians may define the standards of medical care applied in medical negligence litigation [6,7].

Cases of laparoscopic bile duct injury exemplify this principle. In the case of bile duct injury, the expert witnesses representing the patient and the operating surgeon attempt to persuade the lay jury that a violation of a standard of care generally used in the operation under review either did, or did not, occur. Ultimately, the strengths or weaknesses of the expert's arguments, as interpreted by the jury, determine the legal outcome of these cases. Because, in a paradoxical fashion, the outcome of these legal actions may redefine a clinical standard, surgeons are justified in their intense interest in the medicolegal aspects of bile duct injury. In particular, surgeons should follow carefully the arguments set forth by surgical expert witnesses regarding the definition of standards of care in cases of bile duct injury undergoing litigation. The same philosophy holds equally true for other areas of laparoscopic surgery.

Several factors might explain the increased frequency of litigation surrounding laparoscopic surgery. Medicolegal studies of why patients sue show that negligence litigation is most likely to accompany complications of surgery under the following conditions: 1) the injury results in significant economic loss to the patient; 2) the injury causes major organ dysfunction, overall disability, or death; 3) the injury will result in a substantial indemnity payout from litigation; and 4) the injured patient believes the injury resulted from negligent medical practice [8]. Unfortunately, laparoscopic injuries (in particular, laparoscopic bile duct injury) tend to fulfill all four criteria.

CHAPTER

21

For example, the median age of patients sustaining laparoscopic bile duct injury is 35 years (mean age, 44 years) [9], whereas the median age of patients with similar injury from open cholecystectomy is 52 years [2]. Thus, patients in the prime of their working or family years are subjected to reoperations, repeat hospitalizations, and the potential for chronic and permanent harm (*eg*, biliary cirrhosis and subsequent portal hypertension). Such has been the fate of many patients sustaining bile duct injury in the past during open cholecystectomy; a similar fate may await patients with bile duct injury from laparoscopic surgery. In our medicolegal study of bile duct injury from open cholecystectomy [2], the average number of reoperations was two (range, one to eight). We recently reported that a similar number of reoperations was required to repair bile ducts injured during laparoscopic cholecystectomy [5••].

Yet it is how patients view laparoscopic surgical injuries, in terms of a lay understanding of negligent surgery, that sets laparoscopic injury apart from similar injuries caused by open surgery. Laparoscopic bile duct injury is an excellent case in point. Clearly, the negative media coverage of laparoscopic injuries has contributed to the litigious nature of these complications. For example, in 1992, *The New York Times* began a front page article reporting laparoscopic complications by stating that "Surgeons who *rushed* to use a new technique to remove gallbladders *without adequate training* have *botched* many procedures . . ." (italics added) [10]. This statement leaves little room for doubt in the mind of the public that laparoscopic injuries are negligent, because the statement immediately links injuries to a surgeon's inadequate training and lack of deliberation, rather than to complexities of surgery or to specific patient factors. Indeed, the article fails to explore the actual mechanism of laparoscopic injuries. Further, the article does not correlate the number or type of injuries to the amount of training, nor does it discuss the problem of bile duct injury occurring when surgeons are adequately trained and clinically experienced.

This widespread negative publicity resulted in a rapid decrease in the time to file negligence claims for laparoscopic bile duct injury. In 1990, the average time to file a claim from the date of a surgical complication was 26 months, or approximately 2 years [6,7]. By June of 1992, I calculated that the time to file negligence claims for nine cases of laparoscopic bile duct injury, surveyed by me, had fallen to 6 months (Kern, Unpublished data). This filing time appears to be the fastest rate at which a laparoscopic injury can enter the process of negligence litigation.

Given the intense medicolegal scrutiny faced by a case of laparoscopic injury, surgeons should strive to understand the overall impact of litigation resulting from these injuries. Common bile duct injuries are an excellent model for the medicolegal fate of laparoscopic injuries in general. Surgeons will gain several specific benefits by reviewing medicolegal data on laparoscopic injuries to the bile ducts and other organs. First, this understanding will prevent unwarranted assumptions about the medicolegal fate of a bile duct injury, as well as other laparoscopic injuries. For example, many surgeons believe a bile duct injury automatically falls under the category of self-evident negligence (*res ipsa loquitur*), without regard to the circumstances of the injury. Given the successful legal defense of many cases of laparoscopic bile duct injury brought to trial, this assumption is clearly false. Second, in the event a surgeon injures a bile duct or other organ, specific knowledge of litigation outcomes will allow the defendant surgeon to make more informed decisions during malpractice proceedings. Third, and perhaps most importantly, a medicolegal analysis of bile duct and other injuries educates surgeons in preventing, recognizing, and repairing injuries. The latter is of particular significance in this era of laparoscopic surgery, because when injuries of high magnitude are contrasted with the usual uncomplicated course of a laparoscopic cholecystectomy, the deviation from the standard for clinical outcome suggests a deviation from the standard for surgical care. Resolving this conflict, and determining the factual basis for claims of deviations from standard surgical care, forms the essence of medicolegal actions.

Because of the prolonged litigation times involved in medical malpractice, data on malpractice litigation resulting from laparoscopic injuries are only now available for review. For medical malpractice claims in general, the median time to resolution of litigation by settlement is 36 months and for resolution by jury verdict, 61 months [6,7]. Sufficient time has now elapsed from the occurrence of laparoscopic cholecystectomy injuries to the filing of lawsuits and completion of civil litigation to enable a medicolegal analysis of an initial set of data. These data are derived from a variety of sources, including insurance carrier surveys, historical reviews, and legal sources. We forewarn the reader that this medicolegal review focuses on medical factors of laparoscopic injury, derived from an empirical analysis of past negligence litigation. As befits our role as an interested clinician only, we do not attempt to be advisory or complete on matters of case law.

OVERVIEW OF LAPAROSCOPIC LITIGATION

Recently, we reported on the medicolegal outcomes of 44 cases of injury resulting from laparoscopic cholecystectomy [5••]. This chapter focuses on a review of these data. Our method of medicolegal analysis has been described in several previous reports of injuries associated with open and laparoscopic cholecystectomy [1,2•,3,4,5••]. Stated briefly, using medicolegal data we created a taxonomy of injuries by type and severity, tabulated costs, and quantitated legal verdicts. We also attempted to define the medicolegal rationale for why cases settled or were brought to trial.

The malpractice actions described in this chapter resulted from injuries sustained during the earliest days of laparoscopic cholecystectomy, specifically during the 40-month period between February 1, 1989 and June 30, 1992. The cases completed litigation in the 39-month interval between January 1, 1993 and April 30, 1996. In 14 cases, the specific dates of laparoscopic injury could be identified and were compared with the dates of resolution of litigation. For these 14 cases, the average time to resolution of litigation by trial or settlement was 34 months. There was no statistical difference in the time interval of litigation for nine cases proceeding to trial (mean, 31) versus five cases settling before trial (mean, 27).

Types of laparoscopic injuries

The 44 cases of injuries comprised four main categories. These categories include bile duct, bowel, major vascular, and other (Table 21-1).

Bile duct injuries

Bile duct injuries (*n* = 27) involved the following structures: common bile duct (*n* = 18 of 27 [67%]), common hepatic duct (*n* = 4 of 27 [15%]), hilar hepatic ducts (*n* = 3 of 27 [11%], and cystic duct leaks (*n* = 2 of 27 [7%]). The types of injuries to major bile ducts were as follows: common bile duct (15 transections, three excisions), common hepatic duct (two transections, two complete clip ligations), and hilar hepatic duct (one transection, two excisions). Cystic duct leaks both involved slippage of clips used to ligate the cystic duct. One

Table 21-1

Types of injuries associated with laparoscopic cholecystectomy

Major category of injury	Subtype of injury	Cases, *n*(%)
Bile duct		
	Common bile duct*	18 (41)
	Common hepatic duct	4 (9)
	Hilar hepatic duct	3 (7)
	Cystic duct	2 (5)
	Total	27 (61)
Bowel		
	Small bowel	4 (9)
	Duodenum†	2 (5)
	Colon	1 (2)
	Total	7 (16)
Vascular		
	Iliac artery	2 (5)
	Aorta	1 (2)
	Iliac vein	1 (2)
	Total	4 (9)
Other		
	Bile spill with peritonitis	2 (5)
	Retained intra-abdominal gallstone	1 (2)
	Lip burned by cautery	1 (2)
	Postoperative bleed with cerebral anoxia	1 (2)
	Conversion to open cholecystectomy with delayed hemobilia	1 (2)
	Total	6 (14)

*One case of combined major common bile duct injury and minor small bowel injury.

†One case of combined major duodenal injury and minor cystic duct leak.

Adapted from Kern [5••]; with permission.

case of common bile duct injury was accompanied by a minor injury to the small bowel.

The median number of additional reoperations to correct bile duct injury was two, with a range of two to nine reoperations. Five cases reported rehospitalizations to dilate recurrent postoperative strictures; one case required four such readmissions. The average delay in diagnosis of seven bile duct injuries was 11 days (median, 13 days; range, 3 to 21 days). Bile duct injuries (*n* = 9) completed resolution of litigation in an average time interval of 42 months. In three separate cases, injuries occurred during the operating surgeon's first, third, and 15th case.

The 27 cases of bile duct injuries were resolved by 13 jury trials and 14 out-of-court settlements. Of the 13 civil trials, 12 were closed with jury verdicts for the defense, and one was closed by a jury verdict for the plaintiff. Thus, the defensibility rate for cases of bile duct injury taken to trial was 92% (12 of 13 successful defense cases). Clearly, these successful defense cases demonstrated that a bile duct injury is not considered by juries to be self-evident negligence. The average cost of a bile duct injury to settle (*n* = 13) was $506,000 (range, $175,000–$1,000,000). A single jury verdict in favor of the plaintiff was accompanied by an award of $250,000.

Bowel injuries

Bowel injuries (*n* = 7) involved three cases of trocar perforation of the small bowel (43%); one case of cautery injury to the small bowel (14%), two cases of cautery injury to the duodenum (29%), and one case of cautery injury to the colon (14%). One case of major duodenal cautery injury was accompanied by a minor cystic duct leak. In two cases of small bowel trocar injury, the number of perforations to the small bowel ranged between two and four.

One case of trocar small bowel injury occurred in a 75-year-old woman who died 3 days postoperatively from septic peritonitis, confirmed by autopsy. The lawsuit alleged that the surgeon failed to respond to phone calls from the patient in the 3 days before her death (result: confidential settlement). In another case of trocar perforation of the small bowel, a 72-year-old man was initially diagnosed with atelectasis (fever and pulmonary failure), but a CT scan revealed a large intra-abdominal abscess. The patient died hours after an exploratory laparotomy to repair multiple perforations of the small intestine (result: $650,00 settlement). In a third case of small bowel injury, extensive cautery dissection was used to lyse dense adhesions. Postoperatively, severe abdominal pain and respiratory failure developed; reoperation was performed 3 days later, with the finding of two perforations of the small bowel. The patient claimed informed consent had not been obtained to perform lysis of adhesions prior to laparoscopic cholecystectomy, and a delay occurred in return to the operating room (result: defense verdict).

In one case of unrecognized perforation of the duodenum, cautery was used to separate the omentum from the gallbladder because of dense, postinflammatory adhesions. The patient complained of severe pain during the evening of surgery, and died the next day of sepsis and respiratory failure. An autopsy confirmed a perforated duodenum (result: jury verdict for $248,547). In another case of perforated duodenum, cautery was used to control bleeding from a torn cystic artery; however, open cholecystectomy was required to control the bleeding. An unrecognized duodenal injury resulted in septic shock the following day. The plaintiff expired 2 weeks later despite a second operation to repair the duodenal leak (result: defense verdict). The cautery injury to the colon occurred after dissection at the hepatic flexure, in which a quarter-sized perforation occurred. A temporary colostomy was created for 7 months, with successful reversal at a later time (result: $225,000 settlement).

The average age of four female patients and one male patient with bowel injuries was 69 years (median, 72 years; range, 64–75 years), which is significantly older than the group as a whole (49 years; $P < 0.01$ [t-test]). Bowel injuries ($n = 3$) completed resolution of litigation in an average time interval of 24 months (SD, 13; range, 12–37; median, 24). The cases were resolved through four civil trials, concluding in three jury verdicts for the defense and one jury verdict for the plaintiff. The average cost of a bowel injury to settle ($n = 2$) was $437,500 (range, $225,000–$650,000). A single jury verdict in favor of the plaintiff was accompanied by an award of $248,547.

Major vascular injury

Major vascular injury ($n = 4$) all involved significant lacerations into major retroperitoneal vessels during trocar placement, causing injury to the following structures: iliac artery ($n = 2$ of 4 [50%]), iliac vein ($n = 1$ [25%], and aorta ($n = 1$ of 4 [25%]). In one case of iliac artery injury, rapid bleeding resulted in hemorrhagic shock, hypotension, and cerebral anoxia leading to permanent brain injury (result: defense verdict). A second case of iliac artery injury occurred during placement of the umbilical trocar using manual lifting of the abdominal wall. The trocar was placed in a lateral direction, resulting in a trocar laceration of the artery with hemorrhage and an additional injury to the femoral nerve (result: settlement $125,000). The iliac vein injury followed two unsuccessful attempts to place the umbilical trocar. On the third, more forceful attempt, the trocar lacerated the junction between the left iliac vein and the inferior vena cava. The injury resulted in a 10-unit blood loss and required an emergency repair of the left iliac vein. The vein repair strictured and thrombosed, resulting in permanent swelling of the left leg (result: defense verdict). The aortic injury involved a through-and-through trocar puncture of the anterior and posterior walls of the aorta by the umbilical trocar. The trocar had been inserted at a 90° angle to the abdominal wall, at a depth of its entire length of 10 cm (result: plaintiff verdict for $131,539). The patient survived the aortic repair without long-term complications.

The sole known length of time for a vascular injury to complete litigation was 9 months. Litigation for vascular injuries involved three jury trials and one out-of-court settlement. The jury trials resulted in two verdicts for the defense and one verdict for the plaintiff. The cost of one known vascular injury to settle was $125,000; a single jury award for the plaintiff resulted in a payment of $131,539.

Other injuries

Other injuries ($n = 6$) included the following five categories: 1) bile peritonitis secondary to intraoperative spillage of bile and stones ($n = 2$ of 6 [33%]); 2) retained "painful" gallstones free in abdomen ($n = 1$ of 6 [17%]); 3) conversion to open cholecystectomy with delayed hemobilia ($n = 1$ of 6 [17%]); 4) cautery burn to lip ($n = 1$ of 6 [17%]); and 5) postoperative bleed with cerebral anoxia ($n = 1$ of 6 [17%]).

One case of bile and stone spill occurred in a 56-year-old woman with insulin-dependent diabetes, who died on postoperative day 5 after early discharge despite a high fever. An autopsy revealed widespread infected bile peritonitis and free gallstones within the peritoneal cavity (result: $225,000 settlement). A second case of bile spill resulted in peritonitis occurring in a severely depressed, mentally ill patient, who was found dead at home from infected bile peritonitis on the third postoperative day. The plaintiffs claimed that the surgeon failed to instruct the patient and her home nursing aides about postoperative follow-up and possible complications (result: defense verdict).

The "painful gallstones" were incidentally discovered at the patient's cesarean section delivery, many months after laparoscopic cholecystectomy. The patient claimed that 1) she had not been told about the remaining gallstones in the abdomen, and that the gallstones were the cause of her painful pregnancy; and 2) the painful gallstones led to the sterilization procedure (result: defense verdict). In another case requiring conversion to open cholecystectomy because of bleeding during laparoscopic cholecystectomy, the patient developed hemobilia 3 weeks postoperatively and underwent embolization followed by a second open reoperation to effect a repair. Three months later the patient again developed hemobilia, and underwent a third open operation to correct the hemobilia (result: defense verdict).

The cautery burn to lip involved an electrified dissector resting on the patient's lip through the surgical drapes; the injury required a plastic surgical reconstruction and residual permanent scarring (result: $95,000 settlement). The postoperative hemorrhage after laparoscopic cholecystectomy was caused by continued bleeding in the gallbladder bed. The patient was left in a hypotensive state for 8 hours without medical intervention, culminating in a hypotensive stroke, residual brain damage, and partial permanent paralysis (result: settlement $1,097,000).

The sole known length of time for a bile spill to complete litigation was 21 months. Litigation was resolved through three jury trials, all resulting in defense verdicts, and three out-of-court settlements. For this group of injuries, the average payment for three settlements was $472,333 (range, $95,000–$1,097,000).

Profound complications of laparoscopic cholecystectomy are listed in Table 21-2. There were seven deaths ($n = 7$ of 44 [16%]) overall, resulting from either septic or bile peritonitis. In four cases of septic peritonitis, complications resulted from the following injuries: small bowel injury with unrecognized leak ($n = 2$ of 4 [50%]), duodenal injury with unrecognized leak ($n = 2$ of 4 [50%]). In three cases of bile peritonitis, the following complications resulted: spillage of bile and stones during resection of the gallbladder, without bile duct injury ($n = 2$ of 3 [67%]) or cystic duct leak without bile duct injury ($n = 1$ of 3 [33%]). There were no deaths from injury or repair of main bile ducts (common, hepatic, or hilar). The death rate in bowel injury during laparoscopic cholecystectomy was 57% ($n = 4$ of 7). Of the seven

Table 21-2

Profound complications of laparoscopic cholecystectomy

Age/gender	Injury	Complication	Outcome	Verdict
41/NA	Trocar puncture iliac artery	Intraoperative hypotension, anoxic CVA	Permanent brain injury	Defense verdict
56/F	Bile spill from gallbladder; insulin-diabetic	Bile peritonitis	Death	Settlement ($225,000)
62/F	Bile or stone spill from gallbladder; mental illness	Bile peritonitis	Death	Defense verdict
64/F	Cystic duct leak	Bile peritonitis	Death	Settlement ($175,000)
64/F	Perforation of duodenum	Septic peritonitis	Death	Defense verdict
68/F	Postoperative hemorrhage	Intraoperative hypotension, anoxic CVA	Permanent partial paralysis	Settlement ($1,097,000)
72/M	Perforation of small bowel	Septic peritonitis	Death	Settlement ($650,000)
75/F	Perforation of small bowel	Septic peritonitis	Death	Settlement (N/A)
NA/F	Perforation of duodenum	Septic peritonitis	Death	Plaintiff ($175,000)
NA/F	Trocar puncture iliac vein	Iliac vein ligation	Venous edema	Defense verdict

Adapted from Kern [5••]; with permission.

CVA—cerebrovascular accident; N/A—not available.

deaths, ages were known in six patients. The average age of patients who died was 66 years. The patients who died were older than the group as a whole (66 years vs 49 years; $P = 0.004$ [t-test; mean difference in age, 30 years]). The average cost of settlement of four deaths from bowel injury was $536,750 (range, $175,000–$1,097,000).

The total liability payout for all 44 cases was $9,679,586, but only 25 cases (57%) completed resolution of litigation with a payment to the patient. Of these 25 payments, 21 (48%) were by out-of-court settlements, and the remaining four (9%) were by jury verdict awards. The mean payout for injuries of all types was $437,822, with a minimum payout of $95,000 and a maximum payout of $1,097,000. The average settlement was $469,711, with a total settlement for all cases of $8,924,500 (range, $95,000–$1,0970,000). By type of injury, the total and mean liability payments for trials and settlements combined are shown in Table 21-3.

Of the 44 cases, 23 (52%) proceeded to trial. In 19 of these 23 cases (83%), the jury rendered a defense verdict in favor of the doctor. The remaining four cases ended in jury verdicts in favor of the plaintiff, resulting in an overall plaintiff win rate for all types of laparoscopic cholecystectomy injury of 17% (four of 23). The total plaintiff verdict was $755,086, with an average of $188,772 (range, $125,000–$250,000).

LAPAROSCOPIC TECHNOLOGY AND MEDICAL LIABILITY

The technical innovation of laparoscopic surgery has opened up new avenues in medical liability. Although some types of injuries (eg, common bile duct injury) were well recognized as possible complications of open surgery, other injuries were unheard of during open surgery. In many cases, these injuries were unusual and came as a complete surprise to the laparoscopic surgeon, having only become evident because of laparoscopic technology. These new injuries, including trocar enterotomy, laceration of vessels, and cautery burns to segments of the intestinal tract, are a direct result of laparoscopic technology, which uses a puncture method of access to the peritoneal cavity and electrical cautery–dissection techniques. Interestingly, prior to laparoscopic surgery, the most costly iatrogenic injuries in general surgery also involved both inadvertent enterotomy (154 paid claims, total $16 million) and major vascular injury to vessels of the abdomen or pelvis (64 paid claims, total $12 million). However, the mechanisms of injury are completely different, and rarely if ever noted during open cholecystectomy [2]. Based on the present study, payments for these types of injuries are likely to remain high in the era of laparoscopic surgery. In the present study, the total payment combined for all injuries exceeded $9 million, whereas the average payment per case for bile duct, bowel, and vascular injuries was $488,214, $374,516, and $128,270.

One of the major goals of this medicolegal analysis is to determine the unique features of laparoscopic injuries that lead to malpractice litigation. In terms of the types and frequency of injuries in these malpractice cases, there was no difference in the spectrum or proportion of injuries compared with data from clinical reports of laparoscopic complications. For example, Deziel and coworkers [11] reviewed complications of laparoscopic cholecystectomy in 77,604 cases operated on by 5358 surgeons in 1140 hospitals. The ratios between the types of injuries in Deziel and coworker's clinical study were similar to those of

Table 21-3

Liability payments for laparoscopic injury*

Category	Payments, n	Total payment	Mean (SD)
Bile duct	14	$6,585,000	$488,214 ($303,000)
Bowel	3	$1,123,547	$374,516 ($239,000)
Vascular	2	$256,539	$128,270 ($4,624)
Deaths	5	$2,322,000	$536,750 ($430,000)
Other	3	$1,417,000	$472,333 ($545,000)

*Payments include trial verdict awards and settlements combined.

the present medicolegal study: bile duct 76%, bowel 18%, and vascular 6%. However, we noted an additional category of litigation of 14% covering injuries unique to laparoscopic surgery, and not specifically identified by the Deziel and coworkers study, including lip burn by cautery or retained gallstones. Wherry and coworkers [12], in an extensive audit of 5642 laparoscopic cholecystectomies performed in 89 military medical facilities, also noted a ratio of organ injury similar to this medicolegal study. In Wherry and coworker's study, the bile duct injury rate was 0.57%, the bowel injury rate was 0.5%, the cystic leak rate was 1%, the major vascular injury rate was 0.02% (aorta), and the death rate was 0.04%. Larson and coworkers [13] noted a 2% complication rate in 1983 laparoscopic cholecystectomies. Of 41 complications, 29% were bile duct injury, 2.5% were duodenal injury, and 2.5% were trocar vascular injury. There were no operative deaths from these injuries. Thus, aside from our smaller category of unusual injuries, the types of laparoscopic injuries resulting in malpractice litigation are no different from the usual reported types of laparoscopic injuries. These data indicate that additional factors must accompany the laparoscopic injury to result in the filing of a negligence claim.

One method of resolving the issue as to whether technical misadventures in laparoscopic surgery represent normal iatrogenic risk, or medical negligence, is to define the degree to which these injuries deviate from the standards of customary practice held by the average practitioner [6,7]. It is important to note that laparoscopic injuries are a worldwide phenomenon, and have been reported from all countries where the technology is applied, including England (bile duct injury, 0.2%) [14], The Netherlands (bile duct injury, 0.8%–1.1%) [15], and Norway (bile duct injury, 0.6%; bowel injury, 0.38%) [16]. Given this frequency of laparoscopic injuries worldwide, it is possible that the absolute prevention of technical misadventures, although proposed as a standard of care in the medicolegal environment, may never be achieved completely in clinical practice. For this reason, some cases of laparoscopic injury may not represent a violation of the customary, local, or community standard of medical practice, but instead may demonstrate the technical limitations and unavoidable clinical complications of the laparoscopic approach.

Based on the present data, it appears that technical misadventures in laparoscopic surgery are a necessary cause of litigation, but they do not appear to be a sufficient cause of litigation. A second vital issue regarding standards of surgical care is related to the management of complications themselves, and how far deviations from the standard clinical course are created by mismanagement of the complications of the injury. As a clinical standard of practice, Lee and coworkers [17] reviewed over 7000 patients from five major clinical series. They noted that the standard postoperative course for laparoscopic cholecystectomy was 1 day, with a return-to-work time of 8 to 10 days. The readmission rate in these 7120 cases was 1% or less. This rapid return-to-work interval stands in stark contrast to that of disability intervals from open cholecystectomy, in which out-of-work intervals average 41 days. Unfortunately, in some types of laparoscopic injury, out-of-work times may greatly exceed this interval.

Deviations from the standard clinical course of a laparoscopic cholecystectomy raise the question of deviations from the standard of surgical care. Several factors have been strongly correlated with surgical negligence litigation, including chronicity of injury, failure to achieve the attainable goals of a surgical procedure, and diagnostic errors [8]. Diagnostic errors are especially prone to litigation: in the study by Weiler and coworkers [7], 75% of these diagnostic errors were associated with negligence litigation, despite these errors accounting for only 8% of the pool of adverse events. The cases in the present series consistently demonstrate these three factors leading to litigation. For example, the median number of reoperations to correct bile duct injury was two, with some cases requiring biliary reconstruction up to 4 years after injury. Others have reported that an average of 3.4 hospital admissions are required in the repair of bile duct injuries [18]. The promise of a "noninvasive approach" was always compromised in these patients, because all the patients had reoperations through standard laparotomy incisions to correct surgical injuries, either immediately (as in the case of some bile duct injuries and vascular injuries), or in a delayed fashion. Lastly, delays in diagnosis of surgical complications were common. The average delay in diagnosis of bile duct injuries was 11 days. Bowel injury, bile leaks, bile spills, and other injuries were delayed in diagnosis, allowing the development of severe and often fatal infection. Delays in diagnosis of bowel injury and bile leak are common [11,13,17,19–21]. However, unlike the present series, in which the mortality rate from bowel injury is 57%, other clinical series report either no or limited mortalities from bowel injury or bile leak [17,19].

In such cases, explanations for the filing of civil lawsuits must reach beyond a focus on the technical failure itself. Based on the data given previously, a picture emerges of the litigated case in laparoscopic surgery in general (and laparoscopic cholecystectomy in particular) as one involving the following features: 1) notable deviations from the standard clinical course postoperatively; 2) a complex technical complication of the surgical procedure, requiring a high degree of skill or a multistage approach to repair; 3) injury leading to chronic illness requiring subsequent hospitalizations or reoperations; and 4) delayed diagnosis of complications resulting from the initial surgical injury.

In this chapter I emphasize that data from actual malpractice cases can be useful in describing the prototype of the litigated case in laparoscopic surgery. In laparoscopic surgery in general, and in laparoscopic cholecystectomy in particular, the litigated case is likely to involve significant delays in diagnosis, complex injury, and chronic illness with incomplete recovery. Unfortunately, even relatively simple bile duct injuries, if not repaired promptly and expertly, may be accompanied by stricture formation, chronic morbidity, and death [1,2•3,4,5••]. Injuries to the bowel or vascular structures may be accompanied by a similar degree of disability and chronicity. Although laparoscopic injuries may not be completely preventable, litigation may be mitigated by maintaining a high index of suspicion for any patient who deviates from the well-defined postoperative course. In such cases, rapid intervention by experienced surgeons offers the best hope of reversing laparoscopic injury. This combination of factors is most likely to lead to a conclusive and swift ending to postoperative complications resulting from laparoscopic injury.

REFERENCES AND RECOMMENDED READING

Recently published papers of particular interest have been highlighted as:

- • Of interest
- •• Of outstanding interest

1. Kern KA: Risk management goals involving injury to the common bile ducts during laparoscopic cholecystectomy. *Am J Surg* 1992, 163:551–552.

2.• Kern KA: Medicolegal analysis of bile duct injury during open cholecystectomy and abdominal surgery. *Am J Surg* 1994, 168:217–222.
A comprehensive review of litigation resulting from open cholecystectomy, to be used as a benchmark from which to compare laparaoscopic injuries. Describes the medicolegal fate of injuries from open surgery, and is useful in predicting the fate of laparoscopic injuries.

3. Kern KA: Medicolegal perspectives in laparoscopic bile duct injuries. *Surg Clin North Am* 1994, 74:979–984.

4. Kern KA: The anatomy of surgical malpractice claims: an overview of 711 general surgery liability cases. *Bull Am Coll Surg* 1995, 80:35–49.
An excellent overview of malpractice actions in the broad field of general surgery.

5.•• Kern KA: Malpractice litigation involving laparoscopic cholecystectomy: cost, cause, and consequences. *Arch Surg* 1997, 132:392–398.
The first paper to describe the medicolegal outcomes from injuries sustained during laparoscopic cholecystectomy.

6. Halley MM, Fowks RJ, Ryan DL: *Medical Malpractice Solutions.* Springfield, IL: Charles C. Thomas; 1989:40–41.

7. Weiler PC, Hiatt HH, Newhouse JP, *et al.*: *Measure of Malpractice: Medical Injury, Malpractice Litigation, and Patient Compensation.* Cambridge, MA: Harvard University Press; 1993:5–6.

8. Localio AR, Lawthers AG, Brennan TA, *et al.*: Relation between malpractice claims and adverse events due to negligence: results of the Harvard Practice Study III. *N Engl J Med* 1991, 325:245–251.

9. Rossi RL, Schirmer WJ, Braasch JW, *et al.*: Laparoscopic bile duct injuries: risk factors, recognition, and repair. *Arch Surg* 1992, 127:596–602.

10. Altman LK: Surgical injuries lead to new rule. *The New York Times* 1992 (June 14):1 (L47).

11. Deziel DJ, Millikan KW, Economou SG, *et al.* Complications of laparoscopic cholecystectomy: a national survey of 4,292 hospitals and an analysis of 77,064 cases. *Am J Surg* 1993, 165:9–14.

12. Wherry DC, Rob CG, Marohn MR, Rich NM: An external audit of laparoscopic cholecystectomy performed in medical treatment facilities of the Department of the Defense. *Ann Surg* 1994, 220:626–634.

13. Larson GM, Vitale GC, Casey J, *et al.*: Multipractice analysis of laparoscopic cholecystectomy in 1,983 patients. *Am J Surg* 1992, 163:221–226.

14. Barton JR, Russell RCG, Hatfield ARW: Management of bile leaks after laparoscopic cholecystectomy. *Br J Surg* 1995, 82:980–984.

15. Schol FPG, Go PM, Gouma J: Risk factors for bile duct injury in laparoscopic cholecystectomy: analysis of 49 cases. *Br J Surg* 1994, 81:1786–1788.

16. Trondsen E, Ruud TE, Nilsen BH, *et al.*: Complications during the introduction of laparoscopic cholecystectomy in Norway. *Eur J Surg* 1994, 160:145–151.

17. Lee VS, Chari RS, Cucchiaro G, Meyers WC: Complications of laparoscopic cholecystectomy. *Am J Surg* 1993, 165:527–532.

18. Asbun HJ, Rossi RL, Lowell JA, Munson JL: Bile duct injury during laparoscopic cholecystectomy: mechanism of injury, prevention, and management. *World J Surg* 1993, 17:547–552.

19. Physician Insurers Association of America (PIAA): Laparoscopic Procedure Study, May 1994. Physician Insurers Association of America: Washington, DC; 1994.

20. Soper NJ, Flye MW, Brunt LM, *et al.* Diagnosis and management of biliary complications of laparoscopic cholecystectomy. *Am J Surg* 1993, 165:663–669.

21. Hebebrand D: Small-bowel necrosis following laparoscopic cholecystectomy: a clinically relevant complication? *Endoscopy* 1995, 27:281.

Index

A

Abdomen, laparoscopic surgery of *see* Laparoscopic surgery
Abdominal aortic aneurysm *see* Aorta, aneurysm of
Abdominal pain, laparoscopy in, 99–103
  acute, 99–102
  chronic, 99, 102–103
  contraindications for, 100–101
  in emergency setting, 100
  indications for, 100
  in intensive care unit, 100
  in pediatric patients, 139
  technique for, 99–100
Abdominal wall retractors, in gasless laparoscopy, 190
Abdominoperineal resection, laparoscopic, gasless, 194
Abscess, in choledocholithotomy, 23
Achalasia, 45–47, 153–154
  in pediatric patients, 138
Acute abdomen, laparoscopy in
  contraindications for, 100–101
  differential diagnosis in, 100, 139
  in gynecologic disease, 101
  indications for, 100
  in intestinal ischemia, 101
  preoperative evaluation in, 101
  in sepsis, 101
  in small bowel obstruction, 102
  technique for, 99–100
  in trauma, 101–102
Adenomas
  adrenal, 91–93, 166
  parathyroid, endoscopic parathyroidectomy in, 117–122
Adhesions, lysing of
  in appendectomy, 55
  in cholecystectomy, 5
Adhesives, tissue, 185
Adnexal disease, laparoscopy in, 101
Adrenal glands, laparoscopic surgery of, 91–93, 166
Anastomosis ring, biofragmentable, 185–186
Anesthesia
  for laparoscopic surgery
    in cardiopulmonary disease, 32–33
    cholecystectomy, 3
    complications of, 35–36
    in elderly persons, 32–33
    in healthy adults, 30–32
    in pediatric patients, 34–35, 137–138
    pneumoperitoneum and, 29–30
    in pregnancy, 33–34
  for mediastinoscopy, 36–37
  for thoracoscopy, 37, 146
Aneurysms, endovascular repair of
  aortic, 128–134
  iliac, 130–132
Anorchia, laparoscopic management of, 140–141

Anterior transabdominal approach, to adrenal surgery, 92
Anthropometry, in obesity measurement, 110
Antiemetic agents, in laparoscopic surgery, 31
Aorta
  aneurysm of, endovascular repair of, 128–134
    aneurysm classification and, 130
    balloon-expandable stents in, 128–129, 132
    graft selection for, 130–131
    hypogastric artery coil embolization in, 131
    Montefiore device in, 131
    multiple component devices in, 129
    patient selection for, 129–130
    self-expanding stents in, 128–129, 132
    single component devices in, 129
    technique for, 131–132
  injury of, in laparoscopic surgery, legal perspectives on, 214
Aortobifemoral bypass, gasless laparoscopic, 198
Aortoiliac occlusive disease, endovascular surgery in, 127–128
Appendectomy, laparoscopic, 53–61
  anatomic hazards in, 57
  in complicated appendicitis, 60
  contraindications for, 54
  vs conventional appendectomy, 58–60
  costs of, 59–60
  equipment for, 54
  in extraperitoneal retrocecal position, 56–57
  historical review of, 53–54
  hospital stay in, 58–59
  indications for, 54
  pain after, 59
  in pediatric patients, 138
  postoperative care in, 57
  in pregnancy, 54, 174
  technique for, 54–57
Arteries, minimally invasive surgery of *see* Endovascular surgery

B

Balloon techniques
  in aortic aneurysm repair, 128–129, 131–132
  in aortoiliac occlusive disease, 127
  in choledocholithotomy, 19
  in gasless laparoscopy, 198
    in aortobifemoral bypass, 198
    in diskectomy, 197–198
    retractors, 190–191, 193
  in urologic disease, 165
Bariatric surgery, 110–115
  adjustable gastric banding, 114–115
  indications for, 110–111
  preoperative assessment for, 111–112
  procedures for, 112–113
  results of, 113
  Roux-en-Y gastric bypass, 114
  vertical banded gastroplasty, 113–114

M

T

U

V

W

Color Plates

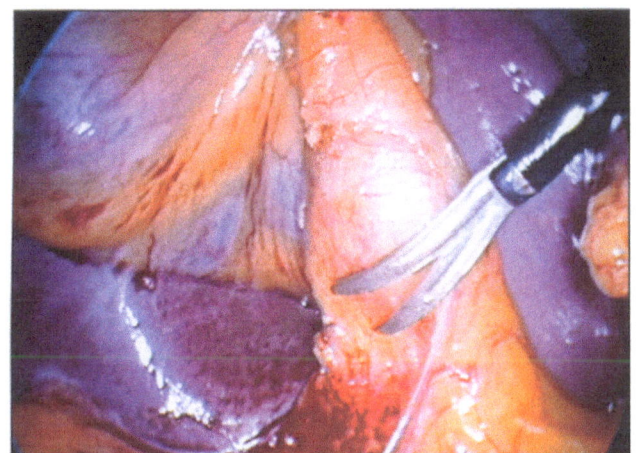

Chapter 2, Figure 2-6, p. 18

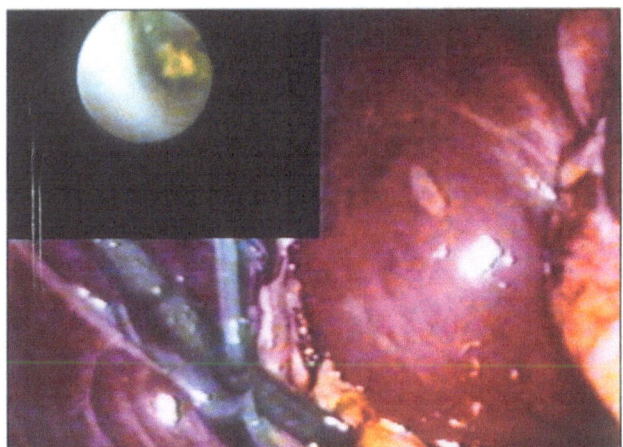

Chapter 2, Figure 2-8, p. 19

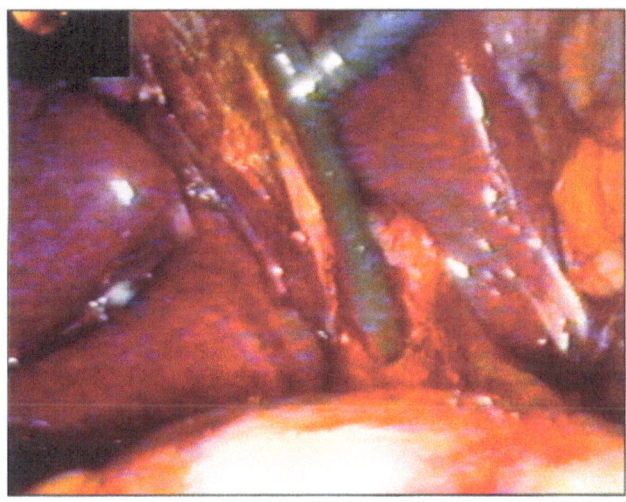

Chapter 2, Figure 2-9, p. 20

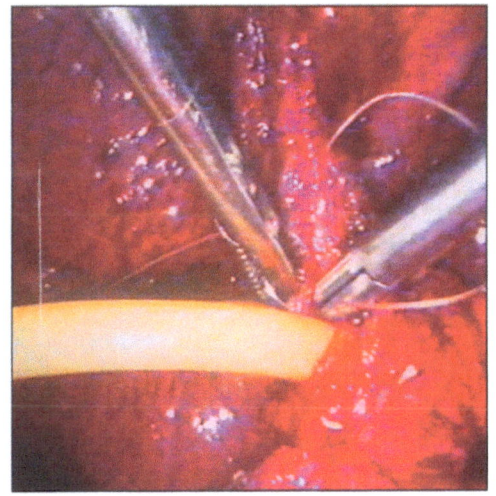

Chapter 2, Figure 2-10, p. 21

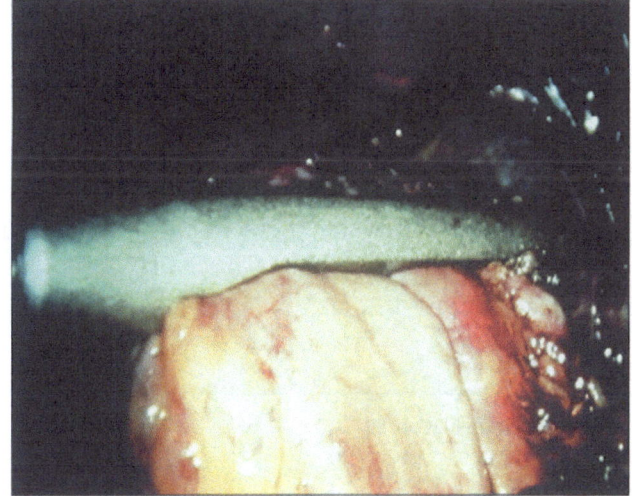

Chapter 6, Figure 6-1, p. 64

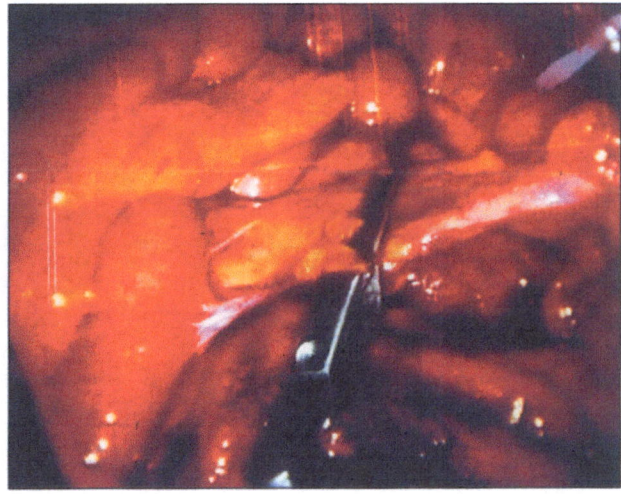

Chapter 6, Figure 6-2, p. 64

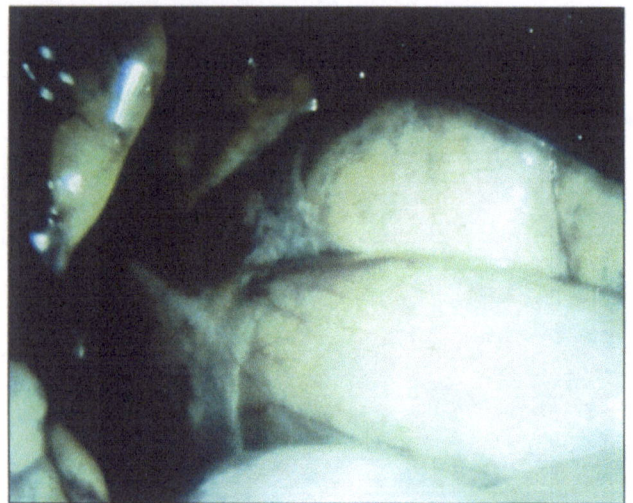

Chapter 6, Figure 6-3, p. 65

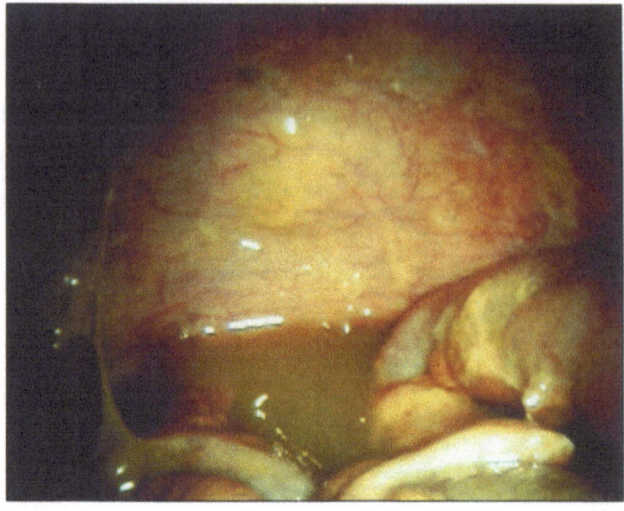

Chapter 6, Figure 6-4, p. 65

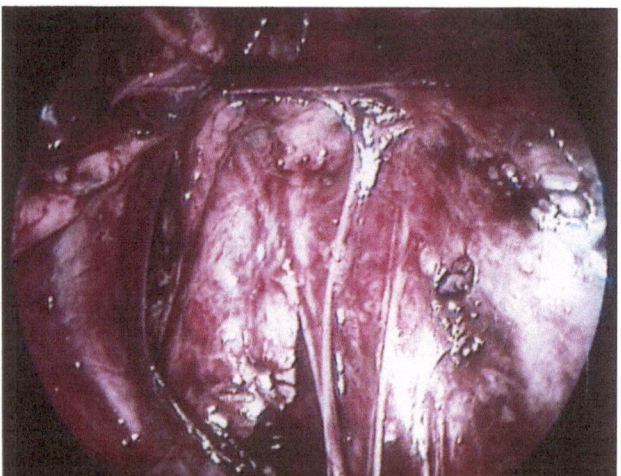

Chapter 8, Figure 8-1, p. 79

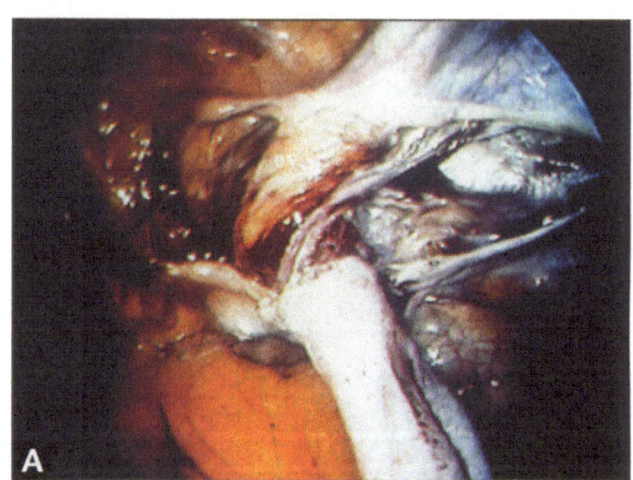

Chapter 8, Figure 8-2A, p. 80

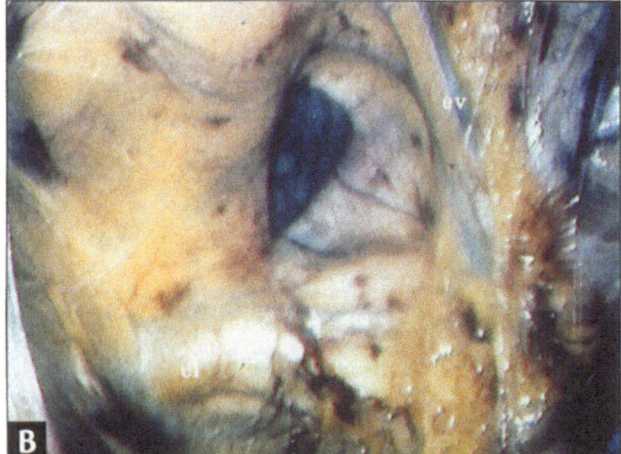

Chapter 8, Figure 8-2B, p. 80

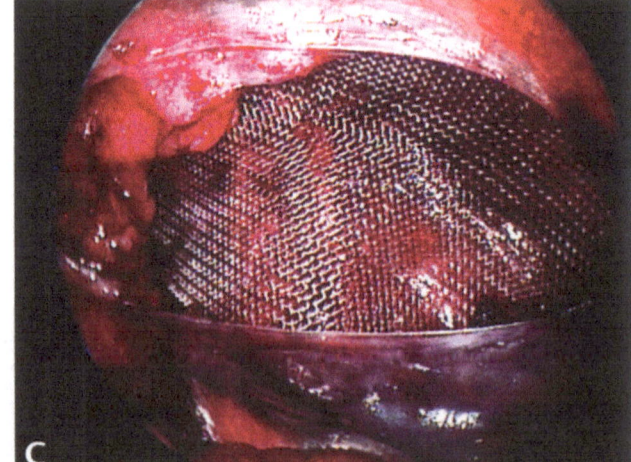

Chapter 8, Figure 8-2C, p. 80

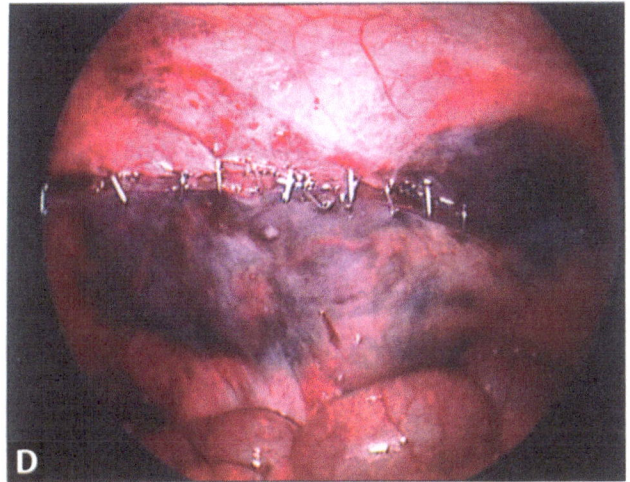

Chapter 8, Figure 8-2D, p. 80

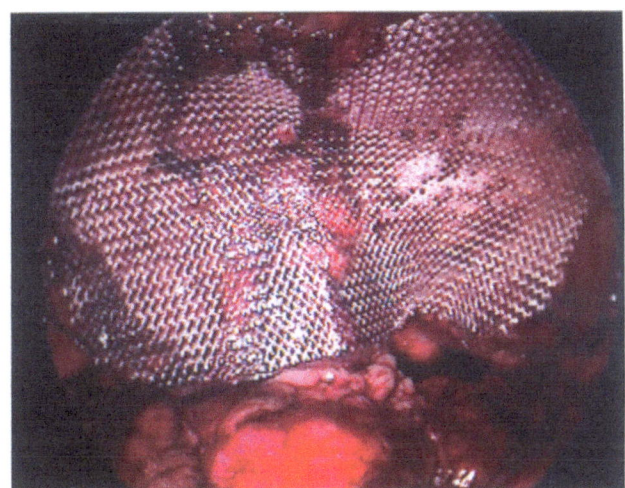

Chapter 8, Figure 8-3, p. 81

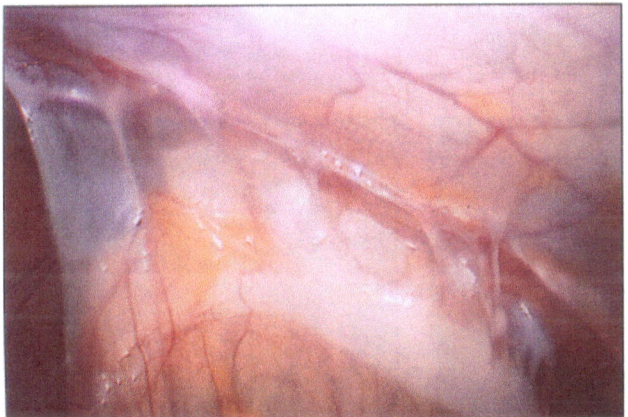

Chapter 10, Figure 10-2, p. 102

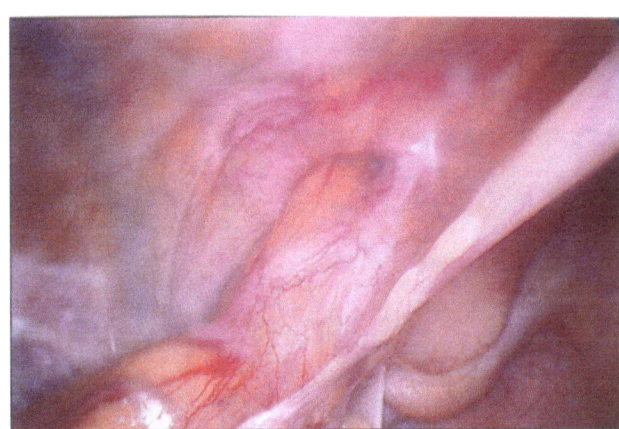

Chapter 10, Figure 10-3, p. 102

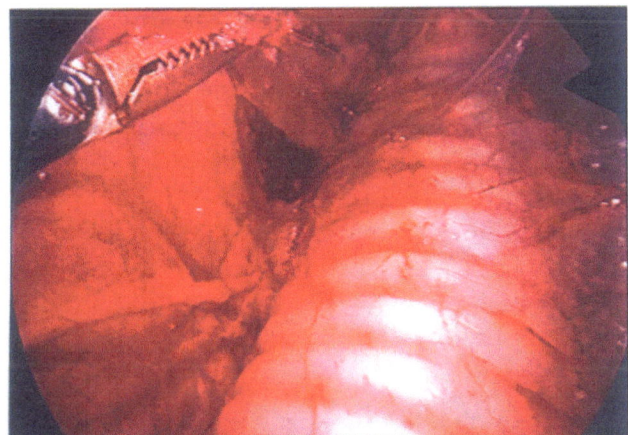

Chapter 12, Figure 12-3, p.119

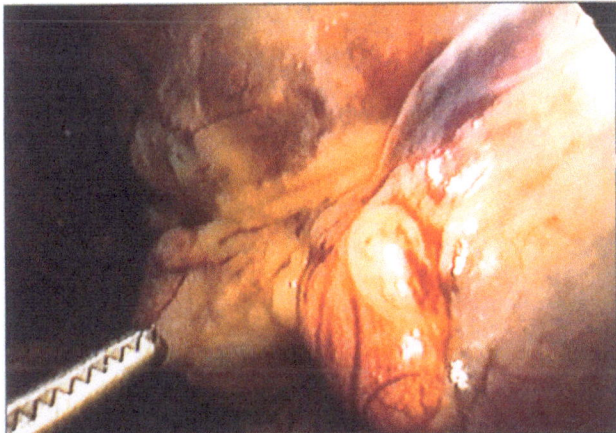

Chapter 12, Figure 12-4, p. 120

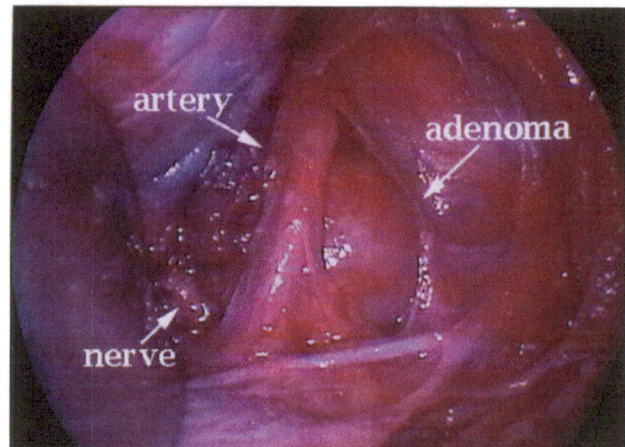

Chapter 12, Figure 12-6, p. 121

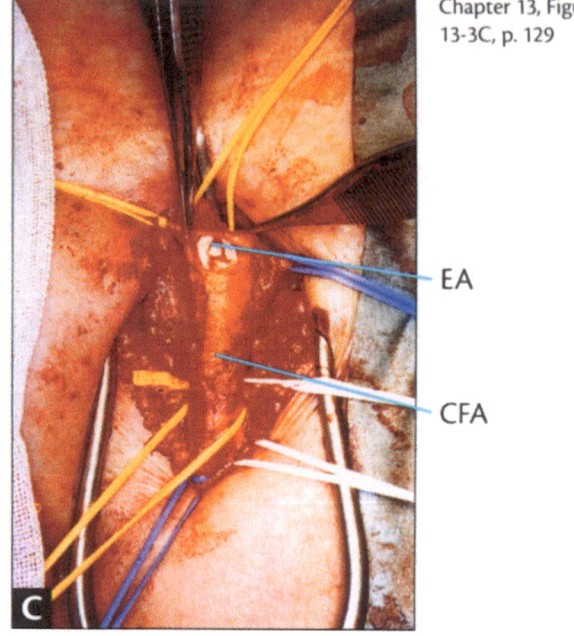

Chapter 13, Figure 13-3C, p. 129

EA

CFA

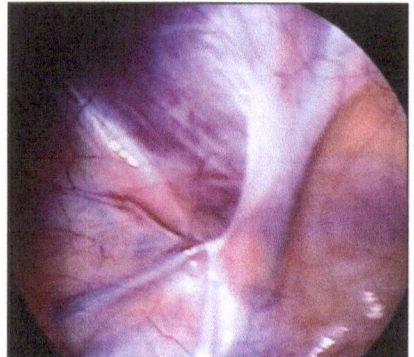

Chapter 14, Figure 14-1, p. 139

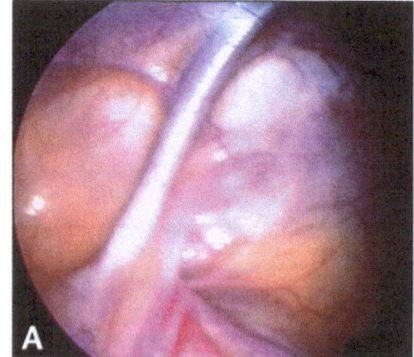

Chapter 14, Figure 14-2A, p. 140

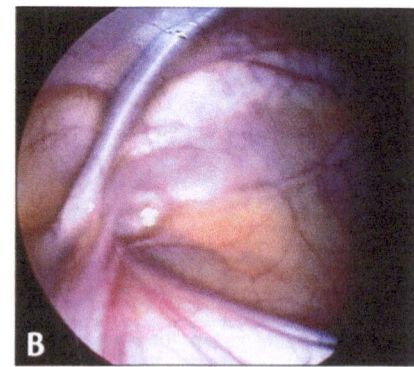

Chapter 14, Figure 14-2B, p. 140

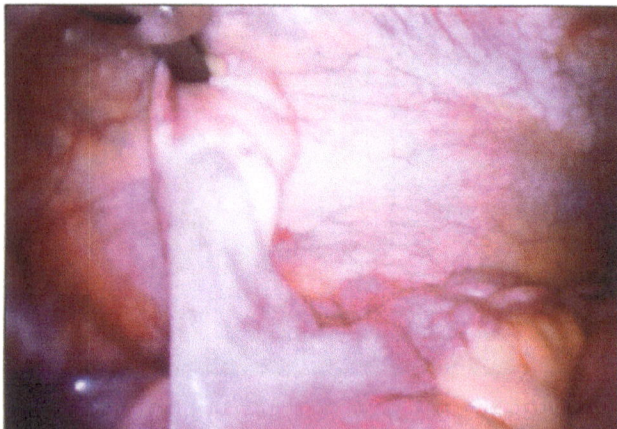

Chapter 14, Figure 14-6, p. 141

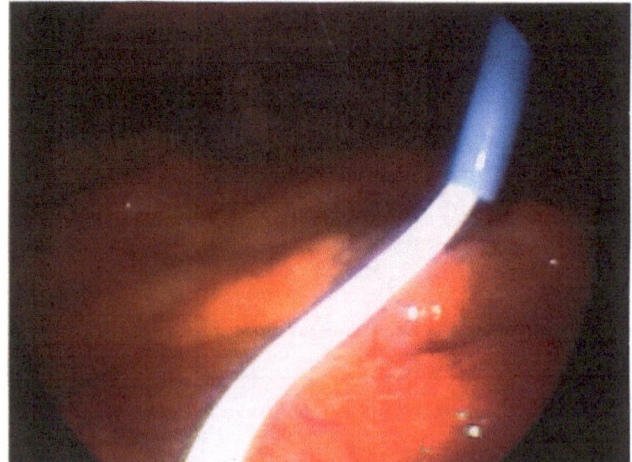

Chapter 14, Figure 14-7, p. 142

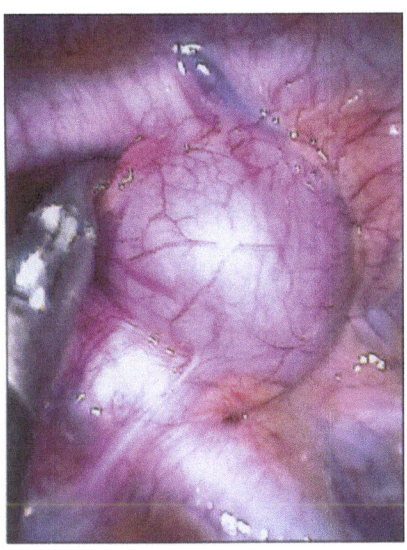

Chapter 14, Figure 14-8, p. 142

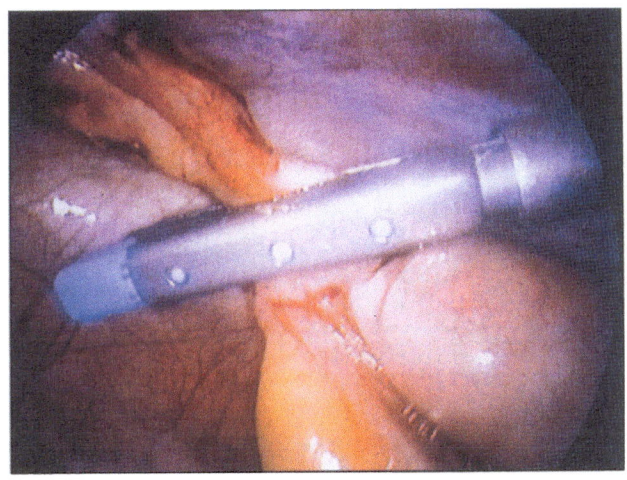

Chapter 18, Figure 18-11, p. 185

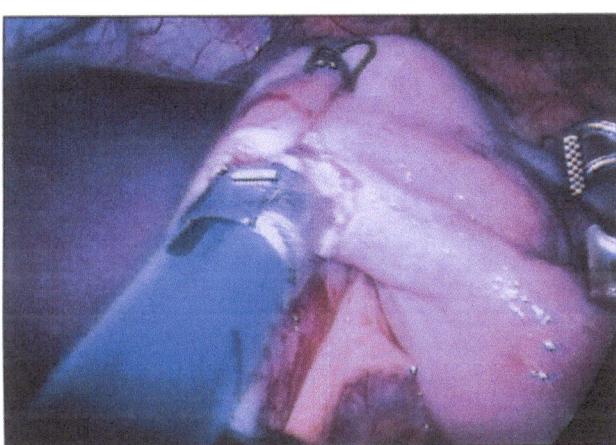

Chapter 18, Figure 18-12, p. 185

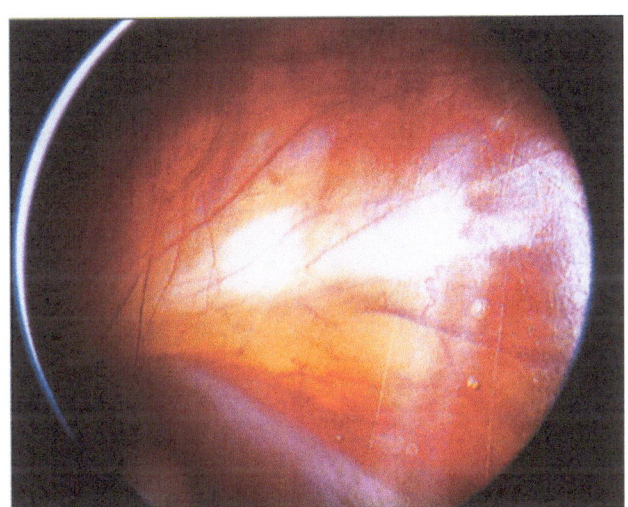

Chapter 19, Figure 19-3, p. 191

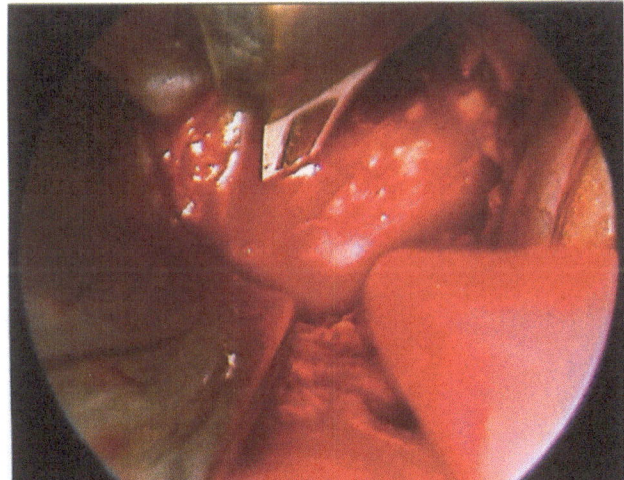

Chapter 19, Figure 19-5, p. 198

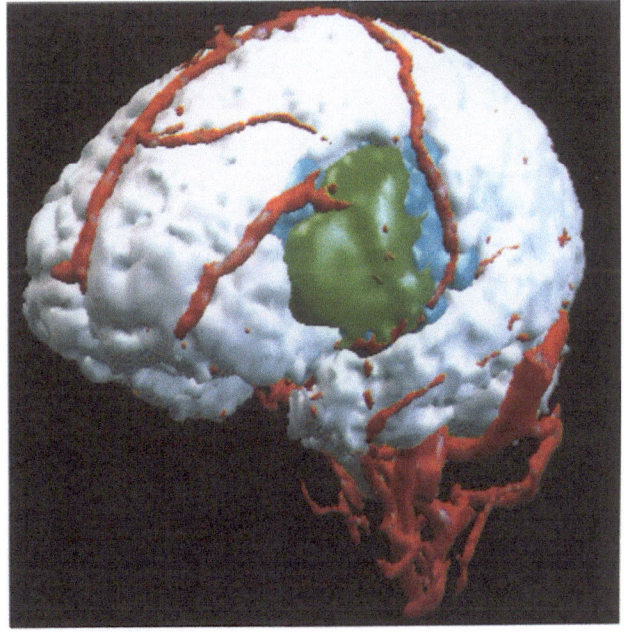

Chapter 20, Figure 20-1, p. 204

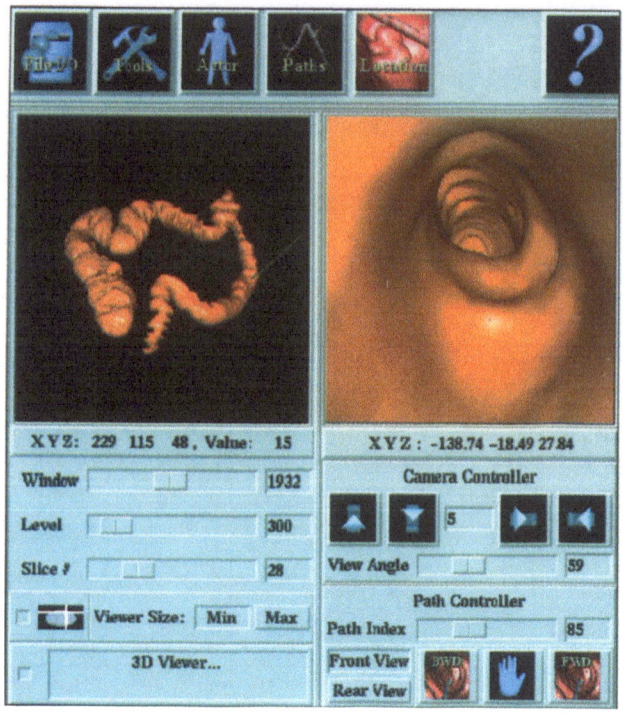

Chapter 20, Figure 20-3, p. 208

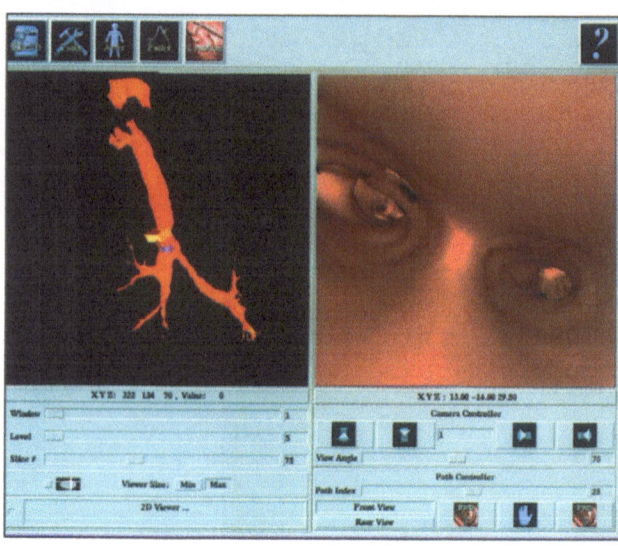

Chapter 20, Figure 20-4, p. 208